Cellular Defects in Disease

To Anna

Cellular Defects in Disease

KENDAL C. DIXON
MA PhD MD FRCPath
Professor Emeritus of Cellular Pathology
University of Cambridge

BLACKWELL SCIENTIFIC PUBLICATIONS
OXFORD LONDON EDINBURGH
BOSTON MELBOURNE

Editorial offices:
Osney Mead, Oxford, OX2 OEL
8 John Street, London, WC1N 2ES
9 Forrest Road, Edinburgh, EH1 2QH
52 Beacon Street, Boston
Massachusetts 02108, USA
99 Barry Street, Carlton,
Victoria 3053, Australia

First published 1982

Typeset by CCC, printed and bound in Great Britain by William Clowes (Beccles) Limited, Beccles and London

DISTRIBUTORS

USA
Blackwell Mosby Book Distributors
11830 Westline Industrial Drive
St. Louis, Missouri 63141

Canada
Blackwell Mosby Book Distributors
120 Melford Drive, Scarborough
Ontario, M1B 2X4

Australia
Blackwell Scientific Book
Distributors
214 Berkeley Street, Carlton
Victoria 3053

British Library
Cataloguing in Publication Data
Dixon, K. C.
Cellular defects in disease.
1. Pathology, Cellular
I. Title
616.07 RB25

ISBN 0-632-00734-6

Contents

Preface

Cellular damage and malfunction are the prime determinants of disease and death. This book discusses the causes and consequences of such pathogenic cellular disorder, as well as some of the cellular aberrations which precede, which accompany and which follow disease.

The aim of the book is directed at giving information which enables medical students and others interested in disease to form a picture of cause and nature of some of the cellular derangements occurring within the body during illness or after injury.

The scope of the subjects treated is necessarily limited by the extent of other readily accessible information. Thus phenomena of inflammation, blood coagulation, immunity and immune processes in disease (such as rejection of transplants) have received such adequate exposition in recently published text books, that these subjects are omitted or only very briefly discussed. Molecular and cytochemical features of disease are, however, emphasised, since progress in cytochemistry is now conjoining anatomy, physiology and biochemistry, and similar knowledge of cellular derangements at a molecular level will assume a cardinal position in the cytopathology of the future.

The basic determinants of cellular disorder responsible for many kinds of malady are obscure, even though the principal lesions may be well defined. We can say with confidence that cardiac arrest following coronary thrombosis is associated with atherosclerosis or that typhoid fever is caused by infection by *Salmonella typhi*; but how cholesterol esters accumulate and induce atherosclerosis or again how *S. typhi* kills cells and also how it produces mental stupor, are questions which are sometimes disregarded because their answers are so imperfectly known. A fair answer to such queries should be a prime concern of cellular pathology and when there is uncertainty this should freely be admitted and frankly emphasised. Indeed, despite continuous and sometimes spectacular advances in knowledge of disease, the actual molecular mechanisms of cellular death are still undetermined: death still is, as Marcus Aurelius so tersely put it 1800 years ago,

> like birth, a mystery of Nature
>
> Meditations IV, 5.

Acknowledgements

This book owes much to the friendship, help and advice of my colleagues in the Department of Pathology in Cambridge University. I wish very specially to thank Professor G. A. Gresham for his dynamic collaboration in selecting specimens given to me over many years. I am deeply grateful to colleagues both near and overseas who have so generously given permission to reproduce figures from their publications. My thanks also go to Mr A. J. King for technical assistance, to Messrs S. W. Patman and P. Curtis for help in photomicrography, and to Dr H. B. F. Dixon, Secretary of the Joint Commission on Biochemical Nomenclature, for advice on some recent changes in biochemical symbols. I have received most valuable aid from my wife in the design of diagrams as well as in secretarial work; I also wish to thank Dr A. K. Dixon for reading the proofs.

The arrangement and sequence of contents in this book partly follow the kind of plan which I have used for teaching cellular pathology. This plan was applied to the chapter on disorders of the cell in *A Companion to Medical Studies Vol. 2.* Some parts of the book are thus concerned with topics discussed in a similar though more condensed manner in the above chapter. I thank Blackwell Scientific Publications for permitting me to use in the book some diagrams and photomicrographs included in this chapter; I also thank the publishers for their continued help and kindness at all phases in the construction of the book.

Note on photomicrographic figures

All tissue-sections illustrated in photomicrographic figures, unless otherwise stated in individual captions, were stained by Harris' (or Ehrlich's) haematoxylin followed by eosin.

CHAPTER 1

Cellular Basis of Disease and Death

All disease is the result of damage, imperfection or malfunction of the cells and tissues of the body. Since the only living things in the body are its cells, the study of their disorder should eventually provide a basic key to the science of disease as a whole.

This book is concerned with:

1. The agents which thus damage cells in disease and the mechanisms of their noxious action.
2. The nature and pattern of cellular defects which may herald, accompany or follow disease.

Chapter 1 gives a brief account of:

1. The nature of cellular lesions including cell death and its relation to bodily death.
2. The principal cellular determinants of disease.

Thereafter the book is divided into Part I, causes of pathogenic cellular disorder (Chapters 2–6), and Part II, nature of cellular disorder in disease (Chapters 7–9).

LESIONS OF THE CELL IN DISEASE

These include:

1. Irreversible cessation of cellular activity and function coupled with irreparable disorganisation of structure, which are together called cell death or necrosis (*νεκρός*, dead); Fig. 1.1a shows necrosis of cerebellar neurones resulting from interruption in their supply of blood (ischaemia).
2. Other less severe changes which indeed may herald necrosis, but which

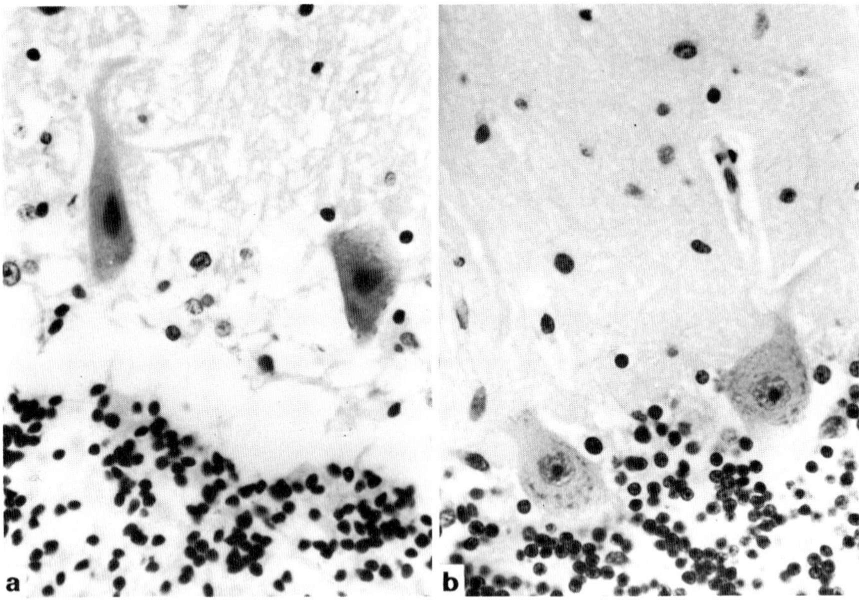

FIG. 1.1a Necrosis with irreparable disorganisation of structure in neurones in cerebellar cortex (*right* side). Owing to heart failure with coincident thrombosis of *right* vertebral artery the supply of blood to these neurones was severely diminished; the cells were therefore killed and the patient suffered from giddiness owing to cerebellar malfunction for two days before death from heart failure. The necrotic Purkinje cells are shrunken and their Nissl substance has disappeared. The nuclei of both the Purkinje cells and of the numerous dead granule cells have shrivelled into darkly staining homogeneous remnants. ×410.

FIG. 1.1b Normal cerebellar neurones from *left* side of same cerebellum as shown in Fig. 1.1a. Nissl substance and nuclear structure are plainly visible in uninjured Purkinje cells, while nuclear chromatin is also clear and well defined in the intact granule cells. ×410.

may alternatively be signs of more temporary or less devastating derangement, e.g.

a. Swelling and enlargement, as in epidermal cells infected by vaccinia (Fig. 1.2) or smallpox;

b. Disintegration or disappearance of cellular constituents, as in spino-medullary motor neurones which lose their cytoplasmic Nissl granules on infection by poliovirus (Fig. 1.3a);

c. Aggregation, deposition or appearance of visible materials within the cell, as when globules of fat appear in the hepatic cells of rats fed on margarine as their sole food (Fig. 1.4);

d. Abnormality of metabolism, behaviour or growth, as when neoplastic cells of a malignant tumour infiltrate and grow along lymphatic vessels (Fig. 1.5).

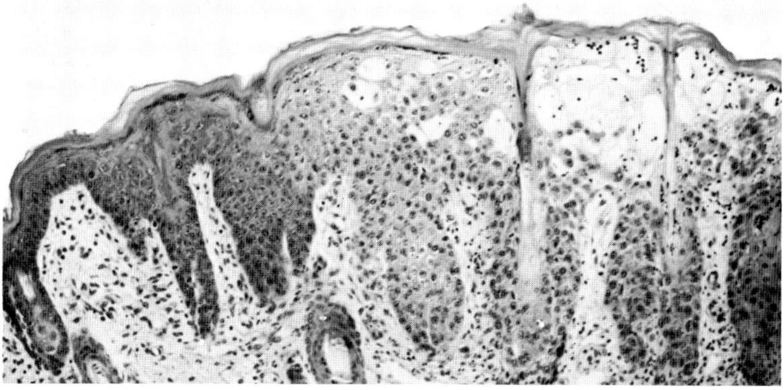

FIG. 1.2 Swelling of epidermal cells following infection by vaccinia virus. Section of epidermis of newborn rabbit: unaffected cells to the left of the field become progressively enlarged towards the centre of the field and ultimately swell into sacs of aqueous fluid. Similar 'ballooning degeneration' occurs in human epidermis both after vaccination and in smallpox. This change results in blistering of skin. ×110. Dixon K. C. (1959) *Amer. J. Path.*, **35**, 249.

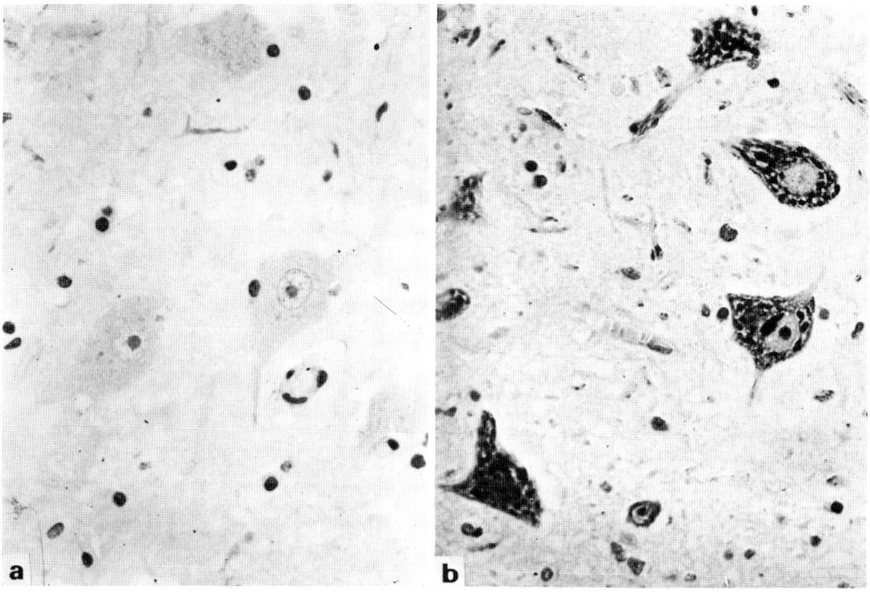

FIG. 1.3a Disintegration and loss of Nissl substance in motor neurones of human hypoglossal nucleus of a patient who died from respiratory paralysis due to bulbar poliomyelitis affecting the medulla and cervical cord. Nearly all the Nissl substance (and its contained RNA) has disappeared from the cytoplasm of the injured neurones, although the nuclei appear undamaged. Pyronin G. ×335.

FIG. 1.3b Normal motor neurones from human hypoglossal nucleus for comparison with Fig. 1.3a. Nissl substance, arranged in streaky masses, is intensely stained by pyronin G which has strong affinity for RNA. Pyronin G ×335.

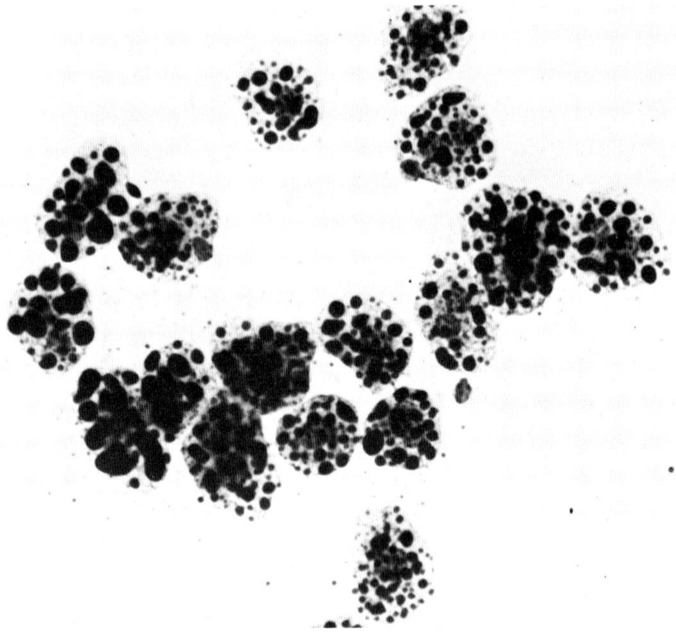

FIG. 1.4 Intracellular deposition of globules of fat in hepatic cells of a rat fed on margarine as its sole food for three days. The coalescent liquid globular fat is coloured intensely by Sudan III and Sudan IV. Rolled film. ×400. Dixon K. C. & King A. J. (1972) *Histochem. J.*, **4**, 111.

CELLULAR DEATH

But death is not a mere slowing down of a machine; it is a total ruin of the supposed machinery.

J. S. Haldane, 1919

We must first consider cellular death in a little more detail and also enquire how far it is related to death of the body as a whole.

Cell death involves both *permanent loss of activity and function* and *irreparable disorganisation of structure*. In this death, therefore, not only do the wheels of life stop turning, but both they and the engine which drives them are so changed that they never turn again. These two aspects of cell death will first be examined.

Permanent loss of activity and function

Abolition of anabolism, autoreplication and division

In death, cellular anabolism, replication of DNA and mitosis are abolished. Transcription of RNA and translation of peptides are also permanently arrested. Such cessation of cell division and replacement is a prominent consequence of injury by ionizing radiation (Chapter 4). This exerts disastrous effect on tissues in which the cells have a short span of life and require constant

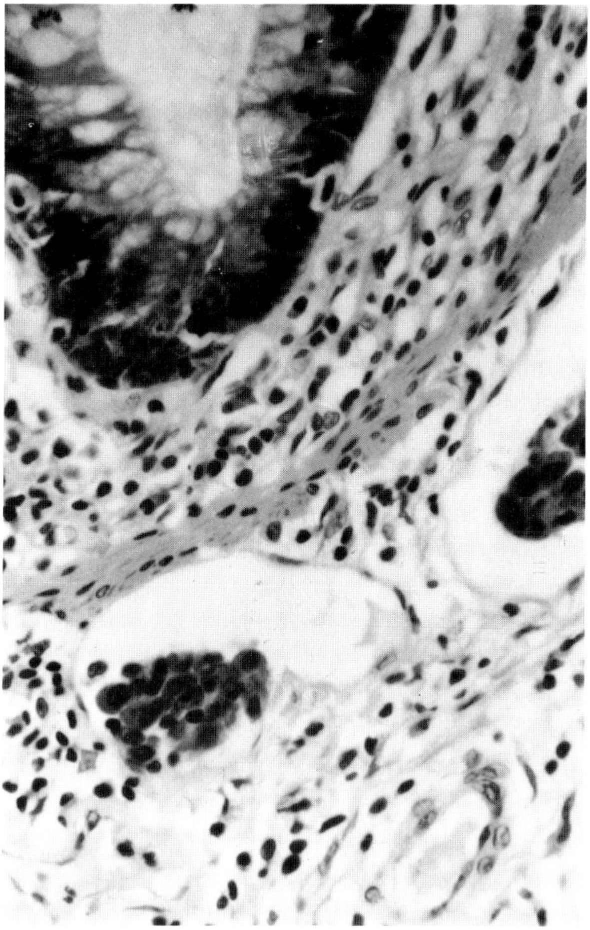

FIG. 1.5 Abnormal behaviour of cells, illustrated by a malignant tumour; lymphatic permeation by cells from a carcinoma of the colon. A normal colonic tubular gland is seen with subjacent muscularis mucosae. *Beneath* the muscularis are two dilated lymphatic vessels, each of which is permeated by a column of malignant cells from the colonic cancer. These cells grow and spread by extension along the lymphatic channels, and thus, although apparently uninjured, display gross abnormality of behaviour; this enables them to penetrate and spread to other organs with disastrous consequences. ×510.

replacement by mitosis. Moreover dividing cells are specially susceptible to injury by radiation. Thus injury to the gastrointestinal epithelium (resulting in vomiting and diarrhoea), the haemopoietic tissues (causing anaemia, infection and purpura), and the epidermis (with ulceration and loss of hair) are typical early effects of exposure to excessive radiation.

Cessation of synthesis of specific cellular secretions

This follows necrosis of specialised fabricator cells. Thus ischaemic necrosis of the anterior lobe of the pituitary gland after post partum haemorrhage (p. 83) abolishes the secretion of essential hormones from its endocrine cells. Similarly bilateral necrosis of the adrenal cortex abolishes the synthesis of corticosteroids and so produces Addison's disease. In this syndrome lack of cortical hormones causes sodium depletion, hypotension, anorexia and wasting. Necrosis of adrenal cells in Addison's disease is usually caused by tuberculosis or by autoimmune atrophy and cytolysis.

Abolition of physical or effector activity

In death cellular motility is irreparably lost. Thus the contractile fibres of cardiac muscle become immobile when killed by ischaemia following occlusion of coronary arteries. Similarly the fibres of voluntary muscle lose their power to contract, when killed by interruption of blood supply following compression of badly applied plaster splints or by infection in gas gangrene of muscle.

When neurones die their electrical activities terminate. Thus the typical waves of electrical activity generated on the surface of the cerebral cortex are abolished when the neurones are killed by electrocoagulation at 80° for 5 seconds. Dead spinal anterior horn cells killed by the poliovirus can no longer transmit impulses received via the axonal terminals of the corticospinal tracts; thus flaccid paralysis of the limbs follows necrosis of these motor neurones during poliomyelitis.

Irreparable disorganisation of structure

This may involve rapid disorganisation and fixation of the cell fabric by exceptionally adverse external conditions (such as exessive heat), or a more gradual progressive and irreparable decomposition which is the usual concomitant of cellular death in disease.

Extremely rapid irreversible fixation

Cells killed by heat, coagulants (e.g. mercuric chloride, ethanol) or protein-linking reagents (e.g. formaldehyde), rapidly become opaque and round up. This fixative effect depends on removal of structured water from the proteins along with disalignment of arrayed proteins and lipids in membranes. The membranes become fully permeable. When polymorphs or macrophages are thus rapidly fixed they become spherical and lose their pseudopodia owing to contraction of their surface. After this rapid fixation immediate denaturation or coagulation of protein impedes autolysis of macromolecules and thus macromolecular components are largely preserved.

Although this rapid fixation is constantly employed in preparing tissues for microscopic examination, it also may occur when cells of the body are killed by injury or disease. Thus epidermal cells are rapidly fixed in burns of the skin while red cells circulating through intensely heated skin are transformed into microspherocytes (see Fig. 4.11). Moreover neurones in proximity to incised wounds of the brain may suddenly contract into darkly stainable cells, which remain unaltered by subsequent autolysis of the damaged tissue [1]; this effect is called *preservation necrosis of Cajal*. Similarly when polymorphs are killed by streptolysin O, they rapidly lose motility and contract into spheres; this change probably occurs in the formation of pus during infection by *Streptococcus pyogenes* (p. 227).

Progressive irreparable disintegration

Cellular death in disease, however, usually involves a sequence of more gradual but spectacular changes in structure, which appear to progress inevitably once sufficiently severe injury has been sustained.

Thus eventual loss of RNA and DNA is a prominent feature of irreparable damage in dying cells maintained at body temperature in a living patient. Cell membranes probably collapse and disintegrate (p. 340), the cytoplasm usually shrivels and becomes homogeneous, while cytoplasmic basophilia due to RNA rapidly disappears (Fig. 1.1a). At first the nuclei may shrink into intensely basophilic spherules (pyknosis, Fig. 1.1a), but ultimately the nuclei dissolve away and their DNA is lost (karyolysis, Fig. 1.6). Fig. 1.1a and Fig. 1.6 illustrate respectively cerebellar neurones and hepatic cells killed by arrest or retardation of their supply of blood (ischaemia). Such necrotic cells usually become fully permeable so that osmotic swelling is largely precluded and later the dead cells shrivel through loss of water. Terminally the cells are transformed into faintly stainable homogeneous remnants, which may persist as ghost cells or else ultimately be consumed by invading phagocytes.

This homogenising change, in which the outline of the dead cells and their cytoplasmic remnants are preserved, is called coagulative necrosis; in it the tissues become opaque and hard and the dead cells retain abundant protein (p. 335). Although micromolecular constituents are lost, the dead macromolecular fabric is largely retained like a building devoid of inhabitants, but which still shows traces of its former grandeur. Coagulative necrosis is the usual sequel to irreparable injury due to ischaemia (Fig. 1.1a, 1.6).

A more severe kind of disintegration of the dead tissue, called caseous necrosis (caseation), occurs in tissues killed by the tubercle bacillus, which of all hostile organisms capable of killing cells is one of the most formidable in causing extensive lethal injury. In caseation the dead tissue including the cells of the inflammatory exudate breaks down into a cheesy mass (L. *caseus*, cheese); the cell outlines and nuclei disappear as well as cytoplasmic structure to leave a

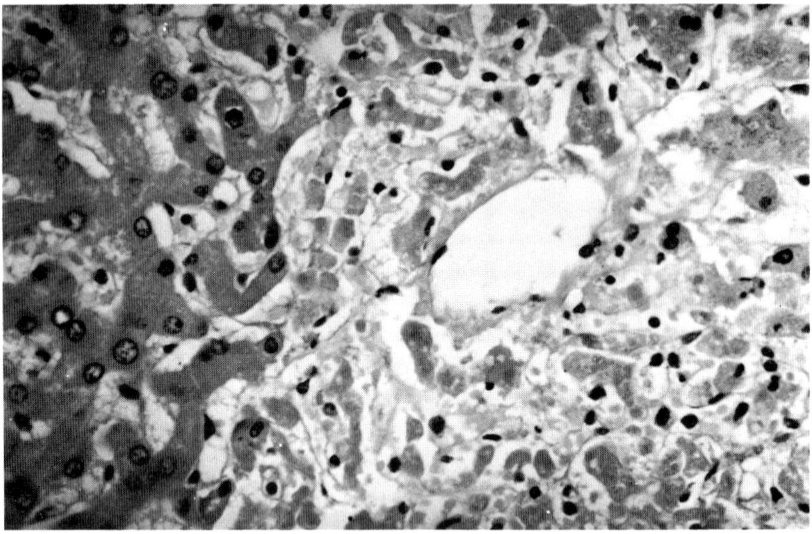

FIG. 1.6 Progressive irreparable disintegration of centrilobular hepatic cells. Liver from patient who died of congestive heart failure. The centrilobular cells around the central vein (to the right of figure) have suffered necrosis due to ischaemia (p. 75); these cells are shrivelled and their nuclei have disappeared while their cytoplasm is faintly stained owing to loss of basophilic RNA. These centrilobular cells show coagulative necrosis. The more peripheral cells to the left of the figure, owing to better supply of O_2 etc. (p. 75), remained alive until the patient died; these peripheral cells retain their cytoplasmic basophilia due to presence of RNA. ×330.

conglomeration of eosinophilic debris rich in protein (see Fig. 7.32, p. 339). Caseation causes complete disintegration of cell structure and is responsible for the extensive devastation of lymph nodes, lungs and other organs affected by tuberculosis. The results of caseous necrosis resemble the rubble of Warsaw rather than the entombment of Pompei.

Nature of irreparable lesions

The exact nature of the irreparable lesions which amount to or lead to cellular death is still obscure. It is possible that:

either the arrangement of arrayed proteins or lipids becomes so disorganised that their conformation cannot be restored, even though the harmful agent is eliminated; ischaemic injury of cells may well be determined by lack of ATP which results in excessive interligation of cell proteins along with irreparable changes in conformation,

or some unique sequence of nucleotides in nuclear DNA decomposes, thus eliminating the potentiality of the cell to translate an essential peptide which normally must be constantly replenished; in this way an irreparable lesion is established which heralds cellular death.

Possibly these kinds of irreparable change may occur simultaneously. Arguments about the exact points of no-return are singularly sterile.

Cellular death and bodily death

for no pulse
shall keep his native progress, but surcease;
no warmth, no breath shall testify thou livest;
the roses in thy lips and cheeks shall fade
to palsy ashes; thy eyes' windows fall,
like death when he shuts up the day of life
William Shakespeare, *Romeo and Juliet* IV, i.

Having considered cellular death we must enquire what happens in the cells of the body when we ourselves die. What indeed do we mean by death of the whole body? In fact we lack a clear definition of bodily death beyond the entirely negative one of cessation of life, and life itself will always defy definition.

Loose notions on death die hard. One is that doctors can with some magic insight immediately pronounce the moment of life's extinction. Unfortunately medical men and women are not endowed with such supernatural power. When is someone dead beyond the possibility of revival? Total immobility coupled with prolonged cessation of heart beat and respiration were the old criteria. To these have now been added others, such as visible changes in the retinal vessels, absence of various brain stem reflexes and of electrical activity in the cerebral cortex. Some of these signs may on occasion be fallacious, especially if observed only over a short period. For instance newborn babes may survive relatively long periods of initial apnoea, and patients have sometimes been revived after electric shock or drowning, even though apparently lifeless as judged by absence of pulse and respiration for considerable periods. Moreover absence of cerebral electrical activity may occur in coma induced by barbiturates and yet be followed by full recovery.

These various signs are, however, of value in trying to assess whether the cerebral neurones are so irreparably injured as to preclude the recovery of consciousness, personality and mental powers. The paramount question is whether or not these essential neurones have been killed.

Physical criteria of human death

Cellular death is not what immediately concerns the man in the street. He wants to know about death of the body as a whole and the conomitant irreparable cessation of thought and mind based on the body. However, since the only living things in the body are its cells, their death or the death of some of them must be crucial determinants of death of the body as a whole and of its internal thinking mechanisms.

Arrest of the heart beat and respiration for more than a few minutes are, as we shall see, usually followed by irreversible injury to the cerebral neurones with permanent abolition of consciousness, memory and thought. Cerebral neurones are of all cells the most rapidly injured by ischaemic anoxia which follows cardiac arrest. Following cessation of circulation these cells are the first to suffer lethal damage. Thus irreversible injury to the cerebral neurones is the most valid physical criterion of death, if we could be absolutely certain that it had taken place. Unfortunately we cannot televise the cytopathology of the brain. But we can be reasonably certain that this damage has taken place when lethal changes occur in other *less* vulnerable cells post mortem.

Post mortem changes

In the pulseless patient irreparable damage to cerebral neurones is thus the first and most disastrous injury; death of other more resistant cells then follows with varying speed. Some cells, such as those of skin and hair, remain alive for days. The changes within the dying cells are less conspicuous than those occurring in *ante mortem* necrosis, as there is no access of flowing blood and autolytic changes are lessened as the body cools after death.

Striated muscles in dead bodies stiffen owing to contraction of their fibres. This condition is called *rigor mortis*. Rigor develops when ATP finally disappears in anoxic muscle; actin and myosin then react together excessively. In the absence of ATP many more attachments develop between actin and myosin than in normal muscular contraction (p. 81). This results in extensive contraction, which occurs with enhanced interligation between molecules of actin and myosin. The muscle becomes rigid and inextensible, and is irreversibly

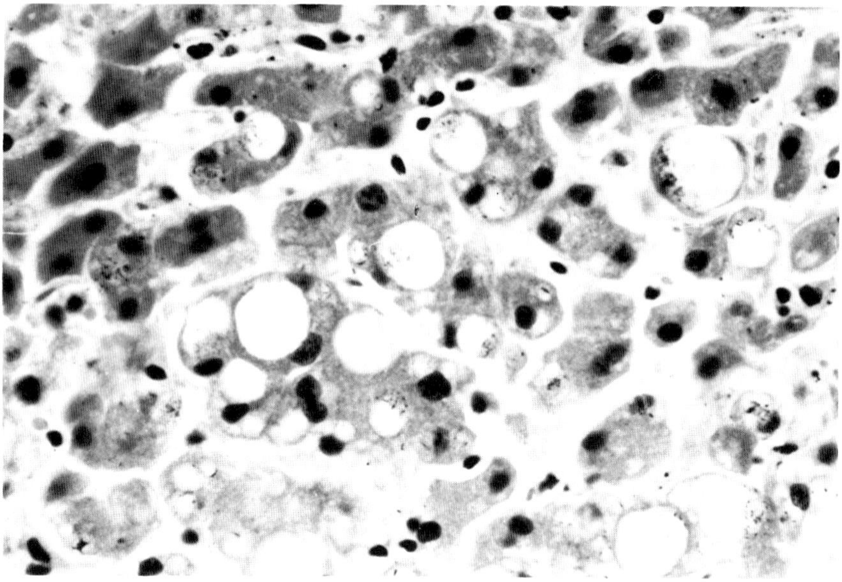

FIG. 1.7 *Post mortem* change in liver. Cellular dissociation and pyknosis of nuclei of liver cells from a body which remained at room temperature for four days after death. Some of the cells contain spherical spaces due to fatty change probably caused by terminal ischaemia during life. × 500.

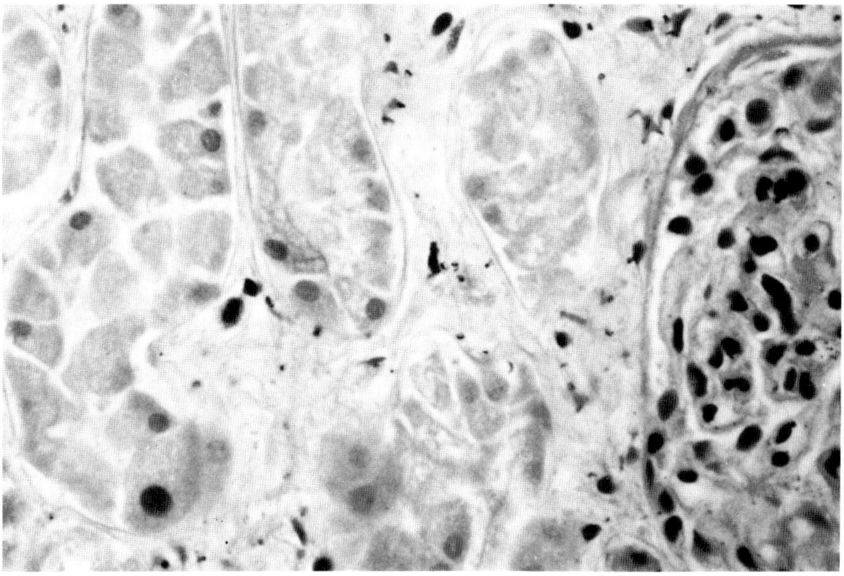

FIG. 1.8 *Post mortem* change in kidney. Cellular dissociation and loss of nuclei among renal tubular cells from a body which remained at room temperature for four days after death. Part of a renal glomerulus is visible at right side of the field; here the nuclei persist as shrivelled remnants. × 500. Fig. 1.7 and 1.8 illustrate sections from specimens kindly provided by Professor G. A. Gresham.

injured. This excessive interligation of proteins may indeed be a general phenomenon of irreversible injury in cells deprived of ATP. Rigor mortis later disappears along with further disintegration of the dead muscle.

Cellular dissociation is another conspicuous change in the liver and kidney of dead bodies. In the liver the hepatic cells separate from one another and their nuclei shrivel into pyknotic remnants (Fig. 1.7). In the kidney the tubular cells also become dissociated and their nuclei disappear (karyolysis), while the nuclei of glomerular cells shrivel into darkly staining spherules (Fig. 1.8).

CELLULAR AND INTERCELLULAR LESIONS

Although intracellular changes in many diseases are so spectacular, as for instance ballooning degeneration of the epidermus in smallpox and vaccinia (Fig. 1.2), in other maladies the most prominent lesion may be intercellular. Thus the fibrinoid change in collagen in rheumatoid arthritis and the deposition of monosodium urate crystals in gout are intercellular events. However many intercellular changes may be initiated by disorders within cells which may influence and determine external aberrations.

This determination of intercellular derangement by intracellular events was first emphasised by Rudolf Virchow [2]. He postulated that 'any given district of intercellular substance is ruled over by the cell which is in the middle of it.'

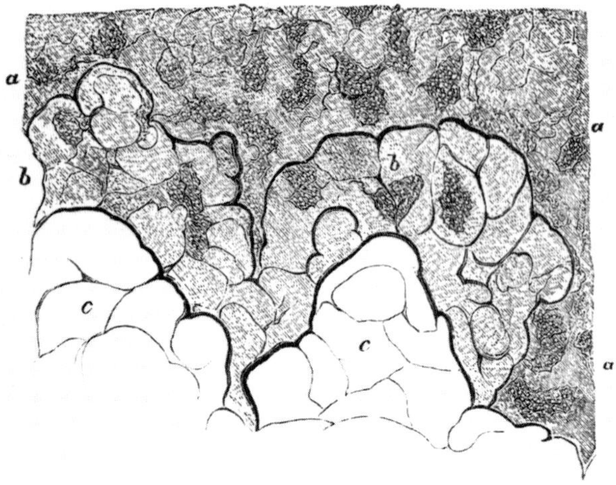

FIG. 1.9 Progressive destruction of cellular territories around osteocytes during necrosis of bone (drawing by Rudolf Virchow, 1860[2]). b shows rarefied degenerate zones which have taken the place of cell territories in the bony matrix around each osteocyte; these zones are finally converted into completely empty cavities (c), each representing a former cell territory. × 300.

Virchow discovered that disease affects such cell territories (*Zellterritorien*) at the same time as the cells which govern each territory. He shrewdly observed that, when bone dies as a result of tuberculous disease, the intercellular territory ('capsule') around each osteocyte ('corpuscle') disintegrates whenever its dominating cell is killed (Fig. 1.9). Virchow's views have since been substantiated by the discovery of the intracellular origin of both collagen and mucosubstances and the present concept of a mucocalyx on the external surface of cells which forms the intercellular material.

It might therefore be supposed that all injury originates within cells and not in the intercellular material secreted by them. This is not so. Fractures of bone for example, are caused by fission of intercellular osseous material. The spicules of broken bone can then lacerate lipocytes in bone marrow and also damage the walls of adjacent veins, so that large globules of liquid fat enter the blood; fat emboli from fractured bone can then later occlude cerebral capillaries and so produce coma and death (p. 106). Thus although rupture of the lipocytes is the basic cause of fat embolism this rupture is itself initiated by fragmentation of bone.

CELLULAR DETERMINANTS OF DISEASE

We would like to be able to account for cellular disorder which leads to disease with the same confidence and assurance as was displayed by the ghost of

Hamlet's father when describing his own treacherous murder by his brother Claudius, who poured poison into his ear:

The leperous distilment: whose effect
holds such an enmity with blood of man,
That, swift as quicksilver, it courses through
the natural gates and alleys of the body;
and with a sudden vigour, it doth posset
and curd, like eager droppings into milk
the thin and wholesome blood: so it did mine;
and a most instant tetter bark'd about,
most lazar-like, with vile and loathsome crust,
all my smooth body.

William Shakespeare *Hamlet* I, v.

Unfortunately our knowledge of the cellular determinants of disease and the exact logical sequence of cause and effect during the injury and death of cells is nowhere near so precise as the ghost's! Until cellular physiology and biochemistry are more perfectly comprehended and the fusion of these sciences with cytology and cytochemistry is achieved, a satisfactory description of even the main causes of cellular disorder will not be possible.

However we do have a partial understanding of the cell's complex membranous fabric and the factors which disorganise it, as well as of the requirements for cellular maintenance and replenishment and the agents which interrupt these vital processes of conservation.

Thus there are two principal origins of cellular disorder which can cause disease:

1. Imperfection or injury of the macromolecular fabric of the cell.
2. Interference with the maintenance and replenishment of this fabric.

Maintenance of the macromolecular fabric depends on the constant supply and interaction of nutrient micromolecules. These micromolecules include:

1. Building units for the cell fabric, e.g. aminoacids, nucleotides etc.
2. Substrates for exergonic reactions, e.g. glucose, oxygen etc., which by their interactions synthesise metabolic initiators of high energy content such as ATP and cytidine diphosphate choline. These high energy compounds are essential for (a) activating the synthesis of macromolecules from their constituent units, as in synthesis of nucleic acids and proteins, and (b) stabilising the proteins in cell membranes and fibrils as well as providing energy for physical activity.

A supply of nutrient micromolecules is thus immediately crucial for the maintenance of cell structure, as well as for the longer term needs of growth and replenishment of loss by catabolism, which would otherwise deplete and injure portions of the macromolecular fabric. Indeed at body temperature catabolism of protein is a continued hazard if replenishment is prevented; as Augustus Waller [3] so ably suggested in 1852 '*le corps de l'animal se compose de parties qui se détruisent et se renouvellent sans cesse .. cela obtient de l'équilibre qui existe entre ces deux actions contraires*'.

To survive and persist the cell thus requires:

1. An intact and permanent self replicating macromolecular pattern.
2. A constant supply of nutrient micromolecules.

The basic mechanisms of cellular disorder may therefore be summarised by recognising that:

either imperfection, abnormality or disorganisation of the macromolecular fabric which constitutes life itself

or, alternatively, interference with the supply or interaction of micromolecular nutrients

can be equally fatal to continued cellular existence.

In fact all forms of lethal or irreparable cellular derangement arise in one or other of these two ways. This is a fairly wide description of the mechanism of cellular disorder; but it is probably comprehensive enough and still definite enough to be helpful in our present state of ignorance.

Initiating agents of cellular disorder

We shall therefore endeavour to summarise the causes of cellular disorder that lead to disease with these two principles in mind (1) that the macromolecular fabric itself may initially be imperfect or become damaged, and (2) that the maintenance and replenishment of macromolecules in this fabric may be disorganised by defect in supply or interaction of micromolecules.

The principal agents which give rise to these two initial kinds of pathogenic cellular lesion include:

1. Genomic imperfection: this may be inherited and thus potentially affect every cell of the body, or may arise from mutation of a single somatic cell as happens in neoplasia.
2. Lack of essential nutriments.
3. Injurious physical conditions.
4. Harmful substances.
5. Living agents: these may be the cells of the body itself acting abnormally or parasitic or hostile foreign cells. Such living agents may act by creating conditions classifiable under 1, 2, 3 and 4 or in some hitherto unsuspected manner.

Indirect and plural causes of cellular disorder

In the ensuing chapters cellular disorder in disease will be considered in relation to these five principal initiating agents. In the origin of disease, however, initial cellular defect or injury often results in secondary or even more remotely dependent effects in the same or in separate cells; these changes may then in their turn be responsible for the paramount symptoms and signs of disease. Indeed more than one of these initiating agents may act in concert or in sequence to produce disease.

Thus genomic defect may be resonsible for the formation of an abnormal type of haemoglobin (Hb) which is inefficient as a carrier for O_2, or which makes the red cells viscous, or which curtails their life span. HbS in sickle cell disease (p. 22) is defective in each of these ways; in this instance therefore a genomic defect indirectly retards the supply of O_2 to cells. Burns of the skin may produce extensive epidermal injuries, but the final lethal effects of burning may be caused by subsequent shock or by even later bacterial infection of the exposed and unprotected subepidermal tissue. Also, injury or malfunction of groups of cells which exert ancillary activity in serving other cells may cause the most harmful effect by damage to cells remote from the initially disabled tissue. Thus the heart may stop temporarily or falter in its beat and thereby produce ischaemic damage in cerebral neurones; these exceptionally vulnerable cells are injured with great rapidity so that consciousness may never return. Thus the initially disabled cells may be far removed from the scene of the final and most devastating catastrophe.

Because of such indirect effects in many disorders only the beginning, or end, or some intermediate phase in a long chain of consequential cellular disturbances is at present understood or even appreciated. Here the disease in question is considered at the points in its aetiology which are best comprehended and in some instances different stages in the pathogenesis of the same terminal lesion have to be discussed separately. This question of indirect injury is discussed further in Chapter 3. We shall now consider in sequence pathogenic cellular disorder initiated by these five principal kinds of agent.

SUMMARY

1. Lesions of the cell in disease include cell death as well as other less severe derangements such as swelling, loss or aggregation of cellular components, and also abnormalities of metabolism, behaviour and growth.

2. Cell death involves irreversible cessation of activity and function coupled with irreparable disorganisation of structure.

3. The irreparable nature of cell death probably depends on disarrangement of arrayed proteins or lipids in cell membranes and organelles, or on disintegration of a unique sequence of nucleotides in an essential DNA code.

4. Cellular disorder in disease results from two kinds of basic derangement:

   a. Imperfection or direct disorganisation of macromolecular fabric.

   b. Interference with supply or interaction of micromolecules which are responsible for maintenance and replenishment of cell fabric and also for metabolic activity.

5. The principal agents which initiate these basic derangements are:

a. Genomic imperfection.

b. Lack of nutriments.

c. Injurious physical conditions.

d. Harmful substances.

e. Living agents, which may be the cells of the body itself or hostile foreign organisms.

REFERENCES

[1] Ramon y Cajal S. (1928) *Degeneration and Regeneration of the Nervous System*, Vol. 2 (translated by R. M. May). Oxford University Press, London.

[2] Virchow R. (1860) *Cellular Pathology*, 2nd Ed. (translated by F. Chance), pp. 15 and 418. Churchill, London.

[3] Waller A. (1852) Huitième mémoire sur le système nerveux. *C. R. Acad. Sci.* (*Paris*). **35**, 561.

PART I

Causes of Pathogenic Cellular Disorder

CHAPTER 2

Genomic Imperfection

As man, perhaps, the moment of his breath,
Receives the lurking principle of death,
The young disease which must subdue at length,
Grows with his growth and strengthens with his strength.
Alexander Pope

The healthy growth and development of cells derived from the human zygote depend on the presence within it of all the requisite DNA nucleotides assembled in viable sequences; these units, when conjoined in this manner, can then initiate cellular replication, differentiation and integration, and so produce during embryonic and infantile life the full mental and physical equipment of a normal child.

Abnormality in the sequence, assembly or quantity of these determinant nucleotides is responsible for disabling or lethal aberrations of the embryo as well as for more slowly evolving disorders of postnatal life.

Genomic imperfection may be inherited and so potentially affect every cell in the body, or may arise by mutation of a single somatic cell and so only affect the clone of cells derived from the mutant as happens in malignant tumours.

Genomic imperfection consists of (a) *invisible* (molecular) *abnormality of the genetic code*, or (b) more massive disarray or alteration of genetic material involving *visible change of karyotype* of the mitotic chromosomes; mutant clones of cells in malignant tumours usually display such visible change of karyotype.

INVISIBLE ABNORMALITY OF THE GENETIC CODE

Genetic constitution is determined by the linear sequence of purine and pyrimidine bases in the DNA molecules of the chromosomes. This sequence of nucleotides in genomic DNA transcribes the specific complementary composition to each new molecule of mRNA, and this in turn translates the exact order of amino acids into the peptide chains which compose the structural, effector and enzymic proteins of the cell.

Thus all genetically determined defects involve alteration, absence or addition in these ordered sequences of amino acids, which compose the fundamental peptide assemblies of the cell proteins. Although genomic defects probably only injure the cell by consequent change or failure in elaborating specific proteins, the identity of the altered or deficient proteins and the nature and mechanism of their alteration have as yet been defined only in a very few instances.

Specialised cells, which elaborate one principal functional protein, provide the simplest picture of how genomic defect can injure the cell or alter its behaviour; study of disorder in the synthesis of haemoglobin (Hb) in red cells and their precursors has thus conspicuously illuminated this branch of cellular pathology. A few examples of these haemoglobinopathies will now be considered.

Single substitution in genome: point mutation

Change of only one DNA base pair can result in gross alteration in behaviour and function of the protein ultimately translated by the altered gene, even though this inherited change determines the substitution of only one aminoacid in a peptide chain. Such a substitution of HbA of human red cells is responsible for sickle-cell disease which will now be discussed.

Sickle-cell disease

In this disastrous inherited illness the replacement of glutamic acid by valine as the sixth amino acid in each of the two β-peptide chains of HbA results in the formation of:

$$\text{HbS } \alpha_2\beta_2{}^{6\text{val}} \text{ instead of HbA } \alpha_2\beta_2{}^{6\text{glu}}$$

This change of the principal protein of the red cell is probably determined by inherited alteration of one codon in the DNA of two homologous chromosomes; indeed present evidence indicates that this change is caused by a point of mutation of a single base in the DNA sequence, which results in the substitution of glutamic acid by valine as the sixth amino acid in the β-chain so that HbS ($\alpha_2\beta_2{}^{6\text{val}}$) is formed.

When this point mutation affects both paternal and maternal chromosomes concerned with β-chain translation, then HbS entirely replaces HbA as the principal erythrocyte pigment of the child, as soon as fetal Hb ($\alpha_2\gamma_2$) declines.

Unfortunately the *deoxygenated* form of HbS polymerises from concentrated solution to form aggregates in which the molecules are closely stacked into rod-like structures. When this happens within red cells, they become progressively elongated and 'sickled' into bizarre shapes (Fig. 2.1). This phenomenon of 'sickling' can occur in blood *in vivo*, when it is extensively deoxygenated in the tissues, and also develops readily *in vitro* on incubation of wet films of blood diluted with 2 per cent aqueous sodium metabisulphite (a powerful reducing agent).

This spectacular change probably depends on a peculiarity in the conformation of deoxygenated HbS. The substitution of the non-polar amino acid valine for the polar glutamic acid may make the molecules of deoxygenated HbS in polymerised form adhere more closely together by hydrophobic association than is possible for HbA [1]. Observations by electron microscopy (EM) show a regular spiral arrangement in polymers of HbS in which the molecules are assembled more closely than in polymers of HbA [2]. During the sickling phenomenon within red cells the deoxygenated HbS condenses on one side of the cell, while the other side contracts into a thin membranous veil (Fig. 2.2); by

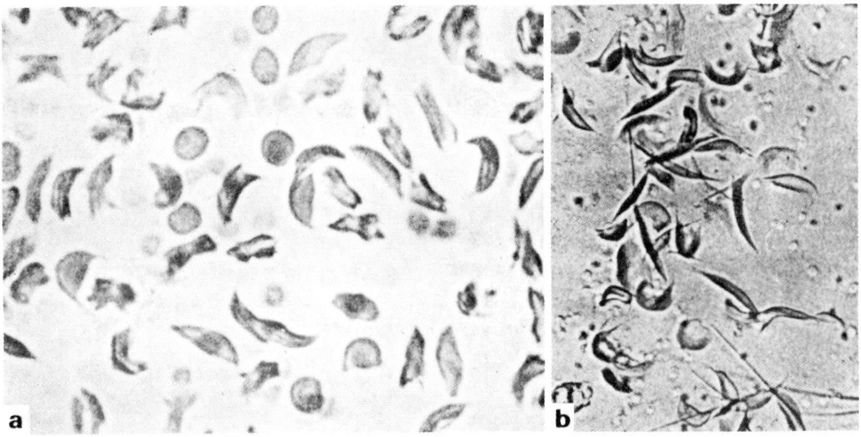

FIG. 2.1 Sickling of red cells containing HbS: wet film of blood mixed with 2 per cent aqueous sodium metabisulphite and incubated for 0.5–1 h.
a. Early stages of sickling.
b. Advanced sickling.
Courtesy of Professor H. Lehmann & Dr R. G. Huntsman. Reproduced from *Man's Haemoglobins*, 1974. North-Holland Publishing Company, Amsterdam.

using scanning EM White [2] elegantly demonstrated this process. In this way, when HbS becomes deoxygenated, the red cells assume asymmetrical sickled shapes.

Patients who are homozygous for this defect suffer from *sickle-cell disease*; in them HbA is entirely replaced by HbS and some sickle-cells are usually visible in fixed films made from circulating blood *in vivo*. Probably many sickled cells

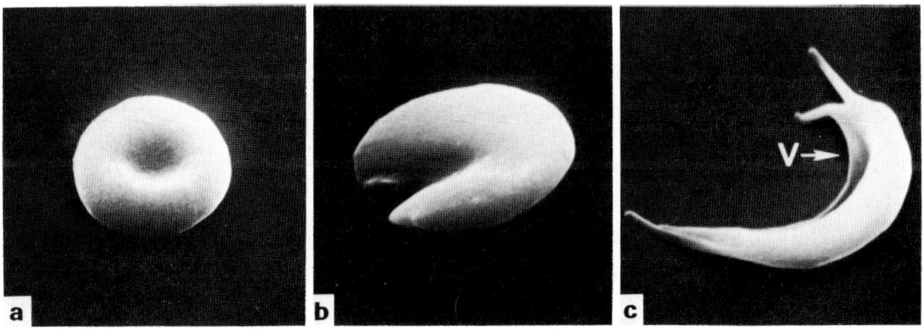

FIG. 2.2 Process of sickling observed by scanning electron microscopy during deoxygenation of Hb.
a. Fully oxygenated erythrocyte (normal in appearance).
b. Commencement of sickling along with deoxygenation.
c. Further stage: one side of cell thins out as a membranous veil (V).
Courtesy of Professor J. G. White. Reprinted from *Archives of Internal Medicine*, April, 1974, Vol. 133, pp. 545–562. Copyright 1974, American Medical Association.

are formed during deoxygenation of HbS in the internal organs of patients with sickle-cell disease; most of these revert to normally shaped cells on reoxygenation, but a few are irreversibly sickled due to membrane damage [3]. These irreversibly sickled cells account for the presence of a few permanently sickled cells in the peripheral blood; the injured cells probably only survive for a few days.

The *Heterozygous* possessors of HbS simultaneously elaborate HbA. For this reason much fewer sickle-cells are formed on deoxygenation of Hb within the tissues and sickle-cells are not seen in fixed films of their peripheral blood. These persons are said to have the *sickle-cell trait* and are usually perfectly healthy. But their red cells, like those of homozygous sufferers from the disease, show sickling on anaerobic incubation *in vitro* with sodium metabislulphite.

The homozygous patients, on the other hand, who have no HbA and much HbS, continually form sickle-cells as their blood becomes deoxygenated in the tissues; this sickling *exerts two gravely harmful effects*;

1. The red cells in these homozygous patients, probably owing to repeated transient sickling, *have a shortened life span*; this is usually diminished from the normal 120 days to about 17 days. Indeed, when cells become irreversibly sickled by membrane damage, their life span may be as low as two days. The rate of metabolism of red cells in sickle-cell disease is greatly increased as shown by augmentation in their emission of heat measured by microcalorimetry [4]. This effect may be a consequence of enlargement in surface area of the red cells which at the same time may increase their vulnerability to ischaemia (p. 92). As the sickle-cells age they are taken up by reticulo-endothelial cells and destroyed. This results in profound haemolytic anaemia and jaundice, sometimes accompanied by formation of pigment stones in the bile duct along with biliary colic and chronic cholecystitis. At first the bone marrow hypertrophies and erythropoiesis is increased; this effect can partially compensate for accelerated loss of red cells. But if the marrow becomes temporarily depressed by an otherwise trivial infection, then, because of shortened life the red cells, a most serious anaemic crisis may develop.

2. The sickled cells are *much more viscous* than normal ones. Therefore, as soon as deoxygenation occurs in capillaries along with formation of sickle-cells, the resultant increase in blood viscosity retards the flow of blood and so induces greater hypoxia and further sickling. Accordingly a vicious cycle may readily develop in the hypoxic tissues, which then die as a result of gross retardation or even complete arrest in flow of blood. Ischaemic necrosis (infarction) may thus occur in various organs, such as bones, lungs, skin, brain or spleen. Infarction in bones of hands and feet causes painful swellings especially in children, while in adults infarcts of the lung produce secondary infection with pneumonia and severe pain. Infarction of skin may produce ulcers on legs. Ishcaemic necrosis in occipital lobes of brain may cause transient or permanent blindness depending on whether other cortical areas can compensate for loss of function. Infarction of the retina may produce permanent blindness. Moreover massive sequestration of the viscous sickle-cells in the spleen and liver of children may

suddenly deplete the blood of red cells leading to grave anaemia and a rapidly lethal state of shock.

In addition to these harmful effects due to sickling of the red cells further disability arises in sickle-cell disease from diminished affinity of HbS for O_2. The excessive binding together of the deoxygenated HbS molecules promotes precipitation of reduced HbS out of solution. This solidification diminishes the concentration of the reduced form in solution and so more oxyhaemoglobin shifts to the deoxy form and releases its oxygen. For this reason HbS possesses a lower affinity for O_2 than HbA [3].

$$\mathrm{HbS} + O_2 \rightleftharpoons \mathrm{HbS\text{-}O_2}$$

$\downarrow$ polymerises and precipitates thus shifting equilibrium to the left

solidified precipitate

This effect probably enhances the action of HbS in diminishing the supply of O_2 to the tissues.

Other Genomic Substitutions

Besides sickle-cell disease other haemoglobinopathies exist in which one amino acid in either the α- or the β-chain is substituted, probably also as a result of point mutation of one DNA base.

Thus in HbC disease substitution of glutamic acid by lysine as the 6th amino acid in the chain results in formation of HbC ($\alpha_2\beta_2{}^{6\mathrm{lys}}$) instead of HbA ($\alpha_2\beta_2{}^{6\mathrm{glu}}$). Patients who are homozygous for this defect may have mild anaemia and jaundice and their spleens are usually enlarged. The disability of HbC disease is so slight that it is usually only discovered by accidental detection of splenic enlargement.

Deficient translation of peptide chains: gene deletion

Abolition or retardation of synthesis of peptide chains in the formation of globin is an important cause of haemoglobinopathy. Such defects are inherited in the various types of *thalassaemia*, in which generally the synthesis of either the *α-chain* or *β-chain* of globin is retarded or abolished as a result of deficiency or absence of the corresponding mRNA. These disorders will now briefly be considered.

β-Thalassaemia

In this type of inherited haemoglobinopathy the synthesis of β-chains of globin is defective.

β-Thalassaemia has a high incidence around the Mediterranean basin and hence the term thalassaemia (*θάλασσα*, sea) was originally applied to it. Defect in the formation of β-chains is not harmful to the newborn, as at birth fetal haemoglobin HbF ($\alpha_2\gamma_2$) is the predominant form of Hb. But in normal children, from about 4 months old, HbA ($\alpha_2\beta_2$) becomes the principal blood pigment; the absence of β-chains then commences to produce serious disability. By this time the formation of γ-chains has declined and, in the absence of β-chains, free uncombined α-chains accumulate in excess. The uncombined α-chains then aggregate *inside* the erythroblasts of the bone marrow to produce large inclusion bodies of 'naked' globin which injure the cells. Many of the erythroblasts never leave the bone marrow, but those which enter the blood are damaged by these inclusions within them and are soon sequestered in the spleen and destroyed by its reticuloendothelial cells. The spleen becomes grossly enlarged.

In homozygous sufferers from this defect very severe haemolytic anaemia (β-thalassaemia major) then develops. The only functional haemoglobin still persisting in the cells is an already diminished amount of HbF ($\alpha_2\gamma_2$). Moreover HbF has such a high affinity for O_2 that its combined O_2 is only slowly liberated. This retardation of liberation of O_2 along with severe anaemia results in profound hypoxia in the tissues. This hypoxia stimulates intense proliferation of red bone marrow which expands to fill the marrow cavities. This expansion causes separation of the tables of the skull with increase of the diploë between them, and also may produce enlargement of the facial bones along with severe disfigurement. Large numbers of erythroblasts enter the blood so as to give a picture of *erythroblastic anaemia*. The anaemia is so extreme that most patients afflicted with homozygous β-thalassaemia (major) die in childhood.

α-Thalassaemia

In this form of inherited haemoglobinopathy synthesis of the α-chains of globin is deficient or absent.

In fetal and neonatal life, *before* β-chains can be formed, deficiency of α-chains results in the accumulation of γ-chains: these free γ-chains aggregate to produce tetramers of γ_4 which combine with haem to produce functional HbBart's (γ_4). If the patient survives infancy then β-chains similarly accumulate because α-chains are deficient; these free β-chains also aggregate to produce tetramers of β_4 which combine with haem to form functional HbH (β_4). HbBart's (γ_4) and HbH (β_4) are both unstable and tend to precipitate as inclusion bodies which severely damage the red cells and diminish their life span; thus haemolytic anaemia develops. Moreover the oxygen-dissociation curves of Hb γ_4 and Hb β_4 do not show the characteristic sigmoid form (Bohr effect) which is necessary for labile transport and release of O_2; thus extreme tissue hypoxia develops in α-thalassaemia.

In the most severe form of α-thalassaemia the affected babies are stillborn because they can produce no *α-chains*. The Hb produced by the fetus is thus entirely HbBart's (γ_4) without *any* normal fetal Hb ($\alpha_2\gamma_2$). the fetus becomes profoundly hypoxic and hydropic. This type of α-thalassaemia is a frequent cause of stillbirth in S.E. Asia and is called *HbBart's hydrops fetalis syndrome*.

When suppression of α-chain formation is not so complete, the child may survive utilising small amounts of HbF ($\alpha_2\gamma_2$) still available in addition to

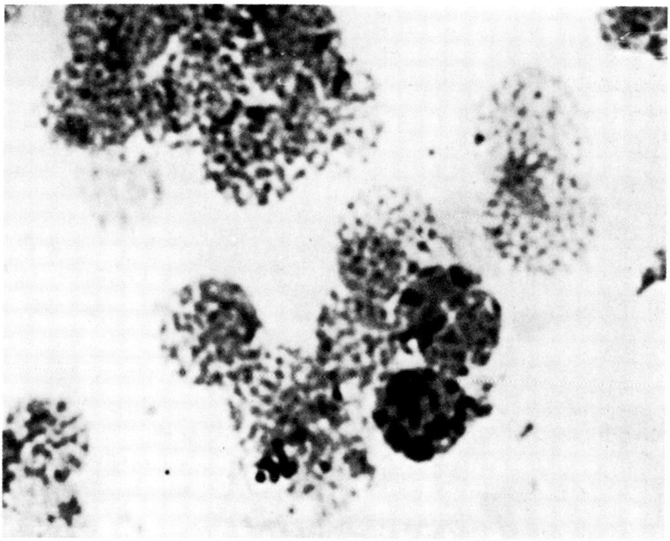

FIG. 2.3 HbH disease, a form of α-thalassaemia. Citrated blood incubated along with brilliant cresyl blue. HbH (β_4) within the red cells becomes denatured to form fine regular inclusion granules stainable by brilliant cresyl blue. These fine granules are visible in most of the cells and differ from coarse granules seen in a reticulocyte (bottom right). Courtesy of Professor H. Lehmann & Dr R. G. Huntsman. Reproduced from *Man's Haemoglobins*, 1974. North-Holland Publishing Company, Amsterdam.

HbBart's (γ_4), until β-chains are fabricated some months after birth. Then functional HbH (β_4) appears and these patients are therefore said to have HbH disease; they have severe haemolytic anaemia along with an enlarged spleen. In children with HbH disease both HbH (β_4) and HbBart's (γ_4) are detectable in the red cells; when these red cells are incubated *in vitro* HbH denatures rapidly to give regular small inclusion bodies stainable by brilliant cresyl blue (Fig. 2.3). The formation of these inclusions *in vivo* is highly injurious to the red cell membranes and shortens the life span of the red blood cells.

Genetic determinants of thalassaemia

The reticulocyctes from patients with α- and β-thalassaemia are found to be deficient respectively in α-mRNA, which translates the α-chains of globin, and in βmRNA, which translates the β-chains [5].

In the most severe form of α-thalassaemia with hydrops fetalis the cause of this lack of specific mRNA has been analysed further [6]. DNAs complementary to α- and to βmRNA were synthesised from mRNAs (using the viral enzyme reverse transcriptase) and these complementary DNAs (cDNAs) were made radioactive by supplying labelled ^{3}H-dCTP as a source of cytosine during this synthesis. The radioactive cDNAs were then used as probes for study of

DNA/DNA hybridisation between them and DNA extracted from normal and thalassaemic human nuclei. DNA was then obtained from the hepatic and splenic nuclei of an infant with α-thalassaemia along with hydrops detalis, who died 20 mins after delivery. The patterns of hybridisation of this DNA (from the hydropic child) with various radioactive human cDNAs, were then compared with similar patterns of hybridisation between normal human DNA and these same radioactive cDNAs. The DNA from the hydropic child was found to contain none of the α-chain genes capable of hybridising with α-chain cDNA. This gene is therefore apparently deleted from nuclear DNA in homozygous α-thalassaemia.

Thus inherited deficiency in mRNAs responsible for translating individual peptide chains in the globin molecule is the general cause of thalassaemia. In the severe homozygous α-thalassaemia with hydrops fetalis the fundamental lesion has been further clarified: in this lethal inherited disability absence or deletion of α-chain gene, or a large part of it, is the basic molecular derangement. But changes involving only single DNA bases are now considered responsible for most kinds of β-thalassaemia; such lesions may interfere with splicing of mRNA precursor units and so inhibit the synthesis of β-globin mRNA [24].

Inherited deficiency of enzymes

Genomic abnormality can result in profound aberration by abolishing or diminishing enzymic activity. Unlike the mechanisms underlying some haemoglobinopathies the genetic determinants of enzymic deficiencies have not yet been interpreted so fully in terms of point mutation or gene deletion, and have therefore to be considered in an empirical manner. Enzymic activity may be absent or diminished.

Absence of enzymic activity

Inherited absence of a normal enzymic protein is well illustrated in *phenylketonuria*. This familial disability occurs in homozygous recipients of a double complement of an abnormal autosomal recessive gene; the phenotypes then suffer from severe mental defect and excrete phenylpyruvic acid in their urine.

The liver of these patients contains no phenylalanine-4-mono-oxygenase. This enzyme, which converts phenylalanine to tyrosine (route A in Fig. 2.4), is a normal component of hepatic cells.

In the absence of phenylalanine-4-mono-oxygenase route A (Fig. 2.4) is eliminated and phenylalanine accumulates, although some of it is diverted along route B to form phenylpyruvic acid. In spite of this diversion the concentration of phenylalanine in blood and in CSF is magnified 15–100 times. This high concentration is harmful to myelination of the developing brain. Zones in which the myelin sheaths fail to stain appear in the cerebral white matter, and later these regions become partly replaced by glial tissue. Similar changes occur in the brain of young animals fed with excess of phenylalanine, while young monkeys fed in this way develop defects of learning. Moreover children with phenylketonuria can achieve normal mental ability if fed from birth on a diet low in phenylalanine.

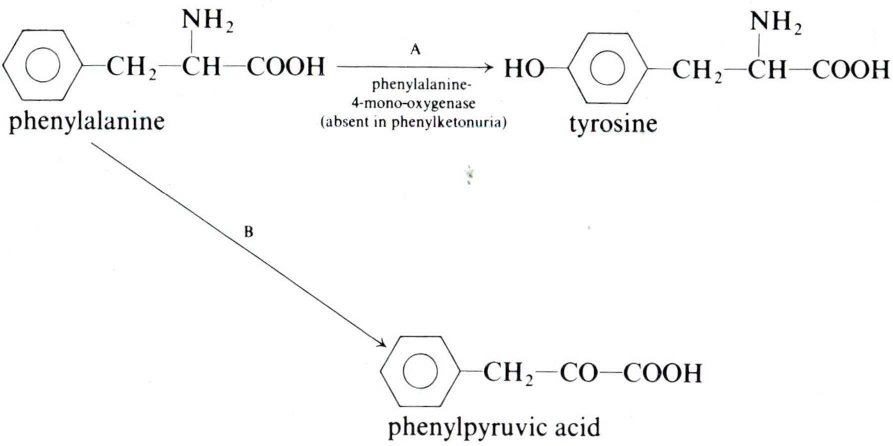

FIG. 2.4 Phenylketonuria. In the absence of phenylalanine-4-mono-oxygenase route A is abolished; phenylalanine then accumulates and its metabolism is diverted along route B to form phenylpyruvic acid which is excreted in the urine. Accumulation of phenylalanine interferes with myelination of axons in developing cerebral white matter and thus is responsible for mental defect.

The mental retardation in phenylketonuria is severe and may be accompanied by epilepsy. The defect in formation of tyrosine from phenylalanine retards formation of melanin which is normally produced from any excess tyrosine; thus fair hair and blue eyes are typical of phenylketonuria. The mechanism by which accumulation of phenylalanine interferes with myelination is obscure.

Many inborn errors of metabolism similarly arise in the homozygous recipients of other defective genes which also fail to elaborate an enzymic protein. In all these cases the substrate of the defective enzyme accumulates.

When this substrate is a soluble and diffusible micromolecule like phenylalanine in phenylketonuria, no visible deposits are formed even though the accumulation is injurious. In some of these disorders the substrate which accumulates is an insoluble or indiffusible macromolecule which forms visible deposits such as:

1. Complex lipids, e.g. ganglioside, in amaurotic family idiocy (p. 405).
2. Mucopolysaccharides, e.g. dermatan sulphate, in gargoylism (p. 408).
3. Glycogen in glycogenosis type 2 (p. 411).

It is unknown whether these defects depend on complete deletion of a whole code for a peptide chain in the abnormal gene, or whether alteration in the sequence of one or more DNA bases results in the eventual translation of peptide chains which are inactive as enzymes: in the latter case a puppet or phantom enzyme may in fact be formed, but it may have no activity.

Diminution in enzymic activity

Genomic defect can also diminish enzymic activity without eliminating it.

Thus in the overtly normal parents of homozygous patients with phenylketonuria the power to oxidise phenylalanine is diminished because the enzyme phenylalanine oxygenase is formed in diminished amount when coded by *only one* normal allele, the other being defective. In such persons harmful levels of phenylalanine are not reached and mental development is normal, although the conversion of phenylalanine to tyrosine is retarded.

In the inherited disease *citrullinaemia* the enzyme arginosuccinic acid synthetase, which normally condenses citrullin with aspartic acid, is defective; this enzyme, in its fully active form, is responsible for removing citrulline from the tissues but in this disorder, although the enzyme is formed, it has only 1 per cent of normal affinity for its substrate. Citrulline therefore accumulates and this partial metabolic block probably determines coincident cerebral defect.

Partial loss of enzymic activity is well illustrated by deficiency of glucose-6-phosphate dehydrogenase (G-6-PD).

Deficiency of Glucose-6-phosphate Dehydrogenase (G-6-PD)

This enzyme catalyses the oxidation of glucose-6-phosphate (G-6-*P*) to 6-phosphogluconolactone in red cells.

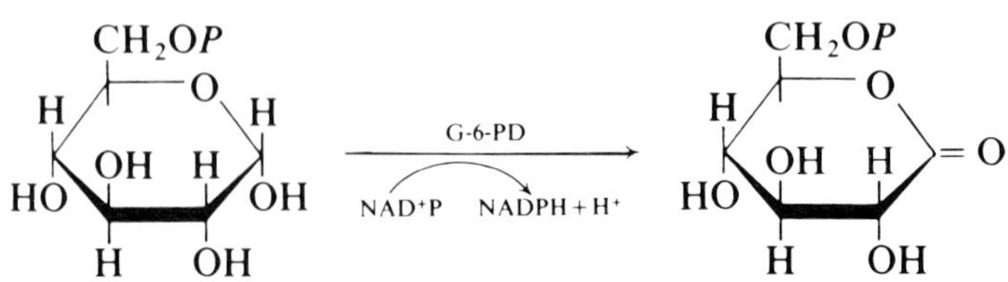

G-6-*P* 6-phosphogluconolactone

The reaction simultaneously results in conversion of $NADP^+$ to NADPH which is needed for stabilization of Hb (see below).

The enzyme G-6-PD occurs in at least 100 different isozymic forms determined by allelic variants of a gene linked to the X-chromosome. These isozymes can be characterised by differences in their electrophoretic mobility; but in some of them this variation in structure can severely impair enzymic activity.

Such defect in structure of G-6-PD coded by this X-linked gene can then produce X-Linked recessive disease; this chiefly affects *males* of certain ethnic groups, who receive this abnormal X-linked gene from their mothers, and who, unlike their sisters, are not protected by another normal allele donated by the paternal X-chromosome.

These male patients, who inherit the defective isozyme, suffer from attacks of haemolytic anaemia precipitated either by treatment with drugs, such as pamaquine or sulphonamides, or by eating broad beans. During these episodes the red cells are found to contain small inclusion bodies composed of *denatured* Hb called Heinz bodies; these adhere to the inner surface of the red cell membranes. The membranes, to which the Heinz bodies are attached, are injured on passage through the spleen and then the red cells become sequestrated and destroyed in splenic and hepatic RE cells; thus very severe haemolytic anaemia may result.

The formation of Heinz bodies is initiated by *oxidative denaturation* of Hb induced by oxidant drugs or by quinones formed from constituents of broad beans. In healthy red cells this oxidation is prevented by high concentration of reduced glutathione (GSH) which is a powerful reducing agent. The high level of GSH is maintained by constant reduction of oxidised glutathione (GSSG) to GSH by NADPH (reaction 1 below), while NADPH is itself continuously replaced by donation of hydrogen to $NADP^+$ from G-6-*P* effected by the enzymic activity of fully active G-6-PD (reaction 2 below).

Thus in normal red cells CSSG is continuously reduced to GSH as follows

$$\text{GSSG} + \text{NADPH} + \text{H}^+ \longrightarrow 2\text{GSH} + \text{NADP}^+ \quad (1)$$

$$\text{G-6-}P + \text{NADP}^+ \xrightarrow[\text{G-6-PD}]{} \text{6-phosphogluconolactone} + \text{NADPH} + \text{H}^+ \quad (2)$$

In this process (reaction 2) G-6-*P* is oxidised by $NADP^+$ and donates hydrogen to reform NADPH, *provided* active G-6-PD is present. But in the red cells of male heterozygotes, with only *one* defective X-linked gene for G-6-PD, the activity of the dehydrogenase G-6-PD may be diminished to low levels (nil to 20 per cent of normal). In this case restoration of NADH is retarded and the concentration of GSH is so low that its protective action against potential oxidants is minimal. Thus, when these patients are exposed to various drugs or bean products with oxidant action, Hb is converted to methaemoglobin by oxidative denaturation and Heinz bodies are precipitated against the cell membranes with resultant sequestration and haemolysis.

In one common form of G-6-PD deficiency, due to allele present among 10–20 per cent of Negroes, haemolytic anaemia occurs among males after treatment with pamaquine. In this disorder the G-6-PD in *young* red cells is a fully active enzyme, which is obtained by separating the young red cells from older ones by differential centrifugation; the activity of this enzyme falls rapidly *as the red cells age* and its half life is then shortened from 62 to 13 days. This suggests that the enzymic protein formed is unstable and suffers denaturation on ageing *in vivo*. In these patients recovery is rapid as young red cells with fully active enzyme replace the older ones which are haemolysed.

In another variant of G-6-PD deficiency, common among Mediterranean peoples, the activity of the isozyme even in young red cells is only 0–7 per cent of normal. This is a particularly dangerous type of disability, as haemolysis does not decrease rapidly when the older red cells are replaced. Attacks of severe haemolysis in these patients constantly follow consumption of broad beans and haemolysis persists so long as the beans are eaten.

Deficiency of G-6-PD thus illustrates genomic aberration in which an enzyme protein is defective although it continues to be formed. The enzyme may initially be diminished in activity or it may be fully active but unstable. Such imperfect or partly sham enzymes probably arise by point mutation in the DNA code rather than by complete deletion of the code for a whole peptide chain.

Inherited loss of structural protein

While many inherited disabilities depend on absence or imperfection of catalytic proteins genomic defect can also determine lack of structural proteins. Inherited absence of a structural protein, responsible for membrane stability and solubilization of hydrophobic lipids, is exemplified by abetalipoproteinaemia.

Abetalipoproteinaemia

In this serious disability, determined by an autosomal recessive gene, there is inherited absence of β-lipoprotein in plasma. The plasma is clear and develops no turbidity after ingestion of fat; chylomicrons, β-lipoproteins (LDL) and pre-β-lipoproteins (VLDL) are absent. The ability to synthesise β-lipoprotein in hepatic and intestinal cells is apparently suppressed. Fat accumulates in the jejunal cells, as the essential solubilising protein is absent and micellar fat (p. 357) cannot be formed.

These patients suffer from malabsorption of fat and later develop ataxia and unsteadiness in walking due to demyelination. They also suffer from loss of visual acuity caused by retinal degeneration.

A spectacular feature of abetalipoproteinaemia is the presence of thorn red cells (acanthocytes) in the blood. These mis-shapen red cells, which have spiny projections, are conspicuous in wet preparations of blood. Probably the apoproteins of plasma lipoproteins are important constituents of red cell membranes which became distorted into spiny projections in the absence of this stabilising component [7]. Plasma lipoprotein may also be incorporated into the plasma membrane of other cells and thus provides structural stability without which retinal nerve fibres and myelin sheaths become defective. This may account for retinal degeneration, and loss of myelin in cerebellum and spinal cord which occur later in the disease. Demyelination produces such severe disablement that these patients, by the age of 30, may be unable to stand upright.

It is possible that absence of β-lipoprotein may cause defective transport of linoleic acid or of vitamins A and E and thus further injure these patients; massive doses of these vitamins have recently been used in treatment [8].

Inherited defects of unknown mechanism

Not only the basic genomic defects but also the cellular mechanisms which account for most inherited diseases are still unknown. A very common disability of such undetermined pathogenesis is cystic fibrosis.

Cystic fibrosis (fibrocystic disease)

This disorder, resulting from an autosomal recessive gene, has the highest incidence of all lethal inherited diseases among European children. Its frequency in parts of Europe is 1 in 2000 live births, which indicates that the determinant carrier gene occurs in about 1 in 20 persons.

Cystic fibrosis is caused by excessive viscosity of the secretion of exocrine glands including pancreas, intestinal crypts, salivary glands and bronchial mucosa. This is due to increase in the concentration of glycoprotein in the fluid formed by the glandular cells (mucoviscidosis). The material which obstructs the glandular ducts is a negatively charged acidic glycoprotein which is coloured by PAS, alcian blue and colloidal iron [9]. The concentration of calcium ions in

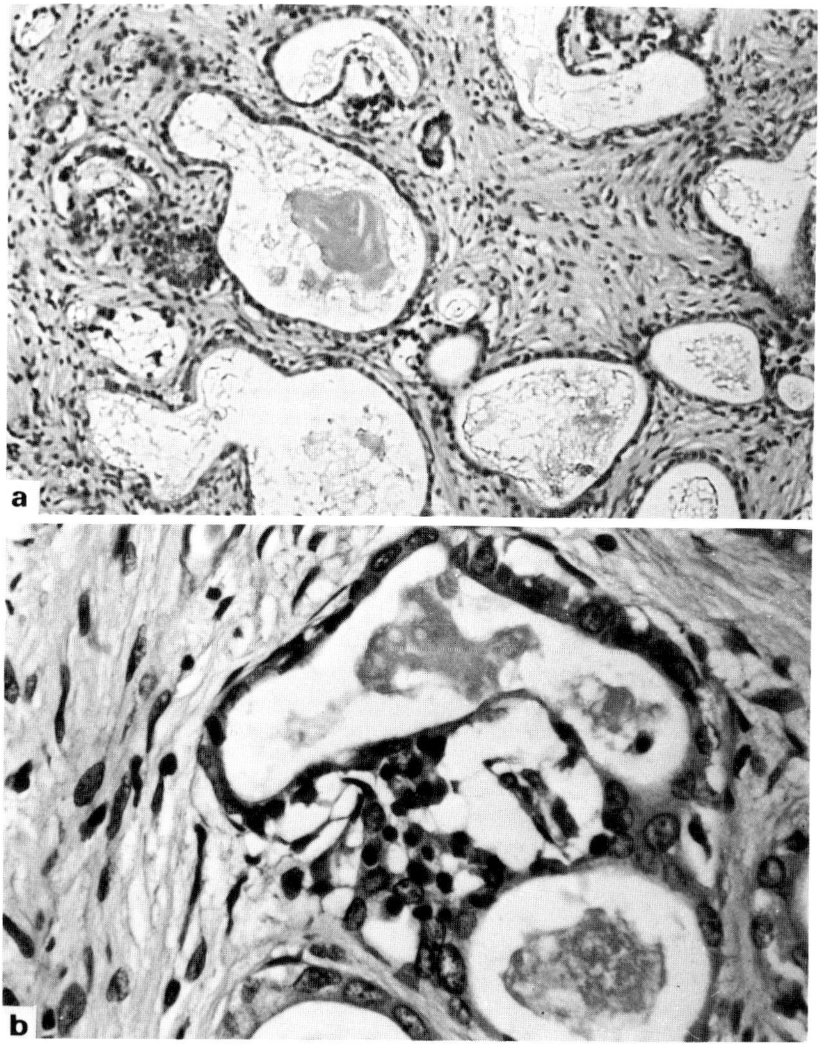

FIG. 2.5a Cystic fibrosis affecting pancreas. Ducts distended into cysts containing viscous eosinophilic secretion. Fibrosis visible between the cysts. × 130.
FIG. 2.5b Cystic fibrosis of pancreas. Enlarged ducts and an acinar remnant, surrounded by fibroblasts. × 500.

these secretions is also excessive and the submandibular saliva is turbid with visible deposits of calcium phosphate complexes, which show the same X-ray diffraction pattern as hydroxyapatite [10]. The sweat of affected children contains higher than normal concentration of NaCl. Excessive secretion of negatively charged glycoprotein may be connected with simultaneous release of Ca^{++} and Na^{+} into the extracellular fluid. But how the determinant genomic abnormality affects the secretions of exocrine cells is at present a complete mystery.

These children may become seriously ill from several causes including meconium ileus, malnourishment and pulmonary infection.

Meconium ileus. In this neonatal defect the terminal ileum of the newborn child becomes blocked by viscid meconium. This obstruction begins before birth and may cause death in early infancy. The increase in viscosity of the meconium is due to excessive concentration of glycoprotein in pancreatic and intestinal secretions.

Malnourishment. The child may fail to thrive owing to malabsorption. Obstruction of pancreatic ducts by viscid secretion prevents digestive enzymes from entering the duodenum. The increased viscosity of the fluid secreted results in obstruction of the ducts and distension of the acini with yellowish eosinophilic mucus; the ducts become dilated into microcysts filled by retained material. Later the acinar cells degenerate and intense fibrosis follows. The pancreas becomes both cystic and fibrous (Fig. 2.5, p. 31).

Pulmonary infection. If the child survives early infancy serious disability may follow because of hyperviscosity of the secretion by the bronchial glands. The bronchioles become occluded by plugs of viscid mucus and zones of emphysema and of partial collapse appear. Infection of these lesions results in bronchitis, bronchopneumonia and bronchiectasis, which are common causes of death in cystic fibrosis.

Huntingdon's chorea

Another inherited disease, in which the mechanism of pathogenesis is undetermined, is Huntingdon's chorea. This very rare disability is probably transmitted by an autosomal dominant gene, so that half the children of affected parents generally develop the disease. The most prominent signs are continuous involuntary movements followed by progressive dementia. These involuntary movements probably depend on loss from basal ganglia of neurones concerned with forming the normal inhibitory neurotransmitter gamma-aminobutyric acid.

The direct determinants of these signs are severe atrophy of the corpus striatum with loss of smaller ganglion cells in caudate nucleus and putamen and also atrophy and loss of neurones in cerebral cortex.

The onset of this distressing disease is usually between the ages of 30 and 45; the patients are therefore likely to have had children before knowing that they have received the fatal gene. How the genomic defect can remain masked for 30 years and then initiate this disastrous cellular degeneration is unknown.

VISIBLE CHANGE OF KARYOTYPE

Visible abnormality of the chromosomes affecting all the cells of the body is sometimes inherited from a similar abnormality in a parent, but more commonly is initiated by errors occurring in gametogenesis, fertilisation, or early mitosis of the zygote. Severe aberrations of this kind are highly lethal to the embryo which may die before implantation or be eliminated by spontaneous abortion. Some lesser degrees of abnormality are compatible with survival and may then be responsible for congenital disability among children born alive.

Localised change of karyotype affecting only a group or clone of cells is also commonly present in cells displaying autonomous neoplastic growth.

Recent refinements in techniques of staining fixed chromosomes with Romanowsky stains (Leishman or Giemsa), following partial denaturation by heat or trypsin, reveal a highly specified banded pattern which appears to be related to the assembly of DNA. These methods enable discrimination between individual chromosomes (1–23) in the principal groups (A–G) among human chromosomes.

Abnormality in appearance of chromosomes at mitosis is called *heteroploidy*: this may be *numerical* (affecting the number of chromosomes) or *structural* (involving change in shape or staining).

Numerical heteroploidy includes:

1. *Aneuploidy* in which there is gain or loss of one or more chromosomes but not amounting to a full haploid set; usually one chromosome is gained (to give 3 allelomorphs in place of a pair—*trisomy*) or lost (to give 1 allelomorph—*monosomy*).
2. *Polyploidy* in which there are more than two full haploid sets of chromosomes; usually three sets (69 chromosomes—*triploidy*) or much more rarely 4 sets (92 chromosomes—*tetraploidy*).

Structural heteroploidy includes deletion of parts of chromosomes, transverse breaks with re-ordering of segments, which may be translocated to another chromosome (translocation), or the presence of bizarre marker chromosomes, which occur in malignant tumours.

Heteroploidy is probably the most usual determinant of spontaneous human abortion. It also accounts for inherited disability among live-born children, and it is an almost universal characteristic among the cells of human malignant tumours.

Heteroploidy and spontaneous abortion

Spontaneous abortion probably occurs in about 15 per cent of human pregnancies, and when natural age is above 44, the incidence is doubled. Chromosomal abnormality is found in approximately 40 per cent of specimens of aborted fetal tissues grown in culture. Moreover, many embryos with chromosomal abnormality probably fail to implant. It is clear therefore that heteroploidy is a major cause or concomitant of embryonic disorder and death.

When abortion occurs early in pregnancy the embryo usually atrophies or disappears before the fetal membranes are discarded; in such cases fused amnion and chorion remain, though sometimes the embryo also persists as a small mass of undifferentiated cells. More than half the successful cultures made from such live aborted fetal membranes show heteroploidy. Chromosomal abnormality is thus probably responsible for early embryonic death followed by rejection of the living fetal membranes.

The abnormalities found in these heteroploid mitoses in cultures of aborted fetal tissue include [11]:

Trisomy	47 chromosomes (often 3 of no. 16)	50 per cent
Monosomy	45 chromosomes (only one X chromosome)	20 per cent
Polyploidy	usually triploidy (69 chromosomes)	25 per cent

Mechanism of rejection of heteroploid fetal tissue

It is uncertain how fetal tissues with chromosomal abnormality are detected by maternal tissues to cause uterine contraction and rejection. Possibly the embryo dies first and abortion follows as a rejection to this dead tissue, even though the fetal membranes are alive [11]. Indeed a limited life span may be an inherent property of heteroploid embryonic cells. Another possibility is that abnormal karyotypes stimulate *immunological mechanisms* which not only kill the embryo but also later cause rejection of the living fetal membranes by the maternal tissue.

Congenital abnormality among autosomes

Human embryos with autosomal abnormality usually perish during antenatal life. However children with trisomy of no. 21 of group G account for 1.5/1000 live births; other autosomal abnormalities are much rarer among live-born children. These changes of karyotype are all accompanied by severe mental and physical disability. Trisomy-21 and its effects only will be discussed here.

Down's syndrome

This type of idiocy is one of the commonest kinds of congenital mental defect. Over 90 per cent of affected children have trisomy of the small acrocentric chromosome no. 21 of group G. They are severely retarded mentally; at age 10 they have a mental age of 2. Their slanting eyes and rounded faces were to some people reminiscent of the mongolian race; hence the singularly inappropriate appellation of mongolism used to be given to this disability. The eyelids are often reddened by highly disfiguring blepharitis. Many infants with Down's syndrome have septal cardiac defects which cause early death from heart failure. Surviving children tend to be short in stature. Their hands are short and broad with small incurving little fingers; usually there is only a single palmar crease in each hand and whorls are absent from the digital markings.

These idiots are usually placid and friendly. The occiput is flattened and the cerebrum is small and poorly differentiated: gyri are often defective and the superior temporal convolution may be contrasted to a ribbon-like structure. The occipital lobes are almost vertical in posterior contour so that the cerebrum is very short. Possibly these abnormalities are impressed on developing brain by retardation of cranial growth. The total number of neurones is probably not diminished, and in parts of the cortex the number of neuronal cell bodies and nuclei per unit volume appears increased. The small size of the brain may thus be due to diminution in number and volume of axo-dendritic arborisations. Such loss in synaptic complexity may account for the mental defect.

In 1959 Lejeuene, Gautier and Turpin [12] made the remarkable discovery that the cells of idiots affected by Down's syndrome have an extra small acrocentric chromosome in group G and that the diploid number of chromosomes is increased from 46 to 47.

This striking addition of one extra of the smallest chromosome is observed in both boys and girls (Fig. 2.6). Thus Lejeune *et al.* observed in affected boys six very small chromosomes, i.e. five acrocentrics and one Y chromosome instead of normal four acrocentrics and one Y; similarly in affected girls five very small chromosomes were found, i.e. five acrocentrics (and no Y) instead of normal four acrocentrics (no Y). More recently introduced techniques, which reveal chromosomal banding with Romanowsky stains and zones that fluoresce on treatment with quinacrine, enable the normal two pairs of small acrocentric autosomes and the small male chromosome to be differentiated into pair-21,

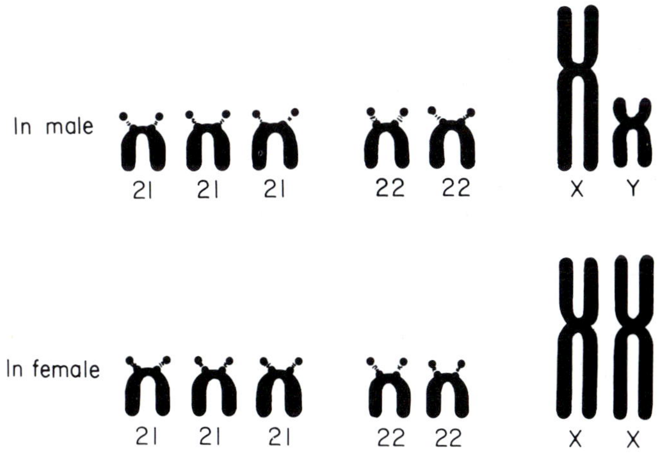

FIG. 2.6 Trisomy-21 in Down's disease. The total number of small acrocentric chromosomes is increased from 4 to 5 in boys and girls by addition of an extra allelomorph to pair-21. Another very small chromosome in boys is the Y chromosome; this has slightly larger short arms than those of pairs-21 and -22 (and also has zones in its long arms which fluoresce with quinacrine: not shown in figure).

pair-22 and Y respectively. The extra small chromosome in Down's syndrome is therefore now known to be allelomorphic to the pair which is designated 21. This karyotype occurs in over 90 per cent of patients with Down's disease, which is thus commonly 'determined' by trisomy-21.

This usual form of Down's syndrome with trisomy-21 becomes more frequent as maternal age advances; indeed, among children born of women over 45, Down's syndrome is 60 times as common as in children of mothers under 30. This fact has led to the view that Down's syndrome is caused by a defect in maternal gametogenesis.

Translocation Down's syndrome

The lesions in Down's syndrome are widespread and affect the development of many organs including brain, skull, heart and hands. One might fairly ask whether these lesions are all determined by a minute genomic imbalance resulting from trisomy-21, or whether the small karyotypic change and the developmental abnormalities alike are consquences of some other fundamental but more esoteric abnormality. The question receives an answer from the discovery that a few patients with Down's syndrome have *not* got an extra chromosome 21, but have the long arms of this chromosome translocated to the short arms of both chromatids of a large acrocentric of D group. These patients have *two* normal chromosomes 21 in G group and also an extra complement of the long arm of the same chromosome attached to a chromosome in D group. Thus an extra complement of the long arm of 21, whether present as an extra chromosome or as a translocated fragment, is associated with the same unique phenotypic lesions. Thus it appears reasonable to assume that triplication of the major genetic contents of chromosome 21 is the basic cause of Down's disease.

Cause of Down's syndrome

Although the inclusion of excessive genetic material derived from chromosome-21 thus appears to be the basic determinant of this distressing disability, the mechanism by which trisomy-21 arises in these retarded children is obscure.

If aberration of maternal gametogenesis with defective disjunction of pair-21 is the prime cause, then monosomy-21 (with 45 chromosomes) might be expected in the resultant zygotes with the same frequency as trisomy-21 (with 47 chromosomes).

One view is that zygotes (45-monosomy-21) are in fact formed but that this karyotype is a 'genetic lethal' and the resultant embryos all perish.

Another possibility is that, following defective disjunction at the first meiotic division in the primary oocyte, the conjoined pair of allelomorphs-21 *always remains* in the central mass, which forms the secondary oocyte and *never migrates* into the minute first polar body. This seems the most likely sequel. The secondary oocyte would then retain 24 chromosomes including pair-21 (as opposed to normal 23 chromosomes), while the first polar body would receive only 22 chromosomes (without chromosome-21). The first polar body then atrophies either directly or after one division. In this way the only fertile female haploid cells have 24 chromosomes including pair-21 and give zygotes (47-

trisomy-21) on fertilisation by a normal sperm with 23 chromosomes, while the possibility of forming zygotes (45-monosomy-21) is eliminated by atrophy of the first polar body with 22 chromosomes (devoid of 21). Thus the normal asymmetric division of female meiotic cells into gigantic secondary oocytes along with minute polar bodies may ensure that defective disjunction of pair-21 is followed by embryos with trisomy and not monosomy.

Congenital abnormality of sex chromosomes

Among children born alive aneuploidy of the sex chromosomes is considerably more common than of the autosomes. Two factors probably diminish the harmful effects of aneuploidy among sex chromosomes and thus permit survival of zygotes with these aberrations [13]:

1. The power to suppress much of the genetic action of X chromosomes, additional to the first by condensation to form Barr bodies.
2. The minute size of the Y chromosome (a small acrocentric) which carries little genetic information apart from determining male characteristics.

Thus an extra X or Y chromosome causes little disability, while absence of Y chromosome is also compatible with life. In contrast trisomy or monosomy among autosomes is lethal or causes very severe disability. Two not uncommon aberrations among sex chromosomes illustrate this power of survival.

Klinefelder's syndrome (karyotype 47, XXY) occurs relatively frequently. Thus Barr bodies, which indicate the presence of more than one X chromosome, are found in the nuclei of one in 600 overt males. Most of these individuals have karyotype 47, XXY. Owing to presence of Y chromosome male genitalia are formed but because of the second X chromosome the testes remain minute and the seminiferous tubules atrophy. The incidence of 47, XXY karyotype, as of autosomal trisomy, increases with maternal age, and it probably also arises from defective disjunction of the primary oocyte nucleus at meiosis.

Turner's syndrome (karyotype 45, X) is probably a frequent embryonic abnormality but most of these embryos die in antenatal life (p. 34) and only a small proportion are born alive. This karyotype occurs in one in 2000 newborn overt females. These individuals never menstruate and are infertile.

The relative frequency of such abnormalities of sex chromosomes thus probably indicates the real incidence of aneuploidy which is usually lethal when it affects autosomes; but similar aberrations among sex chromosomes are more compatible with survival.

Heteroploidy and neoplasia

Human malignant neoplasm

The cells in most human malignant tumours are abnormal in karyotype.

Abnormalities include (1) deviation in number of chromosomes from the normal diploid 46, (2) variation in number of chromosomes from cell to cell (aneuploid spread), and (3) change in chromosomal size and form to visibly mis-shapen, gigantic or bizarre 'marker' chromosomes.

Unlike normal human cells in mitosis, which uniformly possess the diploid number, the mitotic cells in malignant tumours generally have a variable number of chromosomes. Counts reveal a majority of karyotypes grouped around a prime modal number, and a smaller group with range of karyotypes around a mode with double the number of the prime mode [14]. Nearly every tumour can be characterised by its modal number, which is also found in the metastases and thus appears as a dominant stem line. This numerical variation implies that mutations are continually occurring along with division of the neoplastic cells, but that certain karyotypes are the most viable.

Most of these modal numbers fall in the diploid range 40–50, or else in the triploid–tetraploid range of 60–90. Only very rarely is the modal number 46, but modes as low as 37 are quite common in tumours of breast and ovary [14].

Change in size and form include deletion of portions of chromosomes and also translocation of fragments from one chromosome to another. Conspicuously abnormal 'marker' chromosomes may be produced by fusion of fragments to form extremely elongated or mis-shapen forms. Fig. 2.7 shows the karyotype of a cell from a malignant adenocarcinoma (probably of ovarian origin) which

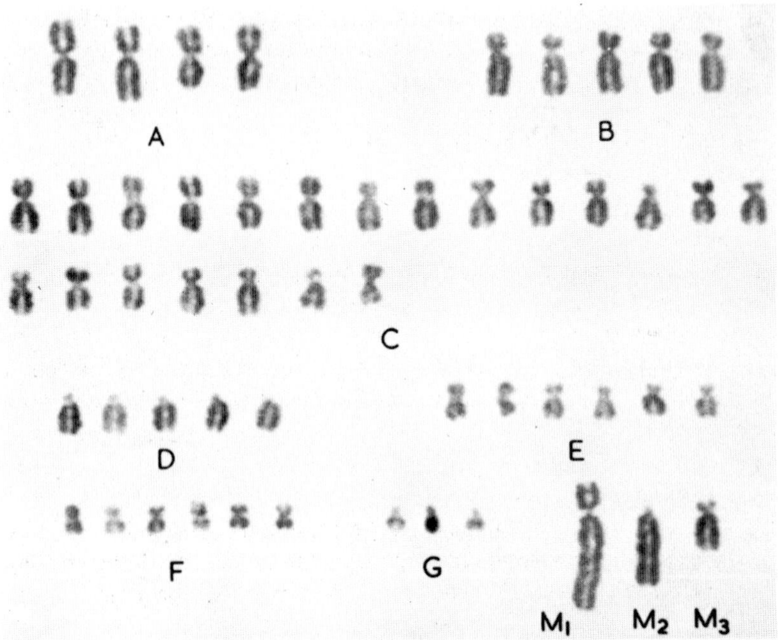

FIG. 2.7 Heteroploidy in human malignant neoplastic cell. This cell came from an infiltrating adenocarcinoma of lower abdomen probably originating in the ovary. This tumour infiltrated into the groin and peritoneum and produced ascites. This cell has 53 chromosomes and a very large marker chromosome M_1 and two smaller markers M_2, M_3. Courtesy of Dr N. B. Atkin and Dr M. C. Baker. Reproduced from *J. nat. Cancer Inst.* 1966, **36**, 539.

infiltrated the groin and peritoneum producing ascites. The dominant modal number of chromosomes was 53–54 and 'marker' chromosomes (M_1, M_2 in Fig. 2.7) were present in most karyotypes of this tumour [15].

Heteroploidy involving abnormality both in number and form of chromosomes is thus a prominent feature of human malignant tumours. The profound alteration in assembly and content of determinant DNA in these grossly aberrant karotypes may, therefore, be responsible for the invasive behaviour of the malignant cells. The similarity of general pattern and the recurrence of the same marker chromosomes both in the primary tumour and its metastases, indicate that all the abnormal cells produced in one tumour are products of a single original clone of deviant cells.

The question then arises whether heteroploidy is a general determinant of malignant neoplastic behaviour, or whether heteroploidy and malignant neoplasia are two separate but concomitant sequels of a more basic but invisible molecular change. Observation on the karyotype of some benign kinds of neoplasm, which are regarded as potential precursors of malignant tumours, throws some light on this problem.

Human benign neoplasms and precancerous states

Some benign tumours are static or grow so slowly that the appearance of their chromosomes at metaphase cannot be observed. When division is more frequent, some of the dividing cells in benign tumours may be *precancerous* in the sense that progression to malignant neoplasia is a common development in these tumours, although they are non-invasive at first. Heteroploidy in such precancerous lesions will now be considered.

Polyps of large intestine

Minor degrees of aneuploidy and some modal spread are usually found in dividing cells of benign tumours of the colon and rectum. Multiple polyps of the colon occur as an hereditary disability transmitted by a dominant gene (multiple polyposis coli, Gardner's syndrome). Nearly always one or more of these multiple polyps becomes malignant; this is a typical precancerous condition. All of these multiple polyps examined contained some cells with abnormal karyotypes [16].

Cervical dysplasia: carcinoma in situ

Dysplasia is a common occurrence in the squamous epithelium of the uterine cervix. The epithelium loses its capacity to differentiate into flattened squamous cells, polarity is lost and the nuclear/cytoplasmic ratio remains at the high primitive level (Fig. 2.8a, b).

When this change is widespread the term *carcinoma in situ* applied to it. It is generally held that dysplasia, which can be detected among cells in cervical smears, can herald progression to invasive carcinoma, although this transformation may be long deferred or may never occur.

The karyotype of dysplastic cervical epithelium is heteroploid and usually shows modal spread with deviation from the diploid number; prominent marker

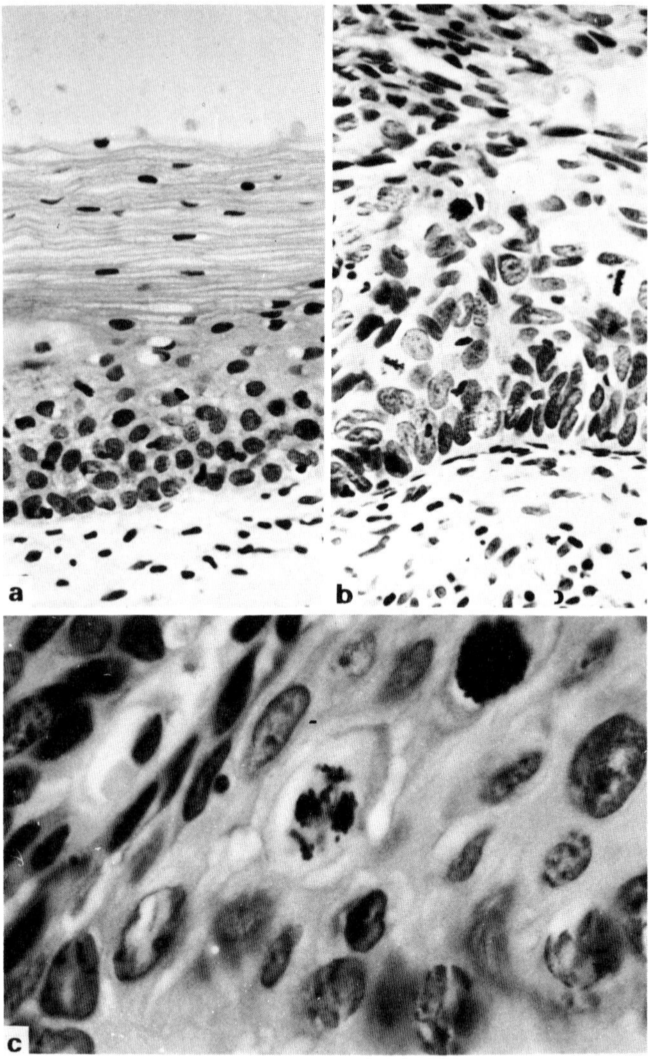

FIG. 2.8 Dysplasia of uterine cervix: carcinoma *in situ*.

a. Normal stratified epithelium of cervix; differentiation to squamous cells. × 400.

b. Cervical dysplasia. Imperfect differentiation; high nuclear/cytoplasmic volume ratio throughout; frequency of mitosis increased. × 400.

c. Cervical dysplasia. Two cells in mitosis; one of these shows a three-group metaphase with chromosomes lagging at poles. × 1000.

chromosomes are sometimes visible [17]. In dysplastic epithelium the frequency of mitosis is increased (Fig 2.8a, b, c) and some of the chromosomes tend to lag at the poles during metaphase to give '3-group metaphases' [18]. Fig. 2.8c shows the effect of lagging at mitosis with incomplete migration of chromosomes from poles to form metaphase plate. This kind of aberration probably indicates instability of karyotype and also potentiality for later progression to maligant neoplasia.

Chronic myeloid leukaemia (CML)

This disease is remarkable as an instance of neoplasia in which the aberrant cells usually display a constant karyotype characterised by a conspicuous marker chromosome. CML also illustrates potential progression towards malignant acute myeloid leukaemia.

Myeloblasts and other narrow stem cells grown in culture from bone marrow or blood patients with CML generally show a uniform diploid karyotype in which one of the small acrocentric chromosomes of pair-22 is replaced by the dwarf-chromosome Ph′ (Philadelphia chromosome). This spectacular pigmy is much more minute than normal small acrocentrics (pair-21, pair-22, and Y) owing to absence of most of the long arms of each chromatid (Fig. 2.9).

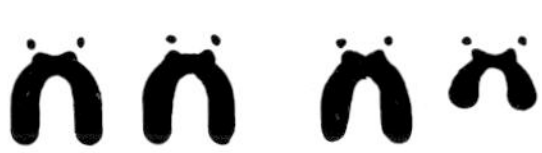

(a) (b)

FIG. 2.9 Comparison of normal chromosomes of pair-22 with those in myeloid leukaemia.

a. Normal small acrocentric chromosomes of pair-22.

b. Pair-22 in chronic myeloid leukaemia. The Ph^1 chromosome is on the right.

The Ph′ chromosome was first observed in two male patients with CML and was then supposed to be an unusually small Y chromosome. Subsequently Bakie *et al.* [19] found the same chromosome in female patients with CML and concluded that the minute marker was an autosome of pair-21 or pair-22. Use of banding techniques later showed that the pigmy chromosome is derived from one of pair-22. More recently Janet Rowley [20], by using both fluoroscence with quinacrine and staining with Giemsa, confirmed that the Ph′ chromosome is formed by deletion of the long arm from one of pair-22, but she also discovered an additional small mass of chromatin consistently attached to the long arm of one chromosome of pair-9 in cells from nine consecutive patients with CML. This suggests that *translation* of the deleted fragment from the long arm of 22 to the long arm of 9 is the dominant event in producing this remarkable karyotype in CML (46, 22q −, 9q +).

When a blastic crisis occurs in CML, a second Ph′ may appear and chromosome counts other than diploid are visible. Such aneuploid spread is, as we have seen, typical of human malignant tumours. In this sense CML may be regarded as an early stage in tumour progression, which probably occurs in all neoplastic tissue before they enter the fully malignant phase. Unstable aneuploid karyotype, with spread of chromosome counts around a modal number, is characteristic of acute myeloid leukaemia, whether or not it is preceded by

CML. In the former case Ph′ chromosomes persist in the newly assumed aneuploid karyotype probably as a remnant of the more stable pre-existing pattern.

Thus several precancerous states in man are accompanied by visible changes of karyotype which probably indicate genomic instability and liability to progress to malignant neoplasia. Indeed the conspicuous heteroploidy commonly present in the cells of malignant tumours may develop from the less severe aberrations which have the tendency to mutate to anaplastic types with grossly abnormal chromosomal patterns.

Heteroploidy as a cause of malignant neoplasia in man

Obervations on human benign tumours and dysplasia which can progress to invasive neoplasm indicate that, even during precancerous change, the chromosomes are already visibly abnormal. Instability or change of karyotype appears to be either a constant concomitant or even a cause, but *not* a mere consequence of malignant neoplasia. Moreover karyotypes of human malignant tumours are usually so far aberrant from the normal diploid pattern that their cells could hardly behave and interact in the same way as those of normal tissues [21]. Since karyotype reflects the structure and array of genomic DNA, the cellular activities of these tumours, as determined by their controlling genes, must differ fundamentally from the constant and ordered behaviour directed by a normal karyotype. These differences may thus include the properties of invasiveness and metastasis (p. 460), which constitute the essence of malignant neoplasia. Thus visible change of karyotype appears to be a usual determinant of human malignant neoplasia.

Malignant tumours of animals

Some transplantable malignant tumours of animals show prominent heteroploidy. The Walker carcinoma of rats has a near triploid modal number of 62 (normal diploid 42) and conspicuous large metacentric marker chromosomes (normal rat chromosomes are telocentric or subtelocentric).

However, the cells of some tumours of animals on first appearance may show no visible chromosomal abnormality. Heteroploidy is not discernible in sarcoma of chickens induced by the Rous sarcoma virus (RSV), but small alterations among the 60 microchromosomes and 12 macrochromosomes of the chick might be very difficult to detect.

RSV can also induce sarcomata in rats, in which the cells of the initial tumours show the normal diploid karyotype of 42 chromosomes. But these tumours, on successive transplantation to other rats become anaplastic (p. 458) and more invasive and simultaneously evolve an apparently predestined pattern of chromosomal aberration [22]. Thus Mitelman analysed the progression of karyotype in transplants of two separate sarcomata induced in rats by RSV. Each of these tumours was transplanted sequentially in five parallel series of transplants into other rats. The transplanted tumours from each of these two separate initial tumours developed its own unique stem lines which showed the same independent type of heteroploidy with characteristic initial hyperdiploid modal number and individual marker chromosomes; these individual patterns developed in the parallel transplants from each of these tumours.

Mitelman *et al.* [23] also examined the karyotypes of fibrosarcomata induced in rats by 7,12-dimethylbenz(a)anthracene (DMB); these tumours showed characteristic heteroploid karyotypes in which trisomy of the longest telocentric and addition of a metacentric chromosome were the most characteristic features. This pattern was conspicuously different from that displayed by karyotypes of transplanted sarcomata initially induced by RSV. Mittelman concluded that essentially different pathways towards extreme malignancy are progressively followed in tumours initiated by different agents. He suggested that apparent lack of chromosomal pattern, noticeable in most classes of human malignant neoplasms, may reflect wide differences in causal agents.

Thus, although the cells of some tumours induced in animals by viruses or chemical oncogens may at first not show any *visible* chromosomal abnormality, their genome is probably altered by an initial molecular change which is not detectable by microscropy. This change apparently gives its own pattern of instability, which is determined both by the original genome and by the nature of the oncogenic agent. This instability gives further mutations, which finally cause gross enough rearrangement of DNA to produce visible chromosomal aberration; along with these changes both heteroploidy and anaplasia progressively become more extreme so that conspicuous heteroploidy is generally present in highly invasive tumours. Indeed the close analysis of the initial changes of karyotype, which is possible in observations on animal tumours, strongly suggests that latent molecular changes herald predetermined visible alterations of karyotype, which are the basic determinants of invasive neoplasm. Moreover different oncogenic agents appear to produce individual patterns of chromosomal aberration (p. 472).

Genomic aberrations in malignant tumours differ from genomic aberrations of inherited diseases in that the former are confined to the cells of the tumour and its mestastases, but the latter potentially affect all cells of the body; in fact the aberrant cells of a tumour probably arise from a single clone of mutant cells. (p. 471).

REFERENCES

[1] PERUTZ M. F. & LEHMANN H. (1968) Molecular pathology of haemoglobin. *Nature*, **219**, 902.

[2] WHITE J. G. (1974) Ultrastructural features of erythrocyte and haemoglobin sickling. *Arch. intern. Med.* **133**, 545.

[3] LEHMANN H. & HUNTSMAN R. G. (1974) *Man's Haemoglobins*, 2nd Ed. North-Holland, Amsterdam.

[4] BOYO A. E. & Ikomi-Kumm J. A. (1973) Metabolic activity of erythrocytes as determined by microcalorimetry. In *Protides of the Biological Fluids, 20th Colloquium*, p. 559, ed. by H. Peeters. Pergamon, Oxford.

[5] WEATHERALL D. J. (1974) Molecular basis for some disorders of haemoglobin synthesis. *Brit. med. J.*, **4**, 451 and 516.

[6] OTTOLENGHI S. *et al* (1974) Gene deletion as the cause of α-thalassaemia. *Nature*, **251**, 389.

[7] LANGDON R. G. (1973) Serum lipoproteins as major protein constituents of the human erythrocytic membrane. *Biochim. biophys. Acta* (Amst.) **342**, 213.
[8] LLOYD J. K. (1973) Hypolipoproteinaemia. *J. clin. Path.*, **26**, supplement **5**, 53.
[9] SHACKLEFORD J. M. & BENTLEY H. P. (1964) Carbohydrate histochemistry of the salivary glands and pancreas in cystic fibrosis. *J. Histochem. Cytochem.*, **12**, 512.
[10] WARTON K. L. & BLOMFIELD J. (1971) Hydroxyapatite in the pathogenesis of cystic fibrosis. *Brit. med. J.*, **3**, 570.
[11] CARR D. H. (1971) Chromosomes and abortion. *Advances in Human Genetics*, **2**, 201.
[12] LEJEUNE M., GAUTIER M. & TURPIN R. (1959) Études des chromosomes somatiques de neuf enfants mongoliens. *C. R. Acad. Sci. (Paris)*, **248**, 1721.
[13] FORD C. E. (1974) General mammalian cytogenetics. In *The Cell in Medical Science*, Vol. 2, p. 54, ed. by F. Beck & J. B. Lloyd. Academic Press, London.
[14] ATKIN N. B. (1974) Chromosomes in human malignant tumours. In *Chromosomes and Cancer*, p. 376, ed. by J. German. Wiley, New York.
[15] ATKIN N. B. & BAKER M. C. (1966) Chromosomal abnormalities as primary events in human malignant disease. *J. Nat. Cancer Inst.*, **36**, 539.
[16] MARK J., MITELMAN F., DENCKER R. H., NORRYD C. & TRANBERG K-G. (1973) The specificity of chromosomal abnormality in human colonic polyps. *Acta path. microbiol. scand.*, Section A. **81**, 85.
[17] BODDINGTON M. M., SPRIGGS A. I. & WOLFENDALE M. R. (1965) Cytogenetic abnormalities in carcinoma in situ and dysplasia of the uterine cervix. *Brit. med. J.*, **1**, 154.
[18] SPRIGGS A. I. (1974) Cytogenetics of cancer and precancerous states of cervix uteri. In *Chromosomes & Cancer*, p. 423, ed. by J. German. Wiley, New York.
[19] BAKIE A. G., COURT-BROWN W. M., BUCKTON K. E., HARNDEN D. G., JACOBS P. M. & TOUGH I. M. (1960) A possible specific chromosome abnormality in chronic myeloid leukaemia. *Nature*, **188**, 1165.
[20] ROWLEY J. D. (1973) A new consistent abnormality in chronic myelogenous leukaemia identified by quinacrine fluorescence and Giemsa staining. *Nature*, **243**, 290.
[21] SPRIGGS A. I., BODDINGTON M. M. & CLARKE C. M. (1962) Chromosomes of human cancer cells. *Brit. med. J.*, **2**, 1431.
[22] MITELMAN F. (1972) Predetermined sequential chromosome changes in serial transplantation of Rous rat sarcomas. *Acta path. microbiol. scand.*, Section A. **80**, 313.
[23] MITELMAN F., MARK J., LEVAN G. & LEVAN A. (1972) Tumor etiology and chromosome pattern. *Science*, **176**, 1340.
[24] WESTWAY D. & WILLIAMSON R. (1981) An intron nucleotide sequence variant in a cloned β^+-thalassaemia globin gene. *Nucl. Acids Res.* **9**, 1777.

CHAPTER 3

Lack of Nutriments

From Nature's chain whatever link you strike,
Tenth, or ten thousandth, breaks the chain alike.
Alexander Pope

Unlike unicellular organisms the cells of the body require an elaborate system of entry, transfer and vascular supply so that the nutrient molecules can be absorbed, travel in the circulating blood and then reach and penetrate individual cells and provide them with the initial substrates for metabolism. Then and then only can the cells survive in health and perform their varied activities.

Interference with the supply of nutriments to the cells of the body occurs in many different ways. Not only may the external supply of nutriments be deficient, but injury or defect in the absorptive activity of intestinal and pulmonary cells can retard entry of nutrient molecules. Moreover specialised *fabricator cells* may cease to produce and secrete substances, which they alone can synthesise and which are necessary for the function of other cells. Even when the blood is effectively charged with all these essential nutriments, interruption of circulation may yet deprive cells of necessary supplies; this kind of deprivation is in fact the commonest cause of cellular defect in disease, and it frequently depends on initial damage to *effector cells* such as those of the myocardium, which serve as propellers for the nutrient blood. Thus injury through lack of nutriments may occur in cells far removed from those initially affected: such consequential damage through lack of nutriments illustrates the principle of indirect injury mentioned in Chapter 1. Finally, even though the necessary nutritive substances reach the cell surface, penetration into the cells may be deficient.

The supply of nutriments to the cells of the body may thus be defective owing to:

1. Insufficiency of external food.
2. Defective absorption and transfer of nutriments.
3. Deficiency of internal secretions.
4. Interruption or retardation in flow of blood.
5. Defective penetration of nutriments into cells.

INSUFFICIENCY OF EXTERNAL FOOD

Lack of protein

Of the three major foodstuffs, protein, lipid and carbohydrate, protein alone is commonly deficient to an extent capable of causing human disease.

When the diet of man and animals contains adequate amounts of protein, granules stainable by basic dyes (see Fig. 7.14a) are visible in the cytoplasm of liver cells [1]. These Berg granules, which were discovered in rat liver, contain protein, RNA and phospholipid [1–3]; by EM the granules are seen as massed cisternae of rough-surfaced endoplasmic reticulum arranged as laminated saccules and covered externally by adherent ribosomes. These zones are endowed with capacity for synthesis of protein and are the sites of formation of serum albumin as well as the other essential proteins produced by the liver.

After short periods of fasting these granules disappear from the hepatic cells of rats but reappear on being fed protein [4]. Loss of granules is accompanied by diminution of hepatic content of RNA and phospholipid, while reappearance of granules after ingestion of protein occurs along with restoration of RNA and phospholipid [3]. Ultrastructural changes in the livers of rats fed on diets deficient in protein include loss of ribosomes and mitochondria with dilatation of ER saccules to form large internal 'lakes' [5].

Chronic severe lack of protein in man leads to famine oedema. Deficiency of amino acids retards the formation of albumin in the liver and this no doubt contributes to causing oedema by lowering the colloid osmotic pressure of the plasma. Although fall in concentration of albumin in the plasma does occur in malnourished patients, other factors are probably also concerned in causing famine oedema [6]. Thus diminution in the size of subcutaneous lipocytes may so diminish the cellular mass in the body that the skin cannot shrink enough to fit the reduced volume occupied by cells; for this reason intercellular oedema may be aggravated by a fall in tissue pressure which can draw water out of the cells into tissue spaces especially in dependent parts of the body.

Starvation, when used as a means of treating obesity, can cause sudden death from acute heart failure. In these patients the myocardial fibres are attenuated to half their normal diameter and the individual fibrils (seen by EM) are grossly fragmented [7].

Prolonged partial deficiency of protein gives rise to kwashiorkor, a disease of malnourished children in Africa and America. These children are weaned early and are fed on a cereal diet grossly deficient in protein. They fail to grow, are pot-bellied and suffer from oedema and diarrhoea. The skin shows patches of desquamation and depigmentation ('enamel paint appearance') and punched-out ('nutritional') ulcers may develop. The muscles are severely wasted. The digestive glands cease to fabricate their specific enzymes; there is hardly any pancreatic juice and fluid aspirated from the duodenum is deficient in trypsin. The concentration of albumin in the plasma falls; this probably accounts for the oedema. The livers are enlarged and fatty and are severely depleted of protein and RNA [8]. The fat content of the liver may reach 50 per cent of its fresh weight [9]; this accumulation of fat in the liver is due to a defect in synthesis of very low density lipoprotein by the liver cells (p. 368).

Lack of digestive enzymes is a crucial factor in development of kwashiorkor. This prevents full utilisation of the small quantities of protein still available in the food. At the same time retention of undigested material in the bowel stimulates diarrhoea which still further impedes absorption. In this way the synthesis of protein in the digestive glands becomes even more deficient. Thus a vicious cycle of deficiency, followed by malabsorption and further deficiency, results in gross cellular deprivation of essential amino acids. The contractile proteins are not formed in the wasting muscles just as enzymic proteins fail to be produced in the exocrine glands.

When protein is fed to patients with famine oedema or kwashiorkor recovery occurs if treatment is started soon enough. In any case time is needed to restore the membrane-orientated sites of translation of mRNA and the coordinated ribosomal activity of liver, muscle and endocrine cells before synthesis of cellular proteins can recommence.

Chronic malnutrition due to lack of protein is usually associated with multiple deficiencies of other essentials including vitamins. The resultant disorder of the deprived cells may be extremely complex.

Lack of vitamins

Essential organic nutriments, which cannot be synthesised by the body itself, but which are only required in relatively small amounts, are the accessory food factors or vitamins. These substances are not utilised as a major source of energy by the cell or even as substantial units of its structural composition, but are required as active portions of enzymes or coenzymes or as microconstituents with potent action on conformation or orientation of macromolecules.

The existence of such accessory food factors was demonstrated in a most cogent manner by F. G. Hopkins in 1912 who fed young rats on a synthetic diet composed of casein, lard, starch and glucose supplemented by mineral salts. The rats failed to grow, but rapid growth occurred when a few ml of milk was added to the diet. This shows that microconstituents are necessary for growth in addition to the major food substances. Soon it was realised that more than one accessory factor is necessary for animals to grow on a purified diet. McCollum and Davis in 1915 [10] referred to two factors, 'fat soluble A' and 'water soluble B'. Now it is realised that several fat and water soluble factors are necessary.

Absence of some of these organic microconstituents causes serious disease in man. The nature of some of these substances and the ways in which their absence can cause disease will now briefly be considered. The fat soluble factors will first be discussed.

Retinol (vitamin A)

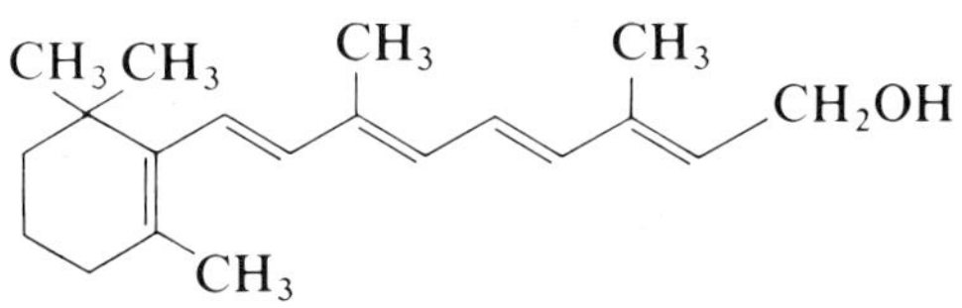

This essential polyenoic alcohol with five conjugated double bonds is frequently deficient in the diet of malnourished children in tropical countries. Retinol is present dissolved in the lipids of eggs, milk and butter and it can also be formed from the plant hydrocarbon β-carotene in passage through the intestinal epithelium. Retinol is principally stored in the liver.

Without sufficient retinol, growth is retarded and moist epithelial surfaces dry up and atrophy and then become replaced by stratified keratinised epithelium. The scleral conjunctiva becomes dry and scaly (xerophthalmia), while the cornea, which is specially susceptible to lack of retinol, softens, opacifies and later becomes infected with subsequent scarring and permanent loss of vision.

Retinol exerts a remarkable effect on explants of embryonic chick ectoderm grown in culture [11]. When grown in a medium lacking retinol, explanted ectoderm rapidly changes into keratinised squamous epithelium; addition of retinol makes the explants develop as a single layer of mucus secreting cells. The vitamin is clearly a necessity for maintaining simple ectodermal epithelium in columnar or pseudostratified form. Without it the epithelium of the upper respiratory tract and cornea develop squamous metaplasia with keratinisation.

Retinol also plays an important part in visual mechanism. Within the eye retinol is isomerised from its usual all-trans form to $\triangle^{11}$-cis-retinol; this is oxidised to an aldehyde, which is then conjugated with the optic protein *opsin* to form *rhodopsin*—the visual pigment in the rod cells of the retina. The action of light probably changes the cis-trans configuration of this polyene-protein complex and thus initiates visual impulses. Without a supply of retinol night blindness develops.

Whether changes in conformation of polyene-protein complexes are also necessary for the development and maintenance of moist epithelial surfaces is uncertain. The principal physiological mechanism of the vitamin is still obscure.

Cholecalciferol (vitamin D_3)

This is a fat-soluble accessory factor derived from steroids, which is responsible for the proper absorption of Ca^{++} from the bowel and the subsequent deposition of calcium salts in bone. Without this substance children are stunted in growth and their bones are imperfectly ossified. In this disorder, which is called *rickets*, calcium salts fail to be deposited in the intercellular material formed by both cartilage cells and osteoblasts. Normal bone is therefore not formed and in its place swollen masses of uncalcified osteoid tissue appear as a product of the still active cartilage cells. These osteoid swellings are formed at the costochondral junctions of the ribs and around joints at the ends of long bones. The legs become bowed owing to bending of the imperfectly ossified skeletal tissues under pressure.

Man has two sources of cholecalciferol:

1. Preformed cholecalciferol, present in animal fats such as milk, butter and fish liver oils, which is absorbed from the intestine.
2. 7-dehydrocholesterol normally present in the skin, which is transformed into cholecalciferol on irradiation by ultraviolet light.

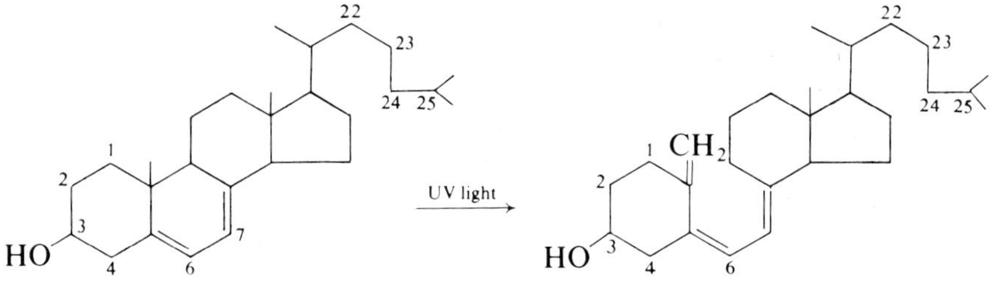

7-dehydrocholesterol cholecalciferol

If both these sources are absent then calcification becomes defective. European children without much sunlight usually obtain sufficient cholecalciferol in their food. Asian children, when living in Europe, may still consume traditional Eastern diets with insufficient animal lipids containing cholecalciferol; hence rickets is more common among immigrant children.

Cholecalciferol is stored in the liver; it is itself probably not the directly active promoter of calcification. But in the *liver* it is oxidized to 25-hydroxycholecalciferol, and this is further oxidized in the *kidney* to 1,25-dihydroxycholecalciferol (1,25-DHCC). 1,25-DHCC is a highly active hormone which is then secreted by the kidney. This hormone acts principally on the mucosal cells of the small intestine which it stimulates to absorb Ca^{++}.

7-dehydrocholesterol in skin
↓ UV light
cholecalciferol in food ⟶ cholecalciferol in tissues and blood
↓ liver
25-hydroxycholecalciferol
↓ kidney
1,25-dihydroxycholecalciferol (1,25-DHCC)
acts on enterocytes in small intestine and promotes absorption of Ca^{++}

The action of 1,25-DHCC [12] is probably exerted in two steps. First this hormone increases the net uptake of Ca^{++} at the surface of the enterocytes and second it accelerates the transport of Ca^{++} across the cells. The latter effect is probably dependent on a special *calcium-binding protein*, which appears in the cells when absorption of Ca^{++} is stimulated by cholecalciferol. 1,25-DHCC probably acts on the enterocyte nuclei so as to induce the transcription of m-RNA specific for translation of this calcium-binding protein. Absence of this carrier protein from the enterocytes appears to be the principal lesion caused by deficiency in vitamin D_3. Ossification may similarly depend on this Ca-carrier.

α-Tocopherol (*vitamin E*)

This fat soluble heterocyclic phenol with an isoprenoid side chain is a powerful antioxidant and it specifically inhibits the oxidation of polyenoic lipids by oxygen. It is present in animal fats and wheat germ oil. Adult rats kept for long periods on a diet deficient in α-tocopherol develop muscular atrophy, ataxia and paralysis, and eventually sink into a stuporous state. These derangements are accompanied by accumulation of abundant deposits of acid fast fluorescent lipoproteins in the muscle fibres and in the neuronal cell bodies of brain and spinal cord [13]. This fluorescent lipid may be formed by lipoperoxidation of phospholipids in cell membranes, a process which is normally suppressed by the antioxidant action of vitamin E.

Similar deposits of lipid appear in the neurones of monkeys fed on E-deficient diets [14]. These granules are intensely coloured by the PAS method and closely resemble the granules of proteolipid which accumulate in human neurones as age advances (p. 400). Einarson raised the possibility that defective utilization of vitamin E might therefore be a concurrent factor in the process of human ageing. It is also possible that time alone exerts an effect in increasing lipoperoxidation of cell membranes which even adequate supplies of the vitamin cannot prevent.

The water soluable vitamins include the numerous vitamins of the B group and also vitamin C. The most important of the B group in relation to human disease are thiamine (B_1), nicotinamide, folate and cobalamin (B_{12}). All these factors have a function as components of coenzymes which cannot be synthesised without precursors supplied by the food; they are active in very small amounts. Vitamin C on the other hand is required in relatively much greater quantity.

Thiamine (vitamin B_1)

This thiazole pyrimidine compound possesses an active group which exerts a crucial coenzymic effect in the normal cellular oxidation of glucose. Meat is a rich source of this vitamin, which is also present in the outer coat of grain but is notably absent from polished rice and is scanty in white flour.

Deficiency of thiamine gives rise to the disease beri-beri, which predominantly affects rice eating people in the East. Beri-beri occurs in 'dry' and 'wet' forms. The dry form is usually a disease of peripheral nerves with weakness, paraesthesia and tenderness in limbs. In early stages the myelin alone degenerates but later the axons disintegrate also. Among British prisoners, who were on poor rice diets in Malaya during World War II, lack of thiamine was one of the most serious causes of illness. They developed an acute cerebral form of beri-beri with disorientation, loss of memory and hallucinations, terminating in semi-coma and death. This condition was rapidly cured by early treatment with thiamine [15]. The wet form of the disease is characterised by heart failure and oedema; the myocardial fibres become swollen and lose their striations. The basic lesion of beri-beri in all its forms is impairment of the normal oxidative decarboxylation of pyruvate, and the concentration of this substance in the blood is consistently raised in patients with beri-beri [16].

The mechanism of this effect was first established in 1932 by Rudolf Peters and his colleagues [17]. They found that pigeons fed on a diet deficient in thiamine develop convulsions and intense head retraction which are rapidly curable by thiamine. Brain tissue from these deficient birds has a lowered O_2 uptake in the presence of lactate; also pyruvate accumulates on incubation of lactate with this tissue. Moreover addition of thiamine to this deficient brain tissue restores the oxygen uptake to normal levels. Excess of pyruvate was also found in the blood of these thiamine deficient pigeons [18].

Lack of thiamine interrupts an essential step in the principal chain of oxidation of carbohydrate in the cell, namely oxidative decarboxylation of pyruvate. This obstruction was most convincingly demonstrated by Lipmann [19]; he showed that slices of cerebral grey matter taken from pigeons, fed on a diet deficient of thiamine, form pyruvic acid from glucose, and that this accumulation of pyruvic is diminished by addition of thiamine.

Thus pyruvic acid, originally formed by glycolysis of glucose, reacts with coenzyme A(HS-CoA) in a process of oxidative decarboxylation in the presence of oxygen to form acetyl-coenzyme A(CH_3CO-S-CoA) along with liberation of CO_2. This oxidative fission is catalysed by the enzyme pyruvic dehydrogenase (P-DH) and requires NAD^+ as hydrogen acceptor:

$$CH_3CO\text{-}COOH + HS\text{-}CoA + NAD^+ \xrightarrow[\text{P-DH}]{} CH_3CO\text{-}S\text{-}CoA + CO_2 + NADH + H^+$$

The reaction is dependent on two other cofactors besides HS-CoA and NAD^+. These are *thiamine pyrophosphate* (ThPP) and *lipoic acid* (6,8-dithio-octanoic acid). The latter is probably joined to lysine in the P-DH enzyme complex by an amide linkage [20, 21].

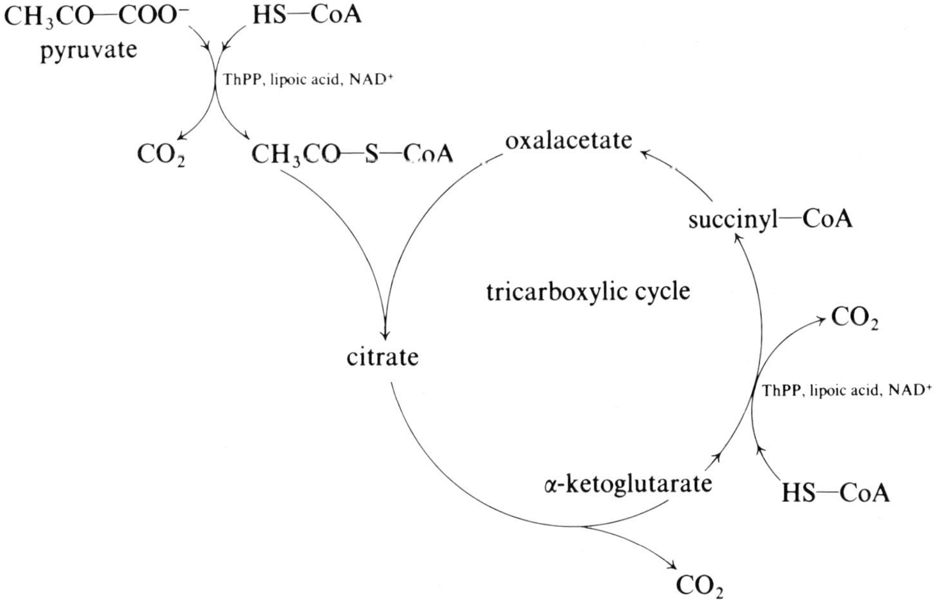

FIG. 3.1 Role of thiamine pyrophosphate (ThPP) in promoting oxidative decarboxylation of pyruvate and of α-ketoglutarate. In the absence of thiamine the tricarboxylic acid cycle is suppressed and pyruvate accumulates.

In this process of oxidative decarboxylation of pyruvic acid thiamine (in the form of ThPP) tears out the elements of acetaldehyde from pyruvic acid and (with them) acetylates lipoic acid, which in turn affects the acetylation of HS-CoA. Thus CO_2 and acetyl-CoA are formed from pyruvic acid; the acetyl-CoA then serves as the basic external substrate for the tricarboxylic acid cycle by which the remaining two C atoms of pyruvic acid are finally oxidised to CO_2 (Fig. 3.1).

ThPP is thus an essential initiator of oxidative decarboxylation of pyruvate and thereby provides acetyl-CoA necessary for reacting with oxalacetate in the tricarboxylic acid cycle (Fig 3.1); ThPP also promotes similar oxidative decarboxylation of α-ketoglutarate to form succinyl-CoA at a later phase in the cycle (Fig. 3.1).

It is clear therefore that deficiency of thiamine can deprive neurones and myocardial fibres of a cardinal coenzyme on which their principal exergonic catabolism depends. The resultant interruption in supply of energy interferes, as we have seen, with both neuronal and cardiac function, and is also responsible for structural changes in the deprived cells. Indeed suppression of the tricarboxylic acid cycle, which is such a dominant component of mitochondrial metabolism, also accounts for shrivelling of mitochondria as well as loss of myofibrils in the cardiac muscle of thiamine-deficient rats [22] (p. 315).

Nicotinamide

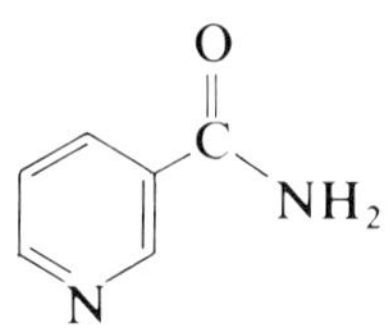

This vitamin is widely distributed in living cells and is a basic component of the coenzymes nicotinamide-adenine dinucleotide NAD^+ and nicotinamide-adenine dinucleotide phosphate $NADP^+$. These substances are coenzymes for numerous oxidoreductions which determine several principal paths of intermediary metabolism (Fig. 3.1). The nicotinamide coenzymes reversibly abstract or donate hydrogen from or to their substrates by virtue of their own potential interconversion between an oxidised form and a reduced form.

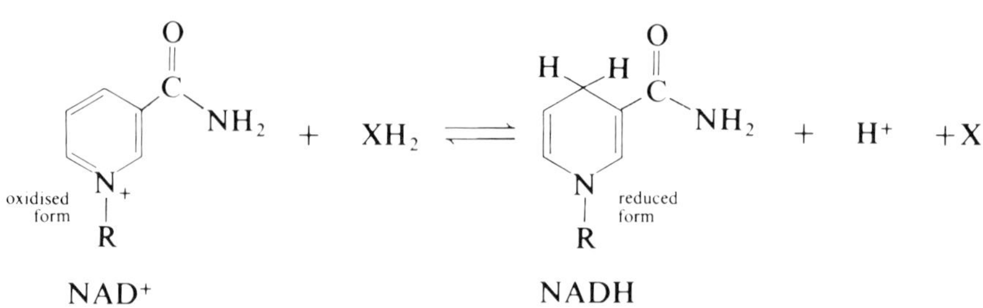

These nicotinamide nucleotides are present in meat, liver and the outer part of grain. Deficiency only occurs in people fed in a grossly impoverished diet principally of maize. Prolonged deprivation from other food leads to the disease pellagra, which used to be common in the Southern USA and still occurs there. This disorder is characterised by irritability and loss of weight coupled with reddening and scaling of skin and soreness of the mouth, finally progressing to diarrhoea and dementia. The oral lesions can determine a vicious cycle of deficiency by preventing the eating of such food as is available.

It is remarkable that pellagra is not more rapidly lethal, since NAD^+ and $NADP^+$ are coenzymes for so many of the principal exergonic reactions of the cell such as glycolysis and oxidation of carbohydrate. Probably small amounts of nicotinamide continue to be available, even to malnourished patients, as a result of bacterial action in the bowel. For this reason deficiency is never complete.

Folates

These derivatives of pteroyl glutamic acid are essential coenzymes required for catalysing specific steps in the biosynthesis of purine and pyrimidine nucleotides in DNA and RNA.

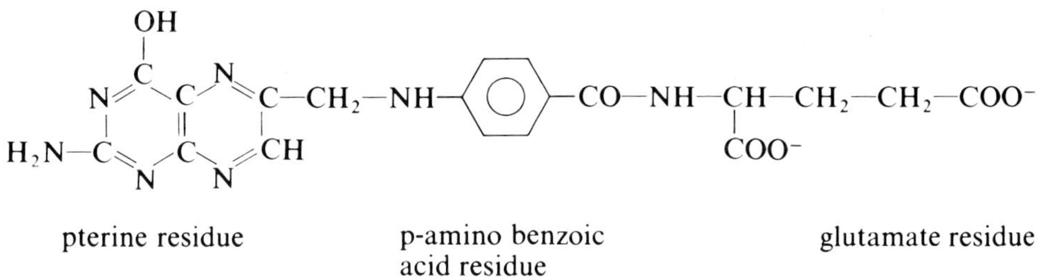

folate (pteroyl glutamate)

Lack of folates is one of the most common human deficiencies today. Because haemopoietic cells require continuous replacement, deficiency of folate usually causes illness by retarding erythropoiesis, which then results in megaloblastic (macrocytic) anaemia.

Folates are present in fresh green vegetables and animal tissues principally as polyglutamates which are broken down in the intestine and then absorbed into the blood as 5-methyl-tetrahydrofolate (methyl-THF).

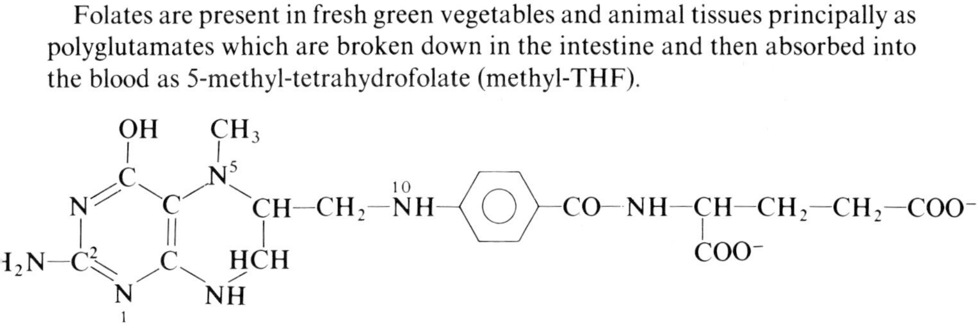

5-methyl-tetrahydrofolate (methyl-THF)

Inside cells methyl-THF is demethylated to tetrahydrofolate (THF) by homocysteine which is simultaneously methylated to methionine.

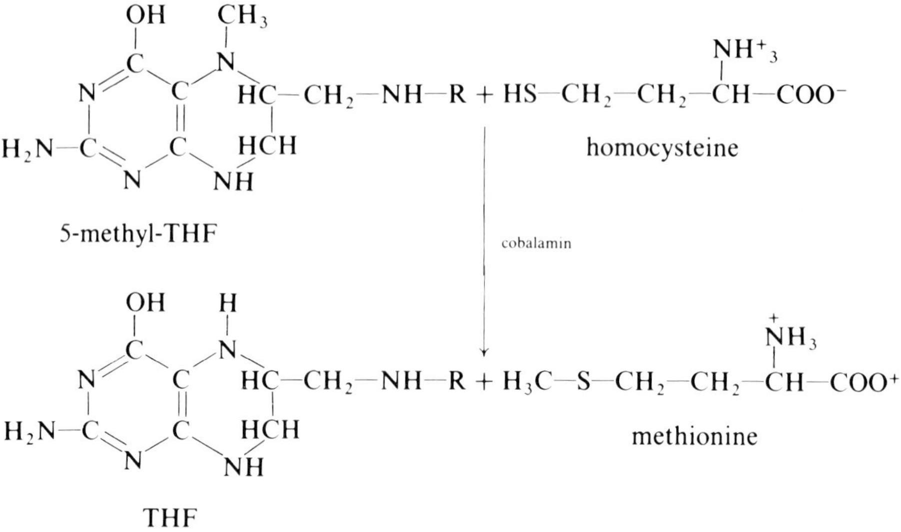

This reaction requires the presence of *cobalamin* (p. 55), without which THF cannot be formed.

THF is an extremely important substance within cells because it can accept and donate molecular fragments containing only one carbon atom. THF can thus accept a hydroxymethyl group from serine to form glycine and 5,10-methylene THF:

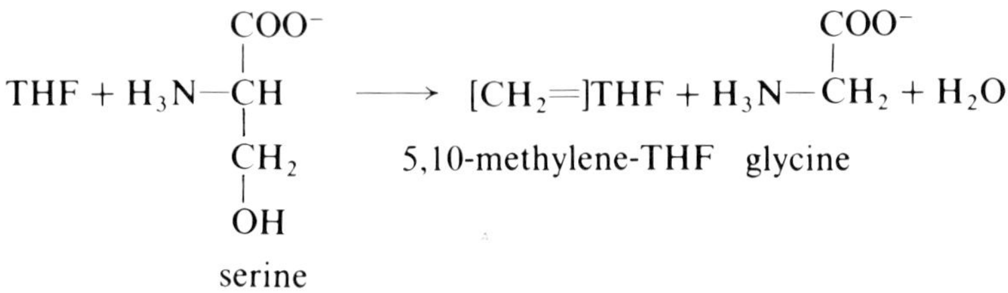

5,10-methylene-THF plays a unique part in cellular life as it induces the methylation of desoxyuridine monophosphate (dUMP) to form desoxythymidine monophosphate (dTMP) and thereby initiates the synthesis of thymine which forms an integral component of DNA:

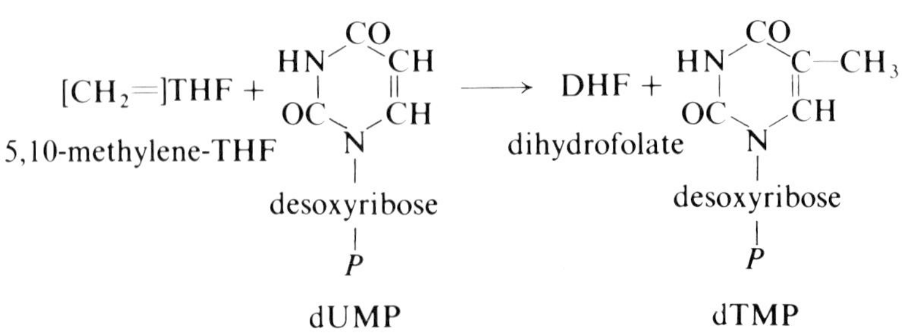

The dihydrofolate (DHF), formed by this reaction, is then reduced by NADPH to regenerate THF. In this way THF acts as a vital catalyst in the biosynthesis of DNA by mediating the formation of dTMP.

By similar acceptance and donation of other 1-C fragments THF is converted into 5-formyl-THF, which then introduces C2 and C8 into precursors of the purine group, and thus contributes to synthesis of another essential part of both DNA and RNA [23].

Intracellular THF becomes deficient in two principal ways, (1) from lack of folates, and (2) from lack of cobalamin, which is necessary for converting 5-methyl-THF to THF (see above). These deficiencies retard the synthesis of DNA in the same way, and both produce macrocytic anaemia as their most immediate harmful effect.

Lack of folate in the diet causes severe macrocytic anaemia among malnourished inhabitants of tropical countries; this disability is often called *tropical nutritional anaemia*. Like nicotinamide, folate can be produced by bacteria in the small intestine; this may explain why lack of folate retards mitosis more conspicuously in bone marrow cells than in the enteroblasts of intestinal crypts, which may be able to utilise folates formed by local bacterial action. The macrocytic anaemia induced by lack of folate is considered on p. 58.

Cobalamin (vitamin B_{12})

This is a corrinoid complex containing a core of four reduced pyrrole rings; these are linked to form one macrocyclic ring around a central atom of cobalt, to which each of the reduced pyrrole rings is individually ligated. Some closely allied corrinoids of this type, which occur in living cells and catalyse the demethylation of methyl-THF to THF (p. 54), are given the general name cobalamin or vitamin B_{12}. Without this catalysis by cobalamin THF is not formed and the synthesis of DNA in the haemopoietic cells of the bone marrow inhibited; mitosis of erythroblasts is thereby retarded or arrested and macrocytic anaemia ensues. Defect in absorption of cobalamin, normally present in the diet, is responsible for human pernicious anaemia (p. 57).

L-Ascorbic acid (vitamin C)

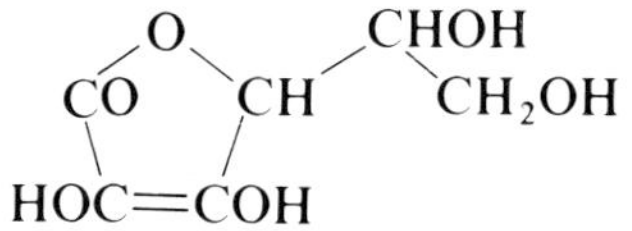

This enolic lactone occurs in all healthy animal cells and is also present in fresh fruit and vegetables. The human body contains as much as 5 g of the vitamin. Ascorbic acid is required daily in relatively large amounts by men and guinea pigs; other animals are able to synthesise it for themselves in the liver.

Deficiency of this factor in the human diet leads to scurvy. This disease is characterised by bleeding into skin and gums, imperfect development of bones and teeth, and defective formation of scar tissue. Vitamin C appears to be essential for the development of properly constituted collagenous connective tissue.

In the normal formation of *procollagen* within fibroblasts the peptide chains are first translated and then some of their proline units are oxidised to hydroxyproline units, probably within the endoplasmic reticulum. Subsequently

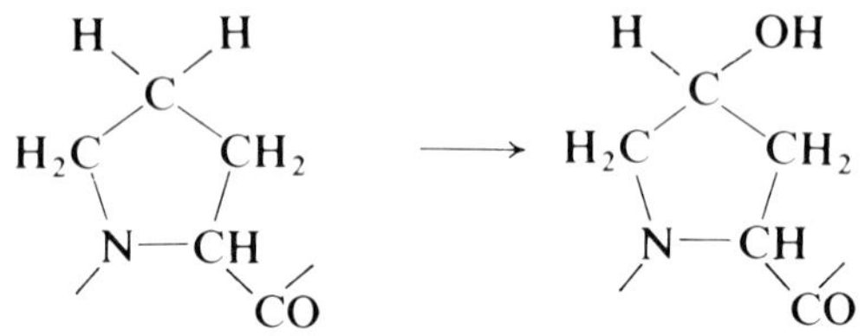

proline unit in peptide chain — hydroxyproline unit in peptide chain

the procollagen molecules are split by a peptidase and then secreted out of the fibroblasts as microfibres of *tropocollagen*; these later become further interlinked by lateral attachment to other fibres to form *collagen* itself.

It is likely that ascorbic acids takes an essential part in this initial oxidation of proline to hydroxyproline in the newly coded peptide chains of procollagen. In the final product (collagen) hydroxyproline accounts for as much as 4 per cent of the total protein. As hydroxyproline is not initially coded in transcription and translation but is formed by this secondary oxidation of the coded peptide, this latter process must consume a considerable amount of the oxidizing agent. Indeed the human requirement for ascorbic acid amounts to about 30 mg/day, far higher than that of any other vitamin.

This effect of ascorbic acid on the formation of hydroxyproline is observable in mouse fibroblasts grown in culture. When ascorbic acid is added to the culture fluid the quantity of hydroxyproline formed both in the cells and their surrounding fluid is greatly increased [24]. However, ascorbic acid does not affect the total amount of protein formed. It thus appears that, without ascorbic acid, collagen continues to be synthesised, but with a grossly diminished content of hydroxyproline. This defect is retained in the finally formed collagen molecules and doubtless is responsible for their altered physical properties which result in weakness of connective tissue and rupture of capillaries by separation of their endothelial cells. Possibly the microfibres which lack hydroxyproline cannot form effective interlinkage and thus tear under tension or trauma. Lack of ascorbic acid during the assembly of procollagen in the cells probably results in the formation of extracellular collagen which is defective in its tensile and cohesive properties. This defect accounts for the lesions of scurvy, in which capillary haemorrhage and tissue softening are such prominant features.

DEFECTIVE ABSORPTION AND TRANSPORT OF NUTRIMENTS

This kind of defect is illustrated by deficient absorption of nutriments from the intestine as well as by retardation of absorption of oxygen from the lungs into the blood.

Deficient absorption by the intestine

Defective absorption frequently arises, as we have seen, as a sequel to malnutrition. In this case proteolytic enzymes are not formed in the pancreatic and intestinal secretions and preabsorptive digestion of proteins and fats is inhibited. Consequently undigested intestinal contents stimulate fatty diarrhoea which further impedes absorption of available protein.

Inherited defect in absorption of fat occurs in hereditary *abetalipoproteinaemia*. In this disability absence of β-lipoprotein in the intestinal cells prevents transport across the cells and so determines defect in absorption (p. 30). Similar defect in a transport mechanism results in the inefficient absorption of Ca^{++} in the absence of cholecalciferol (p. 48).

In *tropical sprue*, which is characterised by fatty diarrhoea, extreme emaciation and macrocytic anaemia, chronic bacterial infection probably interferes with absorption of fat and also of folates and cobalamin.

Atrophy of gastric or intestinal mucosa is also a serious cause of intestinal malabsorption; *pernicious anaemia* and *coeliac disease*, which are conspicuous examples of such disorder, will briefly be considered.

Pernicious anaemia

In this disease absorption of cobalamin (vitamin B_{12}) is defective. The basic lesion is atrophy of the gastric mucosa. The normal elongated glands, composed of specialised peptic and parietal cells, are replaced by lymphoid cells. Both peptic and parietal cells are lost. *Intrinsic factor* and HCl disappear from the gastric juice.

Antibodies to gastric parietal cells are usually present in the serum of patients with pernicious anaemia; also antibodies to intrinsic factor are found in the gastric juice. The presence of these gastric antibodies as well as of lymphoid cells in the gastric mucosa suggests that the gastric atrophy may be caused by autoimmune injury. Possibly the lymphocytes in the mucosa destroy the gastric cells by delayed hypersensitivity (p. 214). Moreover, relatives of patients with pernicious anaemia have an increased incidence of autoimmune Addison's disease and of circulating antibodies to gastric and thyroid epithelial cells [25]. This suggests that the gastric lesion in pernicious anaemia may be determined by inherited defect in immune tolerance so that an autoimmune reaction to liberated gastric components results in destruction of gastric epithelial cells.

Normally intrinsic factor, a glycoprotein secreted by the parietal cells, forms a complex with cobalamin. Only then can cobalamin be absorbed by the small intestine. Without intrinsic factor therefore the cells of the body become deprived of cobalamin. This results in (a) macrocytic anaemia and (b) subacute degeneration of the spinal cord.

This *macrocytic anaemia* is a consequence of disorder of mitosis in the bone marrow. Indeed deficiency of either cobalamin or of folates retards the synthesis of DNA by interfering with formation of THF necessary for catalysing anabolism of purine and pyrimidine bases, which are essential components of nucleic acids (p. 54). Cell division is therefore retarded at S phase and G_2 phase (p. 130). This effect is at first mainly exerted on the bone marrow, so that erythropoiesis is severely slowed and nuclear condensation to form normoblasts is consequently postponed. Instead of normoblasts (with intensely pyknotic nuclei) large nucleated erythroblasts called megaloblasts accumulate in the bone marrow; these cells are 20–30 μm in diameter and have primitive stippled nuclei. Some of these megaloblasts show abnormal mitosis in which chromosomal fragments are visible (see below). Many megaloblasts die in the bone marrow but some with more condensed nuclei (Fig. 3.2a) escape into the blood; some of these late megaloblasts seen in the blood contain spherical remnants of chromosomal fragments called Howell-Jolly bodies (Fig. 3.2b).

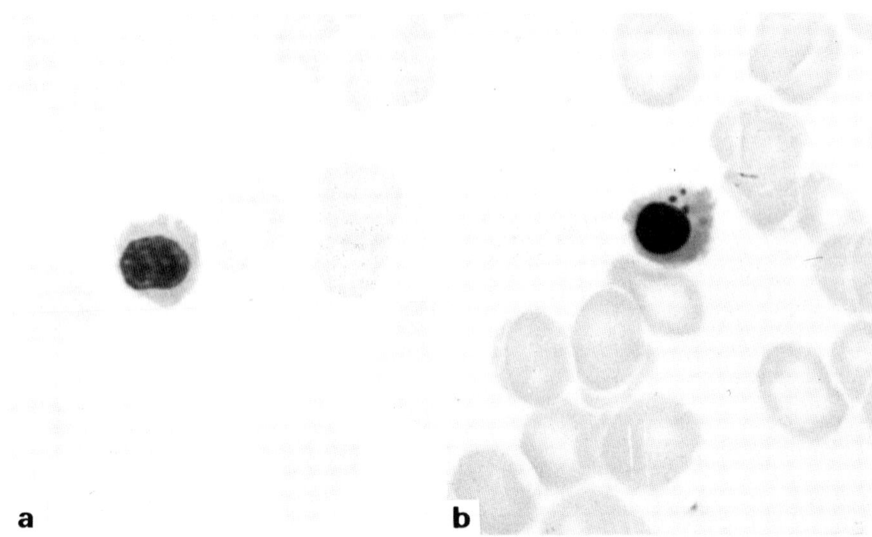

FIG. 3.2 Blood films from a man of 70 with pernicious anaemia (red cells 1.2×10^{12}/litre, white cells 3.6×10^9/litre, Hb 5.5 g/dl). Leishman. × 1300.
a. Megaloblast: traces of chromatin structure still present in nucleus.
b. Late megaloblast condensed pyknotic nucleus and three Howell–Jolly bodies (chromosomal fragments).

The formation of red cells is thus grossly diminished and those which enter the blood are, on the average, enlarged (macrocytosis: MCV 110—140 fl). The enlarged red cells include macrocytes without nuclei and usually a few nucleated late megaloblasts (Fig. 3.2a). The red cells show conspicuous inequality in size (anisocytosis) and deformity in shape (poikilocytosis). Synthesis of Hb in the enlarged cells proceeds normally so that the amount of Hb/cell is increased, although the amount of Hb/litre of blood is much diminished because of extreme diminution in the number of red cells. The anaemia is further aggravated by shortening in life span of the deformed cells.

Retardation of synthesis of DNA in haemopoietic cells due to lack of cobalamin or folates, which interferes with the process of mitosis, also causes chromosomal fragmentation [26]. Thus, when bone marrow cells from patients with B_{12} or folate deficiency are treated with colchicine so as to arrest mitosis at metaphase, conspicuous breaks are visible both in chromatids and in whole chromosomes. These changes doubtless reflect genomic lesions which cause the death of many of the dividing cells in bone marrow and so contribute greatly to the resultant anaemia. Disorder of maturation with retardation of cell division also affects the myeloblastic cells in the bone marrow; this probably accounts for the leucopenia and the presence of enlarged granulocytes with highly segmented nuclei (macropolycytes) which are characteristic features in the blood of patients with macrocytic anaemia (Fig. 3.3).

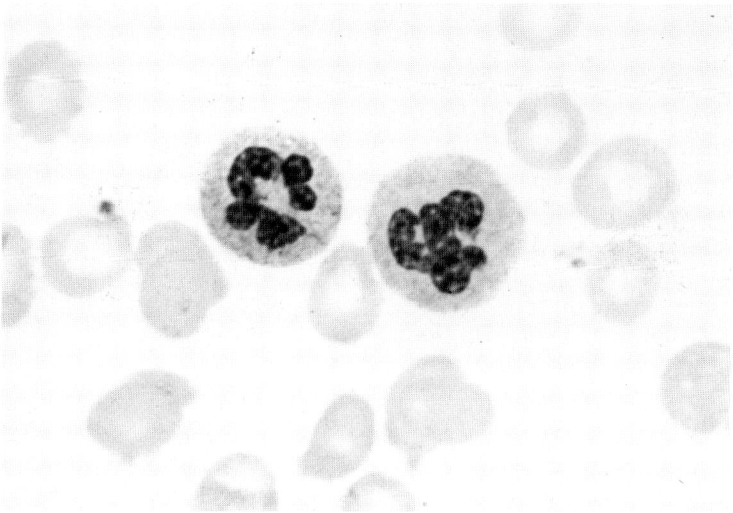

FIG. 3.3 Same blood film as shown in Fig. 3.2 (pernicious anaemia). Two enlarged neutrophil granulocytes (macropolycytes) with highly segmented nuclei

The second consequence of lack of cobalamin in human patients with pernicious anaemia is *subacute combined degeneration* of the spinal cord. This results in ataxic paraplegia affecting the legs and trunk with bilateral paresis and paraesthesia. The white matter of both posterior and anterolateral columns of the spinal cord degenerates; at first fusiform swellings appear in the myelin sheaths and later the axons degenerate [27]. This degeneration is relieved by cobalamin but *not* by folate. The pathogenesis of these neural lesions is obscure.

Cobalamin is thus necessary for maintenance of the long myelinated tracts in a manner independent from its other essential effect on metabolism of folates. Provided cobalamin is absorbed at the rate of 3 μg/day both these needs are satisfied.

Coeliac disease (gluten-sensitive enteropathy)

This is an inherited disorder of enterocytes in the mucosa of the small intestine caused by abnormal sensitivity of these cells to the toxic action of gluten, the principal protein of wheaten flour. The mechanism of this action is obscure.

The most prominent lesion is flattening of the jejunal mucosa with loss of villi so that the orifices of the intestinal crypts become plainly visible. The life span of the enterocytes is shortened, the intestinal villi disappear and the columnar epithelium is replaced by flattened cuboidal cells. The enteroblasts of the intestinal crypts become hyperplastic and their frequency of mitosis is increased; the enterocytes formed from the hyperplastic enteroblasts are flattened and their microvilli are irregular and distorted [28].

As a result of severe diminution in the absorptive surface, consequent upon loss of villi, absorption is gravely retarded; fatty diarrhoea develops, and this then interferes with absorption of carbohydrate, fat, protein and vitamins. The disordered enterocytes are rapidly exfoliated from the flattened epithelium and this increase in turnover causes loss of protein, iron and folates from the body. This effect summates with malabsorption to produce very severe malnutrition.

The disease often starts in children a few months after weaning to a mixed diet rich in gluten. Affected children fail to thrive and their muscular and subcutaneous tissues become wasted. Although the mechanism which determines the extreme sensitivity of the enterocytes to gluten or its products is uncertain, adoption of the gluten free diet by these patients is rapidly followed by restoration of the cytoarchitecture of the jejunal mucosa and also by clinical improvement [28, 29]. Moreover peptic-tryptic digests of gliadin (a protein in gluten) are toxic to organ cultures of intestinal epithelium from patients with active coeliac disease, but cause no injury to similar cultures from normal persons [30–32]. The toxic effect is not exerted by digests of gliadin on cultures taken from patients during temporary remission from the disease; this may indicate that an allergic mechanism is involved in the injurious action of gliadin-digests on the mucosa of patients with the active disease.

In coeliac disease, therefore, the elimination of a large part of the effective absorptive surface is the basic cause of malabsorption.

Defective absorption and transfer of oxygen

Even when normal air at atmospheric pressure is breathed, sufficient oxygen may not be absorbed by the pulmonary capillaries because of (1) diminution in pulmonary ventilation and access, or (2) defective transfer of oxygen into the blood.

Diminution in pulmonary ventilation and access

Drowning or occlusion of the larynx by foreign bodies directly prevents ventilation. Paralytic poliomyelitis may destroy lower motor neurones in the brain stem and cervical cord and thus weaken or arrest respiratory movement. Reduction in pulmonary ventilation may result from excess of drugs such as barbiturates which depress the respiratory centres.

Inflammatory exudate in acute or chronic pulmonary infections or pulmonary oedema can also interrupt access of oxygen to the alveolar surfaces. Alveolar structure may be disorganised by chronic fibrosis in silicosis, asbestosis or pulmonary tuberculosis, or the alveoli may be invaded by new growth. In these circumstances the alveoli may both be underventilated and underperfused.

Access of oxygen is also severely impaired in *respiratory disease of the newborn*. This is the commonest cause of death in live-born premature infants. In these children the fluid covering the immature alveolar cells is deficient in pulmonary surfactant; the air spaces therefore collapse at each expiration owing to the high surface tension at the air/liquid interfaces on the alveolar surface. The collapsed alveoli then fail to re-expand on inspiration and plasma leaks out to form a pinkish *hyaline membrane* composed of fibrin, red cells and necrotic alveolar epithelium. This membrane covers the surface of the alveoli and their ducts and further precludes the possibility of expansion and aeration of the collapsed alveoli. Access of oxygen is grossly diminished and this results in death from anoxia. This lethal pulmonary defect is often called *hyaline membrane disease*. These babies suffer from intense respiratory effort and distress, leading to tachypnoea and intercostal recession [33].

Such alveolar collapse is prevented in normally developed newborn children by the presence of surfactant phospholipid in the fluid secreted by more mature alveolar cells. When the normal fetus reaches term, two types of cell compose the alveolar epithelium. Type 1 cells are flattened and permit diffusion of oxygen; type 2 cells are spheroidal and contian numerous osmiophilic bodies which are concerned with storage of lecithin, a surfactant phohpholipid synthesised in these cells [34]. The fluid secreted early in gestation contains only small quantities of lecithin but, as the type 2 cells develop, lecithin becomes much more abundant in the alveolar fluid. This lecithin is a powerful surfactant and lowers the surface tension of the air/liquid interface on the outside of the alveolar cells and so prevents collapse of the alveoli as they contract in expiration. In premature children lack of lecithin in the alveolar fluid permits collapse and so precludes normal pulmonary expansion during inspiration, thus causing hyaline membrane disease.

Defective transfer of oxygen into the blood

Even when pulmonary ventilation and access of oxygen to the alveolar surface are both adequate, transfer of oxygen into the pulmonary capillaries may still be deficient. Thus *heart failure*, by retarding pulmonary circulation, diminishes absorption of oxygen and so produces anoxic anoxia. Moreover *anaemia*, by lowering the content of Hb in the blood, severely reduces the capacity of blood to absorb O_2 and promote trans-alveolar diffusion. Such deficiency of Hb results from defects in globin synthesis (pp. 20–26), from lack of Fe^{++} in diet, or from defect in maturation of red cells as in pernicious anaemia (p. 58). CO also eliminates functional Hb and so prevents absorption of O_2 with particularly injurious consequences (see Chapter 5). The mechanism by which anoxia injures cells is considered along with cellular injury produced by ischaemia (pp. 84–86).

DEFICIENCY OF INTERNAL SECRETION

Even though the blood receives nutriments from the bowel and oxygen from the lungs in sufficient amounts, it may still not contain all the substances required by many of the cells of the body. An adequate complement of cellular nutriments includes numerous substances internally secreted by fabricator cells.

These substances may be added to the blood in *large amounts*, such as glucose liberated by the liver or fatty acids by adipose tissue. When glucose is not secreted by the liver, as in children with glycogenosis 1 (von Gierke's disease), severe hypoglycaemia develops; the blood sugar may even fall to 10 mg/100 ml (see p. 410), and this may deprive cerebral neurones of their principal exergonic substrate and so cause convulsions and mental retardation.

Other substances secreted by fabricator cells, particularly by those of the specialised endocrine organs, may be intensely active, and are therefore only required in *minute amounts*, such as the hormones thyroxine and insulin. To illustrate deficiency of internal secretion some effects of lack of each of these two hormones are briefly considered; for defects of internal secretion in general, text books on endocrinology should be consulted.

Deficient formation of thyroxine is exemplified by the adult type of hypothyroidism or myxoedema. In this disorder the thyroid gland atrophies and becomes fibrotic probably in many cases as a result of autoimmune disease (p. 203). The acinar cells of the thyroid are destroyed or replaced by inactive clear cells, and thyroglobulin and thyroxine are no longer formed. Thyroxine ceases to be liberated into the blood. The protein bound iodine in the serum, which is largely composed of iodine *in* thyroxine molecules, is normally of the order of 4–8 μg/100 ml but in myxoedema this value falls to level of 0–3.5 μg/100 ml. Lack of thyroxine depresses cellular metabolism, because thyroxine is necessary for activating the transcription of RNA and the consequent synthesis of enzymic proteins. The BMR therefore falls. Early signs include fatigue and mental dullness. Speech becomes slow. Subcutaneous accumulation of watery mucin causes thickening of the skin; this phenomenon has not been satisfactorily explained, although from it the word myxoedema is derived. Later these patients develop severe hypothermia owing to diminution in cellular metabolism and terminally they pass into coma.

Lack of insulin, secreted by the β-cells of the pancreatic islets into the blood, causes the *'juvenile onset' type of diabetes mellitus*. During the onset of this disease the number of β-cells in the pancreatic islets is greatly diminished and the islets become largely composed of α-cells or atrophic fibrous tissue; later the β-cells disappear entirely [35]. In patients with this kind of diabetes, therefore, insulin ceases to be formed and no longer enters the blood. Without insulin very serious metabolic derangements follow including failure of transport of glucose into various kinds of cell such as muscle fibres and lipocytes (p. 96). Diabetes and its metabolic lesions are considered in Chapter 9.

The blood thus receives, by the secretion of fabricator cells, supplements which are not supplied by the food. Many of these additions are of paramount importance to the nutritive value of blood and other extracellular fluids.

INTERRUPTION OR RETARDATION IN THE SUPPLY OF BLOOD

Although the blood may contain adequate amounts of all the numerous nutriments required by the cells, yet sufficient blood may fail to reach them. Insufficiency in the supply of blood is by far the most frequent cause of lack of nutriments affecting the cells of the body, and is in fact the most important single determinant in the pathogenesis of cellular injury in human disease as a whole.

Insufficiency in the supply of blood to a tissue is called ischaemia (*ἴσχω*, stop, check; *αἷμα*, blood).

Ischaemia may arise from general or from local retardation of circulation or from a combination of both.

General ischaemia

This may follow (1) heart failure, (2) occlusion of pulmonary artery, (3) acute haemorrhage, or (4) vasomotor failure.

Heart failure

When the heart fails to expel sufficient blood to maintain an adequate supply of oxygen and other nutriments to the tissues ischaemic cellular injury follows. Heart failure then causes *ischaemic anoxia* in the deprived cells; it can also cause *anoxic anoxia* (p. 61) by impeding pulmonary absorption of oxygen and so directly producing hypoxaemia. Indeed such defective absorption by the lungs is itself determined by retardation in the flow of blood and so is also a result of ischaemia. The commonest cause of heart failure is occlusive disease of coronary arteries; thus local cardiac ischaemia by injuring the myocardium results in general ischaemia.

Acute heart failure. This follows cardiac arrest, ventricular fibrillation or rapid diminution in the volume of systolic output. Arrest and ventricular fibrillation are common sequels of acute coronary occlusion and are the most usual causes of sudden death. Ventricular fibrillation also arises from accidents with anaesthetics and from drowning by *fresh* water (p.194). After cardiac arrest or ventricular fibrillation consciousness is rapidly lost owing to cessation in supply of oxygen and glucose to the brain but, provided normal cardiac rhythm can be re-established within a few min by sternal compression or defibrillation, there is a chance of full recovery. However interruption of circulation for more than 5 min is generally succeeded by irreversible injury to the cerebral neurones (p. 87). Fibrillation or arrest accompanied by visible injury to myocardial fibres may occur during the toxaemia of severe diphtheria (p. 223). Typhoid fever similarly causes toxic myocardial injury culminating in cardiac arrest. Acute heart failure with cyanosis due to general ischaemia or pulmonary congestion is also a sequel to myocardial damage in children caused by Coxsackie B virus. This may be particularly serious in the newborn.

Acute coronary occlusion of less severe degree may not initially injure sufficient ventricular muscle to cause cardiac arrest or ventricular fibrillation, but may, however, seriously diminish systolic output and so also result in acute heart failure. The patient then becomes pallid, breathless and hypotensive with weakened pulse; although conscious he may be in a state of collapse due to general ischaemia, and may frequently suffer from acute cardiac pain. The zone of ischaemic ventricular muscle, previously supplied by the occluded vessel, then becomes fatty or necrotic (Fig. 3.11) and, if the process of coronary occlusion is extended by further coronary thrombosis, cardiac arrest and death may follow. Otherwise the patient may survive with permanent chronic heart failure, or may recover provided coronary anastomotic channels become effective.

Chronic heart failure. Local cardiac ischaemia caused by *gradual coronary occlusion* eventually produces atrophy or fatty change of cardiac muscle fibres followed by chronic deficiency in systolic output. This results in generalised ischaemia often coupled with hepatic and pulmonary lesions characteristic of congestive cardiac failure (p. 75). When local cardiac ischaemia injures the auriculoventricular bundle then *complete heart block* may occur. This is followed by extreme retardation of the heart beat. The ventricle then contracts with its own rhythm of 30/min. This behaviour is associated with episodes during which the pulse becomes even slower still, resulting in bouts of coma succeeded by periods of extreme mental confusion. These episodes are called *Stokes-Adams attacks*. William Stokes in his book *Diseases of the Heart and Aorta* published in 1854, emphasised the occurrence of apoplectic attacks with coma, lethargy and loss of memory in patients with extreme weakness or slowing of the heart beat due to chronic heart failure, often accompanied by fatty change in the heart muscle. He described one of these patients: 'on recovery, after all the comatose symptoms have passed away he remains for half an hour unable to recognise his most intimate friends or relations, even his wife he has mistaken for his mother'. Stokes rightly attributed these attacks of coma and the disorientation and confusion which follow them to defect in the arterial supply to the brain associated with the general ischaemia of heart failure; he even 'noticed one case in which on the occurrence of the premonitory symptoms, the patient by hanging his head so that it rested on the floor, used to save himself from an attack'.

Occlusion of pulmonary artery

Thrombi arising in veins or in the heart itself can be transported as emboli which suddenly occlude the main pulmonary trunk (at its point of bifurcation) or one of its two principal branches. Such embolism can produce almost immediate coma followed by death in a few minutes owing to irreparable ischaemic injury to the cerebral neurones.

Massive pulmonary embolism is usually caused by large thrombi formed in deep veins of the leg; these may develop when the blood is slowed by congestive cardiac failure or by prolonged muscular inactivity from rest in bed.

Acute haemorrhage

Either external or internal haemorrhage may rapidly cause general ischaemia.

The brain is usually the first organ affected so that coma may follow almost immediately. Acute haemorrhage may also injure the anterior lobe of the pituitary gland when this organ is hypertrophied by pregnancy. This happens typically as a result of post partum haemorrhage when enlarged uterine vessels are lacerated during labour (p. 83). Acute haemorrhage into the brain itself is considered in Chapter 4.

Vasomotor failure

Rapid fall of blood pressure resulting from sudden neurogenic shock is responsible for *fainting fits*. In these attacks vasodilation in the splanchnic area accounts for the fall in blood pressure which produces short periods of coma with pallor and feeble pulse. Fainting fits usually cause no harm to a healthy person provided he is placed in a recumbent position or falls down without traumatic injury; the cerebral circulation is then restored and consciousness rapidly returns. But great danger is incurred during a faint, if a patient is retained upright or if his head is propped up. In this case the already retarded cerebral circulation may be further diminished or even arrested by added hydrostatic pressure which may equalise or exceed the lowered blood pressure. Bourne [36] emphasised that severe cerebral ischaemia may occur in this way during dental anaesthesia by N_20, when a patient is propped up in a dental chair. If a patient faints under these conditions the resulting fall in blood pressure and pallor may pass unnoticed but the concomitant ischaemia may cause irreversible injury to the cerebral neurones so that the patient never recovers consciousness even though administration of N_20 is stopped (p. 87). The horizontal position used in modern dental surgery may diminish this serious risk of cerebral damage.

Local ischaemia

External compression of nutrient vessels

Crush injuries to limbs, as we shall see, can produce ischaemic muscle necrosis, while prolonged pressure on skin and subcutaneous tissue can similarly give necrosis with formation of bed sores in recumbent patients. Compression of cerebral capillaries by an expanding extradural haemorrhage results in cerebral ischaemia with 'traumatic coma' and death.

Disease of the vessel wall

Eccentric thickening of the intima by atherosclerosis (p. 377) narrows the vascular lumen of arteries; this change occurs with disastrous effect in coronary and cerebral vessels. Spasm of cerebral arterioles may occur in hypertension and then cause ischaemic injury of the vessel walls leading to cerebral haemorrhage (p. 103).

Proliferation of intimal fibrous tissue of arterioles is a common occurrence in tertiary syphilis which may result in occlusion and contribute to the development of syphilitic necrosis (p. 220).

Capillaries may become occluded by proliferation of their endothelial cells. This happens in the brain in typhus fever and is responsible for stupor followed by death in coma (p. 251).

Occlusion of the lumen
Arteries, when narrowed by atherosclerosis, frequently become occluded by thrombosis. This arises in the slowly flowing blood within or beyond a zone of atherosclerotic narrowing. The site of this kind of occlusion is commonly in the coronary or cerebral arteries.

Capillaries can also become occluded by obstruction of their lumen. Thus in sickle-cell disease the distorted red cells increase the viscosity of the flowing blood and finally effect complete stasis (p. 22). Similarly capillaries are obstructed by red cells parasitised by the schizonts of *Plasmodium falciparum* (see Fig. 6.19, p. 248). These infected red cells are abnormally sticky and thus occlude capillaries in brain or heart to give terminal coma or heart failure in malignant tertian malaria.

Very severe inflammation can promote such substantial loss of plasma from capillaries that stasis results from the greatly increased viscosity of the blood. This happens in the necrotizing inflammation of plague and anthrax, when inflammatory stasis causes ischaemic necrosis.

Combination of general and local ischaemia
Local retardation in the supply of blood may not by itself be sufficiently severe to cause ischaemic injury to cells. Even when an artery is entirely occluded, local collaterial vessels can provide adequate nutriments to avert ischaemic damage. But if *coincident* general ischaemia arises, loss of function and also necrosis are likely to occur in tissues where the local supply is already retarded.

This principle was illustrated by occlusion of the middle cerebral artery in monkeys [37]; this operation by itself did not suppress electrical activity of the cerebral cortex nor cause irreversible damage to the brain but when the artery was occluded and the blood pressure was *simultaneously* diminished by lowering the feet of the animal, the electrical activity diminished and cellular injury eventually followed. Presumably sufficient collateral channels remained open to prevent injury by local ischaemia alone, but the combination of local with partial general ischaemia diminished supply sufficiently to cause injury.

Similarly in human patients prolonged occlusion of the internal carotid artery may produce no permanent cerebral disorder nor injury, because there is sufficient anastomtic supply from the opposite carotid via the Circle of Willis. But in such patients temporary fall in blood pressure produces sufficient general ischaemia superimposed on partial local ischaemia to cause unilateral loss of cerebral function with transient episodes of hemiplegia and aphasia [38].

Such a combination of general and local ischaemia affecting the brain can have disastrous consequences in human patients, as illustrated in Fig. 3.4. This shows a coronal section of brain from a woman of 67 who developed acute cardiac failure with auricular fibrillation resulting from coronary artery atherosclerosis. She rapidly became comatose with left-sided extensor plantar response and died the next day. Her right internal carotid artery was severely narrowed by atherosclerosis and was partly occluded by friable material. Conspicuous zones of haemorrhagic necrosis (red infarction) were present in the frontal cortex of the right cerebral hemisphere, although the left cerebral

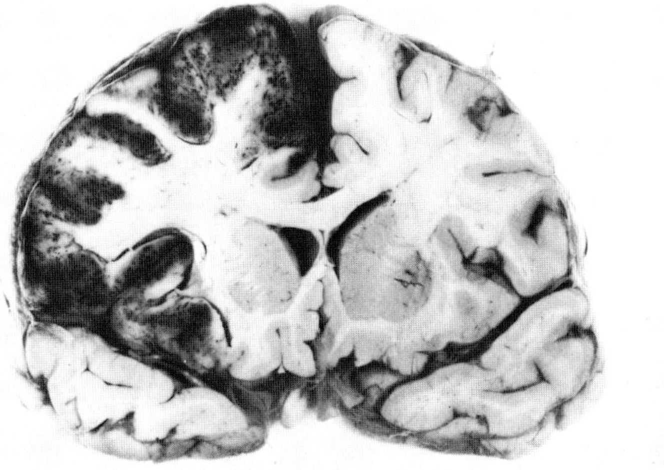

FIG. 3.4 Unilateral red infarction of right cerebral cortex caused by general ischaemia, due to acute heart failure, superimposed on partial local ischaemia, resulting from atheromatous narrowing of right internal carotid artery. Courtesy of Professor G. A. Gresham.

cortex was unaffected. Thus the combined effect of general ischaemia due to acute heart failure, suddenly superimposed on partial local ischaemia, caused by narrowing of the right internal carotid, resulted in extensive ischaemic necrosis in the right cerebral cortex. Under these circumstances the Circle of Willis did not provide sufficient collateral supply of blood to avert injury to the vulnerable ipsilateral grey matter of the right cerebral cortex but the supply by the still patent left carotid was sufficient to maintain the equally vulnerable left cerebral cortex intact (Fig. 3.4.). The less vulnerable cerebral white matter appeared unaffected on both sides.

A combination of general and local ischaemia is also responsible for causing ischaemic necrosis (infarction) in the lungs. Collateral circulation in the lungs is usually so efficient that local occlusion of a pulmonary arterial branch by itself does not result in ischaemic necrosis, unless the pulmonary circulation is already retarded by concomitant heart failure. But when local ischaemia, caused by impaction of an embolus, is superadded to pre-existent general ischaemia then circulation is more completely arrested and necrosis follows (see Fig. 3.7a & b).

Combination of hypoxia and local ischaemia

Severe hypoxia, however generated, may similarly summate with partial local ischaemia to produce anoxic damage. Thus limited local ischaemia, insufficient by itself to cause necrosis, may determine the location of cells which are later killed by superimposed hypoxic or cytotoxic anoxia.

A particularly clear demonstration of this principle was made by Levine [39], who ligated the *right* common carotid artery in rats and then exposed them to

N_2O or N_2 so as to produce hypoxic coma for 10–45 min. After 24 hours or more the animals were killed. Necrotic lesions confined to the *right* side of the brain were found in these rats but no lesions were present in the brain of animals in which one carotid was ligated without subsequent exposure to N_2O or N_2. These lesions were mainly situated in the grey matter of the hippocampus, neocortex, and basal ganglia (p. 84). This type of cerebral injury produced by summation of the effects of generalised hypoxia superimposed on local ischaemia is called *anoxic-ischaemic* encephalopathy.

The severity of injury produced by poisons which cause cytotoxic anoxia may also similarly be increased by localised ischaemia. Thus the extreme sensitivity of the globus pallidus to CO may be related to coincident local ischaemia affecting the pallidal grey matter owing to local arteriolar occlusion (p. 152).

Consequences of ischaemia

Ischaemia interrupts function and it kills cells. When incomplete, ischaemia can induce fatty globulation in the affected cells or they may slowly shrivel (atrophy) and eventually die. But, when ischaemia is complete and permanent, the cells, deprived of all nutriment, are rapidly killed *en masse*.

Ischaemic fatty change and atrophy: fibrosis and gliosis

Partial ischaemia, that does not produce sufficient hypoxia to kill cells, is a potent cause of intracellular fatty change, which can develop rapidly in hypoxic tissues. This visible deposition of fat is a prominent sequel to partial ischaemia both in hepatic cells and in myocardial fibres. Fig. 3.5 shows such fatty myocardial fibres in a partially ischaemic subendocardial zone in the left ventricle of a man who died from acute heart failure due to occlusive coronary disease. This progressed rapidly over a period of four days and terminated in death from cardiac arrest. The most ischaemic parts of the ventricular muscle became necrotic but in the surrounding regions, where ischaemia was incomplete, conspicuous fatty globulation developed in large groups of myocardial fibres.

When gradual in onset, ischaemia can also produce cellular shrinkage or atrophy. Such ischaemic atrophy commonly occurs in centrilobular hepatic cells as a result of congestive heart failure (see below). Similar atrophy occurs in myocardium when coronary arteries become gradually narrowed by atherosclerosis; the most hypoxic fibres then shrink and die. The dead myocardial fibres are later replaced by connective tissue which can survive and lay down collagen fibres in the ischaemic zones. In this way cardiac muscle is slowly replaced by useless fibrous tissue; this *replacement fibrosis* is a common concomitant of chronic ischaemic heart failure.

In the brain partial ischaemia of long duration also results in shrinkage of neuronal cell bodies and loss of their processes. This neuronal atrophy is followed by *replacement gliosis* in which dense fibrous astrocytes and their processes occupy much of the space vacated by their more vulnerable neighbours. Replacement or reactive gliosis also occurs round zones of more severe ischaemia, where neurones are killed *en masse*; Fig. 3.6 (p. 70) shows

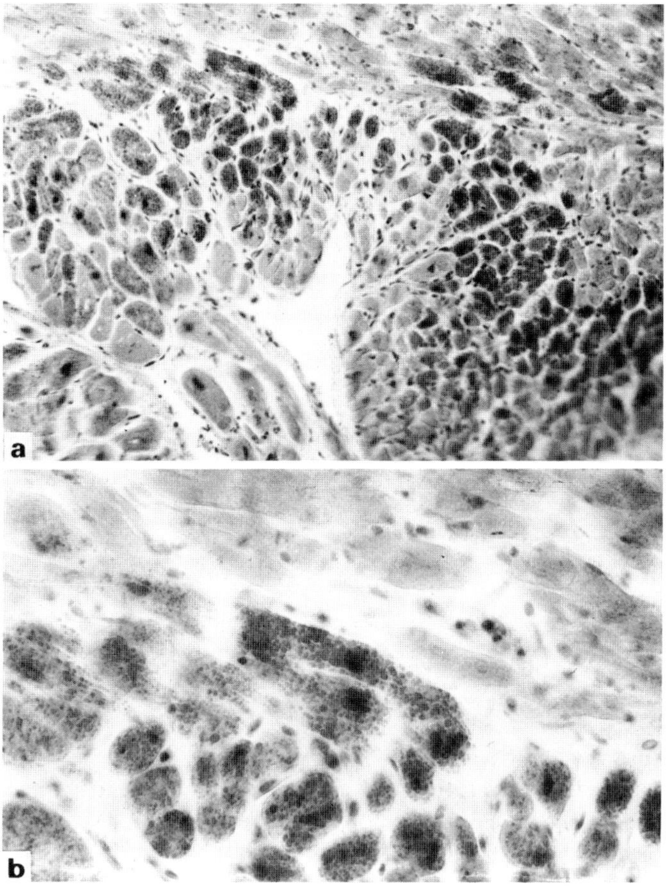

FIG. 3.5 Ischaemic fatty change in cardiac muscle. Myocardium from a man of 75 who died of cardiac arrest five days after onset of acute heart failure due to progressive coronary artery occlusion caused by atherosclerosis. Sudan III & IV and H.

a. Section of ventricular wall showing three zones: (1) immediately around a tubular channel of ventricular cavity the myocardial fibres (lower centre) are unaffected; (2) adjacent to these unaffected fibres is a zone of partial ischaemia where hypoxia was sufficiently severe to cause maximum fatty change; (3) external to these extremely fatty fibres is a zone (top of field) where more complete ischaemia has killed the myocardial fibres before fatty changes could occur. ×125.

b. Part of same section showing extremely fatty fibres (below) and necrotic fibres (above). ×265.

proliferating astrocytes at the margin of such a necrotic zone in cerebral cortex. This gliosis is conspicuous in zones of partial ischaemia, where hypoxia is not sufficiently severe to prevent growth of relatively resistant astrocytic cells and fibres.

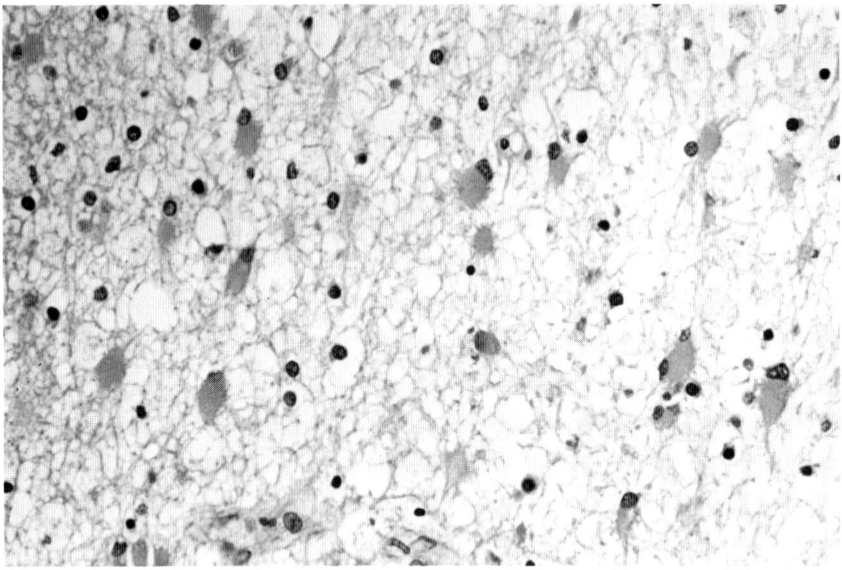

FIG. 3.6 Hypertrophic astrocytes in a zone of partial ischaemia on the surface of an old infarct in occipital cerebral cortex caused by thrombosis of an atherosclerotic posterior cerebral artery. H & E. ×330.

Infarction

When ischaemia is sudden in onset, complete and permanent, it is followed rapidly by death of the cells throughout the affected tissue. When such an event occurs as a result of interruption of blood supply it is referred to as infarction; the dead tissue is called an infarct.

Along with other cells damaged in the ischaemic tissue the endothelial cells of its capillaries are also injured. Accordingly red cells entering the damaged tissue, either through still patent anastomotic arteries or by retrograde flow through the veins, may escape through the injured capillary walls. For this reason the dead tissue may become swollen with blood; this phenomenon gave rise to the word infarction (*L. infarcire*, to stuff). This word has however now come to include all forms of continuous *ischaemic necrosis en masse*, whether or not accompanied by the extravasation of red cells.

If the dead tissue is filled with extravasated red cells, as happens commonly in lung, intestine, cerebral grey matter, and sometimes in the heart, the process is called red infarction (Figs. 3.4 and 3.7). If the necrotic tissue is not haemorrhagic, as is generally the case in ischaemic kidney, spleen, white matter of the brain and frequently in the heart, the term pale infarction is used (Fig. 3.8, p. 72).

The cells of infarcts initially show coagulative necrosis (p. 7). Cellular outline is preserved, but cytoplasmic RNA is lost. The cytoplasm usually becomes homogeneous and eosinophilic, while the nuclei shrivel (pyknosis), break up into granules (karyorrhexis) or become unstainable (karyolysis).

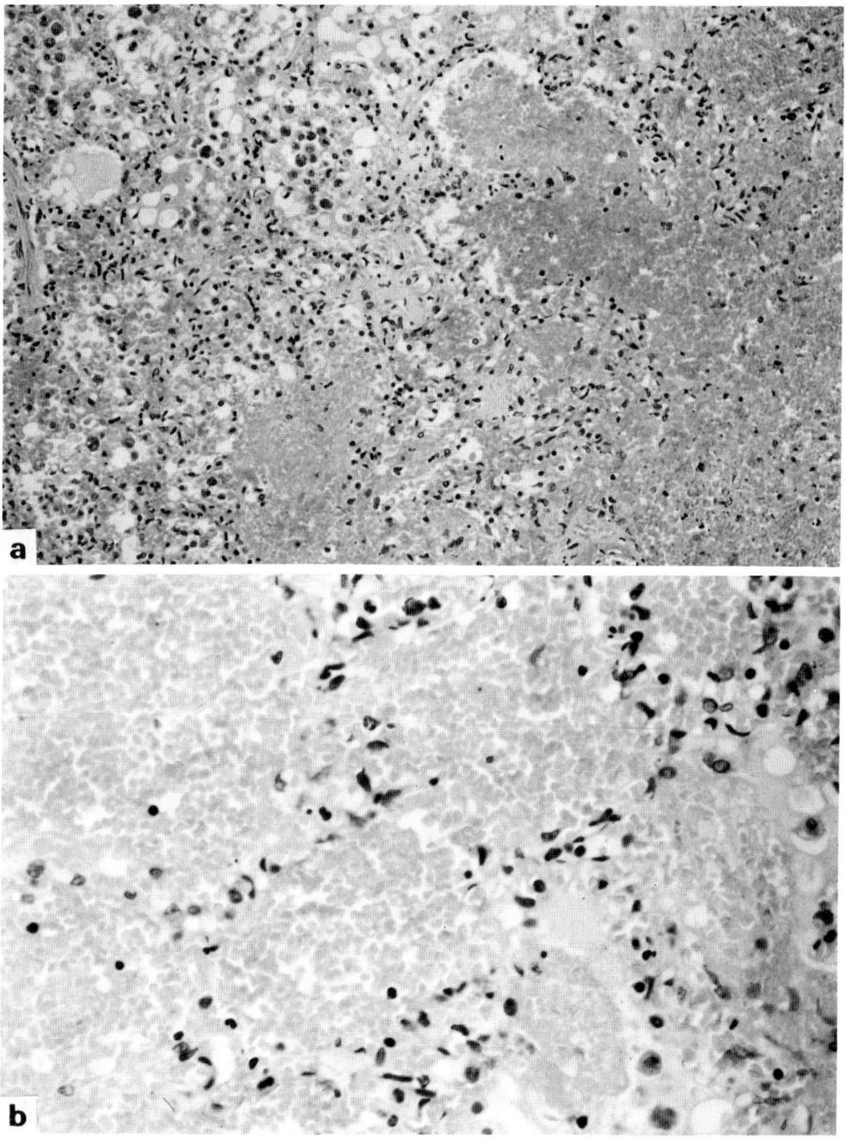

FIG. 3.7 Red infarction of the lung due to combination of general ischaemia due to heart failure with superadded local ischaemia due to a pulmonary embolus. H & E.

a. Low power field, ×130. At left of figure swollen alveolar walls (not necrotic) show congestion due to chronic heart failure; alveoli contain macrophages darkened by haemosiderin. At right of figure superadded local ischaemia has caused necrosis and red cells have filled the alveoli by leaking from the necrotic alveolar capillaries (red infarction).

b. High power field from necrotic zone in same section, ×330. Alveolar walls have disintegrated but their position is revealed by pyknotic nuclear remnants; the alveolar cavities are filled by extravasated red cells.

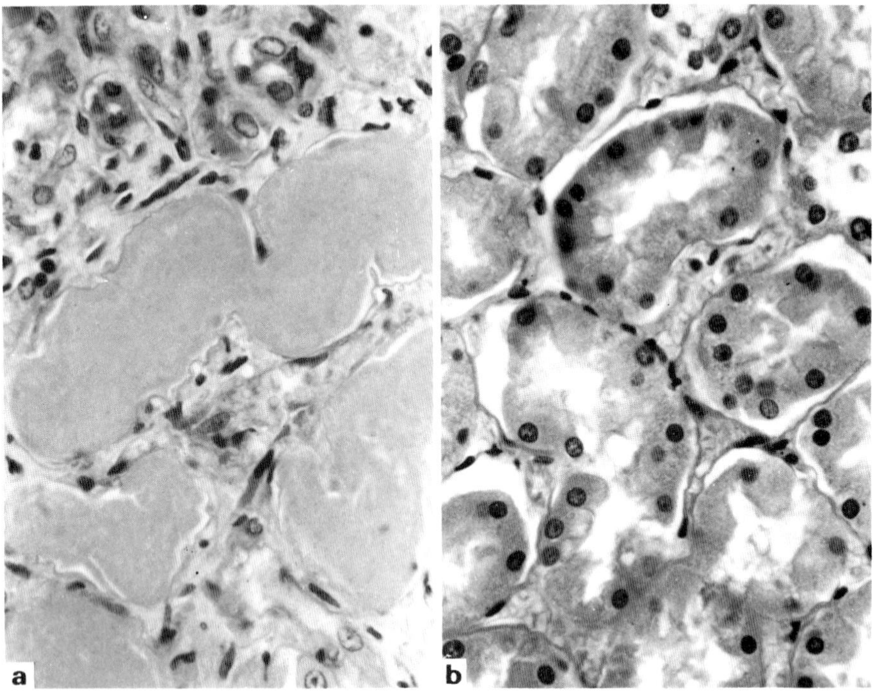

FIG. 3.8 Pale infarct of kidney from a woman of 79 who had suffered from auricular fibrillation for many years. Thrombi present in the left auricle resulted in emboli which produced multiple pale infarcts in kidneys, as well as cerebral embolism which was the immediate cause of death. H & E. ×410.

a. Necrotic renal tubules from pale infarct: there is *no* extravasation of red cells, in contrast to Fig. 3.7. The cytoplasm of the necrotic tubular cells has become homogeneous (coagulative necrosis) and the nuclei have disappeared (karyolysis). These necrotic tubules are situated near the margin of the infarct where sufficient nutriments still penetrate to maintain the interstitial renal tissue; the latter appears uninjured.

b. Unaffected renal tubules outside the infarct.

Differential vulnerability to ischaemia

Cells, tissues and organs differ markedly in power to survive interruption in their supply of blood.

The resistance of some cells depends on local differences in supply which ensure that they are more fortunately situated than their neighbours. But in other cases there are real differences in metabolic requirement and demand for nutriments by different kinds of cell. Indeed nutrient substances provide energy for differing levels of cellular mechanical and electrical activity as well as for maintenance of extensive surface membranes which vary in area and complexity from one type of cell to another.

Local differences in supply

Zonal susceptibility of hepatic lobules

Because of the dual supply by branches of both portal vein and hepatic artery infarction of the liver hardly ever occurs. But although the hepatic cells are thus protected from necrosis *en masse* following local occlusion of a nutrient blood vessel, the liver shows spectacular *zonal susceptibility* to the ischaemia of heart failure (Fig. 3.9).

The blood which supplies the hepatic cells percolates from the terminal branches of the portal vein and hepatic artery along the sinusoids from the periphery to the centre of the lobules, and finally drains into the central vein of each lobule. The cells situated near the centre of the lobules therefore only receive blood which has first traversed the outer parts of the lobules. This fluid has become depleted of some of its nutriments by the more fortunately situated

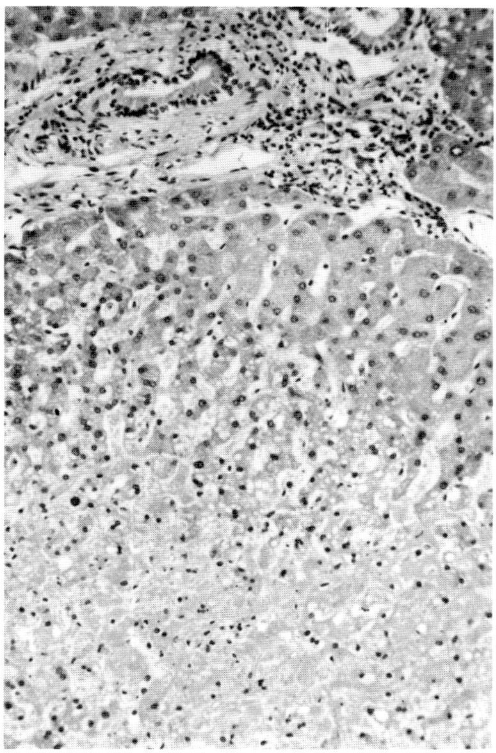

FIG. 3.9 Differential ischaemic injury to hepatic cells. Liver from a patient who died in coma following rapidly progressive heart failure, developing over one week, due to coronary artery thrombosis. In the hepatic lobule shown the uppermost periportal cells are unaffected, the midzonal cells contain spherical spaces due to globular fat, while the centrilobular cells (at lower end of field) are necrotic. H & E. × 130.

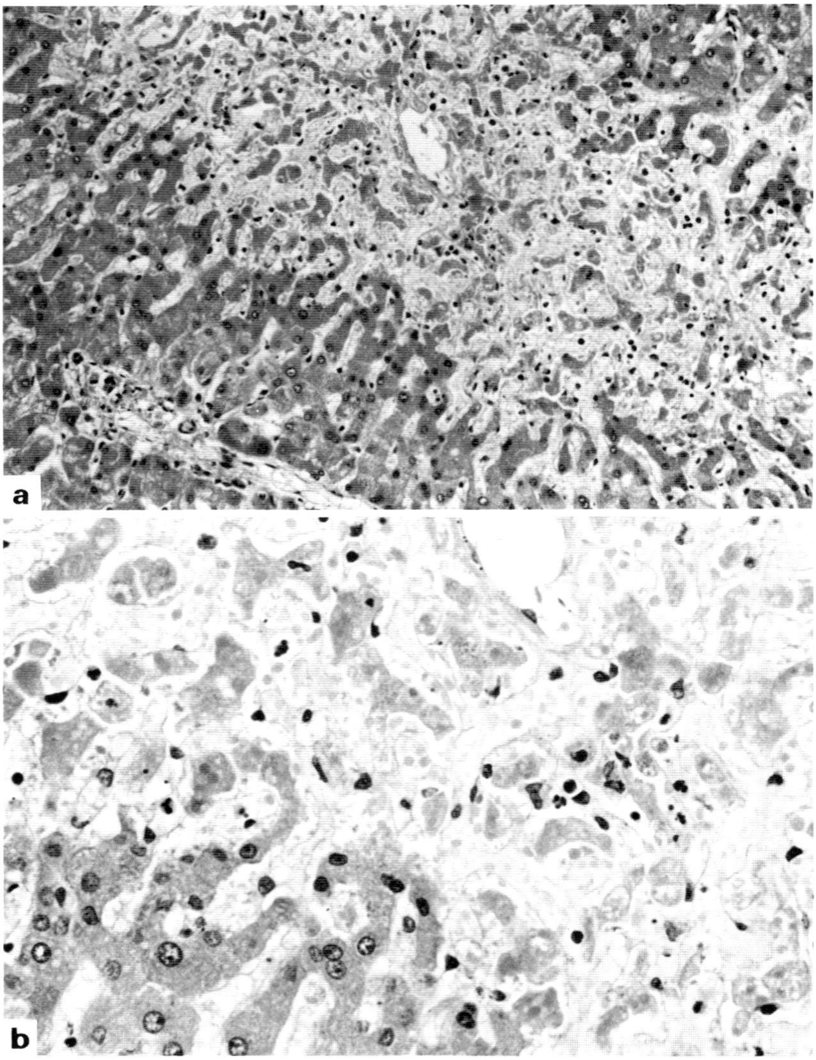

FIG. 3.10 Differential ischaemic injury to hepatic cells (with slower onset than lesions seen in Fig. 3.9). Liver from a diabetic man of 64 who died of recurrent left ventricular failure associated with both old and recent myocardial infarction, produced by progressive coronary occlusion due to atherosclerosis. Liver showed pronounced centrilobular congestion.

a. Liver lobule × 130. The faintly stained centrilobular cells around central vein are shrivelled and necrotic due to a combination of general ischaemia and local hypoxia; peripheral cells are unaffected.

b. Same liver lobule × 330. Shrivelled centrilobular cells have lost their nuclei (karyolysis) and their faintly stained cytoplasm contains vacuolar spaces due to globular fat. The peripheral cells are almost unaffected and retain their nuclei. The centrilobular sinusoids are widely dilated.

external cells. However, if the flow of blood is rapid, the central cells still receive an adequate supply of oxygen and other nutriments.

Along with the general ischaemia of chronic congestive heart failure the rate of percolation of blood through the hepatic sponge-work is grossly retarded. Thus a remarkable zonal distribution of progressively more severe injury develops in the lobules from the outside in. The best nourished peripheral cells are unaffected, the partially maintained midzonal cells may show fatty change (Fig. 3.9, p. 73), while the centrally situated cells shrivel and die; these central cells may also contain fat droplets formed before the onset of atrophy and necrosis (Fig. 3.10). The shrunken centrilobular cells become separated by widely dilated (congested) sinusoids filled by the slowly flowing blood; this gives a characteristic pattern of red mottling to the centrilobular zones so as to form the typical 'nutmeg' liver of congestive heart failure.

Zonal vulnerability of cardiac muscle

The heart also shows zonal necrosis, atrophy and fatty change which result from local disparity in the supply of nutriments to the cells in different regions. During systole the capillaries in the myocardium are narrowed or occluded by the contracting muscle. This effect is more severe and prolonged in the inner parts of the myocardium where the intramural pressure becomes highest [40]. Thus local coronary narrowing or occlusion is likely to cause more serious interruption in the supply of nutriments to the inner than to the outer myocardium. This accounts for the characteristic location of many cardiac infarcts in the inner portions of the ventricular muscle (Fig. 3.11). The more gradual processes of fatty deposition, atrophy and replacement by fibrous tissue

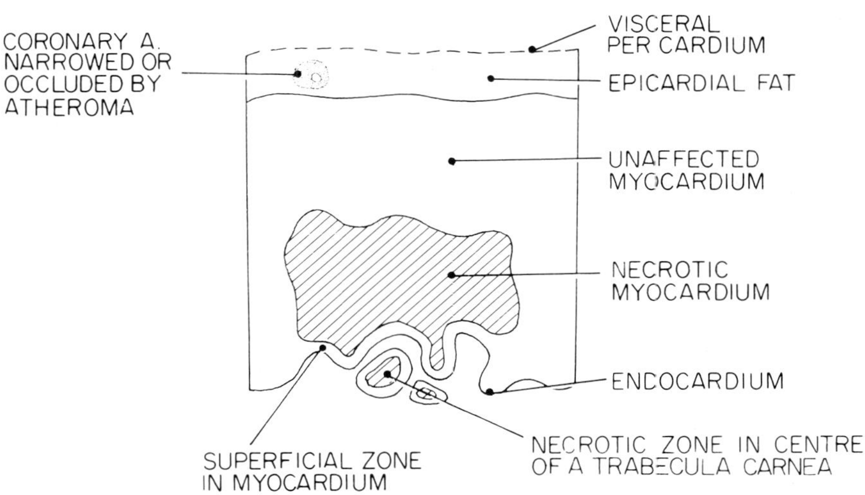

FIG. 3.11 Infarct of myocardium, showing typical location of necrotic heart muscle in the inner part of ventricular wall.

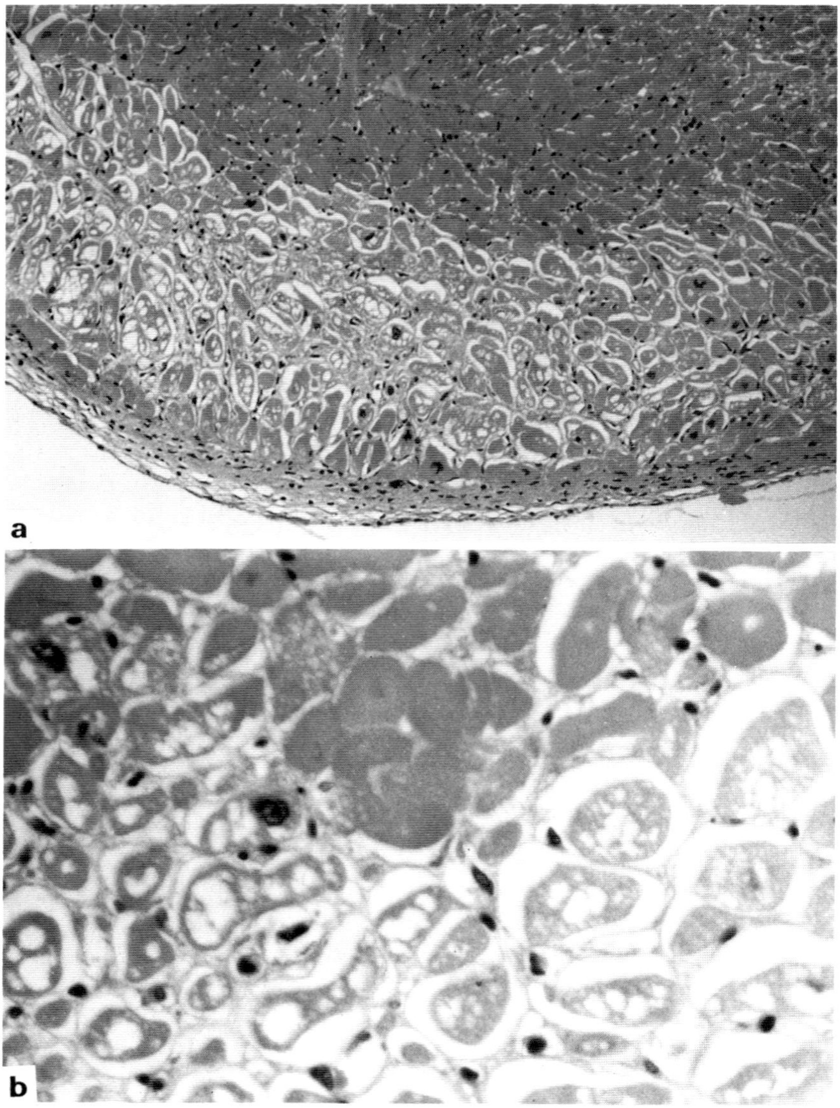

FIG. 3.12 Infarct of inner myocardium associated with acute left ventricular failure commencing about six days before death. Gradation of injury caused by varying degrees of hypoxia. H & E.

a. General view showing inner margin of infarct with uppermost zone of necrotic myocardial fibres, intermediate fatty fibres, and lowest layer of unaffected fibres next to endocardium and ventricular cavity. × 130.

b. Transition from uppermost necrotic fibres (without nuclei) to intermediate fatty fibres (some nuclei visible). × 510.

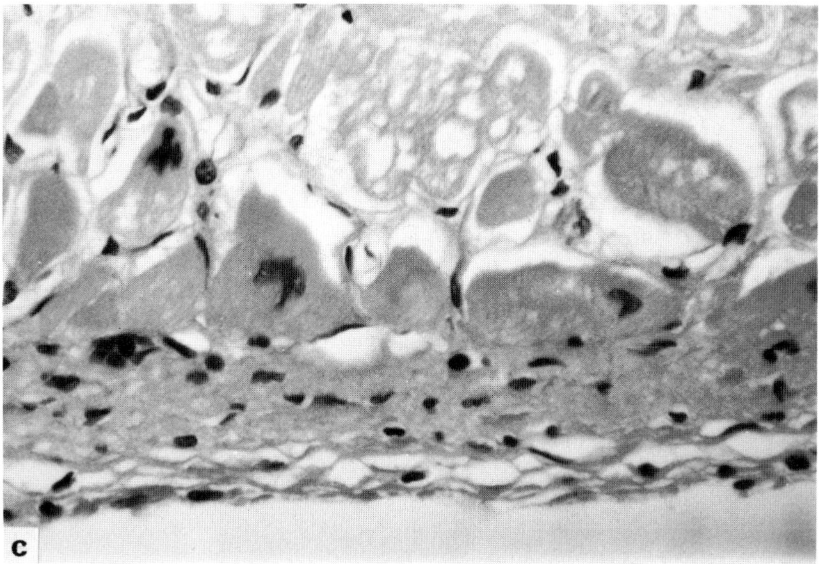

FIG. 3.12 cont.
c. Transition from intermediate fatty fibres to unaffected fibres (with nuclei) next to endocardium. ×510.

are, for similar reasons, more pronounced in the inner than the outer myocardium.

Myocardial infarcts situated in the inner ventricular muscle frequently do not extend to the innermost subendocardial myofibres which may receive sufficient nutriments by diffusion from the ventricular cavity to remain alive. Such survival of the *innermost* myocardium is illustrated in Fig. 3.12a, which shows in more detail the inner margin of a myocardial infarct; this lesion was situated in the inner left ventricular muscle of a man of 56 who died six days after the onset of left ventricular failure due to coronary occlusion. In the upper part of the figure the most ischaemic zone, composed of necrotic fibres, is seen as a darkly eosinophilic mass. Between this zone and the endocardium lies a less prominent region of fatty fibres, in which fat appears as lacunar intracellular spaces. In this intervening zone partial deficiency of oxygen caused fatty globulation in the cells (p. 365), but sufficient oxygen penetrated from the ventricular cavity to prevent necrosis of these fatty fibres. Nearer still to the cavity can be seen a narrow rim of apparently normal fibres immediately subjacent to the subendocardial connective tissue; in this situation cardiac nutrition was unimpaired. Fig. 3.12b and c illustrate at higher magnification this gradation of normal, fatty and necrotic myocardium which probably reflects progressive defect in oxygenation [41]. It is clear that local difference in supply of nutriments exert a profound effect on the fate of myocardial cells.

Real differences in cellular requirements

Differential vulnerability to ischaemia also depends on real disparity in need for nutriments by different kinds of cell.

Brown-Séquard [42] emphasised that of all organs the brain is most vulnerable to lack of oxygen. He showed that cerebral and nervous activity, when temporarily lost owing to cessation of circulation, could be restored by perfusion with oxygenated blood. He was able in this way to restore co-ordinated facial and ocular movements (apparently under cerebral control) by perfusing the carotid and vertebral arteries of a decapitated dog. In numerous similar experiments he revivified spinal and muscular activity of decapitated animals. He concluded that duration of this power of revival was shortest for brain (a few minutes) and was progressively longer for spinal cord, nerves and muscles (several hours).

There is thus a gradation in the susceptibility of cells to ischaemic injury; in considering the action of ischaemia on cells we shall first consider the more resistant cells and then progress to the more vulnerable. The initial events leading to injury by ischaemia will be discussed but the details of ensuing damage will be considered in Chapter 7.

Skin, cornea and subcutaneous tissue

Epidermal cells survive for many hours at room temperature after the heart has stopped. Hair in fact grows for some time after death.

Excised skin and cornea remain alive for some weeks at 2–4°C, if kept in a moist and sterile atmosphere. Cornea can then be used successfully for *allografting*, while epidermis, although rejected by the allograft reaction, if transferred to an *allogeneic* patient can still be accepted by its own donor as an *autograft*. Such autografts of epidermis are most valuable in treatment of burns.

The epidermis of living rabbit skin can thus be used successfully for autografting on the donor animal. Such excised skin used afterwards for autografts survived for four days at 37°C, for 11 days at 22°C and for 35 days at 0°C [43].

Skin and subcutaneous tissue are seriously injured when their blood vessels are occluded by prolonged external compression. This happens in bedridden patients when left too long in one position. The resultant ischaemia causes extensive necrosis and ulceration affecting epidermis, dermis and subcutaneous tissue and thus creates the *bed sores* which are such ominous sequels to inefficient nursing.

Macrophages and microglial phagocytes are also exceptionally resistant to ischaemia. Thus, when ischaemia in congestive heart failure kills the centrilobular hepatic cells, macrophages filled with brown granules survive among the dead hepatocytes in the central hypoxic zones. Similarly when neurones in the cerebral cortex are killed by ischaemia, microglial phagocytes, which consume the remnants of the more vulnerable neurones, survive and prosper for many months. Fig. 7.36 (p. 344) shows these spherical microglial cells eroding neuronal remnants long after the neurones have died from partial occlusion of their nutrient vessels.

Fibroblasts and astrocytes
The extreme resistance of fibroblasts to defective supply of nutriments is evident from the remarkable capacity of these cells to survive in ischaemic tissue where more specialised cells are destroyed. Thus, after ischaemic atrophy or infarction of cardiac muscle, fibroblasts continue to form collagen fibres which in part repair the zones vacated by the necrotic cells.

Similarly astrocytes, in the central nervous system, proliferate at the borders of areas where neurones have been destroyed by ischaemia. The zones which are softened and converted into cystic spaces by microglial destruction of the dead neurones are surrounded by an accumulation of astrocytes which invest the necrotic foci by dense canopies of astroglial fibres (Fig. 3.6).

Renal tissue is readily injured by ischaemia. Excised kidneys rapidly become unsuitable for transplantation unless removed immediately after death of donor and then cooled in iced saline and perfused with cold fluid; this treatment probably diminishes metabolism and so may avert ischaemic injury which otherwise may prevent recovery of renal function. Renal tubular cells are clearly more vulnerable to ischaemia than the interstitial cells which lie between the tubules; this differential vulnerability is apparent from Fig. 3.8a which shows *necrotic* renal tubules in an infarct of the kidney surrounded by uninjured capillaries and fibroblasts.

Susceptibility of hepatic cells
The liver, as we have seen, rarely develops infarction because of its dual blood supply by both portal vein and hepatic artery, but if both are permanently occluded necrosis inevitably follows.

The sequence of events in ischaemic injury to hepatic cells has been greatly illuminated by the work of Bernelli-Zazzera and his colleagues. Ultrastructural changes caused by ischaemia were observed in hepatocytes after temporary or permanent clamping of pedicles to whole liver lobes in rats and the effects of re-establishment of blood supply were also studied [44]. After ischaemia lasting 15 min blebs and discontinuities develop in the plasma membrane and the microvilli disappear at the sinusoidal borders of the cells, while vacuoles become visible in the adjacent cytoplasm (see Fig. 7.2, p. 287). Prolongation of ischaemia is followed by mitochondrial swelling and fragmentation of the endoplasmic reticulum (ER) into vesicles; polyribosomes are simultaneously detached from the rough-surface ER and became disaggregated into monosomes. All these changes are reversible provided duration of ischaemia does not exceed 1 h; re-establishment of circulation restores normal structure. But after initial ischaemia lasting 2 h, the cells lose their capacity to recover after reassumption of blood supply and structural changes then become progressively more conspicuous.

Ischaemia incurred by clamping pedicles of hepatic lobes of rats *in vivo* also changes the subsequent activity *in vitro* of *homogenates* made from the ischaemic cells [45]. The homogenates from previously ischaemic liver contain fewer ribosomes than their normal counterparts and the ribosomes become disaggregated from polysomes to form monosomes. Moreover the ribosomes from ischaemic liver are less efficient than normal ribosomes in their capacity to promote polypeptide synthesis *in vitro*. The normal polysomal pattern in homogenates and their capacity to promote polypeptide synthesis are restored after re-establisment of blood supply to ischaemic liver, provided the duration of ischaemia does not exceed 1 h; but if ischaemia lasts 2 h recovery does not occur [46]. Ischaemic injury also alters the physical nature of the membranes of rough surface ER by diminishing their binding power for added ribosomes during incubation *in vitro*; whether irreversible injury depends on one crucial lesion, such as disintegration of cell membranes, or on the summation of several induced defects is still uncertain [47].

Liberation of hydrolytic proteases from hepatic lysosomes as a consequence of injury by ischaemia, with subsequent enzymic destruction of cellular proteins, was regarded as a possible mechanism of irreversible damage to ischaemic liver, but this type of action is unlikely to be of importance since EM observations on ischaemic liver cells show that lysosomes remain intact in the early phases of irreversible injury (p. 316).

The relative resistance of hepatic cells to ischaemia, which enables them to survive occlusion of vascular supply for up to 1 h probably depends on abundant reserves of intracellular glycogen; this provides a substrate for exergonic catabolism both by aerobic oxidation as well as by anaerobic glycolysis in the absence of O_2. In starvation, however, depletion of glycogen deprives the hepatic cells of this exergonic reserve. Indeed the liver of starved rats is much more susceptible to injury by ischaemia than that of well fed animals. Thus when starved rats are killed by asphyxia their hepatic cells become grossly vacuolated within 20 min, but this vacuolation does not occur in the liver of well fed animals [48] (p. 293). Similarly the livers of well fed rats, when perfused under anaerobic conditions, liberate lactic acid at a constant rate for about 1 h by which time their stores of glycogen are depleted, but the livers of starved rats liberate hardly any lactic acid and rapidly become swollen on anaerobic perfusion [49]; this swelling is probably due to the same kind of vacuolation as described by Trowell [48].

The presence of abundant intracellular glycogen thus contributes to the capacity of hepatic cells to survive substantial periods of temporary ischaemia. When this reserve is depleted more serious irreversible injury occurs in the cell membranes and this may produce swelling and vacuolation.

Ischaemic necrosis of striated muscle

Occlusion of arterial supply to limbs by application of tourniquets for periods of an hour or less does not injure human skeletal muscle, which is relatively resistant to ischaemia.

When victims of air raids were trapped by falling buildings, the muscles in compressed limbs survived ischaemia, if its duration was less than 2 h but occlusion of blood flow for longer periods caused ischaemic muscle necrosis [50].

Burial by debris for longer periods than the minimum to cause muscle death did not further increase the mortality, which was determined by the *extent* of muscle death and the consequent secondary shock and later renal injury. In patients who died about six days after the initial injury the dead muscle appeared swollen and bulged out immediately the fascia was incised. This necrotic muscle is opaque, greyish white and friable, having a 'fish flesh' appearance characteristic of Zenker's hyaline degeneration (p. 315). The pallor of the dead muscle is due to loss of myohaemoglobin, which, along with K^+, escapes from the dying fibres into the blood; the secondary effects of these liberated constituents of necrotic muscle may exert disastrous effects on the rest of the body (pp. 195, 196).

Sometimes ischaemic necrosis of striated muscle develops as a result of overtight splinting or of pressure from haemorrhage following fractures. This injury usually occurs in the flexor muscles of the forearm. The dying muscles contract and produce extreme flexure of the fingers. The dead muscle consolidates into hard homogeneous material; microscopically nuclei and striations are lost and eventually the dead muscle is replaced by fibrous tissue. The fibrosis results in further flexion. This condition produces very severe disability and is called *Volkmann's ischaemic contracture*.

Rigor mortis in striated muscle

The general arrest of circulation that occurs with death specially affects skeletal muscle which develops the spectacular phenomenon of *rigor mortis* (p. 10). The muscles contract and stiffen within 4–10 h after death and so produce the general condition of *post mortem* rigidity which lasts for about 48 h.

Contraction of living muscle is normally prevented by the continuous presence of ATP; this reacts with myosin and so prevents the myosin from combining with actin to produce contraction. In normal muscular contraction Ca^{++} activates the enzymic role of myosin as an ATP-ase. ATP is then split and simultaneously some myosin is freed to react with actin so that contraction occurs.

After death and general arrest of supply of O_2 and glucose to muscles the synthesis of ATP, catalysed by oxidative phosphorylation and by glycolysis of glycogen, ceases in the ischaemic muscle. But hydrolysis of ATP continues slowly so that ATP ultimately disappears. Myosin then becomes entirely freed from ligation with ATP and reacts with actin *en masse*, so that very extensive contraction results and *rigor mortis* develops.

During this complete destruction of ATP after death many more attachments are found between myosin and actin than in normal contraction. In this process of excessive ligation to actin the macromolecules of myosin are rotated so as to allow as many myosin cross-bridges as possible to bind with actin. Observations on X-ray diffraction of frog sartorius during rigor [51] indicate that such a change in cross-bridge arrangement alters a considerable part of the entire helical conformation of the myosin molecules and also destroys the accurate transverse registration of the muscle filaments; this causes the rigid inextensible condition of rigor.

Later rigor passes off owing to breakage of links between Z discs and fragmentation of myofibrils [52].

Susceptibility of myocardial fibres to ischaemia

The myocardium suffers irreversible injury fron ischaemia much more rapidly than skeletal muscle. Like skeletal muscle and liver, myocardium possesses intracellular reserves of glycogen, which enable its cells to survive periods of temporary ischaemia. But the maximum period of survival is much shorter for myocardium, probably because its cells, unlike those of *resting* skeletal muscle, are continuously utilizing their reserves in providing energy for *spontaneous* contraction. This contractility is displayed in the so-called 'contraction bands' which are conspicuous features in ischaemic myocardial fibres (see Fig. 7.7, p. 296). Within 5 min of ligation of coronary arteries in rabbits granular glycogen (visible by EM) disappears from ischaemic myocardium [53]. This rapid loss of glycogen may be stimulated by 'feed back' acceleration of glycolysis caused by depletion of ATP during activity. In any case anaerobic glycolysis, occurring during ischaemia, may not provide sufficient ATP to compensate for that lost by continuous activity. Thus spontaneous contractility of myocardium contributes to its high vulnerability to ischaemia and extreme liability to infarction.

Important observations on the onset of irreversible damage after transient and permanent myocardial ischaemia were made by Jennings and his colleagues [54]. They clamped the circumflex branch of the left coronary artery in dogs for various times and then examined the ischaemic myocardium in the posterior papillary muscle and in other parts of the left ventricular wall. The tissues were fixed either *immediately after* the period of ischaemia, or *after further* periods of reflow, during which the vessel was unclamped and blood was allowed to recirculate freely through the previously ischaemic myocardium. The tissues were examined by chemical methods [54] and by LM and EM [55].

In the myocardium, exposed to ischaemia for 15 min with subsequent reflow for 2 min, no changes were detected apart from a slight increase of intracellular Na^+. Following 40 min of ischaemia, terminated by immediate fixation, the myocardial fibres and their mitochondria were slightly swollen and amorphous densities became visible within the mitochondria but no significant changes were detectable in water content or electrolytes, even though this period of ischaemia apparently produced irreversible injury (see below). After 40 min of ischaemia, followed by reflow for 2 min or more, the myocardium developed explosive swelling, the cell membranes were lifted away from the myofibres forming large subsarcolemmal blebs, and the mitochondria became intensely swollen and dense bodies appeared within them (p. 314). During this rapid cellular swelling striking increases occurred in tissue content of H_2O, Na^+, Cl^- and Ca^{++} [54]. No changes however were detected in the lysosomes during these early phases of irreversible injury.

It is clear from these findings that much of the initial irreparable damage caused by ischaemia is at first masked and only produces the more spectacular sequels when fluid can enter the damaged tissue. Presumably the initial lesions involve macromolecular alterations in cellular membranes or other changes in conformation which are at first not detectable by LM of EM.

After such temporary coronary occlusion for only 40 min, which was long enough to produce irreparable myocardial injury, injection of markers such as carbon black and thioflavines was followed by their complete penetration throughout the previously ischaemic myocardium [56]. But after occlusion for 90 min these markers failed to penetrate the inner half of the myocardium probably owing to development of capillary damage. Irreparable damage to the ischaemic myocardium thus occurs *before* the onset of vascular changes which might prevent reflow of blood into the ischaemic zone. The initial irreparable lesions produced by ischaemia in the myocardium must therefore be determined by changes in the cells themselves and *not* as a consequence of vascular injury.

Secreting cells of the anterior lobe of the pituitary gland

These cells usually receive sufficient nutriments to cope with their various activities, and even generalized ischaemia does not normally single out the pituitary gland as a specially vulnerable organ. But in pregnancy the anterior pituitary cells are hypertrophied and excessively active; under these circumstances their demand for nutriments, including oxygen, is apparently greatly increased. Moreover during pregnancy the swelling of the cells within the rigid confinement of the sella turcica may retard the flow of blood in the vascular sinusoids. The extreme fall of blood pressure caused by severe post partum haemorrhage results in extensive necrosis of these hypertrophied highly vulnerable cells; this effect may be intensified by stasis and thrombosis in the portal venous system which supplies the anterior lobe. The lesion results in pituitary hypofunction with hypothyroidism, gonadal atrophy and amenorrhoea and loss of skin pigmentation due to lack of melanocyte stimulating hormone; this condition is called *Sheehan's syndrome*.

Nerve fibres and axons

Nerve fibres are relatively resistant to ischaemia. Although conductivity is abolished and paralysis follows compression of nerves in the limbs of cats for 10–90 min, full recovery and restoration of both sensory and motor activity without structural damage ensue after release of pressure [57]. This *transient* interruption of function is apparently due to local ischaemia and not to trauma, since it does not occur in cold blooded animals.

Pressure applied to nerve fibres for longer periods (two hours or more) results in more lasting paralysis with axonal swelling and degeneration of myelin. The axons, however, are only reversibly injured and the fibres with their myelin sheaths recover completely in structure and function in about eight weeks. Longer periods of ischaemia are followed by complete degeneration of both axons and myelin (Wallerian degeneration). This is the same irreversible process which also follows axonal section (p. 108); recovery can then only occur following regrowth of living nerve from above the zone of injury. This regeneration takes many months.

Cell bodies and dendrites of neurones

The cell bodies and dendrites, as opposed to the axons, show unique vulnerability to ischaemia.

Litten [58] found that compression of the abdominal aorta of rabbits for one hour is followed by permanent paralysis of the lower limbs and he suggested that this is due to injury to the spinal cord. Litten noted that the kidneys which are more susceptible to ischaemia than many tissues are not so rapidly injured as the spinal cord. Ehrlich & Brieger [59] showed that compression of the aorta in fact kills the anterior horn cells of the spinal cord and that the grey matter exhibits microscopic evidence of injury before the white matter. They also found that the living grey matter rapidly reduces alizarin blue to a colourless compound, but the dead grey matter in the spinal cord which has been killed by ischaemia fails to do so. Marinesco [60, 61] showed that the dendrites of the anterior horn cells are also destroyed following occlusion of the aorta and he emphasised that later degeneration of the axons is determined by injury to their cell bodies. More recent work [62, 63] has established that occlusion of the abdominal aorta for as short a time as 20 min is sufficient to kill anterior horn cells of the spinal cord. Neurones of higher centres (as discussed later) are killed by even shorter periods of ischaemia.

Retina

Retinal cells, which are of cerebral origin in their development, are highly susceptible to deprivation of nutriments.

Isolated retina, detached from eyes of rabbits and then incubated in the presence of glucose and O_2, showed no ultrastructural alteration visible by EM after one hour [64]. The zones studied included the rod-inner segments, rod-synapses, and bipolar cell-bodies. Deprivation of glucose and O_2 for only 3 min caused mitochondrial swelling along with swelling and loss of synaptic vesicles. Extension of the period of deprivation caused further mitochondrial swelling and also swelling of ER vesicles. These changes were completely reversible up to 20 min, but were irreversible by 30 min, when multiple discontinuities appeared in the cell and organelle membranes. Anoxia alone caused alterations similar to those resulting from shorter periods of combined deprivation, whereas withdrawal of glucose alone produced only minor changes.

Retina, like brain, is thus highly vulnerable to lack of O_2 and glucose. This susceptibility can be demonstrated in detached tissue suspended in nutrient solution and must therefore be determined by real *cellular* vulnerability and not by any local peculiarity in arterial supply.

Ischaemia exerts a remarkable effect on human retina *in vivo* by causing the appearance of localised whitish zones ('cotton wool spots') due to axonal swelling. These lesions are considered in Chapter 7.

Depression or annulment of exergonic metabolism

Cells vary greatly in their capacity to survive temporary diminution of their supply of nutriments from the blood. Irreversible injury commences when exergonic metabolism is severely depressed or annulled. Although ischaemia can eliminate oxidative metabolism and thus deprive cells of their principal exergonic reactions, anaerobic glycolysis can temporarily provide minor compensation and so postpone the onset of injury caused by deficiency of metabolism. Most rapid injury therefore depends on:

1. *Lack of intracellular reserves*, such as glycogen, which in the absence of glucose can form a substrate for anaerobic glycolysis (Fig. 3.13); cerebral cortex has minimal reserves of glycogen compared with liver and striated muscle and is therefore more rapidly deprived of energy by lack of O_2.

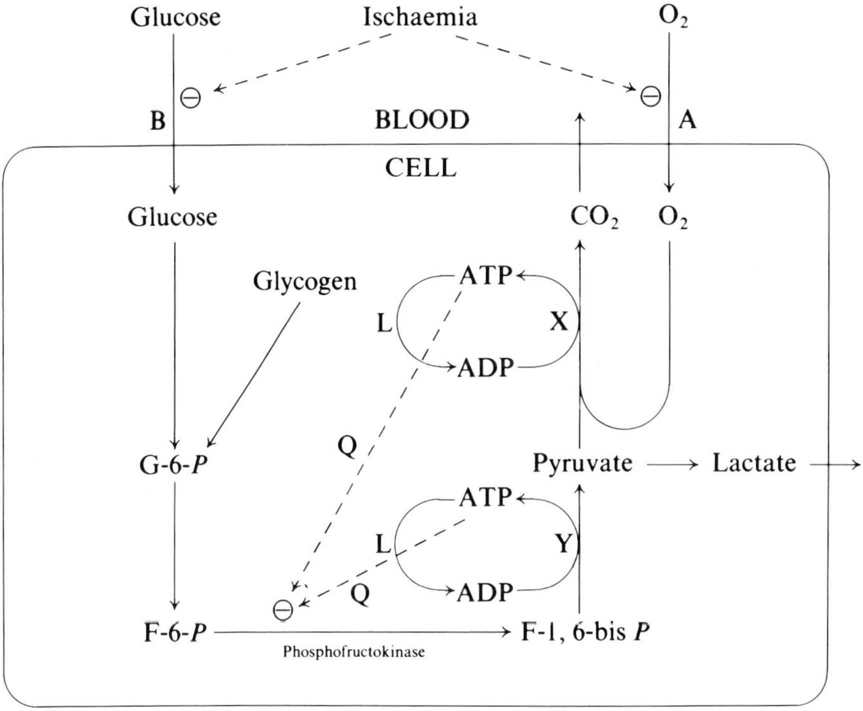

FIG. 3.13 Retardation of formation of ATP in ischaemia. Ischaemia retards entry of O_2 (A) and of glucose (B) into the cell. This results in inhibition of aerobic (oxidative) phosphorylation of ADP to ATP (X) and of anaerobic (glycolytic) phosphorylation of ADP to ATP (Y). X is much more effective in producing ATP than Y. Initially loss of ATP induces a temporary increase in glycolysis probably by diminishing feed-back inhibition (Q), which ATP normally exerts on enzyme phosphofructokinase. But this effect (which temporarily increases Y) cannot compensate for abolition of formation of ATP by X, which is the dominant mechanism of cellular replenishment of ATP. As loss of ATP (L) continues undiminished, retardation of X soon results in serious depletion of ATP; this depletion becomes largely uncompensated when all available intracellular glucose and glycogen are consumed or when anaerobic glycolysis is inhibited by K^+ (p. 92), and Y also is eliminated.

G-6-*P*	glucose-6-phosphate
F-6-*P*	fructose-6-phosphate
F-1,6-bis*P*	fructose-1,6-bisphosphate

2. *High rate of metabolism* which soon consumes all substrates for anaerobic glycolysis; in this respect cerebral cortex and cardiac muscle become depleted of substrates for exergonic metabolism more rapidly than skin, cornea or cartilage.

This rapid onset of irreversible injury in cerebral grey matter as a result of ischaemia doubtless depends both on deficiency of reserves and on high rate of metabolism. The latter reflects the need for abundant supply of energy for cellular processes, but does not explain the basis for this need, nor the mechanism of the damage which so rapidly occurs if this need is not satisfied. As the effects of annulment of exergonic metabolism are likely to be most definite in the most vulnerable type of cell, the unique vulnerability of the neurone will now be considered along with the mechanism of ischaemic damage in general.

Neuronal vulnerability to ischaemia

Ischaemia with great rapidity interrupts the function of neurones and it also destroys their life. These two effects must carefully be distinguished.

Arrest of function

The rapidity with which ischaemia can interrupt cerebral function was early recognised, as we have seen, by William Stokes. He described [65] sudden attacks of coma in patients with extreme slowing or weakening of the heart. He considered these 'seizures are owing to deficient arterial supply. The suddenness of the attack, and, in many cases the rapidity of the recovery are in favour of this view". Stokes [65] was thus responsible for the extremely important concept that rapid, transient and reversible loss of cerebral function is a direct sequel of temporary cessation of cerebral nutrition.

It is now known that arrest of cerebral circulation in man for as short a time as 7 sec produces loss of consciousness, although no permanent damage usually results for even as long as 100 sec [66]. Similarly in dogs very rapid loss of consciousness follows arrest of circulation for 20–30 sec, though no permanent injury is caused by ischaemia lasting for less than 6 min [67]. The availability of O_2 in the cerebral cortex measured by polarograph falls to a minimum after occlusion of middle cerebral artery or inhalation of N_2 for 8–12 sec, and is followed by a corresponding disappearance of electrical activity in another 6 sec [68]. The rate of oxygen consumption of cerebral cortex of cats *in vivo*, recorded by polarographic changes in electrodes placed over cerebral arterioles, is inhibited after 30 sec of ischaemia caused by arterial compression [69].

Ischaemia thus with unique rapidity interrupts cerebral function and electrical activity. All these changes are at first reversible and are followed by full recovery of neuronal function provided reflow of blood is restored within a few minutes.

Onset of permanent damage

Irreversible damage due to ischaemia also occurs much more rapidly in neurones than in other cells. Thus the pyramidal cells of the cerebral cortex are irreparably injured by ischaemia lasting for a few minutes, while striated muscle can survive arrest of circulation for more than an hour and epidermal cells are unharmed by deprivation of blood supply for many hours.

The onset of irreversible neuronal damage is, however, considerably less rapid than the inhibition of neuronal activity and function. Thus episodes of coma in human fainting fits occur without any permanent loss of cerebral power including thought and memory. Similarly occlusion of middle cerebral artery in monkeys, along with lowering of blood pressure for minutes, abolishes rythmic electrical activity in parts of the cerebral cortex without producing any permanent damage, provided the circulation is rapidly re-established, but on prolongation of the period of inactivity irreversible damage with neuronal death follows [37].

The minimum period of ischaemia which results in irreparable cellular injury differs in various types of neurone as well as in different species. Controlled experiments on animals have provided more consistent results than the necessarily less systematic observations on man. Weinberger *et al* [70] interrupted the entire circulation of cats by occluding the pulmonary artery with a clamp for varying periods. This procedure induced coma with convulsions after 20 sec. Occlusion lasting 3 min was followed by complete recovery without any visible microscopic changes in the brain, but when the period of ischaemia was extended to 3.5–6 min, neurones in the frontal cortex were destroyed and the intelligence and character of the animals changed so that they did not recognise their keeper nor purr when stroked; they were, however, able to eat the food which they were offered. These experiments showed that the frontal neurones are the most rapidly injured and that 'higher' functions such as the power of recognition are the most vulnerable. Arrest of the circulation for more than 8 min produced necrosis of the entire cerebral cortex with permanent and complete dementia, while progressively longer periods of ischaemia also injured the basal ganglia thereby establishing irreversible coma, and finally the most resistent medullary centres were damaged by vascular occlusion for more than 10 min. Temporary occlusion of the abdominal aorta in cats and rabbits is similarly followed by irreversible paralysis and necrosis of spinal anterior horn cells provided the period of ischaemia exceeds 15 min [62, 63, 71, 72].

In man more variable results have been described. Occlusion of aorta and pulmonary artery in open heart operations for nearly 2 min [73] is followed by full recovery, but if this time is extended to 3 min the brain suffers permanent damage. Brock also discovered that the circulation can be arrested in these operations for up to 7 min without causing any cerebral injury, provided body temperature is lowered to 28°C by perfusion of venous blood through a cooling coil. The resultant depression of cerebral metabolism apparently diminishes neuronal requirements and so enables the cells to survive longer periods of hypoxia. Bourne [36] concluded, from observations on patients who suffered fainting fits accompanied by fall in blood pressure during general anaesthesia, that cerebral ischaemia lasting nearly 2 min is generally followed by full recovery, but that even a small extension of this time may cause permanent damage. Meyer [74] recorded a distressing example of extensive neuronal necrosis in a patient who suffered cardiac arrest under anaesthetic when the period of cerebral ischaemia lasted only 1 min. It seems likely that other factors, such as previous neuronal activity or anoxia, may account for these differences.

The protective action of cooling cerebral tissue to 28°C suggests that irreversible injury due to ischaemia is dependent on depletion of ATP and is postponed when catabolism of ATP is retarded. Moreover the duration of this protective effect can be extended by further reduction of temperature. Indeed the capacity for electrical activity can apparently be preserved indefinitely after arrest of blood supply, if the tissue is kept 'uninjured' in the frozen state. Thus the brain of anaesthetised cats was initially perfused with cooled saline and glycerol and then frozen for some months; on thawing and reperfusion with oxygenated blood the initially frozen brain recovered electrical activity and the Nissl substance in the cerebral neurones was retained [75]. It is possible that depletion of ATP is completely arrested in the frozen state and therefore some of the injurious effects of ischaemia are prevented, but the fabric of the neurones is probably simultaneously damaged by the action of freezing (p. 123).

It is clear, therefore, that cessation of function and of electrical activity due to ischaemia need not produce any permanent damage. The survival of memory and other cerebral determinants of behaviour must therefore depend on preservation of macromolecular patterns in the neurones or their membranes, rather than on more transient changes in electrical potential at neuronal surfaces. Function and memory are only irreparably injured when the macromolecular fabric suffers permanent damage; this happens after longer periods of ischaemia than are necessary to cause temporary suppression of consciousness and electrical activity.

Visible changes in ischaemic neurones

Rapid and reversible loss of function is accompanied by immediate swelling of cell bodies and dendrites and entry of H_2O and Cl^-; these changes as well as the structural alterations associated with irreversible damage are considered along with ischaemic cellular disintegration in Chapter 7.

Selective vulnerability of different neurones to ischaemia

Neurones differ among themselves in this exteme susceptibility to ischaemia. As with other cells these differences partly depend on local variation in the type of vascular supply, but they also are determined by real disparity of vulnerability between different kinds of neurone [76].

We have seen how the cells of the cerebral cortex are more rapidly damaged by ischaemia than the more resistent spinal and medullary neurones. This cellular disparity in vulnerability is particularly well illustrated by ischaemic lesions in the cerebellar cortex of dogs induced by temporary occlusion of the entire cerebral circulation for 8 min by means of cervical cuffs without interferring with respiration [77]; after this temporary ischaemia all the Purkinje cells became necrotic but the granule cells and even the terminal 'boutons' of the presynaptic fibres around the Purkinje cells remain intact.

In human brain also some kinds of neurone are specially vulnerable. Following temporary cardiac arrest produced by accidents with anaesthetics, neurones of the cerebral cortex, basal ganglia and cerebeller cortex are the most frequently injured in patients who die after survival for various periods in coma [27, 74].

These real differences in vulnerability to ischaemia between one kind of neurone and another are probably related to differences in their metabolic requirements.

Utilization of oxygen and glucose by cerebral tissue

The exceptional capacity of cerebral grey matter for utilizing oxygen was clearly demonstrated by Paul Ehrlich [78]. He showed that 'Nadi' reagent (α-naphthol and dimethyl p-phenylene diamine) in the presence of O_2 is oxidised to deep blue pigment indophenol blue by cerebral grey matter and not by white matter.

This reaction is now known to depend on cytochrome oxidase situated within mitochondria of neuronal cell bodies and dendrites. This enzyme catalyzes the oxidation of intracellular reduced cytochrome C by molecular O_2 to oxidized cytochrome C; the latter then promotes the oxidative condensation of the Nadi reagent to indophenol blue which is deposited inside the cells, while the oxidized cytochrome C is itself reconverted to reduced cytochrome C. The reduced cytochrome C is then free to absorb more molecular oxygen in the presence of cytochrome oxidase.

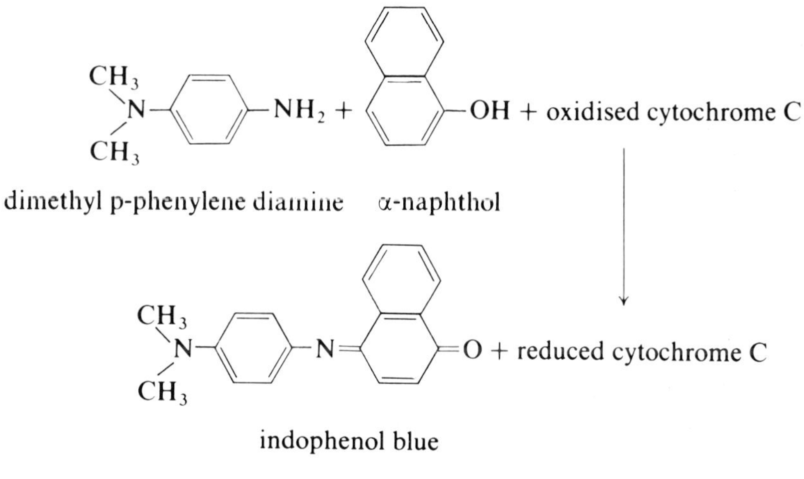

This absorption of O_2 along with deposition of the blue pigment occurs with spectacular intensity in the cell bodies and dendrites of cerebral grey matter and thus enables the grey nuclei of brain and spinal cord to be differentiated with dramatic clarity from neighbouring white matter [79].

The power of grey matter to absorb oxygen is also intense when glucose is provided as the oxidizable substrate. The immediate necessity of glucose for cerebral activity was proved by Mann & Magath in 1921 [80] who showed that dogs lose consciousness after hepatectomy, owing to rapid loss of glucose from the blood. In fact cerebral cortex, unlike many other tissues, contains scanty stores of intracellular substances that can be used for respiration and glycolysis, and is thus directly dependent on blood sugar for its immediate source of energy. The continuous utilization of both oxygen and glucose by human brain was established by observing arteriovenous difference in both content of oxygen and of glucose [81].

Observations on the metabolism of slices of cerebral cortex *in vitro* provide evidence of the unique dependence of cerebral tissue on a continuous supply of oxygen and glucose from the external environment.

Under anaerobic conditions slices of cerebral cortex continuously utilise glucose at a constant rate to form lactic acid [82]; in the absence of glucose this formation of lactic acid ceases within a few minutes, as the cerebral cells contain no appreciable reserve of glycolysable substrate. Much more lactic acid is in fact formed from glucose by cortical slices in anaerobiosis than in the presence of oxygen [82], and anaerobiosis also increases the consumption of glucose by this tissue.

In the presence of oxygen slices of cerebral cortex, when supplied with glucose or lactate, continuously absorb oxygen at a constant rate for many hours [82] but in the absence of added substrate, although absorption of oxygen continues at a substantial rate for about 0.5 h, this process then rapidly declines [83].

Cerebral cells are thus devoid of stored substrates for anaerobic glycolysis, which depends almost entirely on the continued entry of glucose from the blood and extracellular fluid. Aerobic metabolism of cerebral cells can, however, be maintained for relatively short periods by oxidation of intracellular substrates, provided the supply of oxygen is not interrupted. Cerebral tissue is thus exceptionally deficient in stored substrates for exergonic metabolism.

Observations on the metabolism of slices of cerebral cortex *in vitro* thus show that the gross metabolic changes, which follow deprivation of oxygen and other substrates, are determined by the cerebral cells and are not merely a result of alteration in vascular permeability or degree of arterial occlusion. Moreover the metabolism of cells in slices of cerebral cortex, like that of living brain *in vivo*, is uniquely dependent on continuous supply of oxygen and glucose from the external environment.

Deficiency of substrate in ischaemic brain

Ischaemia deprives the brain of two cardinal nutriments, glucose and oxygen. Which of these is paramount?

In the brain there are scanty reserves of substrates for exergonic catabolism. Cerebral function is suppressed by ischaemia or anoxia lasting for more than a few seconds but cerebral tissue probably contains sufficient glucose and glycogen to support anaerobic glycolysis for considerably longer than this [84]. Although the glucose within cerebral tissue can be very substantially diminished within 30 sec of the onset of ischaemia, lactic acid continues to be formed for at least 2 min [85]. On the other hand the quantity of O_2 dissolved in the brain is only sufficient to maintain cellular respiration for about 10 sec [86].

It is clear therefore that lack of oxygen and not lack of glucose is the immediate cause of the rapid loss of consciousness, which follows arrest of cerebral circulation. Indeed deprivation of glucose from brain slices *in vitro* does not rapidly arrest absorption of oxygen, as would happen if lack of glucose external to the cells could with the same rapidity as lack of oxygen, prevent intracellular oxidation [87]. This does not however prove that lack of oxygen rather than lack of glucose is the sole determinant of permanent damage which follows more prolonged ischaemia. It may be significant that irreparable injury occurs more slowly than loss of function and only takes place after a period of circulatory arrest of the same order as would be required to deplete the brain of both glucose and glycogen as well as oxygen, and thus eliminate all exergonic reactions available to the cells.

Lack of oxygen alone without lack of glucose can of itself cause coma followed by irreparable neuronal injury; this happens in aviators exposed to rarefied air at very high altitudes [88], and also results from poisoning by CO (p. 151). Similarly deprivation of glucose alone without lack of oxygen, as occurs in patients who have received excessive doses of insulin, can produce coma followed by neuronal necrosis [89], but these effects are much slower in onset than those due to lack of oxygen.

We may conclude that the sudden coma which occurs in a few seconds after arrest of cerebral circulation is determined by cellular hypoxia, but that deprivation of glucose in addition to deprivation of oxygen is likely to contribute to the succeeding irreversible neuronal damage resulting from ischaemia lasting for longer periods.

The question then arises as to why cessation of exergonic reactions within the neurone is so rapidly followed by irreversible damage; this can best be answered by considering the course of events within ischaemic brain which inevitably leads to depletion of ATP within the cerebral cells.

Depletion of ATP: the prelude to ischaemic damage

In less than 15 sec after arrest of circulation the oxygen within cerebral cells is exhausted. There is then a sudden switch to *anaerobic metabolism.*

In brain under these circumstances glycolysis of glucose to lactic acid is at first much accelerated. In fact the rate of utilization of glucose is initially greatly magnified and the formation of lactic acid increases rapidly (p. 90). In spite of this much less free energy is liberated than during oxidative catabolism of glucose so that rate of formation of ATP diminishes (see Fig. 3.13). This acceleration in anaerobic utilization of glucose may be regarded as a vain effort on the part of the cells to obtain energy from the uneconomic process of anaerobic glycolysis. This stimulation of anaerobic glycolysis may depend on such factors as removal of normal feed-back inhibition of phosphofructokinase (see Fig. 3.13) when the concentration of ATP declines [90]. For a short time this acceleration of glycolysis may avert a catastrophic fall in level of ATP and thus provide temporary compensation, but, since the formation of ATP/mol glucose glycolysed to lactic acid is only about a twentieth of that formed per mol of glucose oxidised to CO_2, a fall in concentration of ATP is inevitable (Fig.

3.13). Indeed more than 80 per cent of ATP in mouse brain is lost 1 min after decapitation [85].

Another factor which may curtail exergonic reactions available to ischaemic neurones is possible local accumulation of K^+ ions. K^+ may be released from neurones by preceding hyperactivity or injury, and they may be liberated by lysis of extravasated red cells after haemorrhage (p. 104). But K^+ exerts a profound inhibitory effect (see Fig. 6.1, p. 195) on the anaerobic glycolysis of slices of cerebral cortex and the onset of this retardation of glycolysis by K^+ is extremely rapid [91, 92]. If this inhibition begins after disappearance of oxygen from ischaemic brain, then the neurones would be deprived of their one alternative source of energy capable of providing ATP to the depleted neurones.

Depletion of ATP may thus be a basic determinant of irreparable cellular damage produced by ischaemia. Such injury, as we have seen, is likely to develop with particular rapidity in brain owing to lack of intracellular substrates for anaerobic glycolysis and possible inhibition of anaerobic glycolysis by K^+. Another factor which may precipitate depletion of ATP in brain is the exceptionally high active surface area of cerebral neurones in relation to cell volume which may determine a uniquely high rate of *consumption of ATP* (see below).

Dependence of susceptibility to ischaemia on high neuronal surface/volume ratio

The remarkably elaborate axo-dendritic arborisations of cerebral neurones give them the highest surface/volume ratio of all cells.

The extreme susceptability of cerebral neurones to damage by ischaemia may depend on this high ratio of active surface to volume [93]. The vastly extensive neuronal surface still *consumes* ATP when its formation is arrested by ischaemia; in fact most of the cerebral content of ATP is lost within 1 min of onset of complete ischaemia. The depletion of ATP probably occurs most rapidly in cerebral neurones where there is this exceptionally expansive surface containing abundant membrane-bound ATPase (see below); here the number of sites which consume ATP is greatest in relation to the volume of cytoplasm and mitochondria capable of restoring the level of ATP by exergonic phosphorylation. Injury of membranes through lack of ATP is thus most likely to occur with greatest celerity where ATP is most rapidly consumed by these uniquely extensive surfaces; the membrane structure then breaks down and with it stored memory and learning are gone for ever.

Such dependence of extreme susceptibility to ischaemia of cerebral neurones on their high surface/volume ratio well correlates with:

1. The remarkable resistance of neonatal brain to ischaemia. Thus newborn animals and babies can, without harm, survive periods of ischaemia and anoxia which are lethal to adults [81, 94, 95]. But at birth the dendrites of many neurones in mammalian cerebral cortex are rudimentary consisting of a few short extensions from the cell body. Within a few weeks of birth, however, the primitive dendrites and axons undergo explosive multiplication into a vast and complex labyrinth of dendritic and axonal arborisations with a most extensive

membrane surface [96–98]. At this time there is an equally spectacular increase in vulnerability to ischaemia. Thus the onset of vulnerability coincides with rapid expansion of dendritic, axonal and synaptic surface. This same correlation between vulnerability to ischaemia and dendritic complexity probably also applies in man; although the dendrites of some human neurones are more advanced at birth than those of most animals, the pattern of human dendritic ramification like that of animals increases enormously in complexity during early postnatal life.

2. The lesser vulnerability of neurones in the lower parts of the brain where the axo-dendritic ramifications are less complex and their surface is less extensive.

3. The relative insusceptibility of myelinated nerve fibres where the active surface, which consumes ATP, is restricted to the nodes of Ranvier.

Thus ischaemic injury due to lack of ATP develops more rapidly in brain than in other tissues because ischaemic cerebral tissue has a maximum rate of consumption of ATP with a minimum rate of replacement.

Consequences of depletion of ATP: irreversible damage

ATP is an essential intraneuronal constituent; a continuous supply of it is necessary to:

1. Restore molecular conformation and ionic gradients in cell membranes after nervous activity; ATP is itself used in the process of expulsion of Na^+ and intake of K^+ across cell membranes and this effect is catalysed by Na^+/K^+–dependent ATPase [99–101].
2. Maintain structure of cell membranes.
3. Initiate synthesis of macromolecules.

When cells are severely depleted of ATP several changes are likely to ensue:

1. Na^+, Cl^-, and H_2O enter the cells which then swell. Entry of Cl^- and swelling of apical dendrites of cerebral pyramidal cells and cerebellar Purkinje cells can be detected within 5 min of interruption of blood supply [102, 103].

2. The cell membranes become more permeable and finally disintegrate. ATP is held combined to ATPase (an enzymic protein) in cell membranes. When ATP is destroyed through action of this enzyme and the enzyme becomes entirely freed from ligation to its substrate, re-orientation of membrane proteins or changes in their conformation may then occur. Possibly interligation of membrane ATPase with other proteins may then follow, as occurs in muscle between myosin and actin when myosin is freed from attachment to ATP. When this interligation becomes excessive, membrane structure may become irreparably disorganised as happens in myofibrils during the development of rigor mortis produced by profound depletion of ATP. Discontinuities then develop in cell membrane which eventually becomes fully permeable (p. 286).

3. Synthesis of macromolecules is retarded through lack of ATP and other

high energy phosphate compounds, but catabolism goes on unimpeded or is even accelerated by increased accessibility of enzymes to their substrates through membrane change.

As a result of (3) disintegration of RNA and DNA occur. Once one essential nucleotide sequence in DNA is lost, cell injury may become irreparable. Irreversible injury is probably also caused by membrane disintegration (2).

No-reflow phenomenon in brain

Temporary arrest of cerebral circulation can result in permanent closure of cerebral capillaries. This effect may also contribute to the special vulnerability of cerebral tissue to *temporary* vascular occlusion which would thus rapidly cause *permanent* local ischaemia even though flowing blood may re-enter the cerebral arteries [104]. If this phenomenon of no-flow develops most rapidly in brain, then cerebral cells would be most easily injured by temporary interruption of flowing blood.

This view is supported by the observation that, after interruption of cerebral blood supply in rabbits for 15 min, subsequent perfusion of fluid containing carbon fails to inject most of the perfused brain. Moreover, after this vascular closure, the foot processes of astrocytes enveloping the cerebral capillaries become swollen and apparently compress the lumina of thse vessels into mere slits; also blebs are formed on the internal surface of the capillary endothelium [105]. These changes were found in zones of no-reflow. Possibly the astrocytes, which like neurones have a large surface/volume ratio, are also specially prone to injury and swelling owing to rapid depletion of ATP.

Such no-flow, however, cannot be a general determinant of irreversible ischaemic injury. Thus, after temporary ischaemia of heart in dogs lasting for 40 min, the myocardial fibres are irreversibly damaged, although no changes in pattern of vascular flow are visible on reperfusion of blood [56]; longer periods of ischaemia can produce zones which fail to be reperfused. The no-reflow phenomenon also cannot account for the greater susceptibility to ischaemia of Purkinje cells of cerebeller cortex in comparison with adjacent Golgi cells [76], but disparity in surface/volume ratio of these two types of neurone would correlate with such a difference in vulnerability, since the more highly ramified Purkinje cells have the greater relative surface area.

Under some conditions, however, no-reflow may add to the injurious action of ischaemia on cerebral neurones, and thus summate with the effect of high surface/volume ratio in making these gigantic cells so uniquely vulnerable to lack of oxygen. Indeed progressive obstruction of microcirculation appears to be a usual sequel of even temporary closure of cerebral capillaries. Thus, when animals are made permanently comatose by exposure to cerebral ischaemia for 20 min (p. 302) and are then kept alive by respirator, intense cerebral oedema develops over a period of two days. This oedema involves swelling of astrocytes and complete obstruction of capillaries by compression from swollen astrocytes as well as by swelling of endothelial cells; the neuronal processes also swell initially but later disintegrate. Clearly by the time these changes are visible cerebral blood flow is very substantially obstructed. Similar cerebral oedema followed by neuronal autolysis develops in comatose human patients in whom cardiac action is maintained by ventilation with respirators after cerebral death. This condition has been called 'respirator brain' and is dicussed on p. 302.

This progressive cerebral oedema and vascular obstruction, which develop in these patients or in animals maintained on respirators after initial ischaemic damage, greatly extend the zone of injury. But these vascular changes do not explain the special susceptibility of brain nor do they account for metabolic lesions which develop in slices of cerebral cortex *in vitro* when exergonic metabolism is eliminated. Thus rapid and irreversible inhibition of anaerobic glycolysis follows anaerobic incubation in media which lack glucose [106] or which contain excess K^+ [91, 92]. Such lesions clearly arise independently of any capillary obstruction and are likely to be important factors in causing permanent depletion of ATP followed by irreparable damage in ischaemic brain, even when the circulation of blood is re-established after a period of arrest.

Cerebral damage by ischaemia: conclusion

The uniquely rapid onset of irreversible damage in ischaemic cerebral tissue may therefore primarily depend on high rate of depletion of ATP.

This loss of ATP is especially rapid for two reasons:

1. Anaerobic glycolysis is less able to compensate for loss of oxidative metabolism in ischaemic brain than in other tissues owing to lack of intracellular reserve of substrates for glycolysis, and also anaerobic glycolysis may be further inhibited by effect of excess of K^+ liberated from ischaemic neurones; thus the speed of replacement of ATP by anaerobic phosphorylation becomes minimal.
2. The rate of consumption of ATP is, on the other hand, exceptionally high in brain because of the high surface/volume ratio of cerebral neurones, in which membrane-bound ATPase utilizes ATP with maximum rapidity.

These factors combine to produce extremely rapid depletion of ATP, which is followed by irreparable disorganisation of cell membranes or other irreversible damage.

DEFECTIVE PENETRATION OF NUTRIMENTS INTO CELLS

Even though the exacting assortment of substances which the cell requires reaches its surface, one more hazard may deprive it of effective nutrition; sufficient nutriments may fail to enter the cell or penetrate compartments and oraganelles within it, so that the intracellular enzymes may not be supplied with sufficient substrates.

Such a defect in penetration of cell membranes by glucose is probably responsible for much of the harm produced by lack of insulin in diabetes mellitus. In the absence of insulin the entry of glucose and other hexoses into certain cells is severely restricted; insulin removes this restriction [107, 108].

The effect of insulin in promoting transport of hexoses out of the blood into the cellular compartment of the body was assessed by Levine *et al.* by measuring loss of galactose (a sugar which is not readily metabolised) from the blood of eviscerated nephrectomised dogs. In the absence of insulin the concentration of galactose fell to a constant level at which it remained; this level corresponded to penetration of galactose into only 45 per cent of the whole body. But injection of insulin was promptly followed by fall in concentration of galactose to a considerably lower level as the sugar penetrated the cellular compartment. It was concluded that insulin is needed to transport hexoses across cell membranes and that in its absence glucose accumulates in the blood.

More recent evidence [90, 109] indicated that insulin is necessary for the transport of glucose into cardiac and striated muscle fibres and lipocytes and that, without insulin, penetration of glucose into these cells is defective. Moreover excess of fatty acids can apparently suppress the normal action of insulin in transporting glucose into skeletal and cardiac muscle. Thus in diabetes both lack of insulin and excess of fatty acids in the blood may combine to diminish entry of glucose into cells.

In the absence of insulin some cells are thus deprived of glucose, even though their outer surfaces are bathed by excessively saccharine fluid, a striking example of need in the midst of plenty. Lack of insulin may thus impede the entry into cells of an essential component of their food and also subject the outer surfaces of cells to harmful hyperosmolarity (p. 436).

The supply of nutriments to the cells of the body can thus be retarded or obstructed at several stages in the chain of transport, supplementation and entry, which intervenes between the external environment and the interior of the cell. Such interruption is the commonest cause of lethal cellular injury in human disease.

God shield the stock! if heaven send no supplies,
The fairest blossom of the garden dies.
William Browne

REFERENCES

[1] BERG W. (1914) Über den mikroskopischen nachweis der eiweissspeicherung in der leber. *Biochem. Z.*, **61**, 428.

[2] BRACHET J. (1940) La détection histochemique des acides pentosenucléiques. *C. R. Soc. Biol. (Paris)*, **133**, 88.

[3] DAVIDSON J. N. (1947) Some factors influencing the nucleic acid content of cells and tissues. *Cold Spr. Harb. Symp. quant. Biol.*, **12**, 50.

[4] BERG W. (1926) Zum histologischen nachweis der eiweissspeicherung in der leber. *Pflügers Arch. ges. Physiol.*, **214**, 243.

[5] SVOBODA D. & HIGGINSON U. (1964) Ultrastructural changes produced by protein and related deficiencies in the rat liver. *Amer. J. Path.*, **45**, 353.
[6] Passmore R. & DRAPER M. H. (1970) Nutritional disorders. In *Biochemical Disorders in Human Disease*, p. 22, edited by R. H. S. Thompson & I. D. P. Wooton. Churchill, London.
[7] GARNET E. S., BARNARD D. L., FORD J., GOODBODY R. A. & WOODEHOUSE M. A. (1969) Gross fragmentation of cardiac myofibrils after therapeutic starvation for obestiy. *Lancet*, **1**, 914.
[8] WATERLOW J. C. & WEISZ J. (1956) The fat, protein and nucleic acid content of the liver in malnourished human infants. *J. clin. Invest.*, **35**, 346.
[9] GARROW J. S., FLETCHER K. & HALLIDAY D. (1965) Body composition in severe infantile malnutrition. *J. clin. Invest.*, **44**, 417.
[10] HARRIS L. J. (1970) The discovery of vitamins. In *The Chemistry of Life*, p. 156, ed. by J. Needham. Cambridge University Press.
[11] FELL H. B. & MELLANBY E. (1953) Metaplasia produced in cultures of chick ectoderm by high vitamin A. *J. Physiol.* (*Lond.*) **119**, 470.
[12] WILLS M. R. (1973) Intestinal absorption of calcium. *Lancet*, **1**, 820.
[13] EINARSON L. (1953) Deposits of fluorescent acid-fast products in the nervous system and skeletal muscles of adult rats with chronic vitamin E deficiency. *J. Neurol. Neurosurg. & Psychiat.*, **16**, 98.
[14] EINARSON L. (1962) Cellular structure in the central nervous system of vitamin E-deficient monkeys. In *Aging Round the World*, Vol. 3, p. 131, ed. by N. W. Shock. Columbia University Press, New York.
[15] DE WARDENER H. E. & LENNOX B. (1947) Cerebral beri-beri cured by thiamine. *Lancet*, **1**, 11.
[16] PLATT B. S. & LU G. D. (1939) The accumulation of pyruvic acid and other carbonyl compounds in beri-beri and the effect of vitamin B_1. *Biochem. J.*, **33**, 1525.
[17] PETERS R. A. (1963) *Biochemical Lesions and Lethal Synthesis*. Pergamon Press, Oxford.
[18] THOMPSON R. H. S. & Johnson R. E. (1935) Blood pyruvate in vitamin B_1 deficiency. *Biochem. J.*, **29**, 694.
[19] LIPMANN F. (1937) Über den umsatz der brenztraubensaure und den mechanismus der vitamin B_1-wirkung. *Scand. Arch. Physiol.*, **76**, 255.
[20] WILSON J. & THOMPSON R. H. S. (1972) Metabolic aspects of some diseases of peripheral nerves. In *Biochemical Aspect of Nervous Diseases*, p. 1, ed. by J. N. Cumings. Plenum Press, London.
[21] REED L. J. (1953) Metabolic functions of thiamine and lipoic acid. *Physiol. Rev.*, **33**, 544.
[22] DAVIES M. J. & JENNINGS R. B. (1970) The ultrastructure of myocardium in the thiamine deficient rat. *J. Path.*, **102**, 87.
[23] DAVIDSON J. N. (1972) *The Biochemistry of the Nucleic Acids*, 7th Ed. Chapman and Hall, London.
[24] LEVENE C. I. & BATES C. J. (1973) Ascorbic acid and collagen synthesis. In *Biology of the Fibroblast*, p. 397, ed. by E. Kulonen & J. Pikkarainan. Academic Press, New York.
[25] WHITTINGHAM S., UNGAR B. MACKAY I. R. & MATHEWS J. D. (1969) The genetic factor in pernicious anaemia: a family study of patients with gastritis. *Lancet*, **1**, 951.
[26] MENZIES R. C., CROSSEN P. E., FITZGERALD P. H. & GUNZ F. W. (1966) Cytogenetic and cytochemical studies on marrow cells in B_{12} and folate deficiency. *Blood*, **28**, 581.
[27] MEYER A. (1963) *Greenfield's Neuropathology*, 2nd Ed., p. 235 and 288. Arnold, London.
[28] BOOTH C. C. (1970) Enterocytes in coeliac disease. *Brit. Med. J.*, **3**, 725; **4**, 14.
[29] WHARTON B. A. (1974) Coeliac disease in childhood. *Brit. J. Hosp. Med.*, **12**, 452.

[30] BROWNING T. H. & TRIER J. S. (1969) Organ culture of mucosal biopsies of human small intestine. *J. clin. Invest.*, **48**, 1423.
[31] TOWNLEY R. R. W., BHAFTHUL P. S., CORNELL H. J. & MIRCHELL J. D. (1973) Toxicity of wheat gliadin fractions in coeliac disease. *Lancet*, **1**, 1363.
[32] FALCHUK Z. M., GEBHARD R. L., SESSOMS C. & STROBER W. (1974) An *in vitro* model of gluten-sensitive enteropathy. *J. clin. Invest.*, **53**, 487.
[33] KELNAR C. J. H. & HARVEY D. (1977) Respiratory distress syndrome. *Brit. J. Hosp. Med.*, **18**, 232.
[34] AVERY M. E., WANG N. & TAEUSEH H. W. (1973) The lung of the newborn infant. *Scientific American,* **228**, 75.
[35] GEPTS W. (1965) Pathologic anatomy of the pancreas in juvenile diabetes. *Diabetes*, **14**, 618.
[36] BOURNE J. G. (1957) Fainting and cerebral damage. *Lancet*, **2**, 499.
[37] DENNY-BROWN D. & MEYER J. S. (1957) Production of cerebral infarction by ischaemic anoxia and its reversibility in early stages. *Neurology*, **7**, 567.
[38] DENNY-BROWN D. (1960) Recurrent cerebrovascular episodes. *Arch. Neurol.*, **2**, 194.
[39] LEVINE S. (1960) Anoxic-ischaemic encephalopathy in rats. *Amer. J. Path.*, **36**, 1.
[40] PAYLING-WRIGHT G. (1958) *An Introduction to Pathology*. Longmans, London.
[41] DIXON K. C. (1970) Hydrophobic lipids in injured cells. *Histochem. J.*, **2**, 157.
[42] BROWN-SÉQUARD C. E. (1858) Recherches expérimentales sur les propriétés physiologiques et les usages du sang rouge et du sang noir et de leurs principaux éléments gazeux, l'oxygène et l'acide carbonique. *J. Physiol. de l'homme et des animaux*, **1**, 95, 353, 729.
[43] MEDAWAR P. B. (1954) The storage of living skin. *Proc. roy. Soc. Med.*, **47**, 62.
[44] BASSI M. & BERNELLI-ZAZZERA A. (1964) Ultrastructural cytoplasmic changes of liver cells after reversible and irreversible ischemia. *Exp. molec. Path.*, **3**, 332.
[45] RAGNOTTI G., CAJONE F. & BERNELLI-ZAZZERA A. (1970) Structural and functional changes in polysomes from ischemic livers. *Exp. molec. Path.*, **13**, 295.
[46] CAJONE F., RAGNOTTI G., BERNELLI-ZAZZERA A. & BASSI M. (1971) State and function of liver polysomes during recovery from ischemia. *Exp. molec. Path.*, **14**, 392.
[47] BERNELLI-Zazzera A.(1975) Ribosomes in dying liver cells. In *Pathogenesis and Mechanisms of Liver Cell Necrosis*, p. 103, ed. by D. Keppler. University Park Press, Baltimore.
[48] TROWELL O. A. (1946) The experimental production of watery vacuolation of the liver. *J. Physiol.*, (Lond.) **3**, 268.
[49] WOODS H. F. W. & KREBS H. A. (1971) Lactate production in the perfused rat liver. *Biochem.* J., **125**, 129.
[50] BYWATERS E. G. L. (1945) Ischaemic muscle necrosis ('crush syndrome'). *Brit. med. Bull.*, **3**, 107.
[51] HUXLEY H. E. & BROWN W. (1967) The low angle X-ray diagram of vertebrate striated muscle and its behaviour during contraction and rigor. *J. molec. Biol.*, **30**, 383.
[52] BENDALL J. R. (1973) Post mortem changes in muscle. In *The Structure and Function of muscle*, Vol. 2, p.243, 2nd Ed., ed. by G. H. Bourne. Academic Press, New York.
[53] CAULFIELD J. & KLIONSKY B. (1959) Myocardial ischaemia and early infarction: an EM study. *Amer. J. Path.*, **35**, 489.
[54] WHALEN D. A., HAMILTON D. G., GANOTE C. E. & JENNINGS R. B. (1974) Effect of a transient period of ischemia on myocardial cells. 1. Effect on cell volume regulation. *Amer. J. Path.*, **74**, 381.
[55] KLONER R. A., GANOTE C. E., WHALEN D. A. & JENNINGS R. B. (1974) Effect of a transient period of ischemia on myocardial cells. 2. Fine structure during the first few minutes of reflow. *Amer. J. Path.*, **74**, 399.

[56] KLONER R. A., GANOTE C. E. & JENNINGS R. B. (1974) The 'no-reflow' phenomenon after temporary coronary occlusion in the dog. *J. clin. Invest.*, **54**, 1496.
[57] DENNY-BROWN D. & BRENNER C. (1944) Paralysis of nerve induced by direct pressure and by tourniquet. *Arch. Neurol. Psychiat.* (*Chic.*), **51**, 1.
[58] LITTEN M. (1880) Untersuchungen über den haemorrhagischen infarct und über einwirkung arterieller anaemie auf das lebende gewebe. *Z. klin. Med.*, **1**, 131.
[59] EHRLICH P. & BRIEGER L. (1884) Über die ausschaltung des lendenmarkgrau. *Z. klin. Med.*, **7**, Supplement, 155.
[60] MARINESCO G. (1896) Lésions de la moelle epinière consécutives à la ligature de l'aorte abdominale. *C. R. Soc. Biol.* (*Paris*), **3**, 250.
[61] MARINESCO G. (1909) *La Cellule Nerveuse*, Vol. 1 & 2. Doin, Paris.
[62] TUREEN L. L. (1936) Effect of experimental temporary vascular occlusion on the spinal cord. 1. Correlation between structural and functional change. *Arch. Neurol. Psychiat.* (*Chic.*), **35**, 789.
[63] KROGH E. (1945) Effect of acute anoxia on the large motor cells in the spinal cord. *Acta Jutlandica* aarsskrift for Aarhus Univ, suppl **17**.
[64] WEBSTER H. DE F. & AMES A. (1965) Reversible and irreversible changes in the fine structure of nervous tissue during oxygen and glucose deprivation. *J. Cell Biol.*, **26**, 885.
[65] STOKES W. (1854) *The Diseases of the Heart and the Aorta*. Hodges and Smith, Dublin.
[66] ROSSEN R., KABAT H. & ANDERSON J. P. (1943) Acute arrest of the cerebral circulation in man. *Arch. Neurol. Psychiat.* (*Chic.*), **50**, 510.
[67] KABAT H., DENNIS C. & BAKER A. B. (1941) Recovery of function following arrest of the brain circulation. *Amer. J. Physiol.*, **132**, 737.
[68] MEYER J. S., FANG H. C. & DENNY-BROWN D. (1954) Polarographic study of cerebral collateral circulation. *Arch. Neurol. Psychiat.* (*Chic.*), **72**, 296.
[69] GRENELL R. G., DAVIES P. W. & BRONK D. W. (1948) Effects of brain anaemia on cortical oxygen consumption *in vivo*. *Fed. Proc.*, **7**, 44.
[70] WEINBERGER L., GIBBON M. H. & GIBBON J. H. (1940) Temporary arrest of circulation to the central nervous system: physiological effects. *Arch. Neurol. Psychiat.* (*Chic.*),**43**, 615 & 961.
[71] TUREEN L. L. (1938) Effects of experimental temporary vascular occlusion on the spinal cord. 2 Changes in mineral salt content of cells. *Arch. Neurol. Psychiat.* (*Chic.*), **39**, 453.
[72] KROGH E. (1950) The effect of acute hypoxia on the motor cells of the spinal cord. *Acta. physiol. scand.*, **20**, 263.
[73] BROCK R. (1956) Hypothermia and open cardiotomy. *Proc. roy. Soc. Med.*, **49**, 347.
[74] MEYER A. (1956) Neuropathological aspects of anoxia. *Proc. roy. Soc. Med.*, **49**, 619.
[75] SUDA I., KITO K. & ADACHI C. (1966) Viability of long term cat brain *in vitro*. *Nature*, **212**, 268.
[76] SCHOLZ W. (1953) Selective neuronal necrosis and its topistic patterns in hypoxia and oligaemia. *J. Neuropath. exp. Neurol.*, **12**, 249.
[77] KABAT H. & SCHADEWALD M. (1941) The relative susceptibility of the synaptic terminals and of the perikaryon to arrest of the circulation of the brain. *Amer. J. Path.*, **17**, 833.
[78] EHRLICH P. (1885) The requirement of the organism for oxygen. In *Collected Papers of Paul Ehrlich*, Vol. 1, p. 433, ed. by F. Himmelweit (1956). Pergamon, London.
[79] MARINESCO G. (1919) Recherches histologiques sur les oxidases. *C. R. Soc. Biol.* (Paris), **82**, 98.
[80] MANN F. C. & MAGATH T. B. (1921) Studies in the physiology of the liver. II The liver as a regulator of the glucose concentration of the blood. *Amer. J. Physiol.*, **55**, 285.

[81] HIMWICH H. E. (1951) *Brain Metabolism and its Disorders*, pp. 10, 13, 125. Williams & Wilkins, Baltimore.

[82] WARBURG O., POSENER K. & NEGELEIN E. (1924) Über den stoffwechsel der carcinomzelle. *Biochem. Z.*, **152**, 309.

[83] DIXON K. C. (1935) The oxidative disappearance of lactic acid from brain and the Pasteur reaction. *Biochem. J.*, **29**, 973.

[84] DIXON K. C. (1965) Ischaemia and the neurone. In *Neurohistochemistry*, p. 558, ed. by C. W. M. Adams. Elsevier, Amsterdam.

[85] LOWRY O. H., PASSONNEAU J. U., HASSELBURGER F. X. & SCHULZ D. W. (1964) Effect of ischaemia on known substrates in the glycolytic pathway in brain. *J. biol. Chem.*, **239**, 18.

[86] KETY S. S. (1950) Circulation and metabolism of the human brain in health and disease. *Amer. J. med.*, **8**, 205.

[87] DIXON K. C. (1937) The carbohydrate metabolism of the cerebral cortex. *Irish J. med. Sci.*, May.

[88] TITRUD L. A. & HAYMAKER W. (1947) Cerebral anoxia from high altitude asphyxiation. *Arch. Neurol. Psychiat. (Chic.)*, **57**, 397.

[89] LAWRENCE R. D., MEYER A. & NEVIN S. (1942) The pathological changes in the brain in fatal hypoglycaemia. *Quart. J. Med.*, **11**, 181.

[90] NEWSHOLME E. A. & START C. (1973) *Regulation in Metabolism.* Wiley, London.

[91] ASHFORD C. A. & DIXON K. C. (1935) The Effect of potassium on the glycolysis of brain tissue with reference to the Pasteur effect. *Biochem. J.*, **29**, 157.

[92] DIXON K. C. (1949) Action of potassium ions on brain metabolism. *J. Physiol.*, **110**, 87.

[93] DIXON K. C. (1967) Cerebral vulnerability to ischaemia. *Lancet*, **2**, 289.

[94] KABAT H. (1940) The greater resistance of very young animals to arrest of the brain circulation. *Amer. J. Physiol.*, **130**, 588.

[95] TIZARD B. M. (1980) Cerebral palsies. The Croonian lecture 1978. *J. roy. Coll. Phycns. Lond.*, **14**, 72.

[96] SCHADÉ J. P. & BAXTER C. F. (1960) Changes during growth in volume and surface area of cortical neurones in the rabbit. *Exp. Neurol.*, **2**, 158.

[97]SCHADÉ J. P. & FORD D. H. (1965) *Basic Neurology*, p. 130, 1st Ed. Elsevier, Amserdam.

[98] SCHADÉ J. P. & FORD D. H. (1973) *Basic Neurology*, p. 28, 2nd Ed. Elsevier, Amsterdam.

[99] GLYNN I. M. (1962) Activation of ATPase activity in a cell membrane by external K and internal Na. *J. Physiol.*, **160**, 18P.

[100] WHITTAM R. (1962) The asymmetrical stimulation of membrane ATPase in relation to active kation transport. *Biochem J.*, **84**, 110.

[101] OPIT L. J. & CHARNOCK J. S. (1965) A molecular model for a sodium pump. *Nature*, **208**, 471.

[102] VAN HARREVELD A. & SCHADÉ J. P. (1959) Chloride movements in cerebral cortex after circulatory arrest and during spreading depression. *J. cell. comp. Physiol.*, **54**, 65.

[103] VAN HARREVELD A. (1961) Asphyxial changes in cerebellar cortex. *J. cell comp. Physiol.*, **57**, 101.

[104] AMES A., WRIGHT R. L., KOWADA M., THURSTON J. M. & MAJNO G. (1968) Cerebral ischaemia. II The no-reflow phenomenon. *Amer. J. Path.*, **52**, 437.

[105] CHIANG J., KOWADA M., Ames A., WRIGHT R. L. & MAJNO G. (1968) Cerebral ischaemia. III Vascular changes. *Amer. J. Path.*, **52**, 455.

[106] DICKENS F. & GREVILLE G. D. (1933) The metabolism of normal and tumour tissue: the effects of lactate, pyruvate and deprivation of substrate. *Biochem. J.*, **27**, 1134.

[107] KNOWLTON F. P. & STARLING E. H. (1912) Experiments on the consumption of sugar in the normal and diabetic heart. *J. Physiol.*, **45**, 146.

[108] Levine R., Goldstein M. S., Huddleston B. & Klein S. P. (1950) Action of insulin on the 'permeability' of cells to free hexoses, studied by its effect on the distribution of galactose. *Amer. J. Physiol.*, **163**, 70.

[109] Randle P. J., Garland P. B., Hales C. N. & Newsholme E. A. (1963) The glucose fatty acid cycle: its role in insulin sensitivity and the metabolic disturbances of diabetes mellitus. *Lancet*, **1**, 785.

CHAPTER 4

Injurious Physical Conditions

So as to illustrate pathogenic cellular defects caused by injurious physical conditions, damage initiated by trauma, heat, cold and radiation will be considered.

TRAUMA

Physical violence more often separates cells from each other than it tears individual cells asunder. Rupture of blood vessels with consequent haemorrhage is therefore the commonest lesion produced by external trauma or by increase in blood pressure *within* the vessels.

Contusion

When trauma dissevers small vessels, blood leaks out into the tissues between the separated endothelial cells of the vessel walls. In loose connective tissue such contusion or bruising, although visibly spectacular, generally produces little damage to the surrounding cells. The extravasated red cells, however, are ingested by macrophages and then lysed within them, where the iron of the contained haemoglobin is converted to brown granules of haemosiderin (a ferric protein complex). This pigment together with tetrapyrrole derivatives of disintegrating haematin account for the kaleidoscopic colour changes visible in bruised tissues.

Cell damage from haemorrhage

When rupture of blood vessels occurs in a confined space, such as within the cranial cavity, the extravasated blood can only cause minimal swelling and so produces substantial rise in pressure which may compress capillaries, and injure the cells by resultant ischaemia or by direct pressure on neuronal processes. This hamorrhage may be extradural, subdural or intracerebral.

Extradural haemorrhage, caused by traumatic rupture of the middle meningeal artery (often following cranial fracture), produces rapid rise in intracranial pressure as extravasated blood spreads in a progressively increasing arc over the surface of a cerebral hemisphere; this results in cerebral ischaemia and rapidly deepening coma.

Subdural haemorrhage, generally caused by trauamatic injury to the walls of venous sinuses, also induces cerebral ischaemia, but with a much more insidious onset.

Intracerebral haemorrhage is a consequence of hypertensive arterial disease. Such haemorrhage is often massive and rapidly lethal, and appears to extend by confluence of small haemorrhages which are commonly present around the principal lesion. Extravasation of red cells probably depends on a combination of hypertension with degenerative loss of smooth muscle, which is usually scanty in cerebral arterioles [1]. Hypertension may also incite arteriolar spasm which can induce ischaemia followed by further vascular injury. Another probable factor in the origin of cerebral haemorrhage is the presence of microaneurysms in the cerebral arterioles of older patients with hypertension [2]. Initial small haemorrhages may at first be formed as dissecting aneurysmal lesions between separated laminae of degenerate arteriolar walls (Fig. 4.1). Finally the extravasated red cells penetrate into the surrounding tissue (Fig. 4.2) and produce further rise in hydrostatic pressure within the confined space of the cranial cavity. This may cause collapse of cerebral capillaries and venules with resultant ischaemic injury to cerebral neurones. This effect may be magnified by

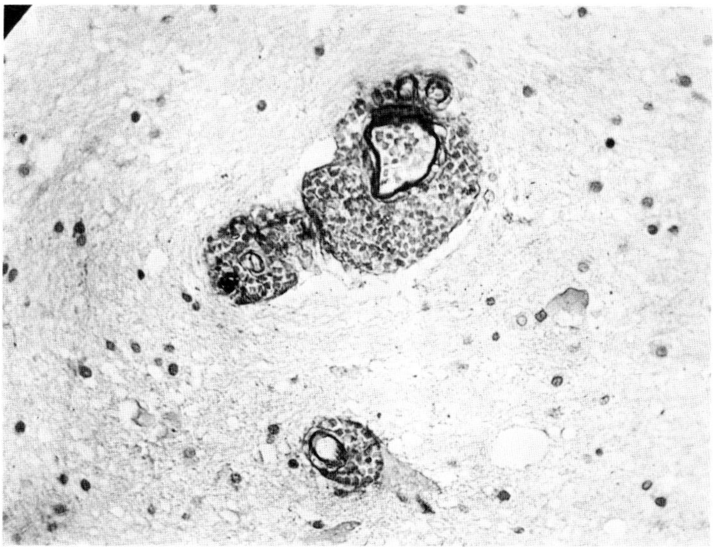

FIG. 4.1 Small haemorrhages around arterioles in cerebral white matter in the vicinity of a massive cerebral haemorrhage. The arterioles are surrounded by extravasated red cells still enclosed by outermost lamina of degenerate vessel wall. From a hypertensive woman of 49 who died following massive haemorrhage into left occipital cortex and adjacent white matter, producing right hemiplegia (BP 300+/170; heart weight 480 g). PAS. ×260.

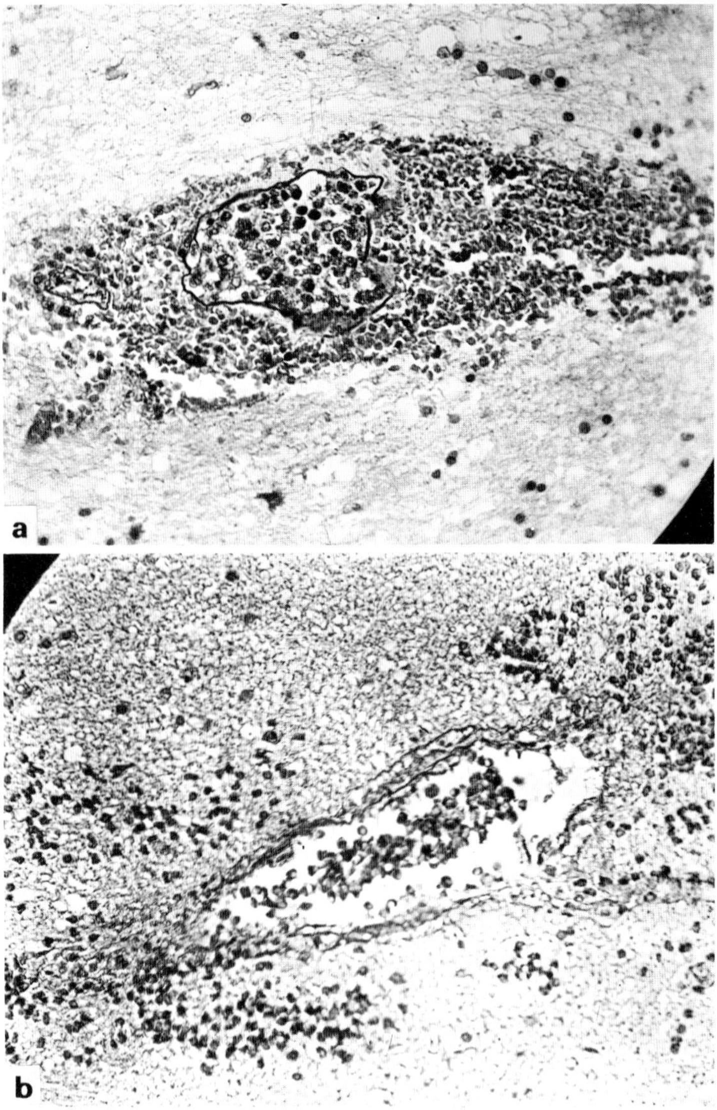

FIG. 4.2 Extension of haemorrhage from arteriole in cerebral white matter (from the same specimen as Fig. 4.1). Red cells have escaped from degenerate small vessels and are penetrating surrounding tissue. ×260.

a. PAS.

b. Coupled tetrazonium method for protein which stains the red cells darkly.

action of K^+ liberated from hypoxic red cells, since K^+ can deprive anoxic neurones of their principal source of energy (see Fig. 6.1, p. 195).

Increase in perineuronal hydrostatic pressure caused by cerebral haemorrhage may also compress neuronal processes sufficiently to interrupt transit of nerve

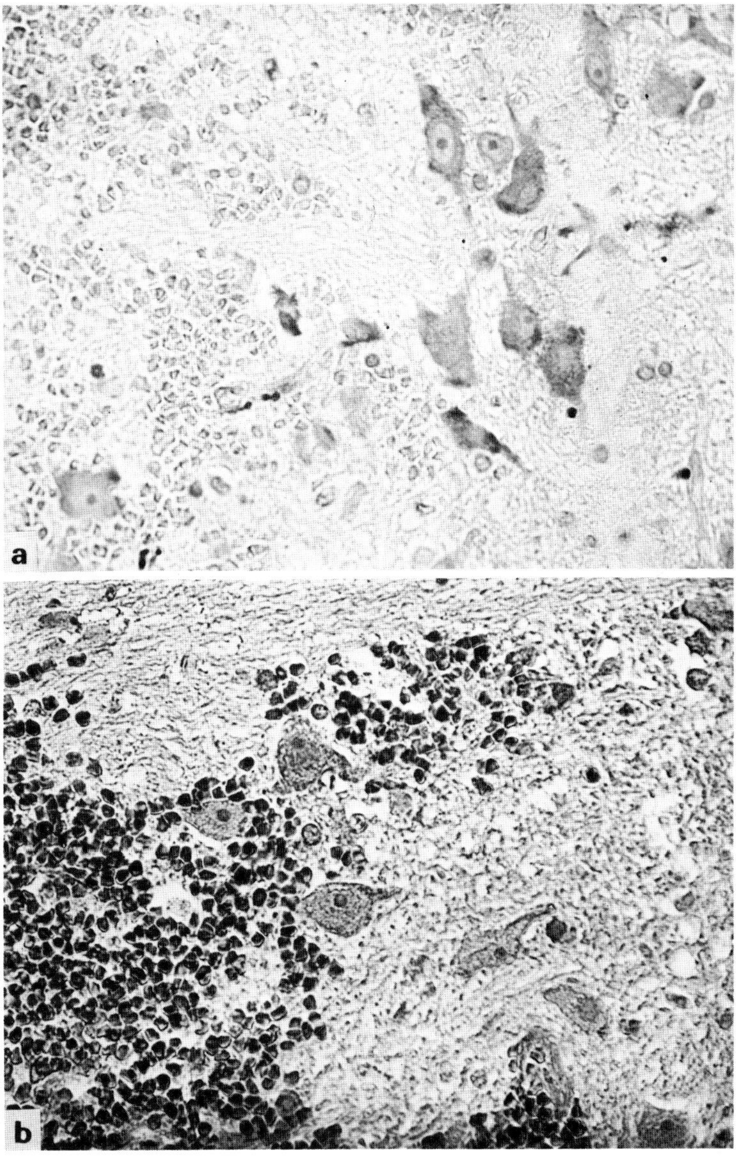

FIG. 4.3 Haemorrhage into pons of a hypertensive man of 46 who collapsed in coma and died six hours later (BP 270/160; heart weight 435 g). Massive pontine haemorrhage with rupture into fourth ventricle. Pontine neurones compressed by extravasated blood. ×260.

a. Pyronin G; Nissl substance visible in cytoplasm.

b. Coupled tetrazonium method for protein; neuronal nucleoli and red cells intensely coloured.

impulses and so become an additional determinant of coma. Such perineuronal extravasation of red cells is illustrated in Fig. 4.3 (p. 105); this shows red cells enveloping neuronal cell bodies in the pons of a hypertensive man of 46, who suddenly collapsed in coma and died in six hours with massive pontine haemorrhage.

Severe and sudden haemorrhage from major blood vessels in any part of the body, or from the heart itself can result in generalised ischaemia which also terminates in coma and irreversible cerebral injury. Rapid deceleration, as in motor accidents or falls from a height, may cause death in this way by *rupture of the aorta* distal to the opening of the left subclavian artery; at this point the attachment of the ligamentum arteriosum may act as a hinge which puts sudden strain on the aortic wall [3]. Usually the lesions consist of transverse slit-like tears in the intima and media with internal haemorrhage into the vessel wall.

Traumatic compression

External pressure on the limbs of patients trapped in accidents chiefly injures by causing ischaemic necrosis of striated muscle (p. 80). However tight clamping of individual nerves gives rise to direct traumatic injury similar to that produced by axonal section. Haemorrhage may also cause neuronal injury by compression.

Laceration and rupture of cells

The cell envelope may be directly disrupted by violence. This happens conspicuously in cells which are bloated by fat and which then consist of liquid globules of lipid covered by tenuous films of cytoplasm. Swelling with water can also rend the surface membrane of the cell.

Laceration of fatty cells: fat embolism

The large lipocytes of bone-marrow are easily ruptured by fractures of bones. When bony spicules perforate both the cell membranes of the lipocytes and the walls of capillaries and venules, droplets of liquid fat are ejected from the lacerated cells and may enter the blood. These fat emboli later occlude capillaries in lungs, skin and brain, sometimes with disastrous consequences.

Fat emboli are always detectable in *pulmonary* capillaries of patients who die soon after severe fractures (Fig. 4.4). Usually these pulmonary emboli do not give rise to clinical symptoms which are mainly determined by systemic fat embolism.

Systemic fat embolism, however, occurs in a small proportion of patients after fractures. This may be fulminating with rapid onset of coma followed by death. Otherwise, there is a *symptom-free period* of 12–36 hours [4] followed by the appearance of a petechial rash on the skin (typically on chest and neck) and the development of confusion terminating in coma; in this event multiple fat emboli are found *post mortem* in the cerebral capillaries of both cortex and white matter and numerous petechial haemorrhages are usually visible in the cerebral white matter (Fig. 4.5). However these petechial haemorrhages may be absent in patients who die rapidly with numerous fat emboli occluding the capillaries. The petechial haemorrhages probably are formed as a result of ischaemic

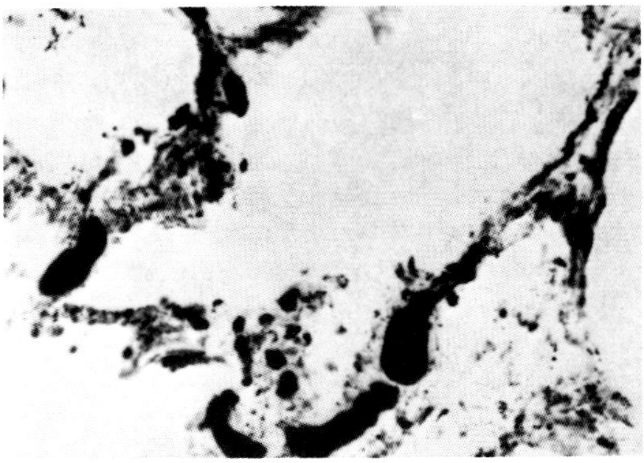

FIG. 4.4 Fat emboli (black) in alveolar capillaries of lung. Frozen section: oil red O. Courtesy of Dr S. Sevitt. *Brit. J. Hosp. Med.* 1973, **9**, 784.

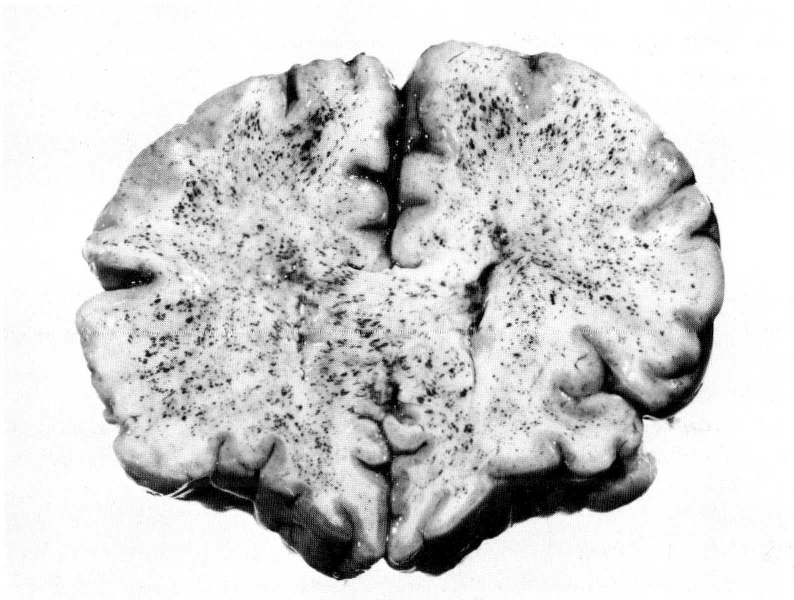

FIG. 4.5 Petechial haemorrhages in cerebral white matter resulting from fat embolism. Coronal view of intensely swollen brain of a man who died 11 days after fractures of femur, tibia and fibula following a blow from a motor vehicle. Fat emboli occluded vessels of cerebral white matter causing ischaemic damage to the vessel walls and focal extravasation of red cells. Courtesy of Professor G. A. Gresham.

necrosis of tissue caused by the fat emboli, followed later by extravasation of red cells through the necrotic capillary walls.

Sevitt [5] suggested that the development of *systemic* fat emboli may result from the opening of precapillary anastomoses between pulmonary arteries and veins in addition to increase in passage of liquid globules of fat through the alveolar capillaries; thus the systemic circulation, including the cerebral and dermal capillaries, is deluged with globules of liquid fat.

Rupture of swollen fatty cells: hepatic cirrhosis

As a result of chronic malnutrition or prolonged alcoholism liver cells may become bloated by excessive quantities of liquid fat. Eventually these swollen hepatic cells burst and collapse. In this way lobules of the liver become replaced by contracted fibrous bands containing remnants of the hepatic cells and compressed vascular sinusoids (p. 374). This condition, which is called *hepatic cirrhosis*, causes serious obstruction of portal circulation and may produce hepatic failure. Cirrhosis of the liver is discussed along with fatty change in Chapter 8.

Rending of cells swollen by water

Swelling of cells by excessive entry of water accounts for rupture of red cells in drowning by fresh-water (p. 194) and also for the ultimate rending of cell membranes following aqueous swelling initiated by action of antibody and complement (p. 291). Indeed many forms of cell lysis depend on rupture by excessive intracellular pressure.

Dissevered neurones

Owing to the great length and tenuity of their processes neurones are some of the few cells which are commonly severed by violence. Transection of nerve fibres or their axons is followed by spectacular changes both distal and proximal to the plane of division.

Changes distal to the plane of injury

The entire length of the nerve fibre which is dissevered from the cell body of the neurone ultimately disintegrates. This process, which is called Wallerian degeneration, involves both axon and myelin sheath and it occurs both in divided peripheral nerves and in severed tracts in the central nervous system. The first clear description of this process was given by Waller in 1850 [6]. In his earliest experiments he cut either the glossopharyngeal or the hypoglossal nerve of frogs on one side and later compared the distal ramifications of the severed trunk in one side of the tongue with filaments of the undamaged contralateral nerves. He discovered that, when continuity with the neuronal cell body becomes interrupted, the severed axon and its myelin sheath below the point of section degenerate. He found that the myelin in the severed distal portion of the divided nerve becomes turbid and 'curdles' into separate ovoid globules some of which show a double contour within 5–6 days (Fig. 4.6a) and are transformed into fine droplets or granules (Fig. 4.6b) in a further two weeks. He also

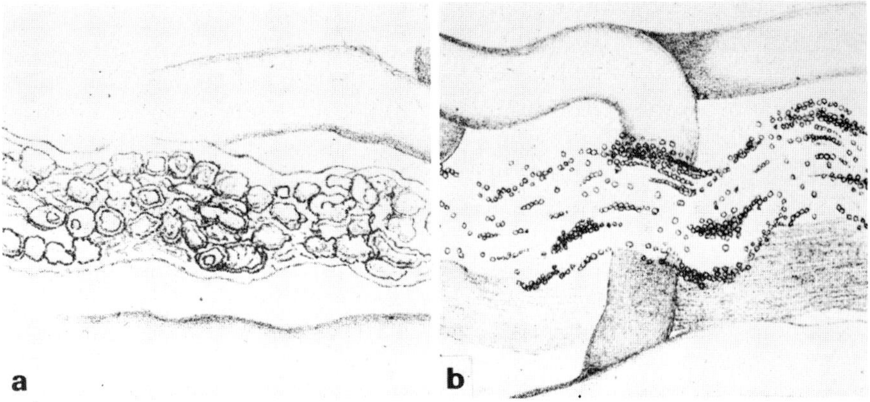

FIG. 4.6 Wallerian degeneration. Illustration by Waller [6] of papillary nerves in frog's tongue following section of glossopharyngeal nerve.
a. 6 days after section: myelin has disintegrated into ovoid globules many of which show a double contour.
b. 22 days after section: myelin has distintegrated into rows of amorphous granules (hydrophobic lipid, p. 397).

discovered similar degeneration in the myelinated fibres of spinal nerves when dissevered from their cell bodies in the spinal cord or posterior root ganglia as well as in the tracts of the spinal cord itself when the myelinated fibres are dissevered from their cell bodies. He thus established that the cell body is the *nutritive centre* of the whole neurone and that axons and their myelin sheaths are dependent on passage of essential nutriments from their cell bodies [6].

This remarkable sequence of events both in myelin sheaths and axons severed from continuity with the neuronal cell body is one of the most dramatic episodes in cell injury and has continued to challenge investigation ever since Waller's time. Knowledge of Wallerian degeneration was greatly extended by Ramon y Cajal [7]; his work as well as more recent observations differentiated changes (a) in the myelin sheath, and (b) in the axon below the point of section of myelinated fibres.

Changes in the myelin sheath. Sixteen hours after section of mammalian peripheral nerves the myelin sheath (as seen in preparation fixed and stained by OsO_4) retracts from the nodes of Ranvier and becomes fragmented into tubules through which extend the still unfragmented axons [7]. Two to three days later these tubules of myelin contract further into ellipsoidal globules (see Fig. 8.29, p. 395) which enclose degenerating fragments of the axons [7, 8]. These elongated globules (called 'ellipsoids' by Ramon y Cajal) possess a central space covered by a double contoured envelope of myelin. EM observations on severed peripheral nerves show that, within one day after section, the contiguous lamellae of the myelin sheath become loosened and appear less mutually adhesive than in normal myelin [9].

More recently Williams & Hall [10], using immersed microscope objectives and oblique incident illumination, examined normal and degenerating myelinated fibres in peripheral nerves of anaesthetised mice *in vivo*. Within 2 min of crushing a nerve the myelin in fibres (distal to the injury) retracted from the nodes of Ranvier and the Schmidt-Lantermann incisurae became widened over a distance of 5 mm from the site of crush; these changes rapidly extended down the nerve and involved all its fibres within a distance 2–4 cm during the next 36 h.

These extremely rapid alterations in the myelin of fibres, distal to the site of trauma, suggest that a self-propagating wave of change affects the conformation of the membrane lipids and extends down the myelin sheath from the point of injury to cause progressive retraction of myelin lamellae. Such a change at molecular level may be a natural consequence of trauma to *single* cell membranes, in which the effect is submicroscopic; but in myelin, which is composed of cell membranes stacked *en masse*, this change or its physical effects are probably magnified sufficiently to become visible by LM with this technique of olbique illumination. Thus a visible alteration in myelin may reflect a molecular change in its individual membranes.

The ellipsoids formed from the retracted tubules of degenerating myelin are finally converted into fine granules after ingestion by phagocytes. The cytochemical nature of these subsequent changes is considered in Chapter 8.

Changes in the severed axon. These changes are clearly revealed by impregnation with $AgNO_3$ and subsequent reduction to metallic silver, a procedure which differentiates the axon and its remnants from enveloping myelin [7]. The axon below the point of section of peripheral nerves becomes varicose or moniliform within 48 h and then disintegrates into granules which finally disappear. Close to the point of section, however, axonal degeneration occurs more rapidly. In the central nervous system axoplasm retracts from this rapidly necrotising zone and contracts into club shaped processes or 'balls' attached at first to the distal degenerating fibre; a similar acute process occurs in the severed stump proximal to the site of injury (p. 112).

The slower degeneration of the axon throughout the length of the severed fibre may be a consequence of interruption in the *flow* of axoplasm. This flow was revealed by the work of Weiss & Hiscoe [11]; they constricted axons *in vivo* and found that axoplasm is dammed up above the constriction to produce axonal swelling. Moreover the flowing axoplasm, which is fabricated in the cell body, is rich in protein and appears to be essential in supplying nutriments for peripheral neuronal metabolism. Interruption of axonal flow may thus deprive the distal portion of the fibre beyond the constriction of necessary replenishments and thus determine axonal degeneration far from the initial site of injury. This arrest of supply of protein may also contribute to irreversible degeneration of the myelin membranes.

Changes proximal to the plane of injury

Above the point of section of a myelinated peripheral nerve fibre degeneration of both myelin sheath and axon only extends a very short distance towards the cell body and is usually arrested at the first node of Ranvier or even more closely to the site of injury [7]. But the cell body of the severed fibre, far removed from the zone of trauma, begins to swell in 24 h and during the next 5–6 days shows spectacular cytoplasmic and nuclear changes which are called *Nissl degeneration*. These changes were first described by Franz Nissl in 1892 [12].

In Nissl degeneration the cell bodies of the severered fibres swell and their perinuclear Nissl substances disintegrates into powdery particles (Fig. 4.7),

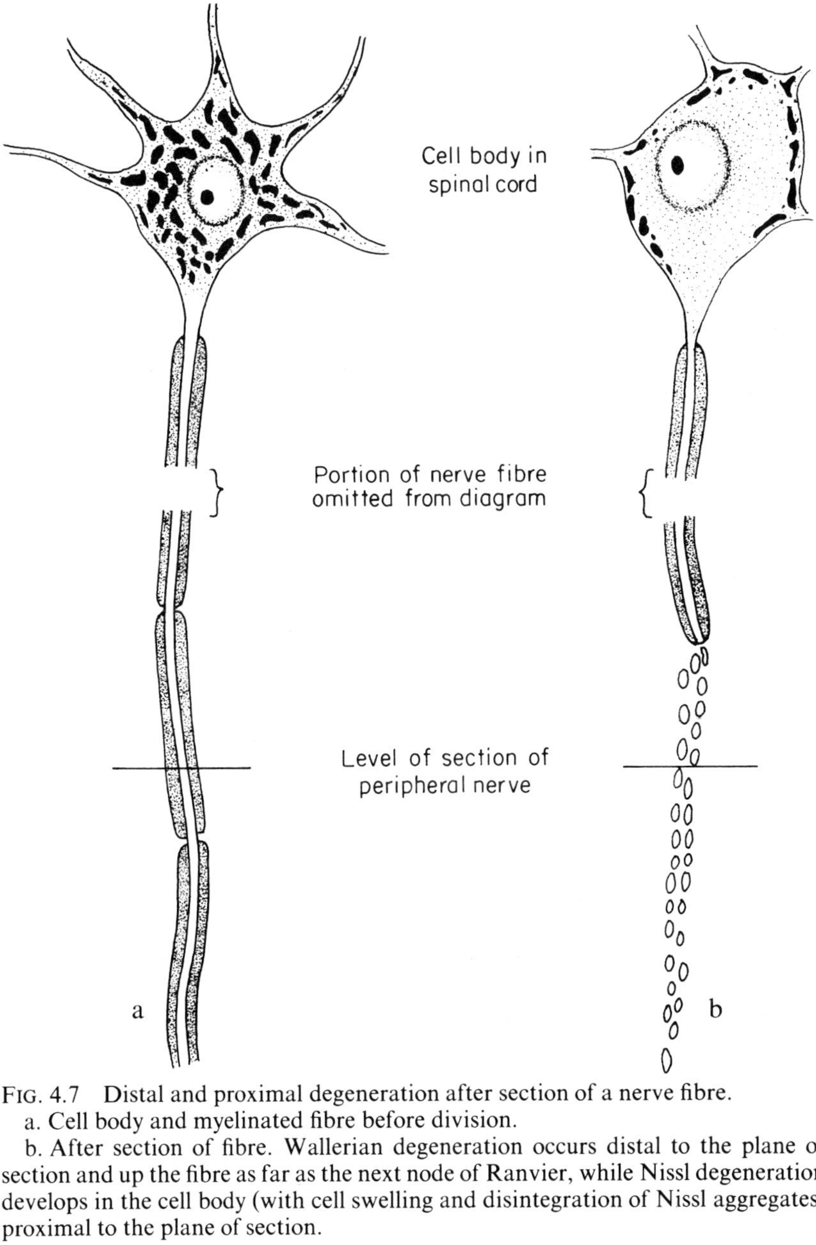

FIG. 4.7 Distal and proximal degeneration after section of a nerve fibre.
a. Cell body and myelinated fibre before division.
b. After section of fibre. Wallerian degeneration occurs distal to the plane of section and up the fibre as far as the next node of Ranvier, while Nissl degeneration develops in the cell body (with cell swelling and disintegration of Nissl aggregates) proximal to the plane of section.

while their nuclei enlarge and move into an eccentric position and in some cases are expelled from the cells. Nissl observed these changes in the cell bodies of the facial nucleus in the medulla of rabbits after tearing out the facial nerve peripherally, and also in spinal anterior horn cells after section of regional spinal nerves such as the radial. Marinesco [13] made similar observations on neuronal cell bodies in the hypoglossal nucleus of the medulla after section of the hypoglossal nerve on the same side. Marinesco emphasised that during this change the Nissl substance disintegrates principally into the cytoplasm around the nucleus; he called this phenomenon *perinuclear chromatolysis.*

The Nissl granules seen by LM in neuronal cell bodies and dendrites correspond to aggregates of rough ER, which are seen by EM as cisternae covered by ribosomes. By LM the granules are intensely basophilic due to their high content of RNA. After axonal section basophilic Nissl substance, rich in RNA, disappears from the perinuclear cytoplasm, although the total content of RNA in cells swollen by Nissl degeneration is undiminished [14]. Observations by EM [15] show that this disintegration of Nissl substance depends on dispersal of ribosomes (rich in RNA) from their attachment to the ER membranes.

This swelling of neuronal cell bodies after section of their axons may be a consequence of continued synthesis of protein which cannot escape into the axonal terminals. When an axon is cut it eventually becomes sealed above the point of section; continued accumulation of axoplasm, which normally flows down the axon, may then increase hydrostatic pressure and so promote swelling of the perikaryon. The swelling and chromatolysis of Nissl degeneration are usually temporary phenomena, but sometimes the eccentric nuclei are expelled from the swollen perikarya and the process terminates in neuronal death.

Acute traumatic degeneration of cerebral and spinal tracts

Following section of nerve tracts in the brain and spinal cord distal and proximal changes proceed in the same way as after division of peripheral nerves to give Wallerian and Nissl degeneration. But section of cerebral and spinal nerve tracts also results in a *much more rapid process* called *traumatic degeneration* in the immediate vicinity of the site of trauma [7]. In this process the severed axons both proximal and distal to the zone of injury disintegrate within a few hours, while apparently uninjured axoplasm retracts from the degenerated remnants and expands on both sides of the wound into club-shaped bodies or 'balls' which are intensely blackened by impregnation with metallic silver. The myelin around these axonal enlargements also swells into bulbous tubules stainable by OsO_4.

At first these clubs or balls are joined to the uninjured axon above and below the point of section. But later these connections are severed by autolysis and the retraction balls become isolated. In the fibres proximal to the site of section this process of retraction continues and clubs develop in continuity with a terminally swollen and varicose axon which retains connection with the cell body. This upper segment of the divided axon then further retracts discarding freshly separated balls of axoplasm each of which arises from a terminal club-shaped varicosity.

Retraction clubs or balls of this kind are formed in human cerebral tracts after head injuries in which the white matter of the brain is exposed to shearing forces. Strich [16, 17] described these retraction balls as eosinophilic argyrophilic swellings on nerve fibres and regarded them as extrusions of axoplasm from the proximal and distal ends of severed axons (Fig. 4.8). She found these bodies in

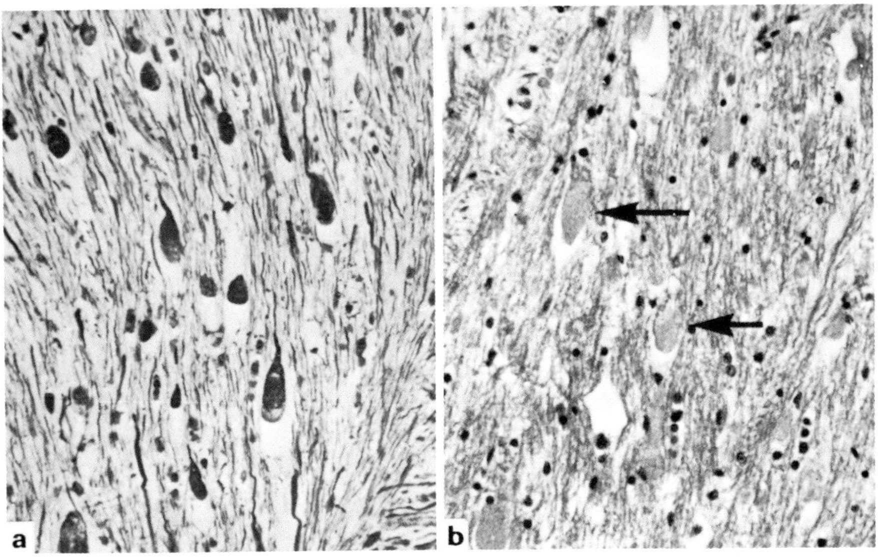

FIG. 4.8 Traumatic shearing of cerebral tracts. Formation of retraction clubs. Section through internal capsule of a woman who died in coma 11 days after a road accident, without recovering consciousness. × 180.

a. Palmgren silver impregnation, showing argyrophil swellings (retraction clubs) at end of ruptured fibres.

b. H & E; retraction clubs (arrows) faintly stained.

Courtesy of Dr Sabina Strich. *J. Clin. Path.* Suppl 4, 1970, **23**, 166.

the cerebral white matter of patients who died 18 h to 6 weeks after head injury. These balls were specially conspicuous in damaged long tracts such as the corpus callosum, internal capsule and superior cerebellar peduncles. These spectacular imprints of axonal damage were usually found in patients who were unconscious after severe head injury and remained in a decerebrate spastic semicomatose state till they died. The presence of these clubs or balls in the injured tracts provides cogent evidence of axonal trauma and suggests that post-traumatic dementia and coma may result from cerebral shearing injury with severance of long tracts. When such patients survived longer and died 2–3 months after the accident, Wallerian degeneration of the myelin in the severed tracts became detectable by the Marchi method for cholesterol esters (p. 391).

Cerebral concussion

Trauma can also interrupt cerebral activity even without severing nerve fibres and without causing any permanent neuronal lesions. This happens in cerebral concussion; this may be defined as temporary post-traumatic coma of instantaneous onset which considerably outlasts the period of violence and is usually attended by amnesia of the moment of accident and of immediately preceding events. On return of consciousness complete recovery is usual.

Concussion probably affects the structure of neuronal membranes and so induces changes in cerebral electrical activity. Williams & Denny-Brown [18] found that electrical activity, recorded by electrodes, applied to the dura mater over the cerebral hemispheres, is conspicuously diminished or suppressed by concussion. Apparently, however, the principal inhibition of electrical activity induced by concussion in the neurones themselves is located in the *reticular formation* of the brain stem rather than in the cerebral cortex [19]. In fact the electrical activity recorded from the reticular formation shows a far greater and longer depression during concussion than that recorded from the cerebral cortex. Moreover during the coma of concussion in monkeys the normal action of sensory impulses in evoking electrical responses from electrodes inserted into the reticular formation is abolished, although similar responses evoked in the medial lemniscus (in the normal sensory pathway) and in the sensory cortex continue uninterrupted by concussion [20].

These observations indicate that concussion blocks the responses of the reticular formation to sensory impulses and that the resultant temporary annulment of reticular activity, which normally arouses and alerts the cerebral cortex, thus determines the coma of concussion. The most frequent and consistent visible cellular change observed after concussion is perinuclear chromatolysis in the cell bodies of the reticular zone of the medulla [21]. Interruption of reticular function and metabolism thus appears to be a prominent event in the phenomenon of concussion. The effects of concussion on neuronal behaviour including memory will be considered in Chapter 9.

INJURY BY HEAT

Thermal injury usually arises from exposure of body surfaces to extremes of temperature which produces burns, or by less extreme but more prolonged overheating of the whole body which causes loss of temperature control with heat stroke.

Burns of body surface

Exposure of body surface to high temperatures can cause irreversible cellular injury as well as transient vascular changes. The most usual irreversible changes in burns involve epidermal damage as well as fission of the dermo-epidermal junction and damage to subjacent capillaries and venules. The degree of damage depends both on the temperature attained and the duration of exposure.

Epidermal damage

Peters and his colleagues [22, 23] studied the effects of applying a burning iron (warmed by circulating hot water at various temperatures) for 1 min to the shaved skin of anaesthetised guinea-pigs and also to human skin. After exposure to a temperature of 45°C the epidermal nuclei begin to swell; this change is reversible. With exposure lasting 1 min the critical temperature for irreversible injury is reached between 50° and 55°C; during this phase the nuclear chromatin collapses into a crescentic mass leaving a residual vacuole, basophilic material (RNA) is lost from the cytoplasm, and spaces appear between the prickle cells along with increase in water content of the epidermis. Above 55°C the nuclei shrivel or split into fragments (Fig. 4.9). These cellular changes are irreversible and may involve transepidermal necrosis with separation of the epidermis from the dermis (with blistering in human skin). At 60°C and above the entire epithelium becomes *coagulated*, and microscopically shows little difference from 'normal' fixed tissues. Although these histological features were usually studied in tissues fixed 2 h after exposure, nuclear swelling and collapse were visible in tissues fixed within 5 min of exposure to 55° for 1 min.

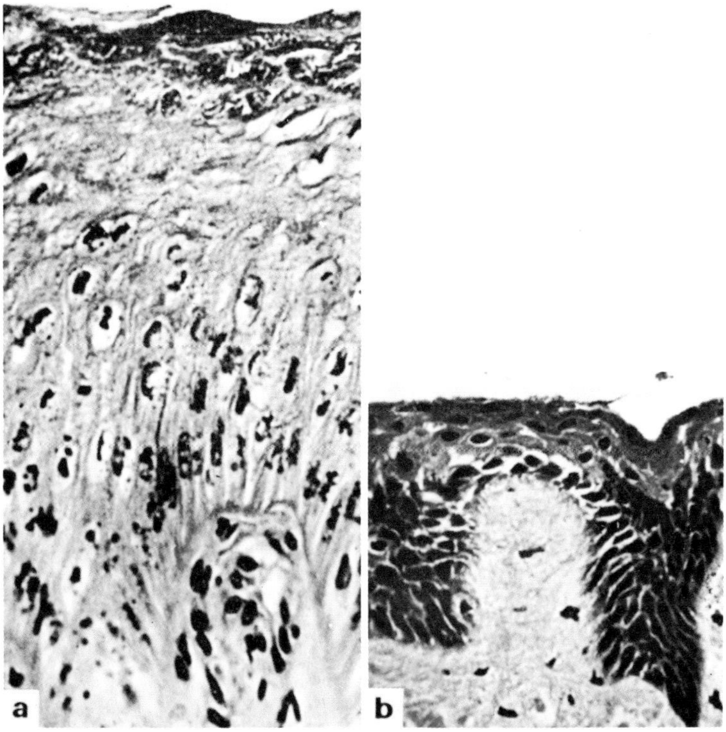

FIG. 4.9 Human skin after accidental burning.

a. Skin of finger cxcised 10 h after burn; in some of the epidermal cells the nuclear chromatin is fragmented (karyorrhexis) or condensed (pyknosis), while other cells have lost their nuclei. H & E. ×450.

b. Skin of forearm excised same day as burn; shrinkage of necrotic epidermal cells and condensation of nuclear chromatin (pyknosis). H & E. ×410.

Courtesy of Dr S. Sevitt. *Burns, Pathology and Therapeutic Applications*, 1957, Butterworth, London, p. 21.

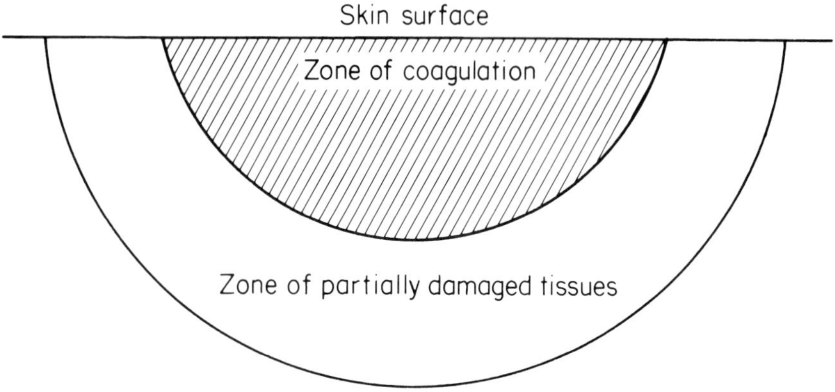

FIG. 4.10 Two zones of thermal injury in a cutaneous burn. Courtesy of Sir Rudolph Peters. *Brit. med. Bull.*, 1945, **3**, 81.

Peters also emphasised that, when skin is locally exposed to temperatures above 60°C, two zones of thermal injury usually become demarcated (Fig. 4.10); first a central zone of complete coagulation where the tissue reached 60°C, and second a surrounding zone of partial damage where the skin temperature attained was lower than 60°C. In the zone of coagulation the cells, if not carbonized, are fixed and show little microscopic change. In the surrounding zone where cell semipermeability and some enzymic activity persist in the damaged cells, the more spectacular changes associated with irreversible damage between 55° and 60° are visible.

Moritz and Henriques [24] and Moritz [25] studied the skin of pigs and men exposed to tangential streams of hot water. The severity of injury between 44° and 60°C increases along with rise in the temperature level attained and also with the time of exposure. The first microscopic evidence of irreversible injury in the epidermal cells consists of swelling of the nuclei in the upper stratum spinosum coupled with change in the distribution of nuclear chromatin. As the nuclei swell their chromatin condenses into compact crescentic segments marginated beneath the nuclear membranes. Then each swollen nucleus bursts and the marginated chromatin contracts into an irregularly shaped central mass separated from the surrounding cytoplasm by a zone of clear fluid and containing a few Feulgen-positive particles of DNA. Further injury results in cellular damage extending through the epidermis to its basal cells, in which the earliest change is cytoplasmic rather than nuclear. The injured basal cells swell and their cytoplasm becomes vacuolated and eosinophilic. With more severe injury there is widespread bursting and disintegration of the lower ends of the basal cells. These changes in the basal cells are the final characteristics indicating complete *transepidermal necrosis*. All these changes, typical of irreversible thermal injury, are extremely rapid in onset and are microscopically visible in epidermal cells placed in fixative immediately after the period of exposure to heat.

These observations on thermal damage of the skin in pigs and men showed that the rate at which irreversible epidermal injury is sustained increases very rapidly as surface temperature is raised. Thus at 44°C transepidermal necrosis only occurs after exposure for 6 h. For each degree rise in temperature between 44° and 51°C the time required to produce irreversible injury diminishes by about one-half. At 51°C transepidermal necrosis develops in 3–4 min.

Fission of dermo-epidermal junction: vesication

Thermal injury also weakens or destroys the attachment of the epidermis to the dermis [25]. At relatively low temperatures this effect is at first latent and reversible. Thus the epidermis is *temporarily* loosened from the dermis in pig skin maintained at 49°C for a time slightly less than the threshold exposure time for transepidermal necrosis at this temperature. This loosened epidermis can then easily be scraped from the dermis by friction; after 18 h this transient state of detachability is lost and firm anchorage is regained.

Rise of temperature for longer periods damages the dermo-epidermal junction *irreversibly*. This damage is an invariable concomitant of transepidermal necrosis. In men and in guinea-pigs this lesion is accompanied by *vesication*, in which a fluid forming a blister separates the epidermis from the dermis (second degree burn). In the pig vesication does not occur, although a similar physical plane of separation (visible by microscopy) permanently dissevers dermo-epidermal adherence so that the epidermis can be wiped away. In the pig insufficient exudation of plasma by coincident injury to dermal capillaries accounts for the absence of blistering, although the basement membrane is destroyed. The mechanism of this separation of epidermis from dermis is obscure; Peters suggested that liberation of a proteinase (which is lost from burnt epidermis) contributes to lysis of the basement membrane. Osmotic rupture of proximal ends of the basal cells however appears to be a more likely cause for this rapid severing of dermo-epidermal continuity.

Transepidermal necrosis with dermo-epidermal separation is thus immediately responsible for increase in transudation of fluid from dermal blood vessels by lowering of intercellular pressure. Blistering of burnt skin is, however, also dependent on exudation of protein-rich plasma caused by increase in permeability of dermal venules and capillaries. Hurley [26] gives a valuable summary of this subject. Mild thermal injury produces a biphasic increase in vascular permeability. At first liberation of histamine from granules discharged by damaged mast cells, causes rapid leakage of plasma from venules which lasts for 15–45 min. This effect probably depends on the action of histamine and other vaso-active substances (p. 193) in causing separation of venular endothelial cells with the formation of small gaps between them. In the second more prolonged phase, which begins about 45 min after mild thermal injury and lasts many hours, *direct injury* to endothelial cells by heat results in leakage of plasma from both *capillaries* and *venules*. This delayed effect is accompanied by the appearance of both small and large gaps (visible by EM) between the endothelial cells and is apparently due to direct action of heat in separating and contracting the cells and not to any chemical mediator. More severe thermal injury at 60°C directly damages both capillaries and venules with immediate and prolonged exudation of plasma; leakage then also occurs from venules in adjacent *unburnt* tissues due to *diffusion* of chemical mediators from the burnt area.

Exudation of protein-rich fluid into burnt skin thus results from changes in the dermal blood vessels as well as in transepidermal necrosis, which together combine to cause the severe blistering characteristic of human burns.

Molecular mechanisms of thermal injury

In cells and tissues damaged by heat the most permanent effects probably originate from changes in the conformation and assembly of macromolecules including protein, DNA and lipid micelles. Injury of this kind occurs rapidly when the temperature reaches 55–56°C and more slowly at even lower temperatures. At higher temperatures (above 60°C) damage is also caused by chemical decomposition and carbonisation of organic molecules.

Belehradek [27] discussed various possible causes of thermal injury including (a) coagulation of protein, (b) destruction of enzymes, (c) 'asphyxiation', (d) 'intoxication', and (e) change of state in lipids. He commented on the sudden break with rise in temperature in curves relating survival-time to temperature of exposure, which for each kind of cell studied, show a sudden break followed by more rapid fall of survival-time above a particular temperature. Belehradek concluded that *at least two processes*, therefore, contribute to thermal injury.

Clearly coagulation of proteins and inactivation of enzymes both depend on the common process of denaturation of protein by heat. 'Asphyxiation', i.e. deprival of oxygen, and similar deficiencies of other metabolites may arise from acceleration of chemical reactions with rise in temperature. Moreover changes in lipid permeability may increase the accessibility of enzymes to their substrates and thus initially accelerate metabolism. How far thermal injury depends on such complex metabolic effects remains obscure. It seems likely however that changes in macromolecular conformation and assembly are the most important initiating events in the damage of cells by heat.

Denaturation and aggregation of protein and DNA

Denaturation of protein attached to DNA may be responsible for the spectacular effects of heat on the nuclei of epidermal cells, in which the dispersed chromatin of the interphase is clumped into a crescentic segment marginated against the nuclear membrane. Removal of structured water bound by hydrogen bonding to histones or to DNA may take part in this denaturation, so that the tenuous helices of partly uncoiled DNA become clumped or coiled into condensed pyknotic remnants.

Enzymic proteins are inactivated by rise in temperature. Enzymes differ in their susceptibility to heat. Thus orientated membrane-bound enzyme complexes associated with anabolism are probably more susceptible than some of the simpler soluble enzymes which cause hydrolytic fission. Indeed some phosphatases remain active in tissues after embedding in molten wax at 56°C. By selective interference with enzymic anabolic processes, while catabolic activity remains unimpaired, a limited rise in temperature may result in increase of intracellular concentration of small molecules. This effect may contribute to osmotic swelling between 44° and 55°C, and also determine loss of cytoplasmic RNA.

Above 60°C cell proteins coagulate. At this temperature water is expelled from hydrogen bonding with proteins. This effect exposes active groups of proteins which then become rearranged by mutual interaction so as to cause coagulation. Damage by water itself also contributes to heat-denaturation of proteins; indeed Greaves succeeded in preventing denaturation by freeze-*drying* proteins before their exposure to heat.

Disintegration of lipid micelles and lipoprotein membranes

Heilbrunn [28, 29] made the important suggestion that heat injures cells by affecting intracellular lipids at temperatures *below* the coagulation point of proteins. He measured the viscosity of crustacean ova by observing the rate at which these cells can be separated into clear and turbid zones by centrifugation. Heating to a temperature (32–33°C), far below the point of coagulation of proteins, caused an abrupt rise in viscosity of the intracellular fluid; after such exposure granules visible in the cytoplasm were unable to move under the influence of strong centrifugal force. Along with this change in viscosity intracellular lipid droplets became more diffuse and ultimately appeared to go into solution. This coagulation of the cytoplasm was at first reversible and preceded irreversible cell death which followed longer exposure to this *same* level of temperature. Heilbrunn suggested that 'heat-death' of cells is determined by this coagulation of the cell contents and is associated with changes in cell lipids and also occurs at temperatures *far below* the level at which proteins coagulate.

It is now realised that thermal injury may primarily be initiated by disarray of micellar lipids in cell membranes. These membranes probably have a semi-liquid consistency, being composed of a fluid mozaic formed by bimolecular laminae of orientated amphipathic lipids in which are suspended partly mobile protein molecules [30]. Rise of temperature increases thermal agitation and thus tends to decompose micellar clusters (or laminae) of lipid amphipathic molecules by increasing repulsion between their hydrophilic terminal groups. Disaggregation of the laminar micelles of lipid in the cell membranes may thus be an initial event in thermal damage. Such disaggregation may initiate lethal disarray of micellar lipids at temperatures *below* the coagulation point of proteins. At higher temperatures expulsion of bound water from membrane proteins may unmask reactive groups which then interact to produce coagulation and more complete disruption of the membrane. The initial changes in lipid micelles may account for increase in permeability followed by entry of water and osmotic swelling of cells injured at 55°C, while more severe micellar disruption coupled with coagulation of protein occurring at 60°C would make cells completely permeable and preclude osmotic swelling at higher temperatures.

Thermal lysis of red cells

Changes in micellar array of lipids in cell membranes are probably concerned in lysis of red cells which occurs in severely burnt patients.

Intravascular haemolysis also occurs in blood of pigs exposed to blasts of hot air at 180°C; some of the red cells disintegrate into small spherical globules called microspherocytes, and haemoglobin released from the lysed red cells appears in the urine [31]. Similar microspherocytes as well as smaller irregular fragments of red cells are visible in blood from patients after severe burns [32] (Fig. 4.11); this change may also be accompanied by haemoglobinaemia and haemoglobinuria [33].

Although thermal fission of red cells is probably a direct outcome of disruption by heat of lipoprotein membranes of the red cells, further indirect haemolysis occurs in burnt patients (after exposure to heat has ceased) and then contributes to later haemolytic anaemia. This is emphasised by observations on survival of red cells in burnt patients. The half life of compatible red cells tagged with ^{51}Cr from non-burnt donors is shortened from 22 to 6 days, when these cells are transfused into burnt patients; moreover similarly tagged red cells from burnt patients have a normal half life after transfusion into blood of non-burnt volunteers [34]. This suggests that, in addition to immediate destruction of red cells by heat, some further mechanism is responsible for later loss of red cells

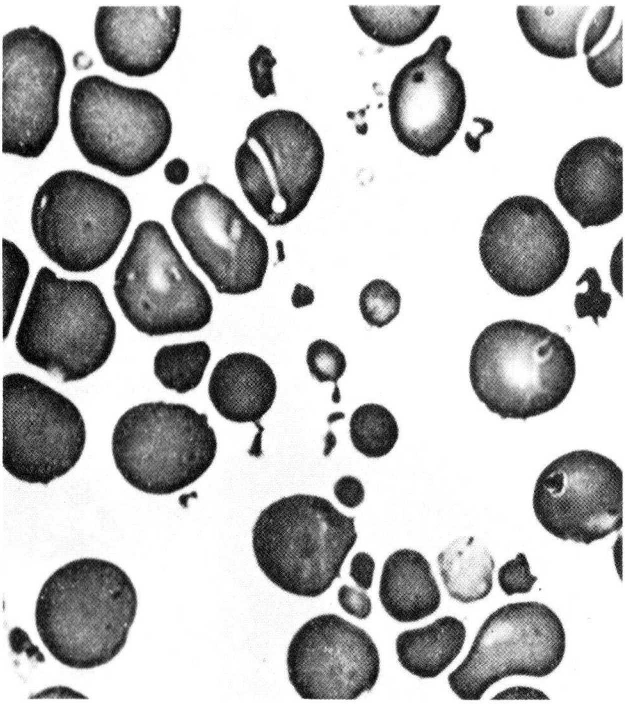

FIG. 4.11 Blood film from a patient with recent extensive burns, showing irregular red cell fragments and microspherocytes. Courtesy of Dr S. Sevitt. *Medicine, Science and the Law*, 1966, p. 36.

after burning; possibly red cells are destroyed by a toxic agent or else are trapped and sequestered by stasis in the burnt tissue [33].

Liberation of K^+ from red cells or other tissues exposed to extreme thermal injury may also contribute to sudden death. Thus anaesthetised pigs immersed for 3–5 min in water at 75°C died suddenly from acute heart failure; simultaneously the level of K^+ in plasma rose from 5 mmol/l to 15 mmol/l [35]. This grossly excessive level of K^+ in plasma was probably responsible for cardiac failure and death of these severely burnt animals. This effect may contribute to sudden death following explosions and conflagrations.

Lethal effects of thermal injury to body surface

Extensive superficial burns cause death in various ways:

1. Transepidermal necrosis coupled with vascular changes in subjacent dermis can together produce devastating loss of plasma from blood vessels in the vesicated and denuded zones. This can lead to hypovolaemic shock followed by death from generalised ischaemia and heart failure.
2. A later highly lethal consequence of transepidermal necrosis is bacterial infection. Colonisation of burnt skin by Gram-positive cocci and by Gram-negative bacilli is frequently followed by terminal septicaemia or bronchopneumonia.
3. When very extensive areas of body surface suffer thermal injury, lysis of red cells in the superficial blood vessels exacerbates hypoxic injury produced by hypovolaemic shock. Extreme thermal injury to erythrocytes and other cells releases intracellular K^+ which can induce sudden hyperkalaemia followed by acute heart failure.

Overheating of body as a whole: Heat stroke

Prolonged high environmental temperature, with failure to adapt to it, can derange the neurones concerned with heat regulation so that body temperature rises to 41°C or more and persists at this extreme level; this condition is called hyperpyrexia or heat stroke.

The most conspicuous signs of heat stroke are sudden collapse with coma, stupor or delirium, often accompanied by convulsions. Death in coma with coincident heart failure may follow in a few hours, but some comatose patients may survive for a few days. In some cases the onset is more insidious with early shock followed by progressive lethargy and rise in temperature terminating in coma.

Malamud *et al.* [36], who studied 125 fatal cases of heat stroke, emphasised that the principal lesion found *post mortem* is necrosis affecting the grey matter of the central nervous system. The brain is heavier than normal owing to oedema. In the cerebral cortex of patients dying within 12 h of onset of coma the neuronal cell bodies are swollen with vacuolar cytoplasm and pyknotic nuclei. But, if survival is longer, the perikarya become shrunken or ghost-like. In the cerebellar cortex the Purkinje cells become swollen and show signs of disintegration within 5 h; they later disappear, although the granule cells persist. If the patients survive for more than a few days intense microglial proliferation occurs in the damaged grey matter.

Necrosis of neurones was found in the brain of all patients who died of heat stroke, whereas degeneration of other cells such as cardiac muscle fibres was only present in some of the patients. Malamud *et al.* considered that most of the lesions in tissues other than the brain can be attributed to coincident anoxia or ischaemic shock rather than to hyperthermia. It is thus probable that cerebral neurones are particularly susceptible to hyperthermia and suffer irreparable damage after exposure to 41°C or above for more than a few hours, and that this damage permanently abolishes the neuronal activity concerned with heat regulation.

The extreme susceptibility of Purkinje cells of cerebellar cortex and of cerebral pyramidal cells to hyperthermia may be related to the exceptionally large surface/volume area posssessed by these cells with complex arrays of dendritic ramifications. This enormous membrane surface may be exceptionally vulnerable to micellar derangement at raised temperatures.

INJURY BY COLD

Cold also causes irreversible cellular injury. Much of the damage produced by cold arises indirectly from ischaemia of the chilled tissues. However, extreme cold also exerts a directly injurious effect.

Indirect damage caused by ischaemia

Immersion of a limb in cold water gives rise to local vasoconstriction and ischaemia. Cellular damage follows as a direct result of defective supply of nutriments to the cells. In limbs the first cells to be injured are those of vascular endothelium. When the temperature rises again the circulation of blood is re-established and plasma leaks out through the damaged endothelium of the small vessels. Oedema and vesication of the skin follow together with necrosis of the skin if the ischaemia has been prolonged. Immersion of limbs for long periods in cold water thus produces swelling and blistering with a variable degree of necrosis; in World War I this condition frequently occurred in soldiers living in water-logged trenches and was called *trench foot*.

More intense cold freezes the exposed parts; this injury is called *frost bite*. The direct effect of freezing is superimposed on the indirect effect of ischaemia, but the ischaemia itself is even more severe after freezing than after mere cooling, since thrombosis occurs in the damaged blood vessels and they may become permanently occluded. The necrotic tissue in frost-bite becomes blackened owing to decomposition of haemoglobin liberated from extravasated blood cells and subsequent deposition of iron sulphide.

Direct damage by freezing

Changes in frozen cells

Rapid freezing followed by slow thawing is highly injurious to cells.

Trump *et al.* [37] compared the effects of rapid and slow freezing on hepatic cells using slices of mouse liver examined by LM and EM. The slices were rapidly frozen by immersion in liquid propane (−174°C) or isopentane (−155° C); slower freezing was achieved by placing the tissue on dry ice (−79°C). The tissues were then thawed for 7 min at room temperature and kept at 0–4°C for 10–30 min before fixation and embedding.

In the rapidly frozen tissue fine reticulation, due to spaces formed by small ice crystals, was visible in cytoplasm and nuclei of the hepatic cells, but no large extracellular ice crystal spaces (ICS) were observed. After rapid freezing also the plasma membrane and mitochondrial membranes showed discontinuities, while the rough surfaced ER was vesiculated and degranulated.

After slower freezing by dry ice no *intracellular* ICS were visible in the centre of the slices where cooling was slowest, but large *extracellular* ICS were prominent. In these more slowly cooled cells mitochondrial membranes appeared undamaged and no ribosomal degranulation of the ER was visible, but the external cell membrane showed discontinuities. There was little intracellular disintegration of the slowly cooled cells, although they appeared shrivelled by abstraction of water into the extracellular ICS. These observations on frozen tissue cooled from without emphasised the highly necrotising action of rapid freezing followed by thawing.

This intensely harmful effect of rapid freezing was also observed in tissues cooled from within by insertion of cryoprobes which initiate freezing from the centre of a group of cells. These probes are cooled to very low temperatures (e.g. −160°C) by rapidly expanding gases, thus utilising the Joule–Thomson effect. Cryoprobes of this kind are used in cryosurgery for killing neoplastic tissues. Under these conditions a spherical zone of frozen tissue ('ice-ball') is formed around the probe where temperature falls to below −20°C. When the tissue is allowed to thaw it gradually becomes oedematous and congested over a few hours to form a cryolesion, in which the most rapidly frozen central cells are irreversibly injured.

Tissues thus cooled from inside by cryoprobes were examined by LM and EM in rat liver [38] and in hamster tongue [39, 40]. In the centre of these cryolesions the ice crystals were predominantly intracellular and occupied the whole cell, while the cell architecture was transformed both in cytoplasm and nucleus into a reticulum composed of ICS. At the periphery of the cryolesions ICS were usually extracellular, and, although the ice spaces produced great distortion of the cells, intracellular structural integrity was retained [40]. Indeed, cells from the most external zones of the thawed ice-balls appeared unharmed [38].

These results confirm the view that rapid freezing is much more lethal to cells than slower freezing. After rapid freezing numerous intracellular icicles appear to be a determinant or a concomitant of irreversible cellular injury. But after slower freezing the ice crystals are larger and mostly extracellular; it is believed that during the formation of these large extracellular crystals pockets of unfrozen hypertonic saline accumulate in the intercellular spaces. Water is then drawn out of the cell by osmosis so that the formation of highly destructive intracellular icicles is inhibited. This sequence of events would account for the relatively less necrotising action of slow freezing.

Causes of cryogenic lesions: molecular changes

The molecular nature of cryogenic lesions is still obscure. Irreversible injury to cells probably depends on macromolecular alterations either in lipoprotein membranes or in DNA. Membrane lesions are likely to be of most immediate import to the rapid death of frozen non-dividing cells.

Traumatic effects of icicles. Intracellular ice is associated with more serious cell injury than extracellular ice. Indeed the outer surface of the cell membrane may be protected by its glycocalyx of glycosaminoglycans from traumatic effects of ice but ice may injure the internal surface of the cell membrane which lacks the protective mucoid covering. Although discontinuities are sometimes visible by EM in cell membranes of frozen cells, recent observations give no evidence of penetration of cell membranes by ice crystals [40].

Damage by hypertonic saline: latent injury. Lovelock [41] introduced the important concept that cell membranes can be damaged by temporary exposure to hypertonic saline during the processes of freezing or thawing. He showed that, when red blood cells are immersed in hypertonic saline (>0.8M NaCl), the cell membrane is injured and the cells are lysed when subsequently reintroduced to isotonic saline ('dilution shock'). During freezing, however, ice crystallises out of the fluid both outside and inside the cell membranes which may thus temporarily be exposed to hypertonic saline before freezing is complete. This may cause latent injury to the membrane which is followed by lysis when the membranes become reexposed to isotonic saline after thawing. However if freezing at first occurs externally the surrounding concentrated saline may extract water by osmosis from the cells, so that, by the time the medium has come to saturation at the eutectic point, the cells are apparently too dry to freeze and may thus survive [41]. Red cells latently injured by hypertonic saline above freezing point may also be lysed by a subsequent fall in temperature ('cold shock') [42] or by mechanical trauma such as centrifugation [41]. Farrant & Morris [42] suggested that during rapid freezing the time of exposure to hypertonic saline may be insufficient to cause this latent injury. However, if intracellular ice is formed, then on thawing hypertonic saline would reappear in a particularly noxious situation within the cells. If thawing is then slow, this saline will act for long enough to cause latent injury to the membrane. Subsequent dilution on complete thawing will then transform the latent damage into irreversible disintegration of membrane micelles.

Removal of bound water. The formation of ice crystals may also injure cell membrane by extraction of bound water into the growing icicles. Karow & Webb [43] suggested that death in freezing is primarily a result of extraction of bound water from vital structures. If water, which is frozen into ice crystals, comes from free water of the cell, no lasting damage may result. But if the water converted to ice crystals is taken from bound cell water, then cell membranes may disintegrate. Normally the —C=O and =N–H groups of membrane proteins form an arrayed complex with a penumbra of bound water, which is attached in a lattice of hydrogen bonding to the cell membrane. This lattice-like extension of the cell membrane may be essential for survival. Karow & Webb supposed that the water extracted from this bonded state and incorporated into growing icicles leaves the membrane protein dehydrated and denatured; they suggested that during slow freezing the membranes are more stable and the lattice structure is preserved, while during rapid freezing not only free water but also bound water is consumed by formation of intracellular ice. Moreover, as we have seen, slow freezing mainly forms extracellular ice and may therefore only remove water bonded from the external surface of the cell. This externally bound water, which is only held to the cell calyx composed of glycosaminoglycans, may be abstracted without disarraying the essential proteins of the cell membrane. But, when *intracellular* ice is formed by rapid freezing, bound water may be removed from the *inner* surface of the cell membrane which is not protected by attached glycans. This irreversible membrane injury may be initiated by the formation of intracellular ice.

The concept of removal of bound water from membrane lattices accounts satisfactorily for the necrotising action of rapid freezing and intracellular ice. However the harmful action of hypertonic saline probably also contributes to these effects. The latent injury induced by hypertonic saline may diminish the stability of membrane array so that bound water becomes more readily removed during freezing. Indeed freezing and hypertonic saline may summate in their effects of destabilising membrane structure, so that a merely latent injury evoked by one noxious agent is rendered irreversible by the subsequent incidence of the other.

Requirements for maximum injury: Crysosurgery

To secure maximum cellular injury by cold, as is needed for cryosurgery, rapid freezing is thus deliberately followed by slow thawing. The rapid freezing secures the presence of intracellular ice which is associated with severe cell disintegration. The slow thawing at first exposes the internal surface of the cell to hypertonic saline for long enough to cause latent injury followed by subsequent dilution 'shock' as the remaining icicles melt. Thus any cells which escape irreversible injury in the initial freeze may succumb to the final thaw.

Requirements for maximum survival

This kind of freezing and thawing is needed for keeping viable cells alive in constant genetic condition over long periods ('sleeping beauty' effect). To secure such survival slower freezing followed by rapid thawing is desirable. The freezing must be slow enough to dry the cells by osmotic action as the external solution becomes concentrated by partial freezing and thus reduces intracellular freezing to a minimum; but thawing must be sufficiently rapid to prevent latent injury by any prolonged exposure to concentrated saline. Protective agents such as dimethyl sulphoxide or serum are added to the medium to give osmotic action without the toxic effects of ions [44]. This object of maximum survival was ingeniously secured by Nagington & Greaves [45] by cooling cell suspensions in dimethyl sulphoxide solution enclosed in ampoules suspended over the surface of evaporating liquid N_2. This procedure secured a cooling rate of 1°C/min down to −25°C and then a slower rate down to −100°C. Thereafter the ampoules were transferred to liquid N_2 and stored in it at −195°C. The cells were reactivated by rapid thawing of the ampoules in water at 37°C. After freezing and thawing in this manner 80 per cent of Hela and human amnion cells survived.

INJURY BY IONIZING RADIATION AND BY ULTRAVIOLET LIGHT

Radiation injures cells by causing chemical changes within them. This injury is generally initiated by displacement of electrons within atoms of cellular molecules; when an electron is displaced by radiation a pair of ions is generated. Ionized molecules are highly unstable and are rapidly converted to free radicals, which either recombine to reform the original molecule or react with adjacent groups in the same or in some other molecules and so result in harmful chemical changes.

Two kinds of radiation are responsible for cellular injury:

1. *Particulate rays.* Neutrons (no charge), protons (+), α-particles (+) and electrons (−).
2. *Electromagnetic waves.* X-rays, γ-rays and ultraviolet light (UVL).

Human exposure to harmful radiation has arisen in several ways. Miners may inhale dust containing radioactive elements such as Ra and U. Nuclear explosions emit neutrons, α-particles, protons, electrons and γ-rays. Routine diagnostic radiography only exposes patients to minute doses of X-rays, but definite human hazard ensues from large doses of X-rays given for radiotherapy and fluoroscopy.

Depth of penetration varies between types of radiation. Fast neutrons, X-rays and γ-rays are highly penetrant and injure both deep and superficial tissues, but electrons can only penetrate a few mm. UVL has even less power of penetration, but unfortunately can seriously injure epidermis and superficial dermis.

Immediate and early effects of radiation

The most conspicuous early effects of radiation usually occur in tissues where the cells have a short life span with a high rate of replacement and also a high frequency of mitosis.

Radiation is specially lethal to cells during mitosis and it also delays onset of mitosis. Hence radiation not only kills tissue with a short life span such as gastrointestinal epithelium but it also impedes their replacement. The special vulnerability of cells in mitosis may be related to the high concentration and aggregation of DNA in mitotic cells. Indeed cells with small nuclei such as lymphocytes which are not dividing but in which nuclear chromatin is closely aggregated are also highly susceptible.

Cerebral injury

All cells are injured by extreme intensity of radiation and even cells with a long life span such as cerebral neurones and cardiac muscle may be damaged by immense doses.

Following doses of 7500 rad X-rays to guinea pigs, cerebellar neurones were irreversibly injured and the animals died within 24 h [46]. Ataxia, nystagmus and bouts of rigidity developed in a few hours followed by death from convulsions and respiratory arrest. In these animals nuclei of the granule cells in cerebellum became homogenised and contracted (pyknotic) and the cytoplasm was vacuolated; these changes were detectable within 2.5 h of exposure and reached a maximum in 8–12 h. Both this damage to the cerebellar granule cells and the acute clinical signs of cerebellar injury were prevented by shielding the hind brain of the guinea pigs during irradiation.

This relative susceptibility of the cerebellar granule cells may be related to the small size of their nuclei with high concentration of DNA which may be more aggregated than in other neurones.

Gastrointestinal injury

After less extreme doses of radiation cerebral injury usually does not occur. Indeed the most serious early sequels to severe exposure usually result from injury to gastrointestinal epithelium.

Within a few hours of intense irradiation of animals mitosis ceases in the enteroblasts of the intestinal crypts. After a few days these dividing enteroblasts become necrotic [47] and their chromatin is clumped; this process of clumping of mitotic chromatin is called *pyknonecrosis* [48, 49]. The mature enterocytes of the villi are then desquamated without replacement and the villi become bared of epithelium. Following smaller doses of radiation some of the enteroblasts are not killed and their mitosis is then followed by epithelial replacement.

Similar changes in the enteroblasts of the human small intestine follow severe exposure to radiation in man. Among victims of atomic bombs injury to intestinal epithelium (through lack of replacement) produced nausea and vomiting in about a day after exposure; some of these patients died within a week with extensive necrosis and sloughing of intestinal epithelium. In patients who survived more than two weeks mitosis of surviving enteroblasts was resumed and epithelium was regenerated [50]. The rapid onset of clinical signs following injury to intestinal cells by severe exposure to radiation depends on two factors:

1. Their high frequency of mitosis which results in high susceptibility.
2. Their short life span which determines ulceration and infection when the mature cells are not continuously replaced.

Haemopoietic injury

After less severe exposure to radiation both human patients and animals may survive the initial gastrointestinal injury and then later suffer the effects of injury to the highly susceptible cells of the bone marrow. These cells are just as rapidly injured or killed by radiation as the enteroblasts of the intestine, but the ill effects of damage to bone marrow cells develop more slowly, as the more resistant *mature cells* of the blood have a longer life span than *enterocytes* of the small inestine and stomach.

In mice following sublethal doses of X-rays red marrow disappeared from femur and vertebral bodies within 10 days [51]. Similarly in human victims of atomic bombs, bone marrow was rapidly depleted of haemopoietic cells. This abolished formation of platelets, granulocytes and erythrocytes; lack of platelets produced severe haemorrhage with purpura, melaena and haematuria, while lack of granulocytes was followed by leucopenia. Death then resulted from combined effects of haemorrhagic ulceration in mouth, pharynx and large intestine, with bacterial infection exacerbated by deficiency of granulocytes in patients already weakened by haemorrhage [50, 52, 53].

The effects of interruption of erythropoiesis among atomic casualties were slower to develop and only became apparent in patients who escaped more intense radiation and survived for two months or more. By this time the life span of many of the resistant mature erythrocytes had terminated and severe anaemia developed owing to lack of replacement; these patients generally recovered after resumption of mitosis and maturation by surviving stem cells in the bone marrow.

Lymphocytic injury

Although lymphocytes in the resting state rarely divide they are killed and lysed by radiation with extreme rapidity.

The necrotising action of radiation on lymphocytes is thus usually exerted on cells in interphase; lysis follows rapidly, and in man the lymphocyte count in peripheral blood usually falls to a minimum 24 h after exposure. Following momentary accidental exposure of a technologist to intense radiation from ^{60}Co, the lymphocyte count fell by 69 per cent in 4 h [54]; full recovery followed later. This swift necrosis of lymphocytes after irradiation is also conspicuous in cultures of thymocytes: in these cells spectacular homogenisation of interphase chromatin accompanies necrosis due to radiation [55].

In victims of atomic bombs who died within 14 days of irradiation the spleen and lymph nodes were diminished in size owing to rapid cytolysis of necrotic lymphocytes: the Malpighian corpuscles were almost completely depleted of lymphocytes and the germinal centres of lymph nodes disappeared [50, 52].

The extreme vulnerability of lymphocytes and thymocytes to radiation may depend on the condensed state of their nuclear DNA even in non-dividing cells.

Epidermal injury

Although not so sensitive to radiation as gastrointestinal epithelium or lymphocytes, epidermal cells are specially liable to injury by radiation owing to their superficial position. They can thus be killed by radiation with very limited power of penetration such as α-particles, electrons or UVL as well as by more deeply penetrating X-rays.

Exposure of human skin to large doses of X-rays is followed by loss of hair and ulceration. Victims of atomic bombs, who survived for more than one week, lost their hair abruptly about two weeks after exposure. This epilation chiefly affected the scalp, producing an appearance like a monk's tonsure [50, 52]. Contamination of human skin by fall-out dust from nuclear explosions also caused epilation and ulceration probably as a result of injury by electrons emitted from ^{60}Sr which is present in the radioactive dust.

In animals small doses of radiation inhibit mitosis in epidermal cells, while larger doses cause epidermal necrosis followed by loss of hair and ulceration [56].

UVL has very limited power of penetration but it can produce severe epidermal necrosis, especially in fair-skinned people. As UVL cannot penetrate more deeply its effects are confined to the skin. The necrotising effect may be due to *direct* alteration of DNA in epidermal nuclei. Immediately after exposure of human skin to UVL an antigenic change can be detected in DNA of epidermal nuclei examined by immunofluorescence in biopsy specimens; this change is revealed by treatment with rabbit antibody (to *irradiated* DNA) followed by fluorescein-conjugated sheep anti-rabbit γ-globulin [57, 58].

Exposure to UVL causes severe epidermal injury in patients with the inherited disorder xeroderma pigmentosum (p. 470), in which repair of DNA chains damaged by UVL is defective.

Late and latent effects of radiation

Radiation can leave latent imprints on cells and tissues which as a result may later die or become neoplastic.

Some of these late sequels appear to arise *de novo* after seemingly complete recovery or absence of any initially visible effect in the irradiated tissue. Thus there is an abnormally high incidence of mammary carcinoma in women 15–20 years after repeated fluoroscopy formerly used in checking treatment of tuberculosis by pneumothorax. Similarly carcinoma of bronchus and thyroid as well as leukaemia are recognised as late effects of radiation among survivors from atomic bombs [59]. Bronchial carcinoma also developed as a late sequel to exposure of miners to radioactive dust in the Schneeberg district of Saxony and Bohemia; oat-cell carcinoma of bronchus (p. 460) developed in many of these miners after 20–30 years of exposure and also in others many years after leaving the mines. Similarly epidermal neoplasia (such as rodent ulcer and malignant melanoma) may occur in fair-skinned people after prolonged exposure to UVL especially in sunny climates.

In some cases latency is not so complete. After repeated exposure of the same area of skin to X-rays burns appear, which heal incompletely and retain thickened collagen and permanently hyperplastic epithelium. Later this collagen may become necrotic, or a maligant carcinoma may arise from the overactive epithelium.

The latency of neoplastic lesions initiated by radiation may be determined by alteration of DNA in cells which are in a state of prolonged interphase; these changes may remain invisible and are only expressed by visible change of karyotype when mitosis is later resumed, possibly owing to some other form of stimulation. Alternatively the initial change induced by radiation may occur in dividing cells, but be entirely at molecular level; this may later lead to neoplasia, when a further mutation occurs after a long latent period to produce a fully visible change of karyotype.

Alterations in nuclei of irradiated cells

Some of these changes, which provide insight into the mechanisms of damage by radiation, will be discussed. As these changes are affected by the stage in the mitotic cycle, at which exposure to radiation occurs, the so-called 'phases' of the normal cycle of mitosis will briefly be summarised.

Phases in mitotic cycle

Among continuously dividing cells, such as human bone marrow, mitosis with its four phases (prophase, metaphase, anaphase, telophase) lasts 1–2 h and is succeeded by interphase lasting 40–45 h before recurrence of another mitosis.

Interphase itself consist of three phases:

1. Pre-DNA synthesis: G_1 (gap 1).
2. DNA synthesis: S.
3. Post-DNA synthesis: G_2 (gap 2).

During G_1 the nucleus has the normal diploid content of DNA (Fig. 4.12). Even in continuously dividing cells G_1 is much longer than S or G_2, and in cells

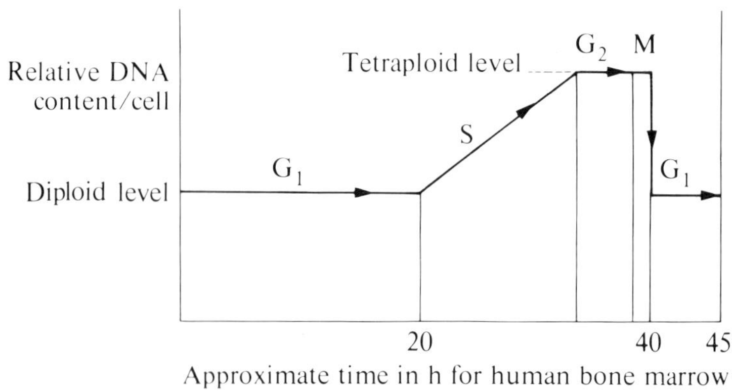

FIG. 4.12 Phases of mitotic cycle in actively dividing cell.

G_1 gap 1 of interphase
S synthesis of DNA
G_2 gap 2 of interphase
M mitosis

In resting cells G_1 is indefinitely prolonged (G_0). From figures given by Davidson [73]. Modified by courtesy of Professor R. C. Curran, Professor D. G. Harnden & Professor J. Stuart from a diagram in *The Pathological Basis of Medicine* (1972), p. 225, Heinemann Medical, London.

which do not divide continuously, such as lymphocytes of peripheral blood, G_1 may be prolonged for years; in the latter situation cells are said to be in G_0 phase which only terminates on stimulation of mitosis. During S phase replication of DNA occurs and its content doubles to reach tetraploid level which persists during G_2. G_2 usually lasts only a few hours (Fig. 4.12) and is immediately followed by mitosis (M in Fig. 4.12).

Inhibition of synthesis of DNA

Radiation inhibits synthesis of DNA. This effect is conveniently studied by observing incorporation of ^{3}H-thymidine (or other radioactive precursors of DNA) into cell nuclei by autoradiography. This incorporation is strongly inhibited by radiation late in G_1 phase just before the commencement of synthesis; but much greater doses are required to inhibit incorporation in S phase once synthesis has started. Observations on incorporation of ^{3}H-thymidine into nuclei of mouse leukaemic cells in culture made by autoradiography, using both LM and EM, indicate that the actual start of synthesis of DNA but *not* the elongation of its chain (seen by EM) is specially sensitive to radiation [60].

Delay in onset of mitosis

This effect is produced by small doses of X-rays which are insufficient to cause cell death. Delay is usually greater after irradiation in S phase, but is also considerable after irradiation in M phase [61]. With larger doses of X-rays fall in mitotic index is almost immediate [62].

Irradiation of individual nuclei during mitosis

The actual process of mitosis is selectively injured by radiation. This is clear from results obtained by irradiating single mitotic cells in cultures of heart muscle cells or chick embryo fibroblasts by microbeams of protons or α-particles [63–66]. In these experiments irradiation generally lasted 0.5–5 min, and the cells were then observed by phase contrast microscopy within 2 min of the end of irradiation.

These studies showed that the chromosomes are the most vulnerable part of the dividing cells. Indeed doses of radiation much larger than those which caused chromosomal injury produced no ill effect if directed on to the cytoplasm or the mitotic spindle. Thus, although passage of a few dozen protons through a metaphase plate regularly resulted in formation of bridges between separating chromosomes, hundreds or even thousands of protons to other parts of the nucleus or cytoplasm produced no detectable effect.

This sensitivity of the chromosomes to irradiation increased ten-fold from prophase to metaphase and appeared to depend on the degree of condensation of chromatin (p. 126). After irradiation of the condensed chromosomes at metaphase the formation of sticky bridges between them retarded or abolished transition to anaphase. With large doses of α-particles the chromosomal material was clumped at metaphase, while the cells failed to divide and died soon afterwards.

Chromosomal aberrations induced by irradiation

Although the chromosomes during mitosis itself are thus immediately damaged by radiation, chromosomal aberrations are also readily induced by irradiation of cells during other phases of the cell cycle. This kind of damage depends on invisible macromolecular lesions which only become revealed as the chromosomes reappear as discrete visible entities with the onset of mitosis.

During G_1 phase of interphase (Fig. 4.13) the DNA of each chromosome is dispersed in an extended double helix visible as a single feebly stainable thread of chromatin, except where it is contracted into tight coils (chromomeres). After replication in S phase each chromosome enters G_2 phase as a *pair* of threads still joined at one point (the centromere). In the prophase of mitosis these paired feebly stainable threads contract and thicken into chromosomes and so emerge at metaphase as the familiar diads comprising two darkly staining paired chromatids still conjoined at their centromere (Fig. 4.13). After splitting of the centromere the two chromatids separate completely in anaphase.

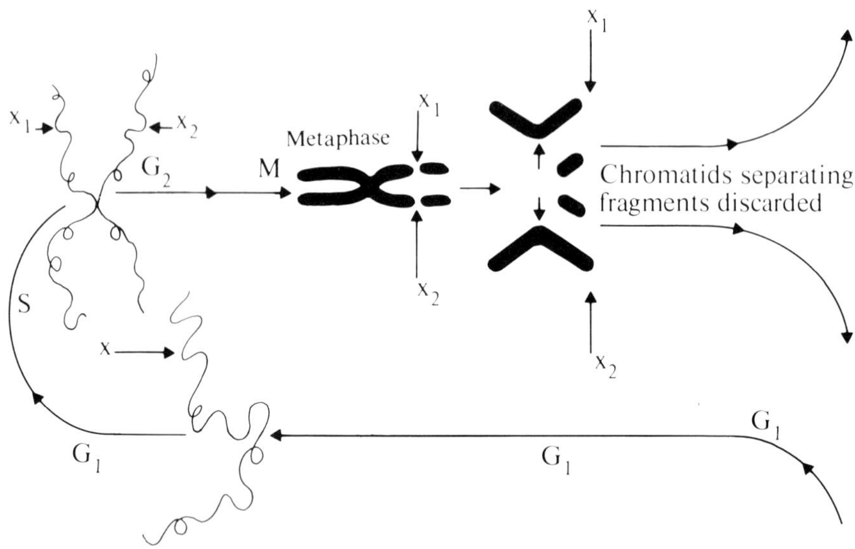

FIG. 4.13 Phases in duplication of a single chromosome during the mitotic cycle (diagrammatic) showing duplication of a lesion inflicted by radiation during G_1 (or G_0) phase. This caused a chromosome-type aberration with formation of a pair of symmetrical fragments.

G_1 interphase gap 1: single thread of chromatin
S interphase DNA synthesis: duplication of each thread of chromatin
G_2 interphase gap 2: duplicated threads of chromatin still joined at centromere
M mitosis: duplicated threads of chromatin condense to form a pair of chromatids (diads) which then separate.
x initial position of a lesion inflicted by radiation during G_1
x_1 and x_2 subsequent positions of the same lesion after duplication during S; x_1 and x_2 are shown first in G_2 and then at two successive stages in mitosis during which these twin lesions cause the release of a pair of identical fragments.
(The double helical molecular structure of each thread of chromatin is not indicated in this diagram.)

Injury by radiation is most commonly initiated during long lasting G_1 or G_0 phase at a locus which later becomes duplicated and thus results in latent identical defects in both chromatids; the latter subsequently condense during mitosis when the injury becomes visible. This damage affecting both chromatids at homologous points is called chromosome-type aberration, and it indicates that damage was initiated *before* replication; this damage includes formation of paired fragments (Fig. 4.13) as well as more complex rearrangements such as translocation and formation of dicentrics when more than one chromosome is fragmented [67, 68].

Injury by radiation during G_2 phase, on the other hand, damages already replicated DNA and the lesion is therefore not duplicated before mitosis. Such lesions affect only one chromatid in a diad and are called *chromatid-type* aberrations; this type of change can only be initiated during a relatively short stage of the cycle and thus occurs much less frequently than chromosome-type injury.

Some of the aberrations appearing in mitotic chromosomes as a sequel to previous radiation cannot survive mitosis [67]. The damaged chromatids may fail to separate at anaphase and cause lagging followed by arrest of mitosis and cell death. The number of abnormalities of karyotype induced by radiation is thus greatest at the first mitosis after exposure, because many of the fragments or even whole cells do not survive long enough to reach a subsequent mitosis. Indeed much of the 'pykonencrosis' produced by radiation among rapidly dividing cells such as intestinal epithelium may be an extreme result of injury to chromosomes which become lethal to the cells as they enter mitosis.

The effects of radiation on chromosomes of human cells are usually observed in lymphocytes of peripheral blood, which are normally in protracted G_1 (G_0) phase and remain in this phase unless stimulated to divide. On treatment of human lymphocytes *in vitro* with phytohaemagglutin (a mitogenic plant lectin) mitosis occurs in about 48 h in culture. When lymphocytes are first exposed to radiation (*in vivo* or *in vitro*) and are then treated with phytohaemagglutin (PHA) *in vitro*, chromosomal alterations become visible at the first mitosis in culture [67]. Since all these cells are in G_1 phase at the time of irradiation, the aberrations are of chromosome-type and are duplicated at identical points in each pair of chromatds at the first mitosis.

Observations of this kind show that chromosome-type aberrations frequently appear in the dividing lymphocytes of patients after exposure to therapeutic doses of X-rays. Moreover lymphocytes taken from the blood of persons who had previously been exposed to atomic explosions developed significantly more aberrations on stimulation to division than lymphocytes from control subjects. Also a higher proportion of chromosomal abnormalities (0.52 per cent of mitotic cells examined) was found among dividing lymphocytes of persons who had been exposed to atomic explosions in *prenatal life* more than 20 years earlier, than in similar cells from control subjects (0.04 per cent). These abnormalities included dicentrics, rings and free fragments, which are usually eliminated from cells in culture before the next mitosis. These cells had probably not divided since the time of prenatal irradiation [59]. The development of these aberrations thus illustrate the extremely long latent period which may occur between incidence of a macromolecular lesion induced by radiation and the first visible genomic abnormality.

Probably these cells which survive with latent karyotypic lesions are only a minute proportion of those in which such damage was initially inflicted. Thus chromosomal aberrations were visible in 70 per cent of the metaphases observed directly in bone marrow cells taken from a man 29 h after he was accidentally exposed to intense γ-radiation from ^{60}Co, while leucocytes from his peripheral blood, during the first day after the accident, developed aberrations in at least 25 per cent of the cells at their first mitosis in culture [54, 69]. Although most of such aberrant cells are discarded after their first mitosis, it is possible that some may later survive division and initiate neoplasia.

Lethal action of radiation: survival of irradiated cells

Measurement of survival on subculture *in vitro* of irradiated cells shows that dividing mammalian cells are most sensitive to killing by radiation during mitosis itself and least sensitive during S phase [61].

The extremely lethal effect of irradiation at mitosis, after synthesis of DNA is complete, indicates that inhibition of synthesis of DNA is not a principal factor in causing cell death after radiation. Moreover small lymphocytes are rapidly killed by X-rays when they are *not* dividing (and are in G_0 phase). This phenomenon of zero-phase death is also displayed (p. 127) by granule cells of cerebellum, which cannot divide but are singled out as targets for most rapid injury by extreme doses of radiation; this may depend on the aggregated state of chromatin in the small condensed nuclei of these cells.

The lethal effect of radiation, when assessed in synchronously dividing hamster cells in culture, correlates with the capacity to induce chromosome aberrations, and both these effects change in unison with phases of the mitotic cycle [70]. Increase in sensitivity (with diminution of survival) is associated with condensation of chromatin which becomes aggregated in M and dispersed in S phase. Possibly the proximity of points of injury ('hits') in closely aggregated DNA of mitotic cells may enable separate sublethal lesions to interact so that a lethal lesion ensues [70].

Damage to chromosomes produced by radiation and observed by phase contrast microscopy can be directly correlated with loss of ability of the same irradiated cells to form colonies in culture [71]. Thus, after irradiation of actively dividing hamster fibroblasts in G_1 phase, the formation of chromosome fragments at the *first* subsequent mitosis proved to be a most reliable indication of future loss in reproductive capacity. Indeed, many of these damaged cells did not divide again, while control cells produced many hundreds of descendants in the next few days.

Damage to chromosomes is clearly a major factor in the necrotising action of harmful radiation.

Mechanism of injury by radiation

When radiation ionizes or excites atoms within cellular molecules free radicals are formed and the molecules containing them tend to decompose. This decomposition may be harmful because *either* the substance destroyed is an essential component on which cellular life and survival depends *or* the products formed are themselves noxious.

The first of these postulated mechanisms is called 'direct' or 'target' action, the second 'indirect' or 'toxigenic' action.

Direct target action

This view supposes that the substance initially altered or decomposed is of such paramount importance to the cell that its alteration or decomposition is directly responsible for cellular derangement. If the ionized or excited atoms or the free radicals, which they form, are part of an irreplaceable target such as DNA, severe or irreparable damage may be inflicted on the cell by chemical change directly affecting only a small part of such a uniquely coded macromolecule.

It is possible, however, that free radicals generated from decomposition of water might be in such proximity to DNA as to initiate similar unique macromolecular lesions. In any case the concept, that change in DNA is the prime cause of injury and death of cells resulting from radiation, receives extensive support from the observed effects of radiation on cells and their nuclei.

Action on cellular DNA

Effects of radiation which almost certainly depend on alteration of cellular DNA will now be summarised.

Delay in onset of mitosis. Small doses of radiation can retard the onset of mitosis without killing the cells, which are most sensitive to this effect during S phase (p. 131). Although delay in onset of mitosis is not in itself lethal to cells, it can be very harmful in arresting replacement of cells with short life span such as enteroblasts of intestinal crypts or haemopoietic cells of bone marrow.

Vulnerability of aggregated DNA to radiation. The sensitivity of cells to killing by radiation in different phases of the cell cycle is highest during mitosis itself when the chromatin is most condensed (p. 134). Moreover chromosomes are much more easily damaged by microbeams of protons or α-particles than other parts of the cell (p. 131). This vulnerability of the chromosomes to particulate radiation increases greatly during transition from prophase to metaphase and appears to depend on the degree of condensation of chromatin. Indeed the action of microbeams clearly pin-points the chromosomes as the principal target for injury by radiation. Small lymphocytes which are in protracted interphase are also extremely sensitive (p. 128); this may depend on the small size of their nuclei with high concentration of DNA in aggregated chromatin. The remarkable correlation between extent of condensation of DNA and lethal potency of radiation points to DNA being the principal locus of damage.

Invisible chromosomal lesions revealed by mitosis. X-irradiation applied in G_1 phase *before* duplication of DNA results in latent lesions, which become revealed as chromosome-type aberrations when mitosis later occurs (p. 132, Fig. 4.13). These lesions affect *both* chromatids of the damaged chromosomes at identical points; this shows that each initial latent lesion must become duplicated as DNA is duplicated, thus indicating that the substance injured by radiation is DNA itself. Moreover, irradiation later in G_2 phase, *after* duplication is finished, causes chromatid-type aberrations in which single chromatids are injured in isolation.

Latent oncogenic effects. Neoplasia induced by exposure to X-rays or to atomic reactions usually occurs after a long latent period (p. 129). Such development of neoplasia probably depends on initial change in DNA, which may be the only cellular constituent capable of persisting long enough in an altered *replicable* state and so be able to produce a clone of neoplastic cells after a long lapse of time.

Changes in cutaneous DNA induced by UVL. Excessive irradiation by UVL causes epidermal necrosis and also induces latent change in the skin of Europeans which increases the incidence of cutaneous neoplasia. UVL also produces rapid antigenic change in DNA of epidermal nuclei (p. 129). UVL probably acts on DNA by forming covalent bonds between adjacent pyrimidine nucleotides [72, 73]. This change involves the formation of dimers composed of two interlinked pyrimidine residues in a DNA chain (Fig. 4.14). Linkage of this kind can profoundly interfere with function of DNA by preventing both replication of DNA itself and transcriptions of mRNA. This may account for the necrotising action of UVL. Normal cells however are able to excise such pyrimidine dimers from DNA and repair the fragmented chain by inserting

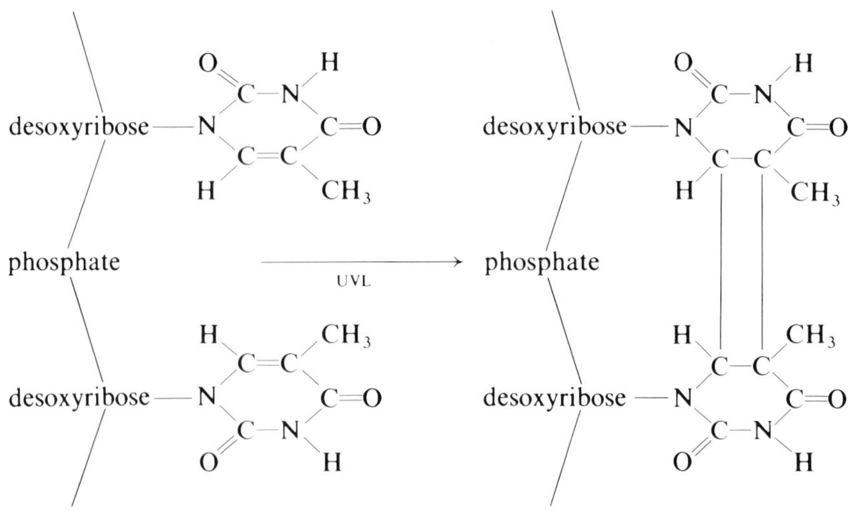

FIG. 4.14 Action of UVL in linking two thymine residues in DNA to form a pyrimidine dimer.

nucleotides into it, using the intact complementary strand as a template for refilling the gap [73]. This mechanism becomes prominent in normal skin fibroblasts in culture which, after irradiation by UVL, incorporate ^{3}H-thymidine into their nuclei at greatly enhanced rate. This process is called *repair-replication* and is readily revealed by autoradiography. The augmentation of incorporation of ^{3}H-thymidine after exposure to UVL indicates that alteration of DNA itself is a central event in cellular injury by UVL. The damaging effect of UVL on DNA becomes much more serious when repair replication is defective (p. 470).

These examples of change in DNA produced by radiation provide unambigious evidence that alteration of DNA is a paramount determinant of cellular injury produced by radiation. The remarkable correlation of susceptibility of cells to radiation with increase in concentration of DNA may depend on the proximity of independently *sublethal* lesions in a DNA strand, which may summate to form lethal lesions when sufficiently close to one another.

Indirect or toxigenic action

Some of the substances initially altered or decomposed may not be of such crucial importance to the cell that their decomposition accounts for all the damaging effects of radiation. Indeed the products of such initial decomposition may be harmful in themselves and so *indirectly* kill or injure cells.

Water, which is by far the most abundant constituent of cells, may act as such an indirect source of toxic products. When water molecules in aqueous solutions are ionized or excited by radiation H and OH radicals are likely to be formed [74, 75]:

$$H_2O \longrightarrow H^{\bullet} + OH^{\bullet}$$

These free $H^{\bullet}$ and $OH^{\bullet}$ radicals react avidly with oxidising and reducing agents respectively. If dissolved O_2 is present, this may react with $H^{\bullet}$ to form a peroxy radical $HO_2^{\bullet}$. Such a radical would be extremely reactive and would almost certainly oxidize SH groups in cells to SS. But in the absence of oxygen most of the free radicals may recombine thus eliminating their toxic potential.

The formation of toxic products by radiolysis of water in the presence of oxygen may thus be of importance in the action of radiation in damaging tissues. This view is supported by the remarkable effects of lack of oxygen in preventing damage induced by radiation.

Newborn mice can survive *anaerobiosis* in N_2 or CO_2 for 10–20 min (p. 92). This treatment causes respiratory and cardiac arrest as well as cooling. On warming these cold asphyxiated mice in *air* they revive completely. When such mice were exposed to X-rays (1500 rad) *during anaerobiosis* and then revived, they survived *entirely unharmed*; but, after exposure to the same dose of X-rays in the *presence of air*, all the mice developed severe oedema with cutaneous burns and died within 12 days [76, 77].

Similar protection was achieved by injecting *reducing agents*. Thus injection of thiourea into mice before irradiation with an otherwise lethal dose of X-rays enabled 50 per cent of the animals to survive [51]. Moreover, pretreatment with thiourea completely annulled the effect of sublethal doses of radiation in eliminating red marrow from the bones of irradiated mice. Thiourea in solution enters equilibrium

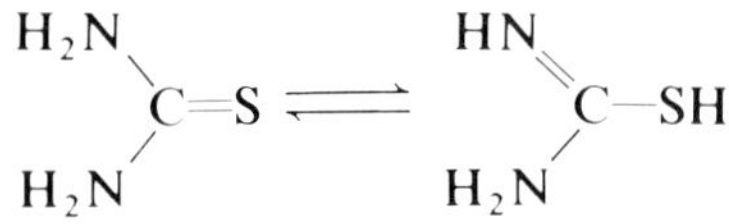

and thus provided —SH groups capable of removing oxygen and other oxidising agents from tissues. These results emphasise that much of the harmful action of radiation is dependent on the presence of oxygen.

The action of radiation in causing *chromosomal alterations* in plant cells and in tissue cultures of animal cells is also diminished by *anaerobiosis* [68, 78, 79]. This effect is cited as evidence that products of radiolysis of water are oxidised to form toxic products responsible for radiation damage. However oxidising agents by *themselves* have not been shown to cause the singularly characteristic aberrations induced by radiation on chromosomes. It seems more likely that radiation causes direct intramolecular changes in DNA, which result in fission to form free radicals or ion pairs. In the absence of oxygen many of these dissevered radicals may recombine. But this protective recombination of metastable dissociated macromolecules may be prevented by oxidising agents formed from water in the presence of oxygen. This view is supported by the fact that some chromosome aberrations can still be induced by irradiation even in anaerobiosis [79]. Direct damage induced by action of radiation on DNA or other macromolecules may thus at first be latent and only become irreversible after subsequent re-arrangements of metastable products especially in the presence of oxygen.

Conclusion

Alterations in structure or conformation of DNA are thus probably the major determinants of lethal and genomic injury induced in cells by radiation. However these alterations may be augmented or finalised by the action of oxidising agents generated by the radiolysis of water in the presence of oxygen; without this additional indirect effect much of the initial damage may be reparable. Free radicals formed by radiolysis of water may, however, also be concerned in producing injurious alterations to the structure of DNA.

REFERENCES

[1] Blackwood W. (1963) Vascular disease of the central nervous systems. In *Greenfield's Neuropathology*, p. 125, 2nd ed. Arnold, London.

[2] Yates P. O. (1976) Vascular disease of the central nervous system. In *Greenfield's Neuropathology*, p. 133, 3rd ed. Arnold, London.

[3] Sevitt S. (1977) The mechanisms of traumatic rupture of the thoracic aorta. *Brit. J. Surg.*, **64**, 166.

[4] Sevitt S. (1977) The significance and pathology of fat embolism. *Ann. Clin. Res.*, **9**, 173.

[5] Sevitt S. (1973) The significance of fat embolism. *Brit. J. hosp. Med.*, **9**, 786.

[6] Waller A. (1850) *Phil. Trans.*, London, 423.

[7] Ramon y Cajal S. (1928) *Degeneration and Regeneration of the Nervous System*, Vol. 2 (translated by R. M. May). Oxford University Press, London.

[8] Wolman M. (1968) Diseases of the myelin. In *Pathology of the Nervous System*, p. 758, ed. by J. Minckler. McGraw Hill, New York.

[9] Lee J. C.-Y. (1963) EM of Wallerian degeneration. *J. comp. Neurol.*, **120**, 65.

[10] Williams P. L. & Hall S. (1971) Prolonged *in vivo* observations of normal peripheral nerve fibres and their acute reactions to crush and deliberate trauma. *J. Anat.* (Lond.), **108**, 394.

[11] Weiss P. & Hiscoe H. B. (1948) Experiments on the mechanism of nerve growth. *J. exp. Zool.*, **107**, 315.

[12] Nissl F. (1892) Über die veränderung der ganglienzellen am facialskern des Kannichens nach ausreissung der nerven. *Allg. Z. Psychiat.*, **48**, 197.

[13] Marinesco G. (1909) *La Cellule Nerveuse*, Vol. 1 & 2. Doin, Paris.

[14] Brattgard S. O., Hyden H. & Sjostrand J. (1957) The chemical changes in regenerating neurones. *J. Neurochem.*, **1**, 316.

[15] Liebermann A. R. (1971) The axon reaction: a review of the principal features of perikaryal response to axon injury. *Int. Rev. Neurobiol.*, **14**, 49.

[16] Strich S. J. (1961) Shearing of nerve fibres as a cause of brain damage due to head injury. *Lancet*, **2**, 443.

[17] Strich S. J. (1970) Lesions in the cerebral hemispheres after blunt head injury. *J. clin. Path.*, suppl., **4**, 166.

[18] Williams D. & Denny-Brown D. (1941) Cerebral electrical changes in experimental concussion. *Brain*, **64**, 223.

[19] Ward A. A. (1958) Physiological basis of concussion. *J. Neurosurgery*, **15**, 129.

[20] Foltz E. L. & Schmidt R. P. (1956) The role of the reticular formation in the coma of head injury. *J. Neurosurg.*, **13**, 145.

[21] Chasen J. L., Hardy W. D., Webster J. E. & Gurdigan E. S. (1958) Alterations in cell structure associated with experimental concussion. *J. Neurosurg.*, **15**, 135.

[22] Leach E. H., Peters R. A. & Rossiter R. J. (1944) Experimental thermal burns, especially at moderate temperatures. *Quart. J. exp. Physiol.*, **32**, 67.

[23] Peters R. A. (1945) The biochemical lesion in thermal burns. *Brit. med. Bull.*, **3**, 81.

[24] Moritz A. R. & Henriques F. C. (1947) Studies on thermal injury. II The relative importance of time and surface temperature in the causation of cutaneous burns. *Amer. J. Path.*, **23**, 695.

[25] Moritz A. R. (1947) Studies on thermal injury. III The pathology and pathogenesis of cutaneous burns: an experimental study. *Amer. J. Path.*, **23**, 915.

[26] Hurley J. V. (1972) *Acute Inflammation.* Churchill Livingstone, Edinburgh.

[27] Belehradek J. (1935) Temperature and living matter. *Protoplasma Monographien (Berlin)*, **8**, 214.

[28] Heilbrunn L. V. (1924) The colloid chemistry of protoplasm. III The viscosity of protoplasm at various temperatures. *Amer. J. Physiol.*, **68**, 645.
[29] Heilbrunn L. V. (1924) The colloid chemistry of protoplasm. IV The heat of coagulation of protoplasm. *Amer. J. Physiol.*, **69**, 190.
[30] Singer S. J. & Nicholson G. L. (1972) The fluid mozaic model of the structure of cell membranes. *Science*, **175**, 720.
[31] Moritz A. R., Henriques F. C., Dutra F. R. & Weisiger J. R. (1947) Studies on thermal injury. IV An explanation of the casualty producing attributes of conflagration. *Arch. Path.*, **43**, 466.
[32] Sevitt S. (1966) Death after burning. *Med. Sci. Law*, Jan, 36.
[33] Sevitt S. (1979) A review of the complications of burns, their origin and importance for illness and death. *J. Trauma*, **19**, 358.
[34] Loebel E. C., Baxter C. B. & Curreri P. W. (1973) The mechanism of erythrocyte destruction in the early post-burn period. *Ann. Surg.*, **178**, 681.
[35] McLean R., Moritz A. R. & Roos A. (1947) Studies on thermal injury. VI Hyperpotassaemia caused by cutaneous exposure to heat. *J. clin. Invest.*, **26**, 497.
[36] Malamud N., Haymaker W. & Custer R. P. (1946) Heat stroke: a clinico-pathologic study of 125 fatal cases. *Milit. Surg.*, Nov, 397.
[37] Trump B. J., Goldblatt P. J., Griffin C. C., Waravdekar V. S. & Stowell R. E. (1964) Effects of freezing and thawing on the ultrastructure of mouse hepatic parenchymal cells. *Lab. Invest.*, **13**, 967.
[38] Smith J. J. & Fraser J. (1974) An estimation of tissue damage in thermal history in the cryolesion. *Cryobiology*, **11**, 139.
[39] Whittaker D. K. (1974) Ice crystals formed in tissues during cryosurgery: I Light microscopy. *Cryobiology*, **11**, 192.
[40] Whittaker D. K. (1974) Ice crystals formed in tissues during cryosurgery: II Electron microscopy. *Cryobiology*, **11**, 202.
[41] Lovelock J. E. (1954) Biophysical aspects of the freezing and thawing of living cells. *Proc. roy. Soc. Med.*, **47**, 60.
[42] Farrant J. & Morris G. J. (1973) Thermal shock and dilution shock as causes of freezing injury. *Cryobiology*, **10**, 130.
[43] Karow A. M. & Webb W. R. (1965) Tissue freezing: a theory of injury and survival. *Cryobiology*, **2**, 99.
[44] Farrant, J. (1975) Cryosurgery: cryobiology. *Brit. J. hosp. Med.*, **14**, 8.
[45] Nagington J. & Greaves R. I. N. (1962) Preservation of tissue culture cells with liquid nitrogen. *Nature*, **194**, 993.
[46] Alvord E. C. & Brace K. C. (1957) X-ray induced pyknosis of cerebellar granule cells in guinea-pigs and its suppression by barbiturate anaesthesia. *J. Neuropath.*, **16**, 3.
[47] Friedman N. B. (1942) Effects of radiation on the gastrointestinal tract including salivary glands, the liver and the pancreas. *Arch. Path.*, **34**, 749.
[48] Dustin P. (1951) Imitation chimique des radio-lésions cellulaires par les agents 'radiomimétiques'. *J. Radiol. Électrol.*, **32**, 333.
[49] Dustin P. (1952) Les poisons mitotiques 'radiomimétiques' et le métabolisme des nucléoprotéines. *Rev. belge Path.*, **22**, 55.
[50] Oughterson A. W. & Warren S. (1956) *Medical Effects of the Atomic Bomb in Japan.* McGraw Hill, New York.
[51] Mole R. H. (1951) Protection from whole body irradiation by chemical means. *J. Chim. phys.*, **48**, 258.
[52] Leroy G. V. (1947) The medical sequelae of the atomic bomb explosion. *J. Amer. med. Ass.*, **134**, 1143.
[53] Cronkite E. P. & Brecher G. (1952) Effects of whole body irradiation. *Ann. Rev. Med.*, **3**, 193.
[54] Vodopick H. & Andrews G. A. (1974) Accidental radiation exposure. *Arch. environm. Hlth*, **28**, 53.

[55] WHITEFIELD J. F. (1967) How radiation causes cell death. *Biomed. Eng.*, **2**, 78.
[56] MILLET P. G., WALKER J. B. & HOUGHTON L. E. (1960) Two-phase ulceration in guinea-pig skin following local irradiation with X-rays. *Brit. J. exp. Path.*, **41**, 160.
[57] TAN E. M. (1968) Antibodies to DNA irradiated by UV light: detection by precipitins & immunofluorescence. *Science*, **161**, 1353.
[58] TAN E. M. & STOUGHTON R. B. (1969) Ultraviolet light-induced damage to DNA in human skin. *J. invest. Derm.*, **52**, 537.
[59] BLOOM A. D. (1972) Induced chromosome aberrations in man. *Advanc. hum. Genet.*, **3**, 99.
[60] WATANABE I. (1974) Radiation effects on DNA chain growth in mammalian cells. *Radiat. Res.*, **58**, 541.
[61] SINCLAIR W. K. (1968) Cyclic X-ray responses in mammalian cells *in vitro*. *Radiat. Res.*, **33**, 620.
[62] KING D. W., PAULSON S. R., HANNAFORD N. C. & KREBS A. T. (1959) The effect of injury on the proteins and deoxyribonucleic acid of Ehrlich tumor cells. *Amer. J. Path.*, **35**, 369.
[63] ZIRKLE R. E. & BLOOM W. (1953) Irradiation of parts of individual cells. *Science*, **117**, 487.
[64] MONRO R. (1957) Alpha-irradiation of parts of single metaphase cells in chick embryo cultures. In *Advances in Radiobiology*, p. 100, ed. by G. C. de Hevesy, A. G. Forssberg & J. D. Abbatt. Oliver & Boyd, Edinburgh.
[65] DAVIS M. I., SIMON-REUSS I. & SMITH C. L. (1957) The irradiation of parts of single cells in tissue culture with micro beams of α-particles. In *Advances in Radiobiology*, p. 114, ed. by G. C. de Hevesy, A. G. Forssberg & J. D. Abbatt. Oliver & Boyd, Edinburgh.
[66] SMITH C. L. (1959) The irradiation of the chromosomes of single cells in metaphase with a microbeam of α-particles 5μ in diameter. *Proc. roy. Soc. B.*, **150**, 372.
[67] AWA A. A. (1974) Cytogenetic and oncogenic effects of the ionising radiations of the atomic bombs. In *Chromosomes and Cancer*, p. 637, ed. by J. G. German. Wiley, New York.
[68] EVANS H. J. (1974) Effect of ionising radiation on mammalian chromosomes. In *Chromosomes and Cancer*, p. 191, ed. by J. G. German. Wiley, New York.
[69] BREWEN J. G., PRESTON R. J. & LITTLEFIELD L. G. (1972) Radiation-induced human chromosome aberration following accidental whole-body exposure to ^{60}Co γ-rays. *Radiat. Res.*, **49**, 647.
[70] DEWEY W. C., NOEL J. S. & DETTOR C. M. (1972) Changes in radiosensitivity and dispersion of chromatin during the cell cycle of synchronous Chinese hamster cells. *Radiat. Res.*, **52**, 373.
[71] GROTE S. J. & REVELL S. H. (1972) Correlation of chromosome damage and colony forming ability in Syrian hamster cells in culture irradicated in G_1. *Corr. Top. Radiat. Res.*, **7**, 303.
[72] BEUKERS R. & BERENDS W. (1960) Isolation and identification of irradiation product of thymine. *Biochim. biophys. Acta* (*Amst.*), **41**, 550.
[73] Davidson J. N. (1972) *The Biochemistry of the Nucleic Acids*, 7th Ed. Chapman and Hall, London.
[74] LIVINGSTON R. (1952) *Symposium on Radiobiology: The Basic Aspects of Radiation Effects on Living Systems*, p. 56. ed. by J. J. Nickson. Chapman & Hall, London.
[75] WALLACH D. F. H. (1972) *The Plasma Membrane: Dynamic Perspective, Genetics and Pathology*, p. 145. English University Press, London.
[76] LACASSAGNE A. (1942) Chute de la sensitivité aux rayons X. *C. R. Acad. Sci.* (*Paris*), **215**, 231.
[77] LATARJET R. (1952) *Symposium on Radiobiology: The Basic Aspects of Radiation Effects on Living Systems*, p. 241. ed. by J. J. Nickson. Chapman & Hall, London.
[78] THODAY J. M. & READ J. (1947) Effect of oxygen on the frequency of chromosome aberrations produced by X-Rays. *Nature* (*Lond.*), **160**, 608

[79] GILES N. H. (1952) *Symposium on Radiobiology: The Basic Aspects of Radiation Effects on Living Systems*, p. 267. ed. by J. J. Nickson. Chapman & Hall, London.

CHAPTER 5

Action of Harmful Substances

Harmful substances injure cells by:

1. Direct effect on cell architecture by disarray or aggregation of orientated macromolecules.
2. Interference with enzymic action.
3. Toxigenesis: some substances, although not themselves directly noxious, react with others already present in the cell to generate harmful substances, or induce the synthesis of enzymes which then form substances with toxic action.
4. Chemical oncogenesis (ὄγκος, swelling or tumour), i.e. initiation or stimulation of neoplasia by harmful substances.
5. Antigenic action: some molecules, that may themselves be innocuous, injure by exciting the formation of antibodies or sensitised cells which can then react with the original antigen to cause harmful effects. The antigen may be a foreign substance or it may be liberated from constituents of the body itself. Harmful agents of this kind are considered in Chapter 6.
6. Toxic idiosyncrasy: the cells of some patients are indirectly injured by drugs such as aspirin which are relatively harmless to the majority of mankind. This kind of effect may be totally unconnected with antigen/antibody interactions and may depend on derangement in activity of intercellular transmitter substances.

DIRECT ACTION ON CELL ARCHITECTURE

Living cells are largely composed of laminated membranes enclosing cavities filled with viscous fluids. Substances that react with specific groups in cell membranes can denature, disorientate or dissolve portions of these complex laminae. Moreover, ligation with even a few loci may initiate widespread conformational changes in the membrane proteins or else promote extensive disarray of the liquid crystalline assembly of the membrane lipids. Harmful substances may also react with nuclear DNA or other unique internal constituents of the cell. Indeed, one substance may react with different portions of the fabric and so injure in more than one way. Lead salts can injure cells by combining with membrane proteins and they also inactivate various enzymes. Similarly folate analogues may act directly by clumping the chromosomes at metaphase but they can also interfere with synthesis of DNA before visible mitosis commences.

Silica

The injurious effects of silica SiO_2 are probably determined by hydrogen bonding of its hydrated form to cell membranes (see below). Crystalline particles of silica, which are inhaled by sandblasters and stonemasons, can cause serious lesions in the lungs. The resulting disease is called silicosis.

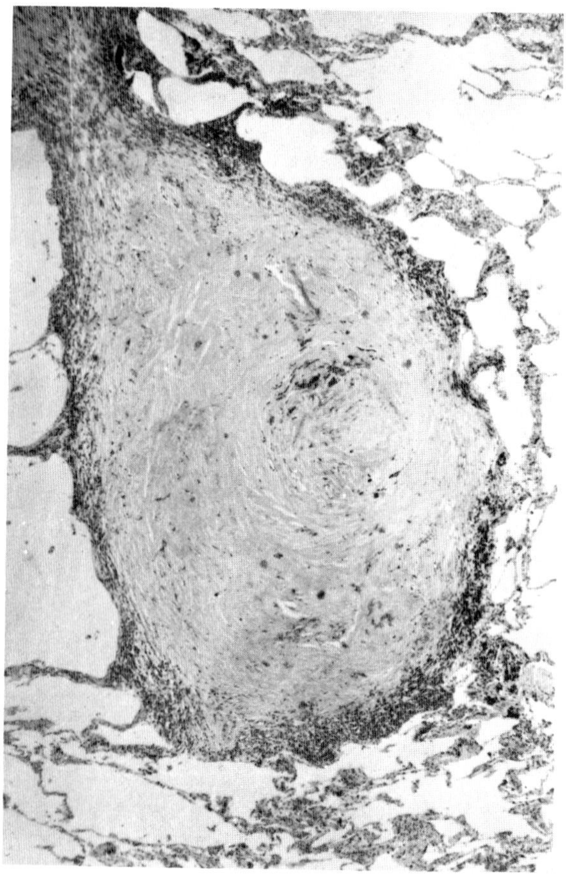

FIG. 5.1 Lung in silicosis. Nodule composed of whorls of collagen fibres in which micelles of hydrated SiO_2 are embedded. This fibrosis results in destruction of alveoli and vascular obstruction. Round the periphery of the nodule there is a dark rim composed of pulmonary macrophages containing black particles of carbon. ×30.

The dominant lesion in silicosis is focal fibrosis resulting in destruction of alveoli and obstruction of pulmonary circulation followed by severe hypoxia. Fibrous nodules also form in the interlobular septa. These nodules are composed of concentric laminae of collagen fibres surrounded by a cellular zone containing numerous macrophages. Fig. 5.1 shows one of these nodules surrounded by a rim of darkened macrophages blackened by ingested particles of carbon, which serve as a useful marker for human pulmonary phagocytes. These peripheral macrophages are visible at higher magnification in Fig. 5.2. The central zone of each nodule is occupied by dense whorls of collagen fibres. Minute angular particles of SiO_2 are present between these fibres which eventually become hyaline.

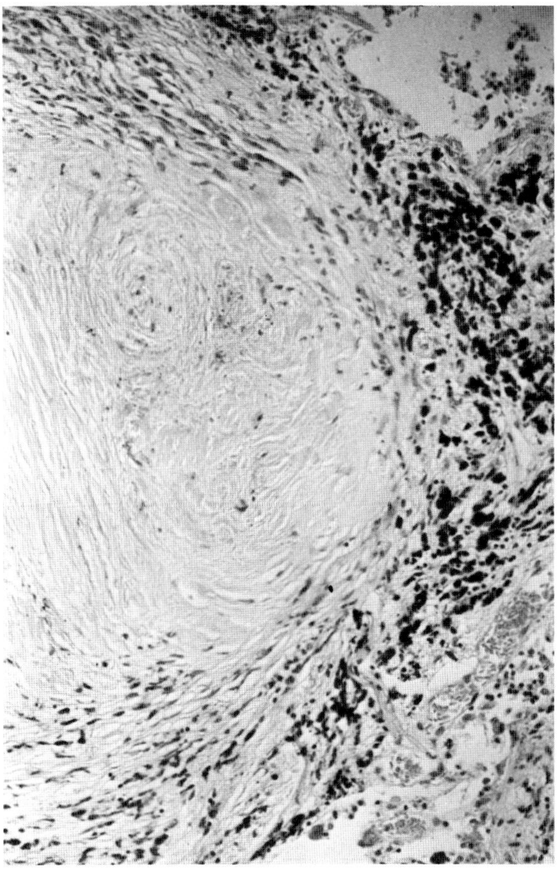

FIG. 5.2 Lung in silicosis. Part of a fibrous nodule showing whorled fibrous tissue surrounded by pulmonary macrophages. The pulmonary macrophages are blackened by previous ingestion of carbon, then are later replaced by fibrous tissue and so the nodules enlarge. ×130.

This actively harmful fibrosis, which is the basis of human silicosis, is probably a sequel to extensive necrosis of macrophages and other cells within the pulmonary tissue. Initially the macrophages have the misfortune to ingest highly toxic polymers of hydrated SiO_2, which are formed in the lungs after inhalation of SiO_2. These polymers probably injure the lysosomes of the macrophages, which are then killed with release of lysosomal enzymes; these liberated enzymes subsequently cause further necrosis of macrophages and other cells and this is followed by intense fibrosis. Thus the nodule expands as necrotic macrophages are replaced successively by fibrous tissue.

The mechanism of the harmful action of silica on macrophages was revealed by EM observations on mouse peritoneal macrophages which ingest fine particles of silica [1]. In medium *containing serum* the particles of silica are probably initially coated by protein and are then taken up by the macrophages without damage to the plasma membrane [2]. Within the cells the particles are first enclosed in membrane bound vesicles (phagosomes). These vesicles then fuse with lysosomes to form compound vesicles called phagolysosomes. Inside the phagolysosomes the protein coating the silica particles is digested by lysosomal proteases and the membranes become exposed to naked hydrated silica; the membranes are damaged and lysosomal enzymes together with free silica particles are discharged into the cytoplasm. Finally the plasma membrane of the cell is also damaged by the freed lysosomal enzymes and the naked particles of silica; the cells are then lysed and lyosomal enzymes along with particles of silica are released from the necrotic cells. After ingestion of silica by macrophages the ultimate lysis of their cell membranes is revealed by release of cytoplasmic enzyme lactate dehydrogenase along with lysosomal enzyme N-acetyl-β-D-glucosaminidase into the extracellular fluid [2]. Release of the enzymes corresponds to death of the macrophages which occurs within about 8 h after uptake of silica in the presence of serum. In the absence of serum the particles of silica are not coated by protein and cell death occurs more rapidly.

The toxicity of SiO_2 may largely result from damage to other cells by lysosomal enzymes released from the necrotic macrophages. The initial injury caused by SiO_2 within the macrophages probably depends on *hydrogen bonding* of *hydrated* SiO_2 to the membranes of the phagolysosomes; this view accounts for the fact that, when macrophages ingest particles of diamond dust which cannot be hydrated, lysosomal enzymes are not nearly so rapidly discharged as after phagocytosis of SiO_2 [1].

SiO_2 can also cause lysis of red cells. During this action of SiO_2 on red cells the hydrated SiO_2 complexes probably combine with protein [3]. Hydrogen atoms of hydrated silica may thus become adducted to arrayed loci of membrane macromolecules, so as to produce internal stress and realignment with consequential lysis or disintegration (Fig. 5.3).

Similar ligation of hydrated silica to the inner surface of secondary lysosomes within macrophages may thus injure the membranes (Fig. 5.3) so that both silica complexes and lysosmal enzymes escape into the cytoplasm. In this situation the hydrated silica may again damage the membrane from *within*, where the cell membrane is not protected by its outer glycoprotein cytocalyx;

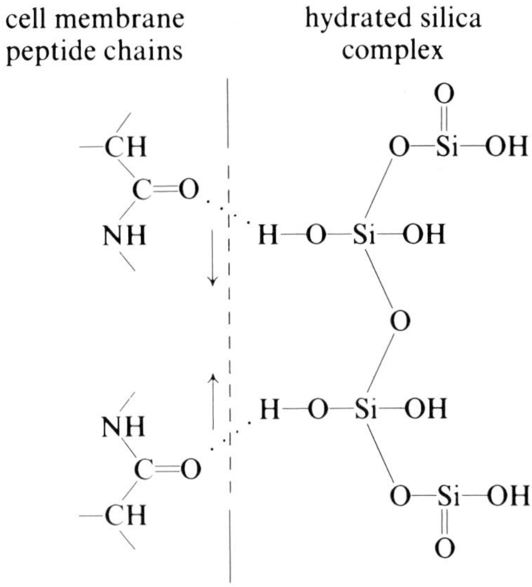

FIG. 5.3 Possible action of hydrated silica on cell membranes. Following adduction of hydrated silica complexes by hydrogen bonding to O atoms in peptide chains (or phospholipids) in membranes of secondary lysosomes and inside the cell surface, the membranes may become perturbed; this stress then may lead to disarray and lysis.

this causes irreversible rupture of the cell membrane and cell death. Once outside the cell the silica particles are again ingested by other macrophages, while the released lysosomal enzymes cause considerable damage to other cells.

The necrotising action of SiO_2 on macrophages is thus clearly an initial event in pathogenesis of silicosis but the later changes are more obscure. Possibly four successive processes occur [4]:

1. Necrosis of macrophages which have ingested SiO_2.
2. Attraction of more macrophages which then ingest SiO_2 liberated from killed macrophages.
3. Fibrogenesis with formation of collagen.
4. Hyalination of collagen.

To these may be added the toxic action of lysosomal enzymes released from the dying macrophages.

Lead salts

Lead ions (Pb^{++}) precipitate proteins by forming bridges between sulphydryl and carboxyl groups in adjacent peptide groups of proteins. They combine with proteins in cell membranes and thus produce direct structural damage. Lead ions may also exert profound effects by interfering with enzymic activity (see below); doubtless this action also depends on combination or chelation of lead with specific metallophil groups in enzymic proteins. Lead thus presents an example of a substance which may injure cells by different mechanisms.

Effects on red blood cells

Lead ions are rapidly taken up by red cells both *in vitro* and *in vivo*. In the blood of patients suffering from lead poisoning more than 90 per cent of the lead is bound to red cells, the remainder being bound to ligands in the plasma [5, 6]. After binding lead the red cells are in fact less easily lysed by hypotonic saline, but they become more fragile to trauma, and lysis occurs as these brittle leaded red cells impinge on each other and against the capillary walls in the flowing blood. This fragility probably depends on disarray of orientated protein molecules in the red cell envelope. Potassium ions as well as haemoglobin escape from the injured red cells [7, 8].

Anaemia in lead poisoning

Anaemia is a characteristic feature in man and animals after chronic ingestion of lead. The red cells show typical basophilic stippling and this is seen also in erythroblasts of the bone marrow; stippling may be due to aggregation of ribosomes by Pb^{++}. The anaemia of lead poisoning depends in part on the increased fragility to trauma of the leaded red cells (see above), which may be ruptured directly and have a shortened life span. Interference with synthesis of Hb also contributes to the anaemia; this interference is partly caused by enzymic inhibition (p. 150), but may also be an outcome of clustering of ribisomes by lead in the erythroblasts of bone marrow.

Lead intranuclear inclusions

A notable feature of prolonged ingestion of lead is the development of acidophilic intranuclear inclusions within the nuclei of renal and hepatic cells. Blackman [9] observed these intranuclear bodies in the convoluted tubules and cells of Henle's loop in the kidneys of children dying from lead poisoning. Similar inclusions form in the nuclei of renal cells of animals fed with lead salts. By EM these inclusion bodies show a dense central core with an outer fibrillar zone.

These intranuclear inclusions contain lead which can be detected by the formation of black particles of PbS on treatment with H_2S. The intranuclear lead is bound to protein as a complex which can be isolated by sonication followed by differential centrifugation; the complex contains 50 μg Pb/mg protein and the concentration of lead in the inclusion body is estimated as 60–100 times that in the kidney as a whole. Goyer & Rhyne [6] emphasised the protective value of this complex of Pb^{++} with protein; this serves as a protective mechanism for maintaining a low concentration of Pb^{++} in the renal and hepatic cell cytoplasm, while Pb^{++} are excreted by the kidney and the liver.

Although these inclusion bodies are found in the kidneys of children dying of lead poisoning, they are also present in the kidneys of rats fed on low doses of lead insufficient to cause any other ill effects. This conspicuous action of Pb^{++} in forming renal and hepatic intranuclear inclusions is probably a valuable protective mechanism in removing soluble Pb^{++}, which would otherwise cause profound damage [6]. Only when the inclusions become saturated with lead and no more complexes can form, does the concentration of Pb^{++} rise appreciably in the cytoplasm. Then and then only can free lead ions combine with enzymes, and mitochondrial swelling follows (see below). Indeed the intranuclear inclusions effectively bind the lead in an *indiffusible* form and thus lower the ionic concentration of lead available for diffusion into the cytoplasm and its organelles. In this way intranuclear inclusion bodies provide a virtually extracellular site for the sequestration of a potential poison.

Lead encephalopathy

The most serious effects of prolonged ingestion of lead occur in children who nibble objects covered by disintegrating flakes of old lead paint. These children lose weight and are irritable; they later develop convulsions, become drowsy and finally lapse into coma. The brain is swollen and is covered by serous perivascular exudate. Similar changes occur in the brain of suckling rats whose mothers are fed lead subacetate. In poisoned children and in these young rats the cerebral capillaries are maldeveloped; thus, possibly the cerebral damage, which includes necrosis and shrinkage of neurones, is due in part to hypoxia [10]. However, recent evidence (see below) suggests that the direct action of Pb^{++} on neuronal adenylcyclase is a basic event in the cerebral malfunction of lead poisioning.

Lead neuropathy

Ingestion of lead salts also causes paresis typified by wrist drop along with sensory loss. This disability is caused by demyelination of the peripheral nerves which undergo *segmental* degeneration. This change is confined to zones between two adjacent nodes of Ranvier and is limited to the myelin formed by single individual Schwann cells. Segmental degeneration thus contrasts with *Wallerian* degeneration (p. 108) which involves the *entire* fibre below the point of injury. In animals poisoned by lead the velocity of nerve impulses is diminished as a result of segmental degeneration [11]. EM observations reveal that lead poisoning causes separation of myelin lamellae with the formation of blebs in the myelin sheath of peripheral nerves. This change may result from reaction of Pb^{++} with the protein covering the arrayed surfaces of the myelin lipids.

Lead ions and enzymes

Pb^{++}can cause profound inhibition of enzyme action by ligation to active loci in enzymic proteins. These enzymic proteins are in some cases situated in cell membranes and then inhibition depends on ligation of Pb^{++} to portions of the membrane. For this reason action of Pb^{++} on enzymes is considered along with other features of lead poisoning, affecting cell architecture.

Pb^{++} conspicuously inhibit several enzymes concerned with the biosynthesis of haem. Thus δ-aminolaevulinic acid (ALA), formed by the condensation of glycine and succinyl-CoA, is normally then condensed to produce the initial haem-forming pyrrole porphobilinogen (PBG) by action of the enzyme ALA-dehydrase:

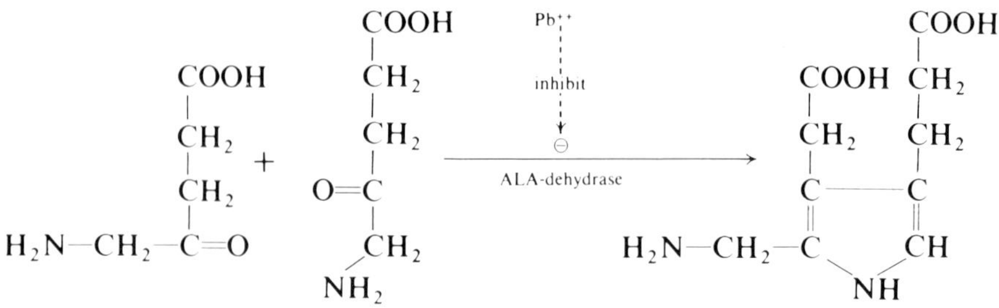

δ-aminolaevulinic acid (ALA) — Porphobilinogen (PBG)

ALA-dehydrase is inhibited by Pb^{++}, and ALA is therefore excreted in the urine in lead poisioning. This inhibition of ALA-dehydrase probably contributes to the anaemia caused by lead poisioning (p. 148).

Pb^{++} also inhibits *ferrochelatase*, which catalyses the final stage in the formation of haem by conjugation of protoporphyrin IX with Fe^{++}. This inhibition retards the whole sequence of interconversion of tetrapyrrole derivatives responsible for forming protoporphyrin, and results in the excretion of coproporhyrin III in the urine.

Interruption in the elaboration of haem thus contributes to the anaemia of lead poisioning in addition to the injurious effects of Pb^{++} on red cells and on the ribosomes of erythroblasts (p. 148).

Holmes *et al.* [12] showed that Pb^{++}, at very low concentration, inhibits adenylcyclase activity in homogenates of brain tissue. They suggested that inhibition of adenylcyclase in brain accounts for the action of lead in causing coma and convulsions as well as defects of behaviour such as hyperactivity and aggressiveness.

Adenylcyclase normally converts ATP into cyclic adenosine monophosphate (3^1,5^1-cAMP). Pb^{++} at a concentration of 3 μ mol/l inhibits this reaction by 50 per cent in homogenates of rat cerebellum.

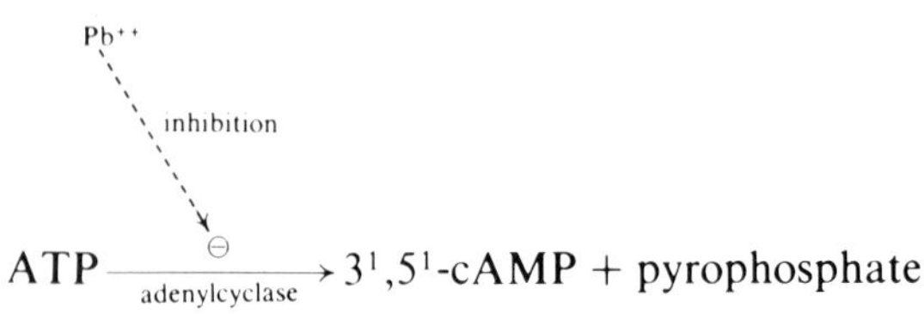

Rats display cerebral hyperactivity when the concentration of Pb^{++} in their brain reaches 3–6 μ mol/l, at which concentration adenylcyclase activity is inhibited by 50–70 per cent. In this way it is suggested that Pb^{++} can annul the action of noradrenaline which normally exerts its central activity by activating adenylcyclase. Holmes *et al.* also found that Pb^{++} markedly inhibits cerebral activity stimulated by noradrenaline.

INTERFERENCE WITH ENZYMIC ACTION

Inhibition of enzymic processes within the cell is harmful when:

1. Enzymic reactions generate energy for synthesising ATP or other exergonic compounds necessary for maintaining cell structure or macromolecular synthesis.
2. The products of enzymic reaction are needed by the cell.
3. The substrates of enzymic reaction are harmful if they accumulate in excess.

Interference with enzymic action by harmful substances depends on:

1. Denaturation of enzymes.
2. Specific disablement of their catalytic sites.
3. Competitive inhibition by mimicry of substrate.
4. Steric exclusion of enzyme from its site of action.

Denaturation of enzymes

Corrosive poisons and heavy metals, which disorganise the fabric of the cell and its membranes, also denature enzyme molecules and may immediately arrest cell enzymic processes. Hence agents such as formaldehyde and Hg^{++} preserve and stabilise partly because they preclude autolytic enzymic action.

Specific disablement of catalytic sites

We have seen how Pb^{++} can injure by combining with active groups in enzymes as well as in other proteins. The harmful action of some other substances, which also specifically combine with active loci in enzymes, will now briefly be considered.

Carbon monoxide: acute poisoning

This poison actively competes with oxygen for haemoglobin and thus causes most profound cellular hypoxia.

Normally O_2 is bound to Fe^{++} at four special sites, one in each of the two α- and β-peptide chains of the haemoglobin (Hb) molecule. These sites are called the 'haem pockets', and in each of them a molecule of haem with its constituent iron atom is accommodated. O_2 becomes reversibly attached to Fe^{++} within these haem pockets.

Like O_2, CO also combines with Fe^{++} embedded in these pockets of the Hb molecule. But CO is ligated more firmly than O_2; HbCO is then formed, from which O_2 can only very slowly displace CO. This accounts for the intense hypoxia produced in poisoning by CO. CO in fact combines with Fe^{++} situated at the same crucial sites in the α- and β-peptide chains of Hb, where normally O_2 is held by looser ligation to Fe^{++}.

CO also combines with other iron-porphyrin complexes besides those of the Hb molecule. Thus CO causes particularly injurious effects by ligation to Fe^{++}

in cytochrome oxidase. This attachment directly precludes the donation of electrons to molecular O_2 by intracellular cytochrome oxidase. The absorption of O_2 *by cells*, as well as by Hb, is in this way arrested by CO.

Thus CO exerts a dual toxic mechanism by:

1. Preventing carriage of O_2 to cells by the blood.
2. Eliminating the power of cells to absorb O_2.

This dual action of CO, in causing both anaemic and cytotoxic hypoxia, produces its most disastrous effects on the central nervous system. Acute poisoning by high concentrations of CO rapidly results in coma followed by respiratory paralysis and death, due to inactivation of the medullary neurones. After exposure to lower concentrations of CO the medullary neurones may survive intact. The patient may then recover completely even after temporary coma, *provided* the more susceptible neurones in cerebral cortex and basal ganglia have suffered no lethal injury. But unfortunately, even though the medullary centres are intact and respiration is maintained, the patient may never regain consciousness or may survive in a stuporous or lethargic state if these higher centres are injured. This tragic outcome of permanent cerebral disability is due to widespread necrosis of neurones in cerebral cortex, basal ganglia and midbrain, which may occur even though the medullary neurones are uninjured. Usually the grey matter of the globus pallidus in the lentiform nucleus of the corpus striatum is specially susceptible to damage by CO, and necrosis of the pallidal neurones is a prominent feature in patients who die after a few weeks of coma due to CO poisoning.

This extreme vulnerability of the pallidal neurones probably depends on the combined effects of toxicity of CO superimposed on local ischaemia. In the pallidal grey matter, as age advances, prominent deposition of iron and calcium salts occurs in the walls of the arterioles (pallidal siderosis); this change is accompanied by thickening of the intima with narrowing of the lumen, which results in local ischaemia.

Fig. 5.4 shows a zone of neuronal disintegration in the globus pallidus of a patient who died three weeks after inhalation of CO, having survived temporarily in stupor. The right side of the figure is occupied by cavities containing cerebral macrophages which are eroding remnants of the necrotic grey matter. The left side shows a branching arteriole with grossly thickened intima infiltrated by Fe^{+++} and Ca^{++} salts which are intensely coloured by haematoxylin; the arteriolar lumen is conspicuously narrowed. The combination of extreme hypoxia due to CO, superadded to the effects of ischaemia produced by local arterial occlusion, thus accounts for the selective necrosis of the pallidal neurones. Many of the dead neurones are rapidly consumed by phagocytes which remain within cystic cavities in the disintegrating grey matter.

Carbon monoxide: chronic poisioning

CO, even in very low concentration, is an insidious cause of chronic cell injury. By its intense avidity for Hb, CO can combine with a substantial fraction of the

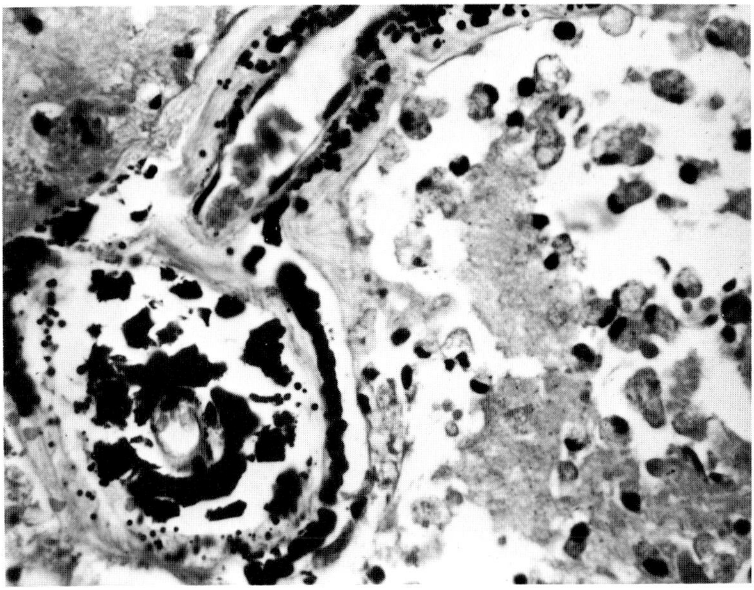

FIG. 5.4 Necrosis of cerebral grey matter in globus pallidus caused by carbon monoxide poisoning. Right side of field shows cerebral macrophages eroding the remnants of necrotic neurones. To the left is an arteriole narrowed by intimal thickening and infiltration with iron salts, which are intensely coloured by haematoxylin. Local ischaemia thus accentuates the necrotising action of CO. ×400. Courtesy of Professor C. W. M. Adams. *Neurohistochemistry*, 1965, p. 561. Elsevier, Amsterdam.

available Hb of the blood and so diminish transport of O_2. Thus about 15 per cent of Hb in the blood of rabbits, kept in air containing 0.17 per cent CO, is in the form of HbCO [13, 14]. Similarly CO, which is an important constituent of tobacco smoke, is inhaled by heavy smokers to an extent which converts 20 per cent of the Hb in their blood into HbCO.

Such chronic displacement of O_2 by CO may be extremely harmful to man and is probably a major determinant in the effect of cigarette smoking in promoting lethal cardiac infarction associated with atherosclerosis. Astrup pointed out that this effect may be increased by the higher affinity of CO for cardiac myohaemoglobin than for Hb. Thus chronic inhalation of CO may induce cardiac hypoxia and hypoxic necrosis in two ways:

1. By stimulating atherosclerosis with occlusion of coronary arteries (p. 389).
2. By replacing O_2 in Hb, in cardiac myohaemoglobin, and in cardiac cytochrome oxidase, by CO.

Cyanide

Cyanide ions (CN^-) also combine with the catalytic iron groups in cytochrome oxidase and, like CO, eliminate the active unit concerned with the transfer of electrons to molecular oxygen; cellular oxidation therefore cannot proceed and the main supply of energy to cells ceases. Without oxidation of glucose neurones convert glucose to lactic acid at a greatly increased rate. In animals poisoned by CN^- the concentration of lactic acid in the brain rises [15] and slices of cerebral cortex exposed to cyanide have an increased rate of aerobic glycolysis although the consumption of oxygen is inhibited [16]. But the supply of energy from this accelerated glycolysis is insufficient to maintain neuronal integrity. Thus small doses of cyanide cause coma and convulsions with irreversible cerebral damage, although the rest of the body is unharmed. Larger doses are followed by arrest of heart and respiration within a few seconds.

Arsenious oxide

Arsenious oxide (O=As—O—As=O) and arsenites act by eliminating the catalytic —SH groups of coenzyme A and of lipoic acid (6,8-dithio-octanoic acid), which are essential coenzymes for the oxidative decarboxylation of pyruvate (p. 51). The arsenite ion (derived from arsenious oxide) forms a stable complex with lipoic acid by ligating to its active —SH groups [17].

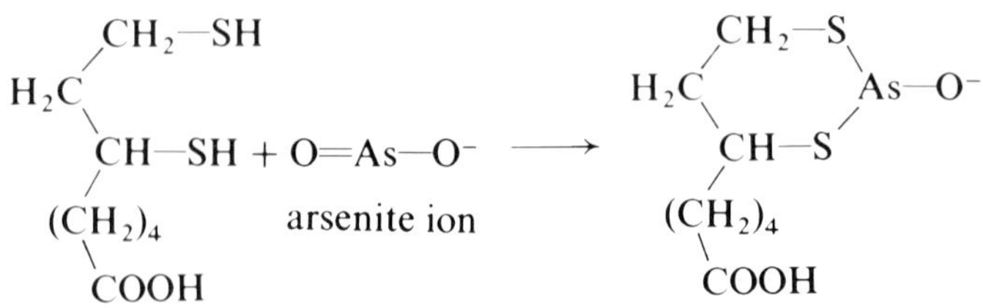

lipoic acid

stable complex of trivalent arsenic with lipoic acid

In the absence of these essential SH groups pyruvate accumulates in blood and tissues.

Thus the concentration of pyruvate rises in the blood of human patients poisoned by arsenic. Similarly substantial increase occurs in level of pyruvate in blood of pigeons and mice two hours after injection of sodium arsenite [18]. Moreover the uptake of O_2 by pigeon brain *in vitro* in the presence of pyruvate is intensely inhibited by concentrations of arsenite, which have little or no effect on respiration in the presence of other oxidisable substrates, such as succinate or α-glycerophosphate. This *selective inhibition* of oxidative catabolism of pyruvate depends on inactivation of lipoic acid by conjunction in a complex with arsenite ions.

Since oxidative decarboxylation of pyruvate is an essential stage in oxidation of glucose, arsenite injures cells by depriving them of their principle source of energy. Such injury affecting epithelial cells in the gastrointestinal tract produces vomiting and diarrhoea in the initial stage of acute arsenic poisoning. This is succeeded by coma and convulsions due to cerebral injury which only develops after the poison is absorbed into the blood. In chronic arsenic poisoning widely disseminated neuronal injury occurs. Thus damage to peripheral nerves causes degeneration of both myelin and axons resulting in paraesthesia and paresis, while injury to cerebral neurones causes terminal 'iditotic apathy'.

Copper salts

Subarachnoid injection of 10–25 μg Cu^{++} into pigeons causes immediate convulsions followed by death [19]. Moreover Cu^{++} *in vitro* at concentration of 20 μM inhibits microsomal ATP-ase from pigeon brain [20]. Cu^{++} at these concentrations do not inhibit the respiration of cerebral tissue. Peters & Walshe concluded that this extremely rapid action of Cu^{++} is exerted upon membrane surfaces: the microsomes show intense avidity for Cu^{++} as detected by binding of $^{64}Cu^{++}$.

Cu^{++} thus probably disables specific catalytic groups in cell membranes in a similar manner to the action of Pb^{++} on membrane-bound adenylcyclase (p. 150). Copper-protein complexes accumulate in the corpus striatum, liver and cornea in hepato-lenticular degeneration (Wilson's disease; p. 415). It is possible that the cerebral and hepatic lesions in this disease are determined by insidious damage by Cu^{++} to enzymic and membrane-bound protein.

Competitive inhibition by mimicry of substrate

Substances with constitution similar to the substrate of an enzyme can inhibit competitively and thus injure cells by retarding or annulling an essential reaction.

Fluorocitrate

This substance inhibits the utilisation of citrate by competitive inhibition of the enzyme aconitase. In this way it interrupts the citric acid cycle in brain and so eliminates the principal source of cellular energy in the cerebral cells. Peters and

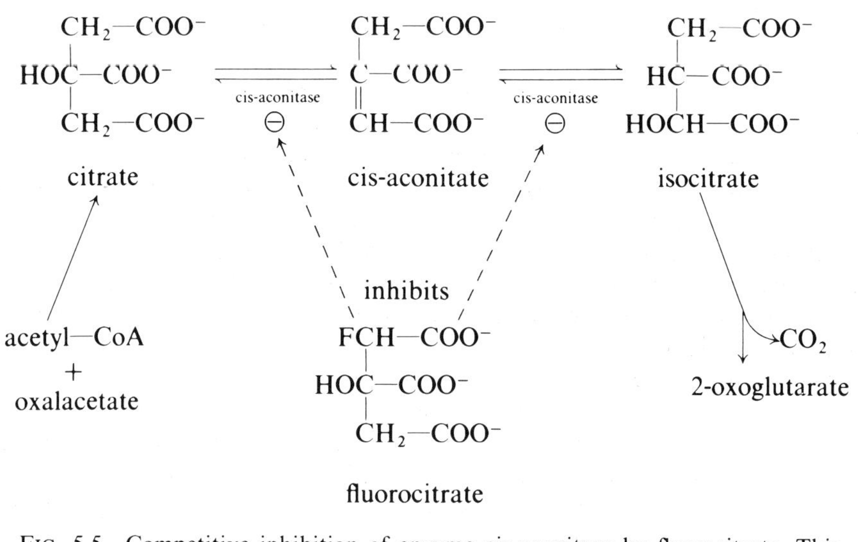

FIG. 5.5 Competitive inhibition of enzyme cis-aconitase by fluorocitrate. This interrupts the conversion of citrate to isocitrate in the tricarboxylic cycle.

his colleagues showed that intracerebral injection of fluorocitrate in minute amounts (less than 1 μg) kills rats in convulsions; it is thus one of the most poisonous substances known [21]. After intraperitioneal injection of fluorocitrate into rats, large amounts of citrate accumulate in brain, kidney, liver and heart [22].

Fluorocitrate specifically inhibits the enzyme cis-aconitase which is responsible for the conversion of citrate to isocitrate in the citric acid cycle of cellular oxidation (Fig. 5.5). This effect is conspicuous in homogenates of kidney, in which the activity of aconitase is 50 per cent inhibited by 10^{-8}–10^{-9}M fluorocitrate. Thus the citrate, formed from acetyl-CoA and oxalacetate during oxidation of carbohydrate or fat, accumulates and isocitrate is not formed. The tricarboxylic acid cycle is therefore arrested and the cells are deprived of their major source of energy (Fig. 5.5).

Fluorocitrate inhibits aconitase competitively by aping citrate in structure. Fluorocitrate thus ligates with the active enzyme sites and thereby annuls the further metabolism of citrate. By interrupting exergonic reactions in brain fluorocitrate can cause coma and convulsions. When animals (poisoned by fluorocitrate) survive up to two hours their renal tubular cells become swollen and show pyknosis and loss of mitochondria [23]. This necrotising effect is also probably due to suppression of essential supply of energy to the cells.

Although arrest of further metabolism of citrate in this way causes injury by depriving cells of exergonic reactions, fluorocitrate may also damage indirectly by causing large accumulation of citrate; this may combine with Ca^{++} within cerebral cells and so cause increase of their excitability.

Folate antagonists

Folate antagonists such as aminopterin (4-aminofolate) competitively inhibit the reduction of DHF to THF by DHF-reductase and NADPH (p. 55). Since THF is an essential catalyst for the biosynthesis of DNA, folate antagonists inhibit formation of DNA during the S phase of the cell cycle (p. 130).

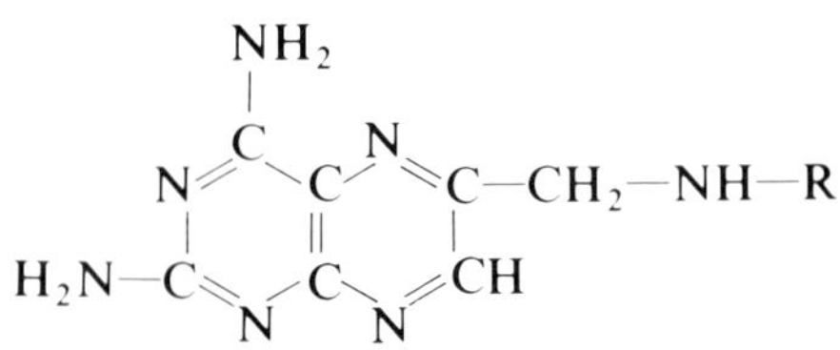

aminopterin
(4-aminofolate)

But folate antagonists also inhibit and arrest the process of mitosis itself (M phase). Thus, following injection of aminopterin into mice the number of mitoses among enteroblasts of the intestinal crypts is grossly diminished and the chromosomes become clumped at metaphase ('pyknonecrosis'); the cells then die instead of progressing to anaphase [24, 25]. This change is so like that produced by radiation that Dustin applied the term 'radiomimetic' to substances which exert this effect.

Aminopterin and its anologues similarly interrupt mitosis at metaphase in embryonic osteoblasts *in vitro* [26], and in bone marrow cells of children with leukaemia [27]. These substances also exert a potent effect in causing remission of some actively growing neoplasms such as acute leukaemia and choriocarcinoma.

Retardation of synthesis of DNA and onset of mitosis by folate antagonists doubtless results from competitive inhibition of reduction of DHF, which these substances so closely resemble in structure. But the mechanism of rapid clumping of chromosomes at metaphase with pyknonecrosis is obscure. It may be significant that radiation and also folate antagonists exert this dual effect.

Steric exclusion of enzyme from site of action: actinomycin

Exclusion of DNA-dependent RNA polymerase from nuclear DNA by a foreign ligand, which also binds specifically to DNA, probably accounts for the harmful effects of the fungal product actinomycin D.

Actinomycin is composed of an oxazine quinone-imine nucleus to which are attached two peptide chains each containing an internal ester linkage. It is a potent antiviral agent and also exerts rapidly necrotising effects on animal cells. Large doses administered to animals are lethal and selectively injure intestinal

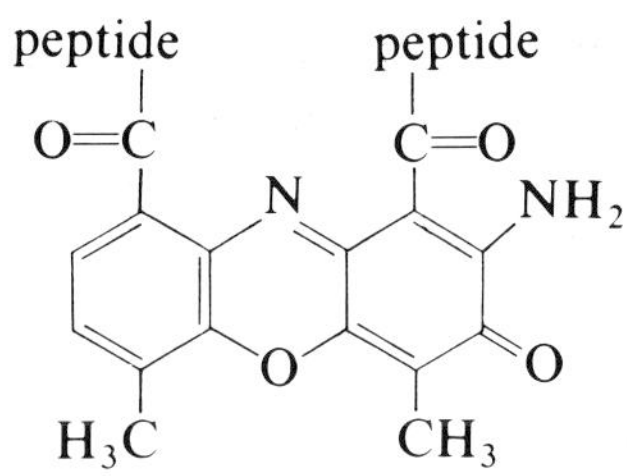

actinomycin D

epithelium, lymphoid tissue and bone marrow causing extensive nuclear karyorrhexis in the dying cells [28].

Actinomycin has a high affinity for DNA with which it forms a non-covalent complex [29]; its structure is similar to that of acridine dyes which also interact with DNA (and *not* RNA) to produce stable but reversible complexes. The quinone-imine group of actinomycin probably becomes bound to the desoxyguanosine in DNA, while the peptide groups may be packed into the small groove of the DNA helix [30]. Actinomycin therefore inhibits both DNA-polymerase and DNA-dependent RNA polymerase but the *latter* is much more intensely inhibited.

This ligation of actinomycin to DNA excludes the enzyme RNA-polymerase, already attached at one site of the DNA template, and prevents it from moving along the template in the process of transcribing and adding successive ribonucleotides to the growing RNA chain. The arrest of transcription is responsible for the necrotising action of actinomycin on rapidly dividing cells and also for its effect in disintegrating polyribosomes by preventing the replacement of mRNA. This latter effect is conspicuous in liver cells of rats treated by actinomycin *in vivo* [31]; presumably the monosomes separate when the supply of mRNA, which strings them together, is cut off.

TOXIGENESIS

Substances, which are themselves not directly noxious, may react with materials present in the body to form other substances which are actively harmful. Thudichum, in 1884, suggested that insanity might be caused by 'effects on the brain substance of poisons fermented in the body'.

In some instances cellular enzymes convert foreign substances which are innocuous into highly toxic derivatives. Such toxigenic enzymes are often situated in the microsomes and form part of the microsomal oxygenase system. In other cases foreign substances can affect the cell genome so as to evoke the previously suppressed synthesis of enzymes, which can then convert the original inducing agent or some other substance into a directly harmful product. The ultimate toxic product may directly injure and kill cells or it may change the genome so profoundly as to initiate neoplasia. Indeed many oncogenic substances are believed to undergo toxigenic conversion from initially innocuous compounds into ultimate direct oncogens.

Examples of toxigenic mechanisms will first be illustrated by the conversion of methanol and fluoracetate within the body to actively harmful agents. The contribution of the microsomal oxygenase system to activation of potentially harmful agents will then be discussed. Finally the action of foreign substances which injure by promoting enzymic induction will be considered.

Toxigenic action of methanol

Methanol would probably be no more poisonous than ethanol but for its intracellular oxidation by alcohol dehydrogenase to the highly toxic formaldehyde, which is then further oxidised by aldehyde dehydrogenase to formic acid:

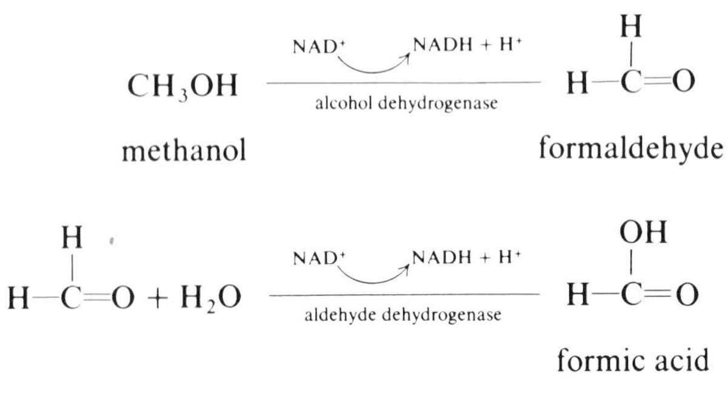

Both alcohol dehydrogenase and aldehyde dehydrogenase occur in liver cells and probably in other tissues as well. Formaldehyde can be detected as a product of oxidation of methanol by alcohol dehydrogenase [32]. When ^{14}C-methanol is fed to rats, it is largely converted to $^{14}CO_2$; this appears in the expired air, while traces of formic acid are found in the tissues [33].

Human poisoning by methanol first produces inebriation presumably due to direct action of this primary alcohol; this may then be followed by violent abdominal pain, blindness, coma and death with respiratory arrest. Patients who recover from coma may be blind owing to destruction of the ganglion cells of the retina with subsequent degeneration of the optic nerves. The optic discs and the nerve fibre layer of the retina become oedematous; the retinal ganglion cells degenerate and their dendrites become unstainable. The cell bodies are swollen and globose, while their cytoplasm becomes frayed and vacuolated and many of the ganglion cells disappear and are completely absent from some areas of the retina [34, 35]. In the brain there is subpial and cortical oedema, but little cellular change is visible possibly owing to the rapidity of death [34]. Microscopically the kidney tubules are well preserved. These retinal changes and the cerebral oedema coupled with good cellular preservation in other tissues may be related to the formation of formaldehyde within the cells where it acts as intracellular fixative with rapidly lethal effects.

Methanol and ethanol are each oxidised to their corresponding aldehyde by the same enzyme *alcohol dehydrogenase*. Ethanol can therefore *prevent* the oxidation of methanol by competitive inhibition. Indeed the oxidation of methanol to formaldehyde by alcohol dehydrogenase of liver is completely suppressed by addition of an equimolar quantity of ethanol [32]. Similarly the ingestion of ethanol by man inhibits the metabolism of methanol, more of which is then excreted unchanged in the urine [32]. Moreover, the expiration of $^{14}CO_2$ by the lungs of rats after feeding ^{14}C-methanol is diminished by simultaneous ingestion of ethanol [36].

This suppression of metabolism of methanol by administration of ethanol is utilised in treating human patients poisoned by methanol; treatment with ethanol averts or delays the onset of symptoms [35]. This effect also implies that the severe lesions produced by methanol depend on its metabolic conversion to a highly noxious agent.

The less immediately harmful effects of ethanol are considered in Chapter 8.

Fluoracetate

This substance is rapidly toxic to animals. About 20 min after injection of 5 mg/kg of fluoracetate to rats they suddenly go rigid in convulsions [37]. The animals may die from asphyxia during a convulsion; otherwise they usually collapse and die from heart failure within 24 hours. Dogs are more susceptible than rats and are killed by 1/100 of the dose that kills rats. In dogs the harmful effect of fluoracetate is principally on the nervous system, but in rabbits the heart is primarily affected.

Fluoracetate is not directly toxic; it inhibits no enzymic action itself, but by entering the citric acid cycle of metabolism in the same way as acetyl coenzyme A (acetyl-CoA), fluoracetate is converted into the highly toxic fluorocitrate, already discussed on p. 155. This view was proposed by Peters, who showed that citrate accumulates in enormous amounts in kidney, heart and brain of rats poisoned with fluoracetate; this suggested that the citric acid cycle is arrested.

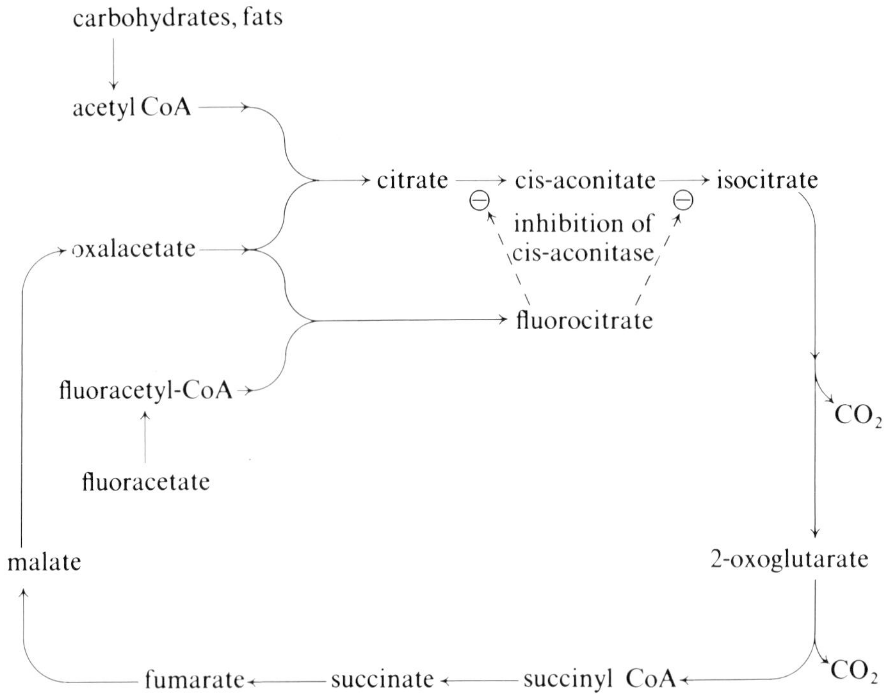

FIG. 5.6 Harmful action of fluoracetate (toxigenesis). Fluoracetate reacts with oxalacetate to form fluorocitrate, which then inhibits cis-aconitase and so prevents conversion of citrate to isocitrate. The tricarboxylic acid cycle is thus arrested and citrate accumulates.

Further investigation [38] showed that:

1. Fluorocitrate is formed from fluoracetate *in vitro* by homogenates made from kidneys of rabbits and dogs, and citrate simultaneously accumulates.
2. Fluorocitrate is highly toxic on intracerebral injection, but fluoracetate is relatively harmless by this route [22].
3. Fluorocitrate inhibits the enzyme cis-aconitase, which converts citrate first to cis-aconitate and then to isocitrate (Fig. 5.5).

Thus the harmful action of fluoracetate depends on its synthesis to fluorocitrate (Fig. 5.6).

Fig. 5.6 illustrates this intrusion of fluoracetate into the citric acid cycle. The highly toxic fluorocitrate is then formed from fluoracetate and oxalacetate by the same synthetic process which normally produces citrate from acetyl-CoA and oxalacetate. In this way, by mimicry of acetyl-CoA, fluoracetate is able to penetrate the citric acid cycle and thus generate a fluoro-derivative of citric acid. The latter then inhibits aconitase and thereby blocks the further metabolism of citrate itself and so heralds disaster from the cell. Peters aptly called this formation of fluorocitrate a lethal synthesis.

Toxigenesis by microsomal oxygenases

Attached to the endoplasmic reticulum in cells of liver and many other tissues are enzymes capable of converting various foreign organic molecules into highly reactive and potentially harmful derivatives. These enzymes occur in the microsomal portion of cellular homogenates and are active only in the presence of molecular oxygen. Their activity is also dependent on NADPH and cytochrome P-450. The action of these enzymes generally involves oxidation and they are conveniently termed microsomal oxygenases. The substrates of these enzymes include aromatic hydrocarbons, carbon tetrachloride (CCl_4), dimethyl nitrosamine and aromatic amines. These substances in their unaltered state and in small amounts are relatively harmless to cells; even in small amounts, however, owing to their solubility in lipids, they may enter cells and become metabolised by the microsomal oxygenases to form reactive derivatives which ultimately may cause cellular injury or abnormality by reacting with complex lipids, proteins or nucleic acids of the cell fabric.

The initial activation of organic substances by these oxygenases [39] probably depends on the formation of activated oxygen (p. 171) by the reaction.

$$NADPH + O_2 \rightarrow NADP^+ + OH^- + O$$

The activated oxygen then oxidises the organic substrate to a harmful product. Cellular disorders caused by the metabolic products of these toxigenic substances include hepatic necrosis (CCl_4, dimethyl nitrosamine), hepatic fatty change (CCl_4), necrosis of bone marrow (benzene) and neoplasia (dimethyl nitrosamine, aromatic hydrocarbons, aromatic amines). This oncogenic action will be considered in the section on chemical oncogenesis.

With some substrates the action of these microsomal oxygenases gives final products in which H is replaced by OH; for this reason the term hydroxylase has been used. Thus hydroxyl derivatives are formed from aryl hydrocarbons by these enzymes. However in this case an epoxide is almost certainly the initial highly reactive intermediary formed by the enzyme; the epoxide is then isomerised to form a hydroxylated hydrocarbon (Fig. 5.11). Thus the term oxygenase is a more appropriate designation of these microsomal enzymes, especially those which oxidise aromatic hydrocarbons.

Carbon tetrachloride

This poison, when inhaled, ingested or injected in toxic amounts, injures hepatic cells, causing necrosis, hydropic change and fatty globulation. The liver lobules of rats injected or fed with CCl_4 rapidly develop extensive centrilobular necrosis, midzonal hydropic change and fatty change affecting both midzonal and centrilobular cells, while the peripheral cells may show no signs of injury (Figs. 5.7 and 5.8). In man inhalation of fumes of CCl_4 or ingestion of fluid CCl_4, used in the treatment of hook-worm infestation, also produces acute hepatic injury, while more prolonged exposure to fumes may eventually be followed by hepatic cirrhosis.

Changes visible by EM in liver cells injured by CCl_4 include swelling of the

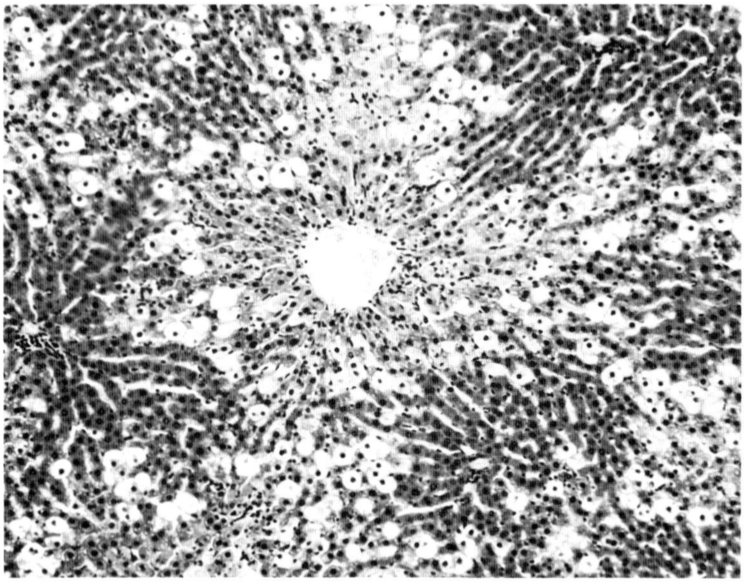

FIG. 5.7 Liver of rat one day after subcutaneous injection of CCl_4 0.75 ml/100 g body weight. Loss of basophilic material stainable by haematoxylin from centrilobular necrotic cells. Midzonal cells hydropic. Peripheral cells unaffected. ×110. Dixon K. C. & McCullagh G. P. (1957) *Quart. J. Exp. Physiol.*, **42**, 104.

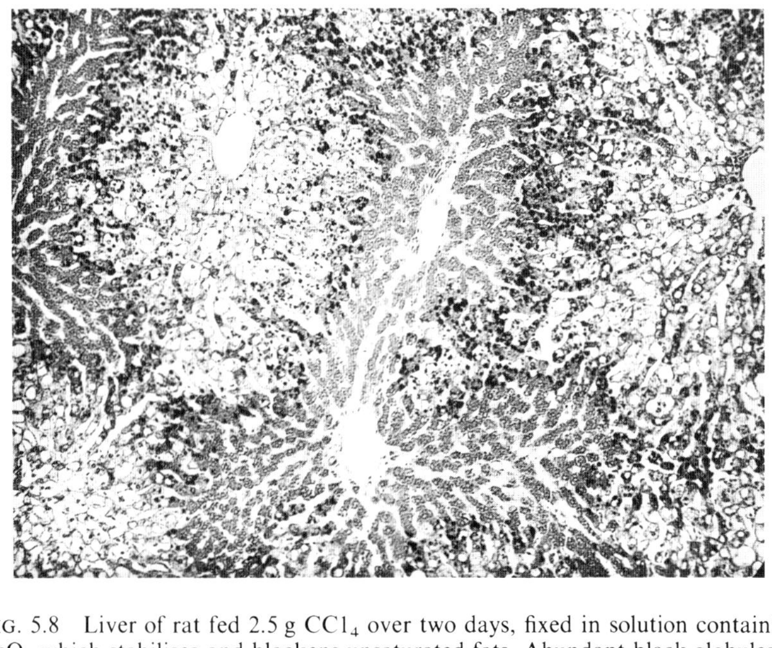

FIG. 5.8 Liver of rat fed 2.5 g CCl_4 over two days, fixed in solution containing OsO_4 which stabilises and blackens unsaturated fats. Abundant black globules of liquid lipid are visible in outer midzonal cells. Central cells appear hydropic and contain some droplets of lipid. Peripheral cells are unaffected. Counterstained by pyronin G. ×90. Dixon K. C. (1970) *Histochem, J.*, **2**, 151.

cisternae of ER, degranulation and loss of ribosomes from rough surfaced ER, with later swelling of mitochondria [40]. The loss of ribosomes from the ER doubtless accounts for the disappearance of basophilic zones of Berg, which is such a prominent feature visible by LM in the cytoplasm of the necrotic centrilobular cells (Fig. 5.7). In the midzonal cells swelling of cisternae of ER and of mitochondria proceeds to an extreme extent and thus produces the grotesquely swollen hydropic cells filled by remnants of these distended organelles. A very early change detectable by EM is aggregation of smooth-surfaced ER tubules; this occurs in the centrilobular hepatic cells of rats within 30 min of feeding CCl_4 by stomach tube [41].

CCl_4 is a powerful solvent for membrane phospholipids, but its specific effect on the liver probably depends on its conversion within centrilobular hepatic cells to an actively harmful intermediary (X in Fig. 5.9). This harmful intermediary is probably formed by the hepatic microsomal oxygenase system [42]. CCl_4 is rapidly bound by microsomal cytochrome P-450, as shown by rapid change in the absorption spectrum of this haem pigment on adding CCl_4 to microsomes. Moreover CCl_4 given to animals is in part oxidised completely and breathed out as CO_2. This oxidation is demonstrated by giving $^{14}CCl_4$ which

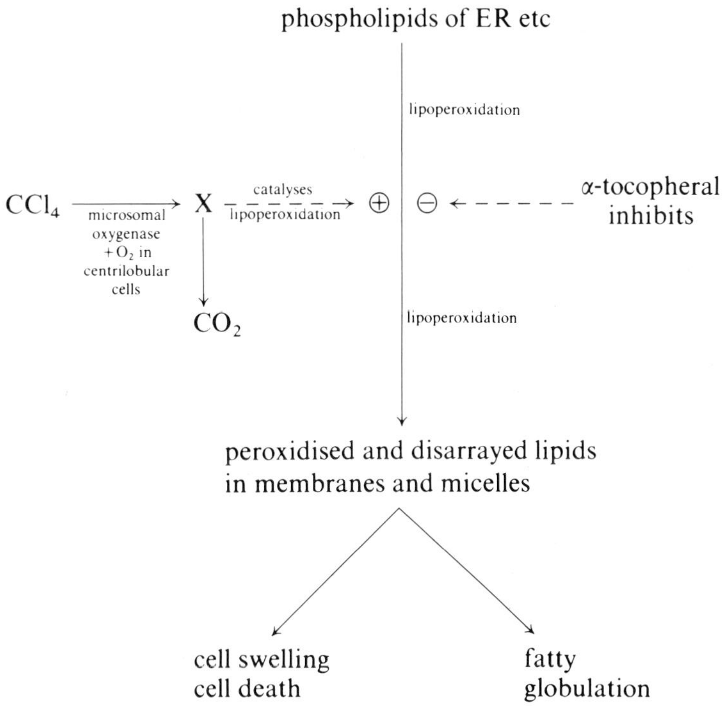

FIG. 5.9 Toxigenic action of CCl_4. Microsomal oxygenation probably oxidises CCl_4 to a harmful and highly reactive intermediary (X), which is ultimately converted to CO_2, but can also catalyse lipoperoxidation of arrayed lipids in cell membranes and hence injures the hepatic cells.

results in expiration of $^{14}CO_2$. The amount of CCl_4 thus oxidised is augmented many-fold by pretreatment with phenobarbitone, which also induces increase in hepatic concentration of cytochrome P450 and simultaneously enhances the lethal action of CCl_4. Thus, McLean [42] found that addition of phenobarbitone to diet of rats diminished LD_{50}/ml CCl_4/kg body weight from 6.45 to 0.5 and at the same time induced a seven-fold increase in hepatic concentration of cytochrome P450.

These observations indicate that CCl_4 is oxidised to an actively lethal agent by hepatic microsomal oxygenase and that this enzyme system is magnified after induction by phenobarbitone. This system is located predominantly in the centrilobular cells where damage by CCl_4 is most severe [42].

The harmful intermediary (X in Fig. 5.9) is probably highly active and is formed in the course of oxidation of CCl_4 to CO_2. Its nature is unknown; it may be a free radical such as $—CCl_3$ liberated by an initial stage in oxidation of CCl_4. Its toxic properties probably depend on the power to catalyse the lipoperoxidation of phospholipids in the membranes of hepatic cells and their organelles (especially the ER) to form more highly unsaturated lipids with changed physical properties. Thus the microsomal lipids, extracted from liver of rats fed CCl_4, show characteristic absorption spectra indicating diene conjugation present in peroxidised polyenoic acids [43]; indeed the diene conjugation in the microsomal lipids triples in the first 15 min after feeding CCl_4 to rats [41]. Moreover, α-tocopherol and other antoxidants, which prevent lipoperoxidation, protect animals from the harmful effects of CCl_4 [44–46]. Thus lipoperoxidation appears to be a crucial event in hepatic damage caused by CCl_4.

Injury by CCl_4, involving this initial oxidation to a toxic intermediary, is most severe in the centrilobular hepatic cells where the microsomal oxygenase system is most abundant. Thus in the centrilobular cells irreversible damage to cell membranes is apparently so rapid that cells become necrotic and fully permeable and *no swelling* occurs; when damage is not so severe, the membranes of the cells and their organelles may at first merely become more permeable, so that Na^+ and H_2O enter (p. 289) and thus cause hydropic swelling [47]; this hydropic swelling is therefore most prominent in the midzonal parts of the hepatic lobules [48]. Coincident fatty change is probably also determined by lipoperoxidation which interferes with solubilisation and excretion of fat [49] (p. 360).

Dimethyl nitrosamine (DMN)

DMN, $(CH_3)_2N—N{=}O$, causes extensive centrilobular necrosis in liver of rats; this appears within one day of intraperitoneal injection [50, 51]. Following administration of DMN labelled with radioactive carbon ^{14}C, the ^{14}C becomes incorporated into protein, RNA and DNA in liver and kidney. Moreover, radioactive foci appear in 7-methyl guanine obtained from hepatic DNA [52]. It is thus possible that DMN exerts some of its harmful effects by converting guanine of nucleic acids into 7-methyl guanine.

The active methylating agent which effects this change is probably formed

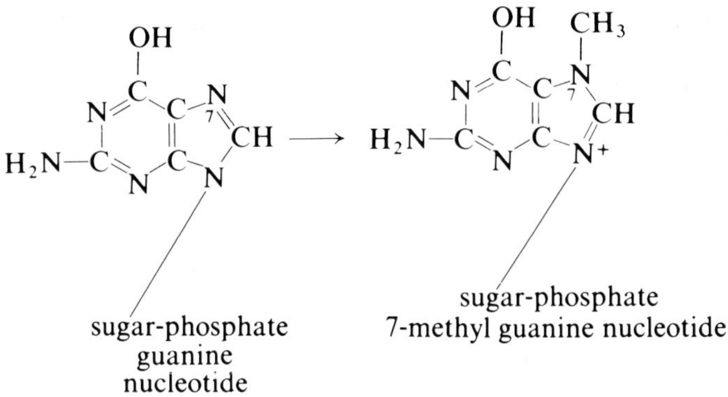

from DMN in centrilobular hepatic cells by the oxygenating system of the ER (microsomal oxygenase). The products of this reaction are powerful alkylating agents which determine the necrosis of the centrilobular cells [42]. In animals depleted of protein the metabolism of DMN in the liver is substantially diminished and the liver lesions are then much less severe [53].

DMN is thus another substance, which is not itself directly noxious, but is converted into an actively harmful agent following oxidation by the microsomal oxygenase system. Toxigenic action of DMN is also probably responsible for its oncogenic effects (p. 182).

Toxigenesis due to enzymic induction

Many of the enzymes capable of catalysing the formation of harmful substances in cells are normally absent or present in insignificant amounts, because their synthesis is suppressed by the action of regulator genes. These genes are believed to direct synthesis of specific proteins called repressors which abolish enzymic synthesis by blocking the genomic complex concerned with expressing a certain group of enzymes. Numerous substances, however, are capable of inducing these repressed enzymes probably by acting on the repressors and altering them so that they no longer block transcription of the mRNAs responsible for translating a specific group of enzymes. Such inducing substances are usually harmless in themselves but by evoking a repressed enzymic reaction they may induce the formation of a highly harmful agent. Foreign substances can initiate such toxigenesis by inducing the formation of enzymes which catalyse the production of toxic products derived from:

1. The inducing agent itself and its homologues.
2. Other foreign substances.
3. Substances already present in the cell.

Toxic products formed from the inducing agent itself (or its homologues)

Benz(a)pyrene (100 μg) administered to rats causes a five fold increase within 12 h of the microsomal enzyme benz(a)pyrene 3-mono-oxygenase in the liver cells [54]. This enzyme is readily detected by its capacity to convert benz(a)pyrene into 3-hydroxybenz(a)pyrene. The latter substance is a metabolite which is readily estimated by its intense fluorescence in UV light. Although it is probable

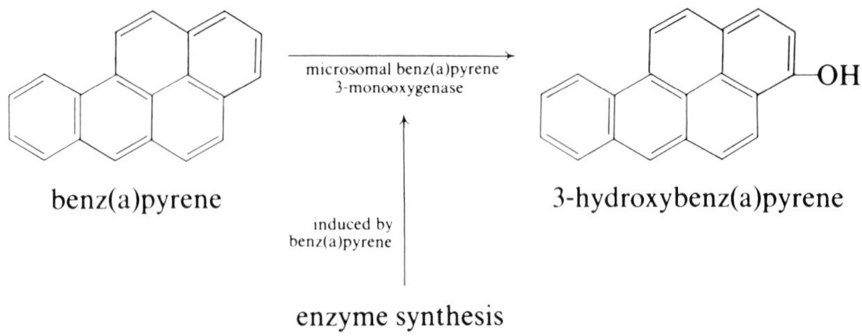

(see oncogenesis) that epoxides are the initial products of this reaction and that these isomerise to phenols, the epoxides are difficult to estimate. For this reason the estimation of arylhydrocarbon oxygenases in the microsomal system of cells is generally based on measuring the rate of the above conversion to 3-hydroxybenz(a)pyrene. But the epoxide is in all probability the initial reactive intermediary formed by the enzyme system, which can then either kill cells or induce neoplasia. This enzyme, in the above instance, can be induced by its own substrate, which it then converts to a directly harmful substance that can cause necrosis or neoplasia.

This same enzyme can also be induced by other polycyclic aromatic hydrocarbons and by other substances such as phenobarbitone (see below).

Toxic products formed from other foreign substances

CCl_4, as we have seen, is oxidised to harmful products by the microsomal oxygenase system of hepatic cells. The formation of this enzyme and of its cofactors is also induced by phenobarbitone. Likewise phenobarbitone induces the formation of microsomal oxygenases which metabolise aromatic hydrocarbons and convert them to reactive epoxides (see below). Indeed phenobarbitone is a most potent inducer of enzymes of the microsomal oxygenase system. This induction is prevented when protein synthesis is inhibited by puromycin or actinomycin D [55].

Toxic products formed from substances naturally present in the cell

Inducing agents may also augment the synthesis of substances naturally formed by the cell in limited amounts, which may then become harmful when present in excess.

The biosynthesis of haem depends on a sequence of reactions initiated by the formation of δ-aminolaevulinic acid (ALA) from succinyl CoA and glycine by the enzyme ALA-synthase present in hepatic cells.

$$\underset{\text{succinyl CoA}}{\text{CoA—S—CO—CH}_2\text{—CH}_2\text{—COOH}} + \underset{\text{glycine}}{H_3N^+\text{—CH}_2\text{—COO}^-} \xrightarrow{\text{ALA synthase}} \underset{\text{ALA}}{H_2N\text{—CH}_2\text{—CO—CH}_2\text{—CH}_2\text{—COOH}} + CO_2 + \underset{\text{coenzyme A}}{\text{CoA—SH}}$$

The extent of this reaction is governed by the variable amount of ALA-synthase in the hepatic cells which is highly susceptible to enzymic induction. Two molecules of ALA are subsequently condensed by the enzyme ALA-dehydrase to form porphobilinogen (PBG).

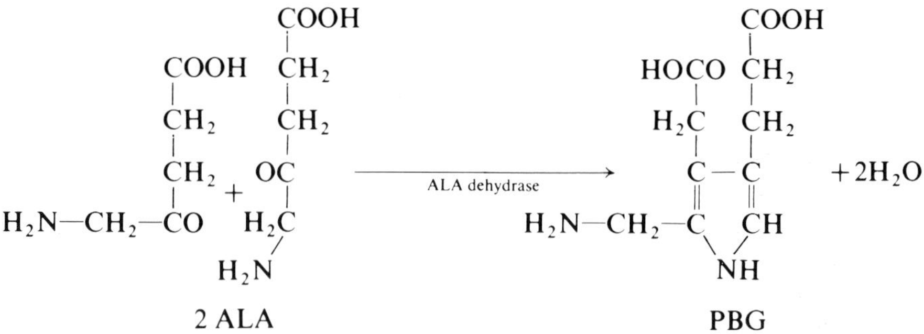

PBG is the initial pyrrol compound, from which porphyrins and finally haem are formed. The synthesis of ALA-synthase is normally limited by repressors. Indeed haem itself acts as a co-repressor and thus indirectly limits its own synthesis (Fig. 5.10).

The pyridine compound 3,5-dicarbethoxy-1,4-dihydrocollidine (DDC), when administered to guinea pigs, induces the synthesis of ALA-synthase; as a result the content of ALA-synthase of the liver is increased 40-fold and large amounts of ALA and PBG appear in the urine. The synthesis of porphyrins is enormously magnified and red brown granules of protoporphyrin appear in the hepatic cells. These granules are 1–3 μm in diameter and give intense pink fluorescence [56]. This accumulation of granular protoporphyrin is harmful to the liver cells and hepatic cirrhosis develops as a consequence.

Similar induction of synthesis of ALA-synthase occurs in cultures of hepatic cells from chick embryo, when these are exposed to DDC or allylisopropylacetamide; the latter substance is particularly potent as an inducer, and pink fluorescence due to intense synthesis of porphyrins develops within 6 h of its addition to cultures [57]. Inhibition of the synthesis of proteins by treatment of the cultured cells with puromycin effectively arrests induction of the synthesis of porphyrin. The action of DDC and allylisopropylacetamide is thus clearly due to induction of enzymic protein *de novo* and not to any kind of activation of a precursor or stimulation by hormones.

Induction of excessive synthesis of ALA-synthase can also occur in man as a result of treatment with barbiturates. Such induction is specially harmful in presence of inherited deflection or retardation in the metabolism of porphyrins. Thus in the disease acute intermittent porphyria (AIP), attacks of confusion and mania occur along with abdominal pain and vomiting, while large quantities of PBG appear in the urine. The urine may turn red on standing owing to condensation of PBG to form porphyrins at low pH. These attacks are

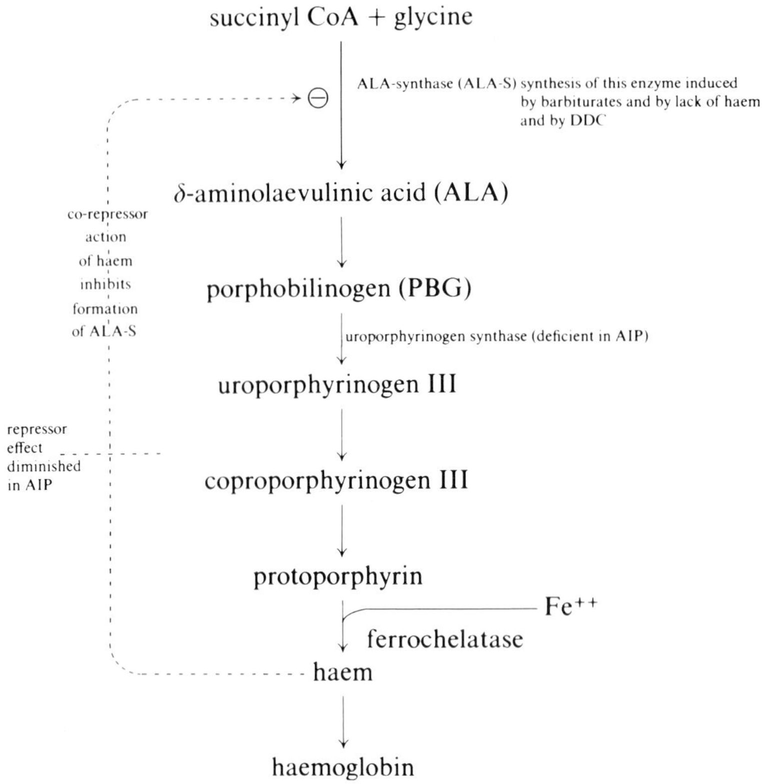

FIG. 5.10 Effect of barbiturates in acute intermittent porphyria (AIP). Barbiturates induce synthesis of ALA-synthase (ALA-S). In AIP the formation of this enzyme is also increased by inherited lack of uroporphyrinogen-synthase; this diminishes formation of haem and so reduces the co-repressor effect of haem on formation of ALS-S. Barbiturates given to patients with AIP raise concentration of ALA-S in liver still higher and therefore cause excessive excretion of ALA and PBG in urine. How this excessive formation of ALA and PBG promotes vomiting, abdominal pain and mania is obscure.

aggravated and precipitated by barbiturates [58], which are potent inducers of ALA-synthase. The actual mechanism of the neuropsychic attacks is unknown, but possibly a neurotoxic metabolite of PBG is responsible. The concentration of ALA-synthase in the liver is greatly augmented. This increase in ALA-synthase is primarily initiated by defect in synthesis of haem owing to inherited lack of enzyme uroporphyrinogen-synthase (Fig. 5.10); this retards the synthesis of haem and so removes its effect as a co-repressor in formation of ALA-synthase (Fig. 5.10). Under these conditions barbiturates or other dietary factors may further increase enzymic induction and so precipitate the attacks [59].

The harmful effect of other forms of porphyria on the skin is considered on p. 196.

CHEMICAL ONCOGENESIS

Harmful substances also injure by causing neoplasia; the development of new growth in this way is called chemical oncogenesis.

In 1775 Sir Percival Pott described carcinoma of the scrotum in chimney sweeps and he suggested that this neoplasm is caused by the harmful action of soot. Since then numerous human and animal neoplasms have been shown to arise from contact with specific substances, and the chemical nature of some of these oncogenic agents has been determined with considerable precision. The action of oncogenic substances will now be considered.

Aoromatic hydrocarbons

Sources of exposure

Neoplasms of the skin occur commonly among men exposed to hydrocarbons formed by thermal decomposition of coal, shale and mineral oil. Usually these tumours begin as benign papillomata which are often highly keratinised and may be multiple. Later malignant change may develop in any of these growths if exposure to the irritant *continues*. Epidermal malignant tumours which thus arise include fully malignant squamous carcinomata as well as rodent ulcers which only infiltrate locally. If exposure to the irritant *ceases* before malignant change has developed, the benign tumours may regress completely, or may become dormant for years but later become frankly malignant.

By painting various pure aromatic hydrocarbons on the skin of mice, Cook, Kennaway and their colleagues showed that many of these substances are oncogenic [60]. They first showed that dibenz(a,h)anthracene produces epithelial

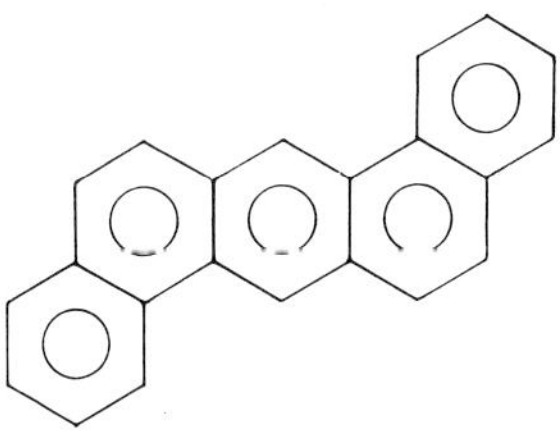

dibenz(a,h)anthracene

tumours and later found that small changes in chemical constitution conspicuously affect the degree of oncogenic activity of these substances. Thus, although benz(a)anthracene showed no activity among the animals tested, 7,12-dimethylbenz(a)anthracene proved to be one of the most highly oncogenic substances known.

Table 5.1 (p. 170) illustrates the effects of changes in chemical constitution on oncogenic activity of derivatives of benz(a)anthracene.

The challenging and elaborate problem of determining the actual oncogenic agents in tar and pitch then followed [61]. Two isomeric pure hydrocarbons were isolated from the products of distillation of gas works pitch. These substances were found to be benz(a)pyrene and benz(e)pyrene.

TABLE 5.1. Influence of chemical structure on oncogenic activity of derivatives of benz(a)anthracene.

Name of compound	Structure	Oncogenic activity
Benz(a)anthracene	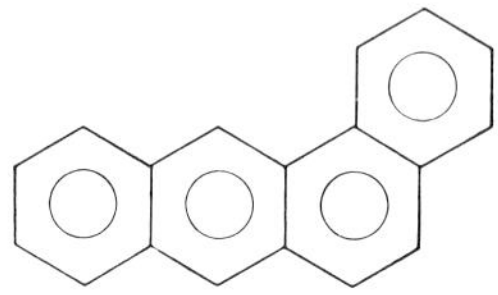	Nil
8-Methylbenz(a)anthracene	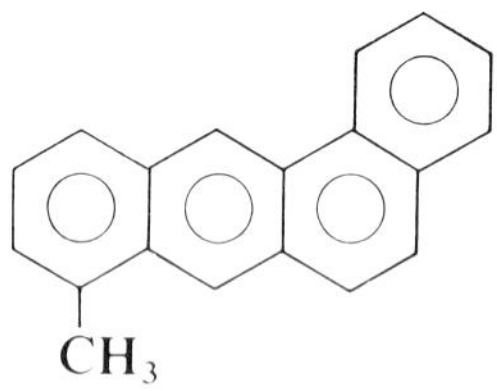	Active
7-Methylbenz(a)anthracene	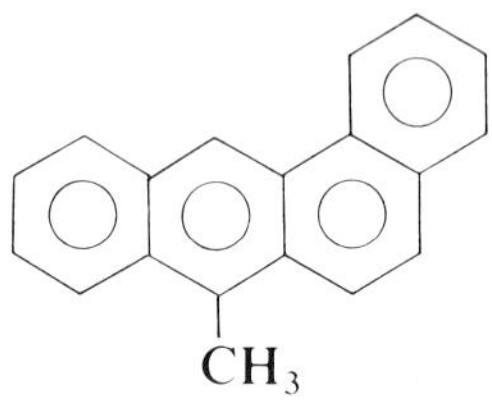	More active
7,12-Dimethylbenza(a) anthracene	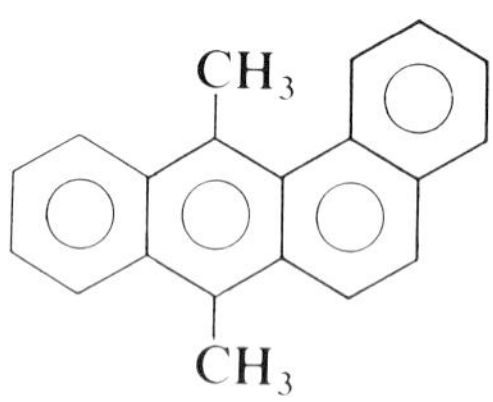	Extremely active
7,12-Dihydro-7-methylbenz (a)anthracene	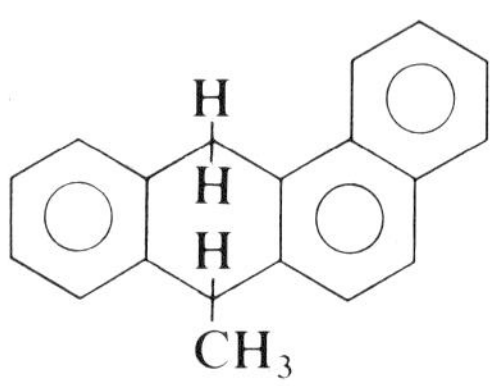	Nil

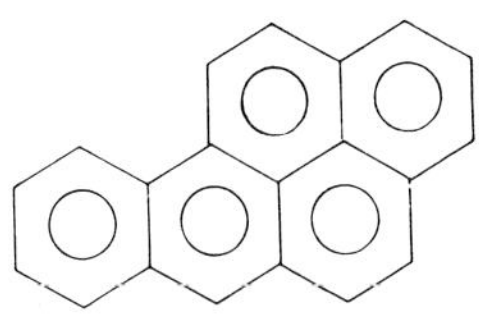

benz(a)pyrene

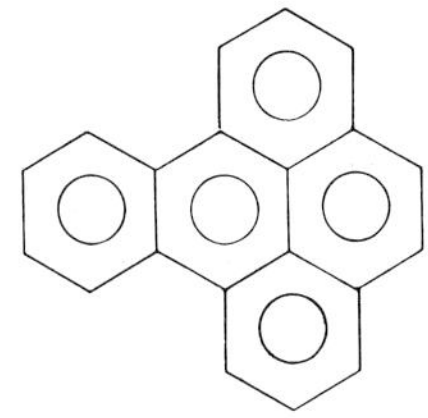

benz(e)pyrene

The former is intensely oncogenic when painted on the skin of mice, while the latter is inactive. Benz(a)pyrene is probably responsible for much of the oncogenic potency of industrial hydrocarbon mixtures such as tar, pitch and machine oil. It is also likely that hydrocarbons play an important part in causing human neoplasms among those not specially exposed to industrial hazards. Benz(a)pyrene is thus an inveterate enemy of man.

Conversion of aromatic hydrocarbons to directly oncogenic agents

Oncogenic activity of aromatic hydrocarbons probably depends on their preliminary conversion by enzymes of the microsomal oxygenase system to highly reactive intermediaries (epoxides). Moreover the aromatic hydrocarbons are potent inducing agents for these enzymes in skin as well as in liver and also in cultured cells. Thus, initial metabolic oxidation appears to be an essential preliminary to oncogenesis by all these compounds [39].

These reactive intermediaries, which are probably epoxides [62], are rapidly converted to stable products such as phenols that are then conjugated to form ethereal sulphates and glucuronides and excreted in the urine. But the unstable intermediaries can disastrously react with DNA and other macromolecules and may thus cause immediate necrosis or latent genomic alterations which are the permanent basis of neoplastic change.

The microsomal oxygenases, responsible for initiating this oxidation of hydrocarbons to epoxides, are NADPH-dependent, and are believed to consist of an electron-transporting system terminating in the oxidation of cytochromes P-448 and P-450 by molecular O_2. The product of this initial reaction is an active oxygen radical (O) which oxidises the hydrocarbon. The initial formation of active oxygen probably occurs as follows:

$$NADPH + O_2 \longrightarrow NADP^+ + OH^- + O$$

Although there is no direct evidence for the formation of this active oxygen atom (O), the existence of such a radical would account for the products formed when naphthalene is oxidised by hepatic microsomes in the presence of $^{18}O_2$ [63]. This results in the formation of 1,2-dihydro-1,2-dihydroxynapthalene, in which one oxygen atom is ^{18}O incorporated from $^{18}O_2$, but the other is ^{16}O derived from water. This observation therefore indicates that *one* oxygen atom *only* is supplied by each molecule of molecular O_2, as depicted above, and that an unstable oxidised compound (epoxide) containing one oxygen atom is first formed and then hydrolysed by water to form a final stable product in the following manner:

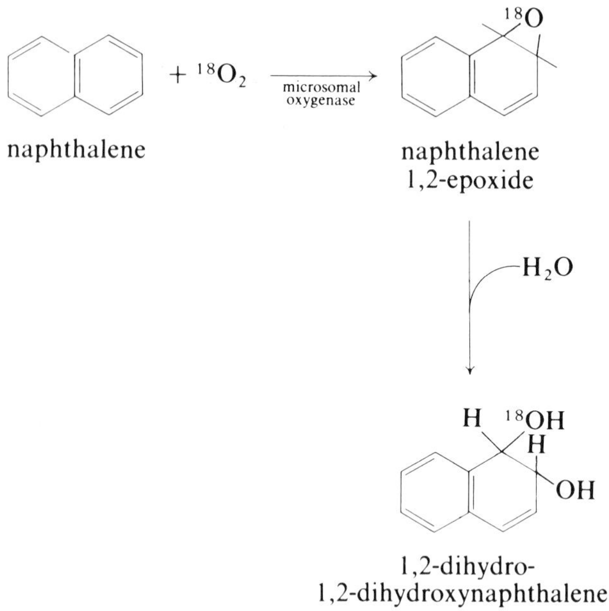

This kind of metabolic sequence ultimately converts aromatic hydrocarbons into stable phenolic esters which are excreted from the body, but in the course of their formation epoxides are produced (Fig. 5.11). These highly reactive intermediaries may then ligate with DNA and thus cause latent change in the cell's genome (see below). Thus an intensely oncogenic hydrocarbon, such as benz(a)pyrene, on treatment with microsomal preparations from liver, lung or embryo cells can undergo a series of changes (Fig. 5.11).

In this sequence the critical stage is the oxidation of aromatic hydrocarbon A to the highly reactive intermediary epoxide B, which binds to cellular macromolecules to form product C. By use of ^{3}H-labelled derivatives and by inhibiting enxymic hydrase, which converts epoxides B to dihydrodiols X, the formation of epoxides B from hydrocarbons A was directly demonstrated in preparations from rat and human tissues [39]. In normal metabolism epoxides are detoxified by conversion to various derivatives such as dihydrodiols X and phenols Y, which in the whole animal are then excreted in the urine after conjugation to form ethereal sulphates and glucuronides (Fig. 5.11). But these mechanisms unfortunately may not prevent some direct linkage of epoxides with DNA and other macromolecules. Upon such ligation of epoxides to DNA the genomic alteration which initiates transformation to neoplastic cells may depend. Indeed, radioactively labelled hydrocarbons become bound to DNA in rat liver preparations in the presence, but not in the absence, of oxygenase-cofactors necessary to catalyse oxidation to epoxides. Moreover in cultures of rodent cells ^{3}H-labelled epoxides are much more extensively bound to DNA

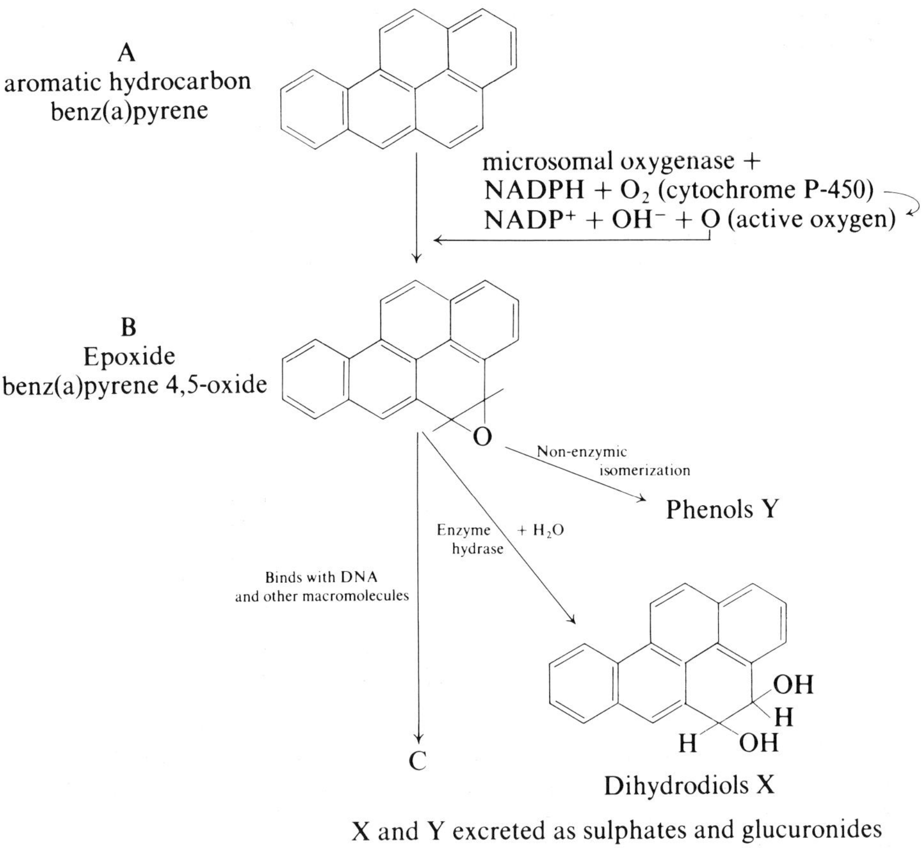

FIG. 5.11 Metabolic fate of oncogenic hydrocarbons. Benz(a)pyrene A is oxidised by microsomal oxygenase system to unstable intermediary epoxide B, which either binds to macromolecules to produce C or is converted to harmless products X and Y which are excreted; product C may then initiate neoplasia.

than the corresponding parent hydrocarbons. Epoxides made from oncogenic hydrocarbons are also potent in causing malignant transformation of mammalian cells in culture and inducing mutation of bacteria. It is possible that the specific effects of chemical structure of aromatic hydrocarbons on their oncogenic activity (Table 5.1) also reflect their capacity for intracellular oxidation to epoxides.

The actual steps in oncogenesis by epoxides of the polycyclic hydrocarbons are still indetermined. But it is likely that these highly reactive substances become ligated to DNA causing conformational changes from which genomic alterations result. Recent evidence suggests that the change in DNA, which follows exposure to benz(a)pyrene, is mediated by a diol-epoxide derivative [64]. This compound 7,8-dihydroxy-9,10-epoxy-7,8,9,10-tetrahydrobenz(a)-pyrene has a very high oncogenic and mitogenic activity.

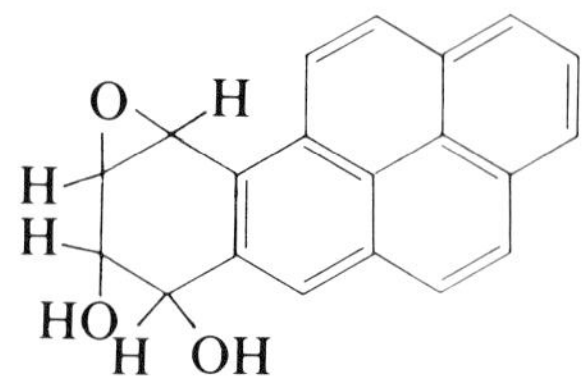

It is strongly ligated to DNA, being bound predominantly to guanine residues in which the N2 or N7 positions of the purine base are the probable sites of junction. The adduction of this diol-epoxide to DNA produces small local zones of denaturation with possible disruption of base-paring in double-stranded DNA. Another effect of binding of the diol-epoxide to DNA is local unwinding of the nucleotide chain. These lesions may give rise to viable neoplastic mutants.

Importance of enzymic induction in oncogenesis

Induction of microsomal oxygenases, which convert polycyclic hydrocarbons to epoxides, is thus probably a crucial event in the action of these hydrocarbons as oncogenic agents.

The formation of epoxides is difficult to measure, but the activity of aromatic hydrocarbon oxygenase in tissues can be assessed readily by estimating the formation of 3-hydroxybenz(a)pyrene from benz(a)pyrene by enzyme benz(a)-pyrene3-mono-oxygenase (p. 166).

The oncogenic agent 3-methylcholanthrene, which is extremely potent in

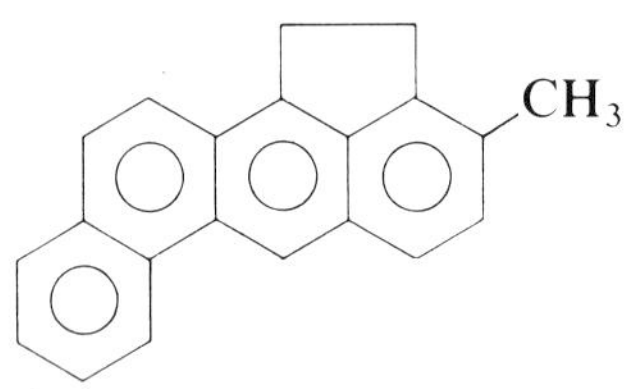

3-methylcholanthrene

causing subcutaneous tumours in mice, is also a highly effective agent for inducing benz(a)pyrene3-mono-oxygenase. The inducibility of this enzyme by 3-methylcholanthrene shows marked differences in various strains of mice. There is, moreover, a close correlation between (1) susceptibility of these different strains to the production subcutaneous tumours on injection of 3-methylcholanthrene, and (2) the genetically controlled inducibility of the oxygenase [65]. Inherited inducibility of enzymes of this kind may thus be an important factor in oncogenesis by aryl hydrocarbons.

Aromatic hydrocarbons and human neoplasia

Prolonged exposure of the skin to aromatic hydrocarbons derived from the thermal decomposition of coal, shale and mineral oil is, as we have seen, a potent cause of human epidermal neoplasia. The apparently fortuitous incidence of these epidermal tumours among those exposed may indicate that other factors, such as genetically controlled inducibility of aromatic hydrocarbon oxygenase or coincident viral infection, may be necessary adjuncts in determining neoplastic growth.

Of even greater significance to human neoplasia is exposure to tobacco smoke of which benz(a)pyrene is a constant constituent. The relation between death from bronchial carcinoma and the smoking of cigarettes was particularly clearly demonstrated by Doll & Hill [66]. They made prospective enquiries commencing in 1951 into the smoking habits of medical men and women and then compared the death rates over a number of years with the number of cigarettes smoked. Among medical men 0.07/1000/year non-smokers died from bronchial carcinoma; with smoking the death rate increased as a linear function of the number of cigarettes smoked, up to the frightening level of 3.15/1000/year among the men who smoked 35 or more cigarettes per day.

This alarming conclusion is tempered by the important finding that men who had given up smoking after the first enquiry showed a dramatic decrease of risk compared with continuing smokers. The disastrous effect of smoking, as revealed by this survey, seems to affect both sexes, though the women had a lower death rate. This analysis indicated that the mortality from this terrible disease might be cut by nearly 90 per cent if people stopped smoking. Indeed, between 1951 and 1965 half of all the doctors included in the study who had smoked before, gave up smoking. Over the same period deaths from bronchial carcinoma among men aged 25–64 in England and Wales rose by 7 per cent, but fell by 38 per cent among male doctors of the same age. On cessation of smoking the decrease in death rate progressed with the number of years which had elapsed since smoking had been discontinued.

In the bronchi of smokers, and notably of those with bronchial carcinoma, areas of non-invasive dysplasia are found in the bronchial mucosa. These lesions are absent in the bronchial mucosa of non-smokers and there is evidence that this dysplasia regresses rapidly when smoking is discontinued [67]. These lesions are probably precancerous zones of neoplasia which are a prelude to progression to irreversible malignant change.

Tobacco smoke contains both benz(a)pyrene and dibenz(*a*,*h*)anthracene. The evidence of the effect of smoking on the incidence of bronchial carcinoma therefore strongly supports the view that aromatic hydrocarbons such as benz(a)pyrene are important determinants of this disease, which is the commonest malignant neoplasm in Britain today. However, not all heavy smokers develop bronchial carcinoma. It is clear therefore that other factors such as concomitant air pollution, exposure to asbestos fibres (see below) and even genetic constitution must play a part in initiating bronchial neoplasia.

Much attention has been given to the possibility that genetic factors affect the induction of microsomal oxygenases which convert aromatic hydrocarbons into directly oncogenic agents. Benz(a)pyrene3-monoxygenase is inducible in human lymphocytes, when they are cultured in the presence of 3-methylcholanthrene (added as inducing agent) together with phytohaemagglutinin which stimulates mitosis. Similar inducibility by benz(a)pyrene itself appears to be under genetic control and the human population is apparently divisible into sections with respectively high, intermediate and low inducibility of the enzyme. Cultured lymphocytes from patients with bronchial carcinoma show significantly higher percentage in the highly inducible group (30 per cent) compared with cultured lymphocytes from control subjects, only 7 per cent of which are highly inducible [39]. Although this inducibility has not been demonstrated in the bronchial epithelium of the patients, the formation of epoxides can be induced in rat lung preparations and benz(a)anthracene 5,6-oxide can be formed by human lung tissue from benz(a)anthracene.

These observations suggest that inducibility of enzymes, which oxidise aromatic hydrocarbons, may be of great importance in causing human pulmonary neoplasia. This inducibility may in part be determined by genetic factors. But other foreign substances including both hydrocarbons as well as totally dissimilar substances may act as inducing agents. This might explain the varied incidence of pulmonary carcinoma among smokers and also account for the remarkable summating effects of other possible oncogens such as atmospheric pollution and asbestos (see below), which greatly increase the incidence of bronchial carcinoma among smokers.

Aromatic hydrocarbons such as benz(a)pyrene, which are present in tobacco smoke and diesel fumes, and which may also be formed by heating cooking fats, are thus a grave potential menace to mankind.

Organic amino compounds

A wide variety of aromatic and aliphatic amino compounds are capable of initiating neoplasia. The danger of such substances to man was first appreciated when it was realised that the incidence of neoplasm of the bladder among workers in the manufacture of aromatic dyes is at least 25 times as great as in the general population.

Although Rehn in 1895 described four patients with tumours of the bladder, who had been engaged in the manufacture of rosanilin (magenta I), this

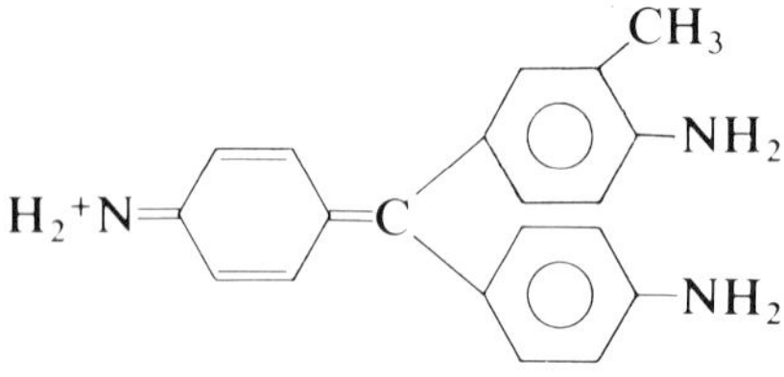

rosanilin

observation was neglected for 50 years. Later work clearly showed that men exposed to 2-naphthylamine and benzidine include a highly significant excess

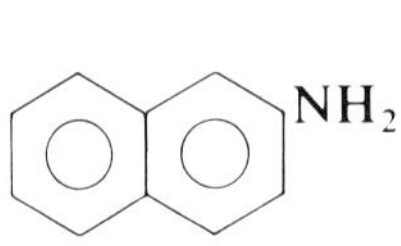

2-naphthylamine

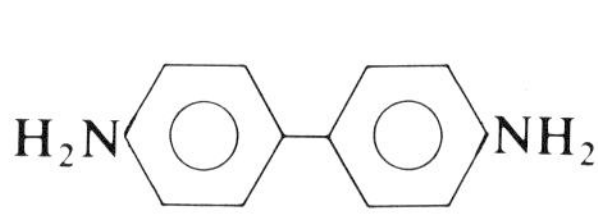

benzidine

of patients with tumours of the bladder, both papilloma and nodular infiltrating carcinoma. These two substances have been specially incriminated as causes of industrial neoplasia in the bladder. The incidence of bladder tumours after industrial exposure to benzidine and 2-naphthylamine is respectively 50 and 200 times that of the general population [69]. Indeed the risk of dying of carcinoma of the bladder among workers employed in manufacture of dyes, utilising 2-naphthylamine, 1-naphthylamine, benzidine and aniline, is about 30 times that of the population as a whole [68].

In considering the action of organic amino compounds in causing neoplasia the effects of 2-naphthylamine, 2-acetylaminofluorene, p-dimethylaminoazobenzene and dimethylnitrosamine will be considered as representing the possible mechanisms involved and also the hazards to man from exposure to these types of compound. Experiments on animals have proved of particular value in averting human risks [70]. For instance, the observation that feeding 4-aminodiphenyl to dogs causes carcinoma of the bladder resulted in prohibition

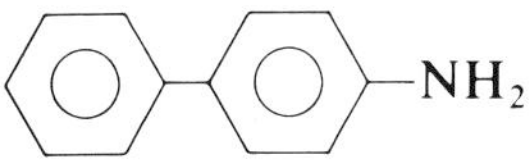

4-aminodiphenyl

of use of this substance in the rubber industry in Britain. But its use in the U.S.A. continued and was followed by the development of 19 bladder tumours among 171 persons at risk.

2-naphthylamine

This compound, which is a dreaded cause of both malignant and benign vesical neoplasm in man, gives variable results on oral administration to different animals. In dogs and rhesus monkeys malignant bladder tumours are readily produced, but in rats usually no vesical tumours develop on oral administration and, even after five years, only papillomatous changes were observed. Indeed 2-naphthylamine itself has very low oncogenic activity at the site of tissue contact on injection into animals. Its potent effects in causing malignant vesical tumours in dogs and man are believed to be due to preliminary metabolic transformation in the liver. The oncogenic action of 2-naphthylamine is thought to be exerted through its derivative 2-naphthylhydroxylamine, which is excreted along with 2-amino-l-naphtholglucuronide in the urine of animals fed or injected with 2-naphthylamine. 2-naphthylhydroxylamine is much more active than 2-naphthylamine in producing abdominal sarcoma on intraperitoneal injection into rats. It is probable therefore that the oncogenic activity of 2-naphthylamine depends on initial hydroxylation in the liver by the microsomal oxygenase system to 2-naphthylhydroxylamine [71, 72]. The latter then becomes isomerised to 2-amino-l-naphthol which is finally detoxicated by conjugation with glucuronic acid in the liver (Fig. 5.12).

The conversion of 2-naphthylamine to 2-amino-l-naphthol (Fig. 5.12) is rapid in dogs, but this change is slow in animals in which vesical neoplasia does not

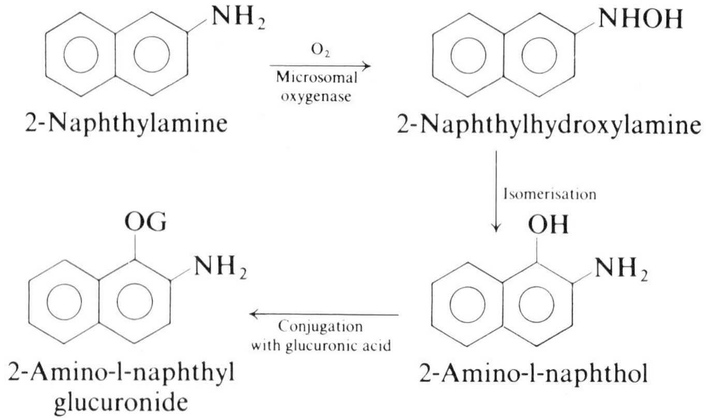

FIG. 5.12 Conversion of 2-naphthylamine to a reactive intermediary 2-naphthylhydroxylamine, which may be the proximal oncogenic agent. This intermediary is then transformed to 2-amino-l-naphthol and its glucuronide, which are excreted in the urine. This formation of 2-naphthylhydroxylamine from 2-naphthylamine is believed to be an essential step responsible for the action of 2-naphthylamine in causing neoplasms of the urinary bladder in man.

develop on feeding the amine. The rapid excretion of 2-amino-l-naphthol and its glucoronide in dogs probably indicates rapid formation of the active intermediary 2-naphthylhydroxylamine. The view that formation of the hydroxyl compound is a prerequisite step in the oncogenic mechanism is supported by observations on the importance of N-hydroxylation in the oncogenic action of other aromatic amino compounds (see below).

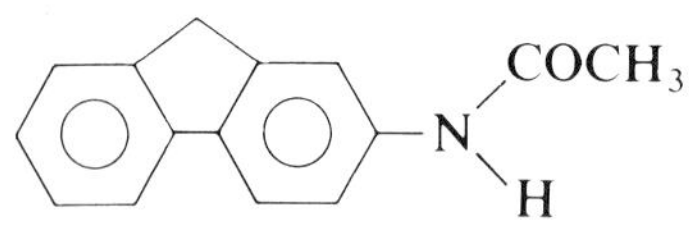

2-acetylaminofluorene

One of the most potent oncogenic substances for animals is 2-acetylaminofluorene (AAF). When it is fed to animals carcinoma develops in skin, eyelid,

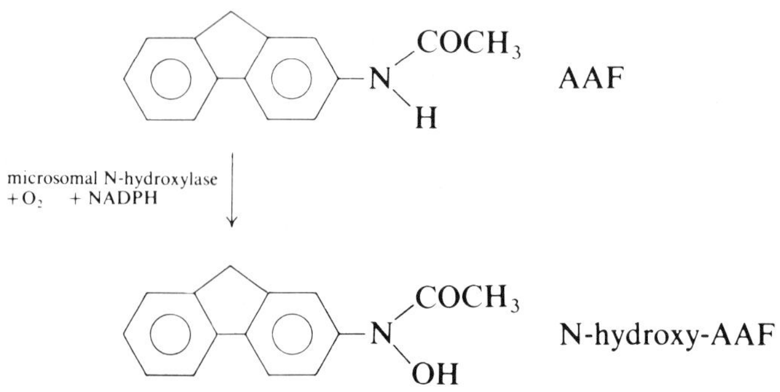

external auditory duct, thyroid and liver, and in breast in females. On injection, AAF produces sarcoma locally and squamous carcinoma on face and in the external auditory duct. Miller and his colleagues discovered that AAF is converted to N-hydroxy-AAF in the liver; this process is called N-hydroxylation and it is catalysed by an enzyme in hepatic microsomes in the presence of O_2 and cofactors such as NADPH.

N-hydroxylation is now regarded as a critical metabolic reaction in the activation of AAF as well as other oncogenic amines. This step [72], takes place in nearly every species and tissue in which these agents exert oncogenic effects. Thus when AAF is fed to rats, in which this substance is highly oncogenic, N-hydroxy-AAF is excreted. But, when AAF is fed to guinea-pigs, which are insusceptible to oncogenesis by AAF, hardly any N-hydroxy-AFF is excreted. Also, the capacity of liver microsomes to convert AAF to N-hydroxy-AAF is substantial in tissue from animals, in which AAF is oncogenic, but is absent or very low in the liver of guinea-pigs which are insusceptible. Pre-treatment of animals by intraperitoneal injection with 3-methylcholanthrene (a potent enzymic inducing agent) 24 hours previously greatly increases *in vitro* hepatic N-hydroxylation in tissue from all animals except the guinea-pig which possesses little or none of the necessary enzymes.

Since neither AAF nor N-hydroxy-AFF appears to be able to react directly with proteins or nucleic acids, Miller [73] suggested that N-hydroxy-AAF is further activated to a directly oncogenic agent which can bind to such macromolecules. N-hydroxy-AAF is, however, even active on cells in culture and can transform rat embryo fibroblasts into cells lacking contact inhibition of growth (p. 465) which produce invasive sarcomata on transplantation into rats.

Azo dyes: derivatives of 4-aminoazobenzene

The aromatic azo dyes include many substances which are potent oncogens when fed to animals. These effects give warning of the inherent dangers which may be incurred by human consumption of artificially coloured foods. Small differences in the structure of azo dyes can cause wide variation in their potency as oncogens.

This relation of structure to activity is well illustrated by the effects of derivatives of 4-aminoazobenzene when fed to rats. This substance, in its unsubstituted form, is apparently inactive as an oncogen. But 4-dimethylaminoazobenzene is highly oncogenic and, when fed to rats, causes the development (within six months) of hepatic tumours, either hepatoma or bile-duct carcinoma. Fig. 5.13 (p. 180) shows the cellular nature of a hepatoma in the liver of a rat fed with 4-dimethylaminoazobenzene. The tumour is composed of large epithelial cells arranged in pseudoacinar masses and trabeculae. The cells have large vesicular nuclei with prominent nucleoli and a high nuclear/cytoplasmic volume ratio; many of the neoplastic cells are in mitosis (Fig. 5.14). At the margin of the tumour its cells are seen to be infiltrating between the adjacent hepatic cells, some of which show conspicuous fatty globulation (Fig. 5.15).

The effect of structure on the activity of derivatives of 4-aminoazobenzene in causing hepatic tumours in rats [74, 75] is shown in Table 5.2.

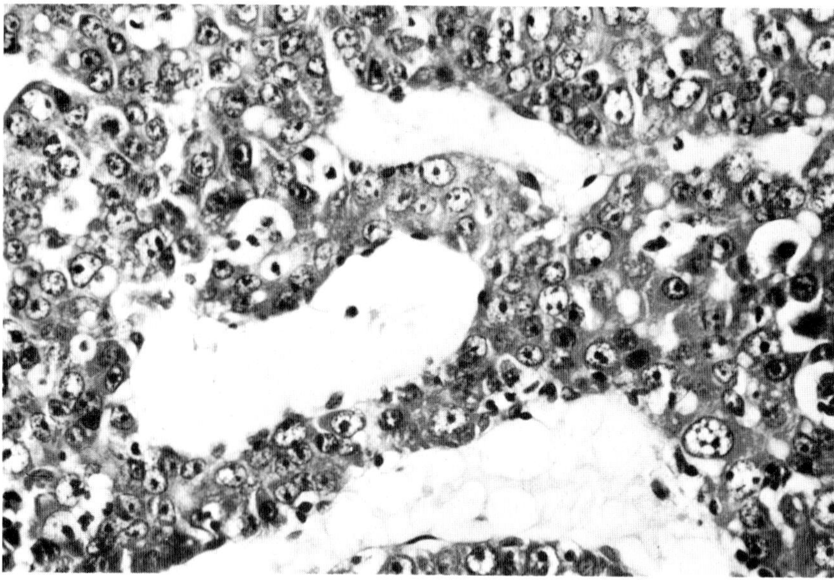

FIG. 5.13 Hepatoma induced in a rat by feeding 4-dimethylaminoazobenzene (butter yellow). Tumour composed of large epithelial cells arranged in pseudoalveolar masses and trabeculae. ×330. From material obtained in collaboration with Dr D. B. Cater.

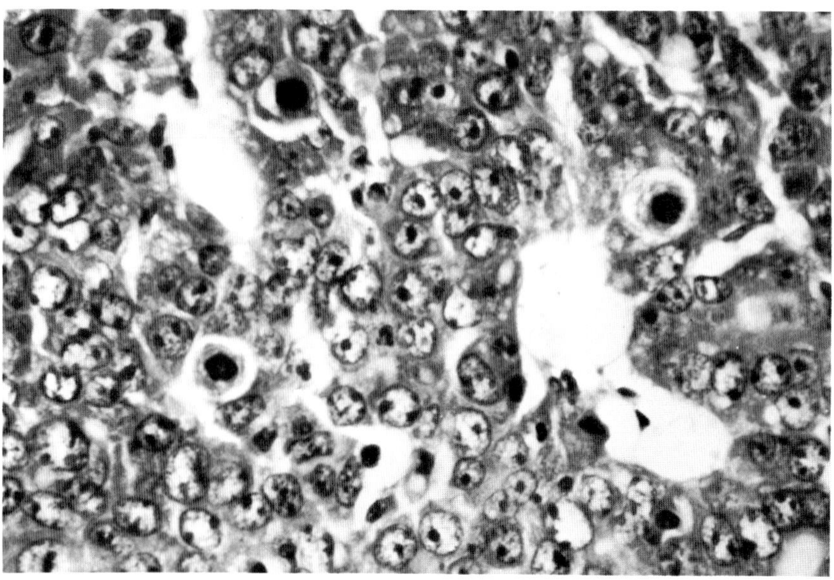

FIG. 5.14 Same malignant hepatoma as in Fig. 5.13 at higher magnification; it shows prominent hyperchromatic nucleoli and numerous mitoses, and high nuclear/cytoplasmic ratio. ×500.

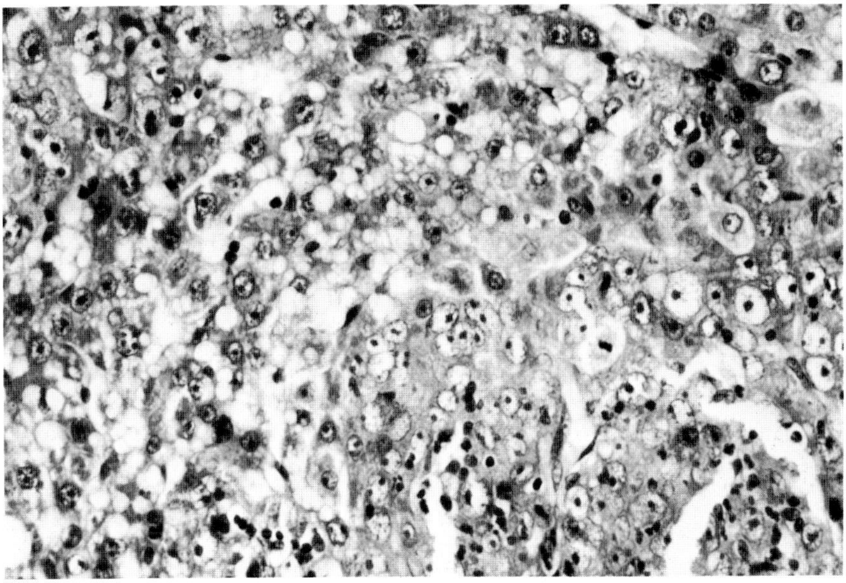

FIG. 5.15 Margin of malignant hepatoma shown in Fig. 5.13. Groups of neoplastic epithelial cells are seen infiltrating among hepatic cells (in upper part of field); the latter show conspicuous vacuoles due to fatty globulation. ×330.

TABLE 5.2. Influence of chemical structure on oncogenic activity of derivatives of 4-aminoazobenzene(4-aminoAB).

Name of compound	Structure	Oncogenic activity
4-AminoAB	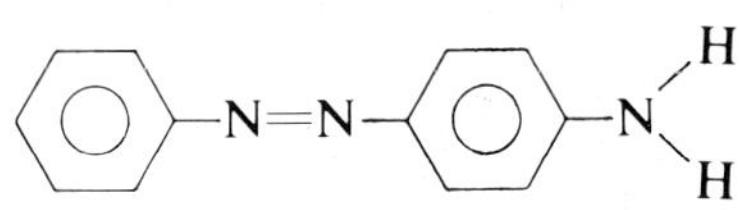	nil
4-DimethylaminoAB	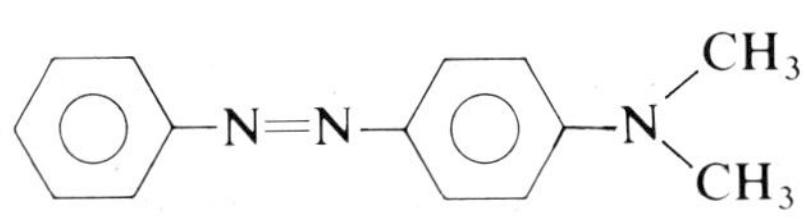	active
2-Methyl-4-dimethylaminoAB	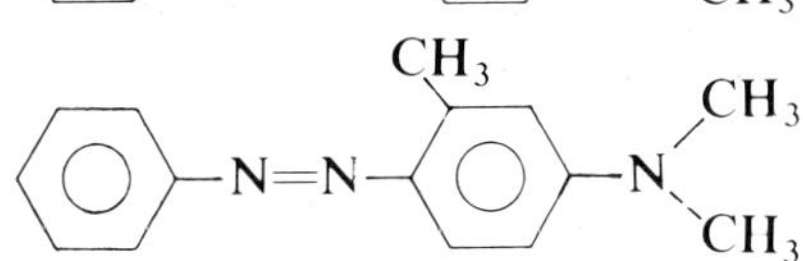	nil
3[1]-Methyl-4-dimethylaminoAB	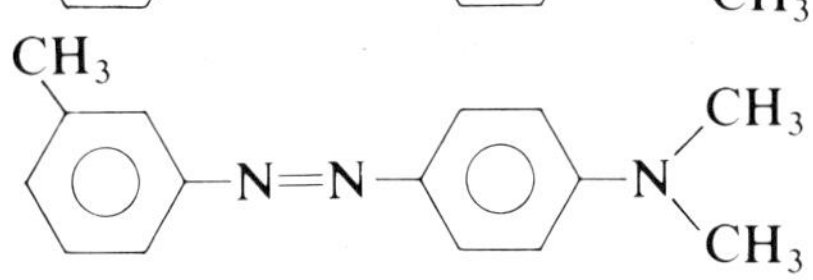	active

It is remarkable that such small changes in structure can so profoundly affect oncogenic activity. Thus introduction of one or two methyl groups on the terminal N atom appears to be a basic requirement for production of neoplasia. But this activity is eliminated by presence of methyl group in position 2 in the proximal benzene ring. On the other hand full oncogenic activity is retained when a methyl group is present at position 3^1 in the distal benzene ring. Such changes however may exert substantial steric effects on the capacity of these substances or their metabolites to become ligated to DNA and thus cause changes in the genomic structure of the affected cells.

This oncogenic activity of the azo dyes emphasises the potential dangers of adding colouring materials to preserved foods so as to give them an attractive appearance of freshness which may stimulate their sale. Such colourants are often said to be safe and to be inactive as oncogens. This can only be a relative statement, since the degree of safety must be expressed in terms of the number of experimental animals fed with a given colourant without development of neoplasia; increase in the experimental population used might well reveal neoplastic potency. Also, since variation in activity may be pronounced in different species, the absence of oncogenic effect in animals can be no guarantee that the same safety can apply when these substances are fed to man. Moreover the long latent period in the appearance of neoplasm in man after exposure to oncogens may mask the real nature of the initiating oncogenic substance. There is thus no valid justification for adding colourants to foods. How much human neoplasia today is caused by coloured contaminants of food is an open question.

Nitrosamines: oncogenic action

The simple nitroso compound dimethyl nitrosamine (DMN) causes hepatic necrosis (p. 164). DMN is also potent as an oncogenic agent and produces hepatic and renal neoplasms when fed to animals. A single oral dose may produce renal tumours in rats [50]. This oncogenic effect of DMN, as with its necrotising action, probably depends on conversion to a toxic alkylating agent (p. 165), which has the capacity to methylate DNA and so kill cells or initiate genomic change giving rise to neoplastic mutants.

This extreme potency of nitrosamines as oncogenic agents may indicate a grave danger to man. Nitrites are added as antibacterial preservatives to many foods and may then react with secondary amines present in the foods to form nitrosamines, which are thus present in some preserved meats and vegetables. It is also possible for fresh foods to be contaminated by nitrosamines. Fish consumed in parts of South China contain both dimethyl and diethyl nitrosamine which may contribute to the high incidence of nasopharyngeal cancer in this part of Asia. The high level of nitrates and nitrites in the environment of Chile and Columbia may also induce formation of nitrosamines and thus be concerned in causing gastric carcinoma which is specially prevalent in these countries.

Oestrogenic hormones

These substances can stimulate neoplasia but usually only when acting in concert with more specific oncogenic agents. Thus mammary carcinoma, basically caused by the Bittner virus, affects most of the females of some strains of mice while the males are unaffected; if the males are treated with ovarian hormones oestradiol or oestrone or with the non-steroid synthetic oestrogen stilboestrol, they also develop mammary carcinoma.

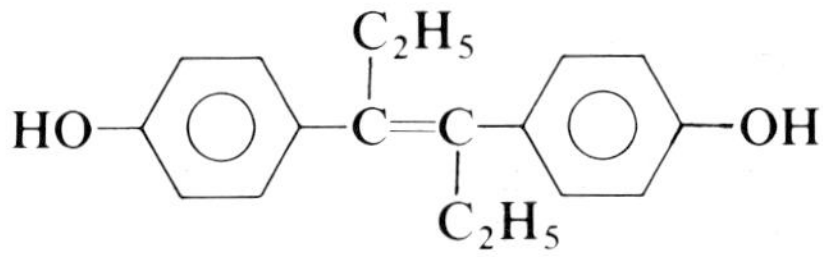

stilboestrol

Stilboestrol by itself can exert a potent oncogenic effect on human embryonic tissue by stimulating adenocarcinoma of the vagina with a uniquely long latent period. This kind of neoplasm hitherto was almost unknown among girls or young women. However, during the last decade clear-celled vaginal adenocarcinoma developed in a number of young females aged 8–25. The history of the mothers of these patients during pregnancy was then investigated. This revealed the fact that the majority of the mothers had been treated with stilboestrol during the first trimester of pregnancy; in an equal number of matched controls none of the mothers had been so treated [76, 77].

This remarkable action of stilboestrol provides a striking example of a latent precancerous lesion. Apparently stilboestrol, given to the mother during pregnancy, passes into the fetus to cause a latent change in some embryonic cells. This change remains masked in vaginal epithelium throughout childhood; later, possibly along with mitosis induced by ovarian hormones, the latently affected cells can progress to overt invasive neoplasia.

Inorganic oncogens

Asbestos

Inhalation of asbestos fibres by workers in the asbestos industry results in chronic diffuse fibrosis of the lungs and also formation of dense fibrous plaques in the pleurae. This disorder is called asbestosis. The inhaled linear fibres of asbestos reach the alveolar cavities and then become coated with brown ferritin and form characteristic radiating masses of thickened filaments shaped like clubs or dumb-bells, which are called asbestos bodies (Fig. 5.16, p. 184). These bodies are composed of small spheroidal masses of ferritin strung like beads along the rectilinear asbestos filaments, which are usually too thin to be visible by LM; thus the deposits of ferritin reveal the site of final arrest of the inhaled fibres of asbestos. These deposits result in fibrous replacement of alveolar tissue as well as interstitial fibrosis with vascular occlusion which combine to produce increasing dyspnoea and cyanosis. The pleural plaques may eventually enlarge to form fibrous masses which fuse the visceral to the parietal pleura. Fig. 5.17 shows a computed tomographic section of the lower thorax of a patient with conspicuous zones of pleural fibrosis caused by asbestosis.

Nearly half the patients with this disease, if they live long enough, probably develop carcinoma of the bronchus or mesothelioma of the pleura. Cigarette

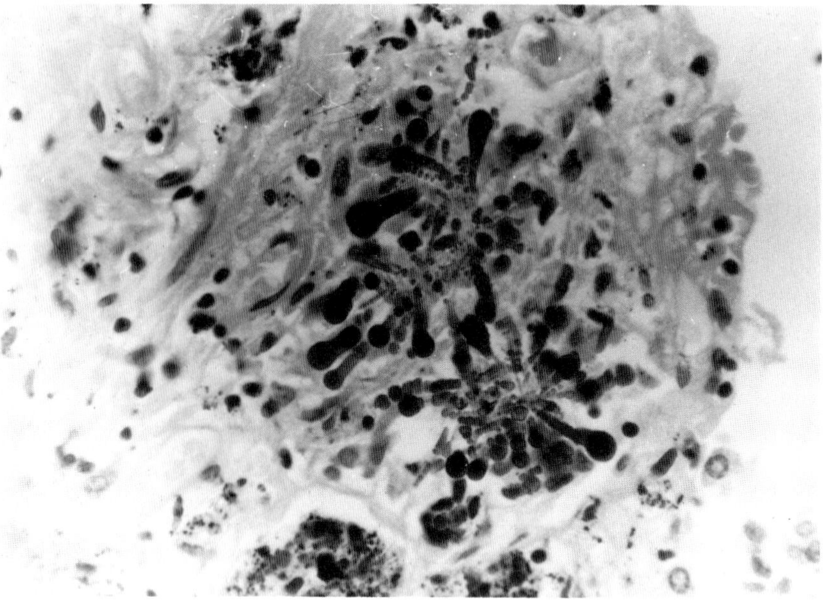

FIG. 5.16 Lung asbestosis. Aggregate of asbestos bodies embedded in collagen of a fibrosed alveolar remnant. The bodies consist of radiating club-shaped and bead-like linear deposits of ferritin which are dark brown in colour. ×520.

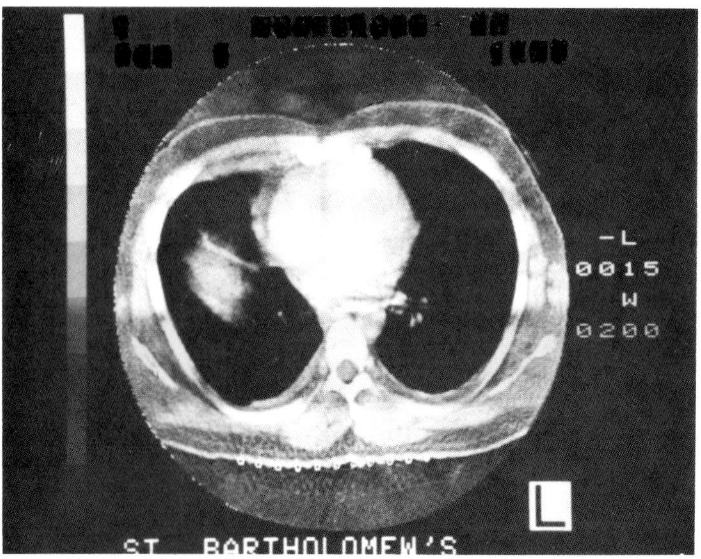

FIG. 5.17 Pleural fibrosis in asbestosis. Computed tomographic section of lower thorax viewed from below. Zones of dense fibrosis are visible on the posterior surface of both lungs as well as on the anterior and the pericardial surface of the right lung. Courtesy of Dr A. K. Dixon.

smokers who are exposed to asbestos have eight times the risk of dying of bronchial carcinoma as cigarette smokers in other occupations. In hamsters, intratracheal instillation of chrysotile asbestos and benz(a)pyrene induces pulmonary carcinoma, while benz(a)pyrene alone causes bronchial papilloma, and asbestos alone has no neoplastic effect. It is possible therefore that asbestos fibres act synergistically with aromatic hydrocarbons to cause bronchial carcinoma in man (see below).

Whether the physical nature of asbestos, as fine cylindrical resistant fibres, or its chemical composition, as complex silicates containing some or all of the metals Na, Mg, Ca, Al and Fe, principally determines its neoplastic action is uncertain. Penetration deep into the lungs and pleura is probably an important factor. Fibres more than 3 μm in diameter tend to fall rapidly and are arrested in the upper respiratory tract and are then removed in the sputum. Finer fibres, such as those of crocidolite (blue asbestos), may penetrate the alveoli and pleura and thus be specially likely to cause mesothelioma of the pleura, which is probably not caused by exposure to the thicker fibres of anthophyllite asbestos [78]. Chrysotile (white asbestos) has long and curly fibres which, although fine, probably cannot penetrate to the same extent as crocidolite and thus carry a much lower risk of causing neoplasia. A further possibility is that asbestos fibres absorb mineral oils and thus introduce oncogenic hydrocarbons and carry them deeply into the lungs.

Arsenious oxide AS_2O_3: *oncogenic action*

This poison in small doses was formerly used in treatment of chronic skin diseases as well as leukaemia. Prolonged medication with As_2O_3 results in the appearance of patches of hyperkeratosis in the skin followed eventually by the development of squamous epidermal carcinoma. Multiple basal cell carcinomata and Bowen's disease (intra-epidermal carcinoma) are also sequels of treatment with As_2O_3. As well as inhibiting oxidation of pyruvate (p. 154) As_2O_3 arrests mitosis at metaphase and causes necrosis of actively dividing cells [24]. Such arrest of mitosis may assist the survival of neoplastic mutants (p. 476) and so induce the development of tumours. Potassium arsenite O=As—OK painted on the skin of mice is also oncogenic.

Other inorganic oncogens include lead acetate, which causes renal neoplasms when fed to rats, and iron-dextran, which apparently can induce sarcomata in human patients following intramuscular injection for treatment of anaemia; also a raised incidence of carcinoma of the bronchus and nasal passages is found among workers in nickel.

Mechanisms involved in chemical oncogenesis

The mode of action of chemical oncogens has not so far been fully explained. The paramount difficulty is to account for the exceedingly wide variety of substances which possess activity. Although small changes in structure may exert large effects on activity, as in substituted benzanthracenes and azo dyes, substances so dissimilar in constitution as As_2O_3 and benz(a)pyrene both lead to squamous carcinoma when applied to the skin. Any valid theory of mechanism should illuminate this paradox of high specificity of some classes of oncogenic substance while other compounds of entirely different composition may generate apparently identical neoplasms. This question is further considered with defects of cell behaviour (p. 476).

It is generally assumed that substances which induce neoplasia initially react with cellular macromolecules such as protein, DNA or RNA and then somehow induce mutation in the cell's genome to produce a genetically altered clone of cells. Indeed there is considerable evidence (p. 471) that many neoplasms are monoclonal in origin. Alteration in DNA following ligation to an activated oncogenic substance may be a cause of mispairing which produces point mutations in genomic replication. Such capacity to alter DNA (p. 173) may explain the power of oncogenic epoxides to transform cells in culture to malignant cell lines and to act as mutagens for bacterial cultures. Moreover, a considerable latent period may intervene between contact of oncogenic substances with cells and the emergence of neoplasia. Such latent change could scarcely remain permanently impressed on cellular constitution unless it affected the genome. But a genomic change may be imposed on a cell during prolonged G_1 interphase and thus no replication of the altered genome can occur until replication of DNA is resumed. In this way the onset of neoplasia might be indefinitely postponed.

Oncogenic substances administered to animals can in fact cause detectable chemical change in cellular DNA. Thus breaks in strands of hepatic DNA develop rapidly in animals treated with dimethyl nitrosamine, AAF or N-hydroxy AAF [79]. Similarly a diol-epoxide formed from benz(a)pyrene by microsomal oxygenase can ligate to guanine residues in DNA and also produce local zones of unwinding in the DNA chain (p. 174). How far such changes are related to the initiation of neoplasia is of course uncertain.

Non-random alterations in kayotype, however, are formed in neoplasms induced by oncogenic substances (p. 43) [80]. Thus a consistent karyotypic pattern was found in sarcomata of rats induced by 7,12-dimethylbenz(a)-anthracene (DMB) which almost always involved trisomy of the longest telocentric chromosome. This picture was entirely different from the karyotype which progressively developed in sarcomata of the same strain of rats induced by Rous sarcoma virus. The constancy of the changes induced by DMB indicates that the oncogen initiates a specific alteration in DNA which is directly related to the oncogenic state. The possibility of oncogenic substances unmasking suppressed oncogenic viruses is considered in the section on behaviour of neoplastic cells in Chapter 9.

HARMFUL ANTIGENIC ACTION

The antigenic action of harmful substances is considered in Chapter 6 along with other mechanisms of disease produced by the cells of the body itself.

TOXIC IDIOSYNCRASY

Some individuals are severely injured by drugs or other substances which are relatively harmless to the majority of mankind. Such exceptional sensitivity is frequently entirely unconnected with antigen/antibody reactions. In some instances idiosyncrasy to a toxic agent is inherited but in other cases toxic effects only follow after repeated and prolonged exposure. A few examples of toxic idiosyncrasy will be considered.

Inherited lack of protective mechanisms

Some substances are toxic when the body lacks an inherited mechanism which normally nullifies their potentially harmful action. Such protective mechanisms frequently depend on enzymic action and are lacking in persons who inherit deficiency of the relevant enzymes.

Inherited lack of glucose-6-phosphate dehydrogenase (GPD) within red cells removes the protective mechanism which causes formation of reduced glutathione and prevents oxidative denaturation of Hb by pamaquine and sulphonamides (p. 29); inherited absence of GPD therefore enables these drugs to cause haemolytic anaemia confined to individuals who lack this enzyme.

Similarly, in phenylketonuria (p. 26) inherited lack of phenylalanine-4-mono-oxygenase abolishes the protective oxidation of phenylalanine which then accumulates with harmful effects on the developing nervous system. In this case a substance normally present in the body becomes harmful to individuals who lack the power to remove it.

Acquired sensitivity to analgesic drugs

Less easily explicable harmful reactions occur in a minority of persons following *prolonged* medication with aspirin and other analgesics.

In these patients wheezing (due to bronchial obstruction) or urticaria may follow almost immediately after ingestion of aspirin or indomethacin, or these symptoms may develop within a few hours. Antibodies to these drugs are not formed in the serum of patients with this kind of intolerance [81]. Patients sensitised to aspirin by repeated exposure almost always show sensitivity to other analgesics of entirely different composition such as indomethacin. Indeed, patients who have become sensitised by repeated ingestion of one analgesic may

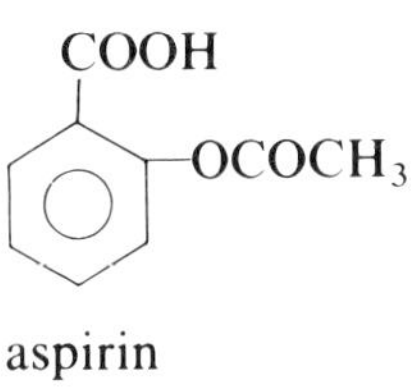

aspirin

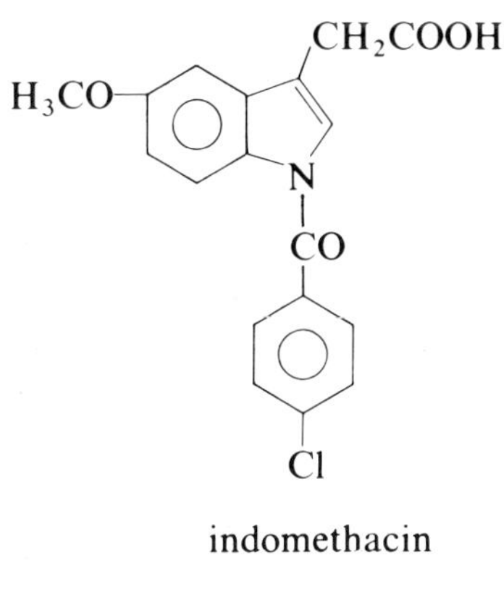

indomethacin

then show identical symptoms on first exposure to another which is chemically unrelated to the original sensitising drug.

Although this kind of intolerance is thus unconnected with antigen/antibody reactions its basic mechanism is obscure. Possibly prolonged medication may alter local chemoreceptors for bradykinin or other active peptides so that blocking drugs themselves cause noxious stimuli. Another possibility is that aspirin etc., which inhibit the synthesis of bronchodilator prostaglandin PGE_2, may ultimately so depress its formation that the antagonist $PGF_{2\alpha}$ exerts effects whenever these drugs are given to sensitised patients.

REFERENCES

[1] ALLISON A. C., HARRINGTON J. C. & BIRKBECK M. (1966) An examination of the cytotoxic effects of silica on macrophages. *J. exp. Med.*, **124**, 141.

[2] ALLISON A. C. (1978) Lysosomes in pathology. In *Recent Advances in Histopathology*, p. 69, ed. by P. P. Anthony & N. Woolf. Churchill Livingstone, Edinburgh.

[3] SUMMERTON J., HOENIG S., BUTLER C. & CHVAPIL M. (1977) The mechanism of haemolysis by silica. *Exp. molec. Path.* **26**, 113.

[4] HEPPLESTON A. G. (1969) The fibrogenic action of silica. *Brit. med. Bull.*, **25**, 282.

[5] MORTENSEN R. A. & KELLOGG K. E. (1944) The uptake of lead by blood cells as measured with a radioactive isotope. *J. cell. comp. Physiol.*, **23**, 11.

[6] GOYER R. A. & RHYNE B. C. (1973) Pathological effects of lead. *Int. Rev. Path.* **12**, 1.

[7] AUB J. C., REZNIKOFF P. & SMITH D. E. (1924) Lead studies: the effects of lead on red blood cells: changes in haemolysis. *J. exp. Med.*, **40**, 151.

[8] HENRIQUES V. & ORSKOW S. L. (1936) Änderung des kaliumgehalts der blutkörperchen bei bleivergiftung. *Skand. Arch. Physiol.*, **74**, 78.

[9] BLACKMAN S. S. (1936) Intranuclear inclusion bodies in the kidney and liver caused by lead poisoning. *Bull. Johns Hopk. Hosp.*, **58**, 384.

[10] CLASEN R. A. *et al.* (1974) Electronmicroscopical and chemical studies of the vascular changes and oedema of lead encephalopathy. *Amer. J. Path.*, **74**, 215.

[11] FULLERTON P. M. (1966) Chronic peripheral neuropathy produced by lead poisoning in guinea pigs, *J. Neuropath.*, **25**, 214.

[12] HOLMES A. M., HESSLEWOOD I. P. & JOHNSTON I. R. (1975) Lead-induced inhibition of brain adenylcyclase. *Nature*, **255**, 421.

[13] ASTRUP P., KJELDDSEN K. & WANSTRUP J. (1967) Enhancing influence of carbon monoxide on the development of atheromatosis in cholesterol-fed rabbits. *J. Atheroscler. Res.*, **7**, 343.

[14] ASTRUP P. (1972) Some physiological and pathological effects of moderate carbon monoxide exposure. *Brit. med. J.*, **4**, 447.

[15] STONE W. E. (1938) The effects of anaesthetics & convulsants on the lactic acid content of the brain. *Biochem. J.*, **32**, 1908.

[16] DIXON K. C. (1940) A study of cortical metabolism in relation to cerebral disease. *Brain*, **63**, 191.

[17] PETERS R. A. (1969) The biochemical lesion and its historical development. *Brit. med. Bull.*, **25**, 223.

[18] THOMPSON R. H. S. (1948) Reactions of arsenicals in living tissues. *Biochemical Society Symposia 2*, p. 28. Cambridge University Press.

[19] PETERS R. & WALSHE J. M. (1966) Studies on the toxicity of copper. I. The toxic action of copper *in vivo* and *in vitro*. *Proc. roy. Soc. B*, **166**, 237.

[20] PETERS R., SHORTHOUSE M. & WALSHE J. M. (1966) Studies on the toxicity of copper. II. The behaviour of microsomal membrane ATPase of the pigeon's brain tissue to copper and some other metallic substances. *Proc. roy. Soc. B*, **166**, 285.

[21] GARATTINI S., MORSELLI P., PETERS R. & VALZELLI L. (1966) The toxicity in rats of intracerebral injections of fluorocitrate. *Information Exchange Group No. 1*, 3 August.

[22] GAL E. M., PETERS R. A. & WAKELIN R. W. (1956) Some effects of synthetic fluoro compounds on the metabolism of acetate and citrate. *Biochem. J.*, **64**, 161.

[23] CATER D. B. & PETERS R. A. (1961) The occurrence of renal changes, resembling lipoid nephrosis in rats poisoned by flurocitrate. *Brit. J. exp. Path.*, **42**, 278.

[24] DUSTIN P. (1950) The action of mitotic poisons on normal and pathological blood-cell formation. *Sang*, **21**, 297.

[25] DUSTIN P. (1951) Imitation chimique des radio-lésions cellulaires par les agents 'radiomimétiques'. *J. Radiol. Electrol.* **32**, 333.

[26] HUGHES A. F. W. (1950) The effect of inhibitory substances on cell division. *Quart. J. Micr. Sci.*, **91**, 251.

[27] JACOBSON W. (1964) Cellular injuries caused by folic acid antagonists and some corticosteroids. In *Cellular Injury*, p. 136, ed. by A. V. S. de Reuck & J. Knight. Ciba Foundation Symposium. Churchill, London.

[28] PHILLIPS F. S., SCHWARTZ H. S., STERNBERG T. C. & TAN E. M. (1960) The toxicity of actinomycin D. *Ann. N.Y. Acad. Sci.*, **89**, 348.

[29] GOLDBERG I. H. & FRIEDMAN P. A. (1971) Antibiotics and nucleic acids, *Ann. Rev. Biochem.*, **40**, 775.

[30] DAVIDSON J. N. (1972) *The Biochemistry of the Nucleic Acids*, 7th Ed. Chapman & Hall, London.

[31] STAEHLIN T., WETTSTEIN F. O. & NOLL H. (1963) Breakdown of rat liver ribosomes *in vivo* after actinomycin inhibition of messenger-RNA synthesis. *Science*, **140**, 180.

[32] ZATMAN L. J. (1946) Effect of ethanol on metabolism of methanol in man. *Biochem. J.*, **40**, lxvii.

[33] BARTLETT G. R. (1950) Combustion of ^{14}C labelled methanol in intact rat and its isolated tissue. *Amer. J. Physiol.*, **163**, 619.

[34] MENNE F. R. (1938) Acute methyl alcohol poisoning. A report of 22 instances with post mortem examinations. *Arch. Path.*, **26**, 77.

[35] ROE O. (1955) The metabolism and toxicity of methanol. *Pharmacol. Rev.*, **7**, 399.

[36] BARTLETT G. R. (1950) Inhibition of methanol oxidation by ethanol in the rat. *Amer. J. Physiol.*, **163**, 621.

[37] PETERS R. A. (1952) The puzzle of fluoracetate poisoning. *Brit. med. J.*, **2**, 1165

[38] PETERS R. A. (1963) *Biochemical lesions and lethal synthesis*. Pergamon Press, Oxford.

[39] SIMS P. & GROVER P. L. (1974) Epoxides in polycyclic aromatic hydrocarbon metabolism and carcinogenesis. *Advanc. Cancer Res.*, **20**, 165.

[40] BASSI M. (1960) Electron microscopy of rat liver after carbon tetrachloride poisoning. *Exp. Cell Res.*, **20**, 313.

[41] REYNOLDS E. S. REE H. J. (1971) Liver parenchymal cell injury. VII Membrane denaturation following carbon tetrachloride. *Lab. Invest.*, **25**, 269.

[42] MCLEAN A. E. M. (1971) The conversion by the liver of inactive molecules to toxic molecules. In *Mechanisms of Toxicity*, p. 219, ed. by A. N. Aldridge. Macmillan, London.

[43] RECKNAGEL R. O. (1967) Carbon tetrachloride hepatotoxicity. *Pharmacol. Rev.*, **19**, 145.

[44] HOVE E. L. (1948) The protective action of vitamin E and certain nitrogenous compounds against carbon tetrachloride poisoning in rats. *Arch. Biochem.*, **17**, 467.

[45] GALLAGHER C. H. (1961) Protection by antoxidants against lethal doses of carbon tetrachloride. *Nature*, **192**, 881.

[46] MEDOLESI J. (1968) Protective effects of α-tocopherol on the hepatotoxicity of carbon tetrachloride: an EM study. *Exp. mol. Path.*, **8**, 225.

[47] Dixon K. C. & MCCULLAGH G. P. (1957) Protein in dying liver cells. *Quart. J. exp. Physiol.*, **42**, 104.

[48] CAMERON G. R. & KARUNARATNE W. A. E. (1936) Carbon tetrachloride cirrhosis in relation to liver regeneration. *J. Path. Bact.*, **42**, 1.

[49] DIXON K. C. (1970) Hydrophobic lipids in injured cells. Histochem. J., **2**, 157.
[50] MAGEE P. N. & BARNES J. M. (1962) Induction of kidney tumours in the rat with dimethyl nitrosamine. *J. Path. Bact.*, **84**, 19.
[51] MCLEAN E., BRAS G. & MCLEAN A. E. (1965) Venous occlusions in the liver following dimethyl nitrosamine. *Brit. J. exp. Path.*, **46**, 361.
[52] MAGEE P. N. & FARBER E. (1962) Toxic injury and carcinogenesis. Methylation of rat liver nucleic acids by dimethyl nitrosamine *in vivo*. *Biochem. J.*, **83**, 114.
[53] MCLEAN A. E. M. & MCLEAN E. K. (1969) Diet and toxicity. *Brit. med. Bull.*, **25**, 278.
[54] CONNEY A. H., MILLER E. L. & MILLER J. A. (1957) Substrate-induced synthesis and properties of benzpyrene hydroxylase in rat liver. *J. biol. Chem.* **228**, 753.
[55] CONNEY A. H. (1967) Pharmacological implication of micorosomal induction. *Pharmacol. Rev.*, 19, 317.
[56] GRANICK S. & URATA G. (1963) Increase in activity of δ-aminolaevulinic acid synthetase in liver mitochondria induced by feeding DDC. *J. biol. Chem.*, **232**, 821.
[57] GRANICK S. (1963) Induction of δ-aminolaevulinic acid synthesis in liver parenchyma cells in culture by chemicals which induce porphyria. *J. biol. Chem.*, **238**, PC2247.
[58] GOLDBERG A. (1959) Acute intermittent porphyria, a study of 50 cases. *Quart. J. Med.*, **28**, 196.
[59] MEYER U. A. & Schmid R. (1974) Intermittent acute porphyria: the enzymatic defect. In *Brain Dysfunction in Metabolic Disorders*, Vol. 53, p. 211, ed. by F. Plum. Raven Press, New York.
[60] HADDOW A. & KON G. A. R. (1945) Chemistry of the oncogenic compounds. *Brit. med. Bull.*, **4**, 314.
[61] KENNAWAY E. (1955) The identification of a carcinogenic compound in coal-tar. *Brit. med. J.*, **2**, 750.
[62] BOYLAND E. (1950) *Biochemical Society Symposia 5*, p. 40, ed. by R. T. Williams. Cambridge University Press.
[63] HOLTZMAN J., GILLETTE J. R. & MILNE G. W. A. (1967) The incorporation of ^{18}O into naphthalene in the formation of 1,2-dihydronaphthalene-1,2-diol. *J. biol. Chem.*, **242**, 4386.
[64] NEIDLE S. (1978) Carcinogen binding to DNA. *Nature*, **276**, 444.
[65] KOURI R. E., SALERNO R. A. & WHITMORE C. E. (1973) Relationships between aryl hydrocarbon hydroxylase, inducibility and sensitivity to chemically induced subcutaneous sarcomas in various strains of mice. *J. nat. Cancer Inst.*, **50**, 363.
[66] DOLL R. & HILL A. B. (1964) Mortality in relation to smoking: ten years' observations on British doctors. *Brit. med. J.*, **1**, 1399 and 1460.
[67] DOLL R. (1965) Cancer: the possibilities. *Brit. med. J.*, **1**, 471.
[68] GOLDBLATT M. W. (1958) Occupational carcinogenesis. *Brit. med. Bull.*, **14**, 136.
[69] BONSER G. A., CLAYSON D. B. & JULL J. W. (1958). Some aspects of the experimental induction of tumours of the bladder. *Brit. med. Bull.*, **14**, 146.
[70] CLAYSON D. B. (1975) The chemical induction of cancer. In *Biology of Cancer*, 2nd Ed., p. 163 ed. by E. J. Ambrose & F. J. C. Roe. Horwood, Chichester.
[71] BONSOR G. (1967) Factors concerned in the location of human and experimental tumours. *Brit. med. J.*, **2**, 655.
[72] ARCOS J. C. & ARGUS M. F. A. (1974). *Chemical Induction of Cancer*, Vol. 2B, p. 9 and p. 253. Academic Press, New York.
[73] MILLER J. A. (1970) Carcinogenesis by chemicals: an overview. *Cancer Res.*, **30**, 559.
[74] MILLER J. A. & BAUMANN C. A. (1945) The carcinogenicity of certain azo dyes related to p-dimethylaminoazobenzene. *Cancer Res.*, **5**, 227.
[75] GREENSTEIN J. P. (1947) *Biochemistry of Cancer*, p. 65. Academic Press, New York.
[76] HERBST A. L., ULFELDER H. & POSKANZER D. C. (1971) Adenocarcinoma of the vagina. *New Engl. J. Med.*, **284**, 878.

[77] HERBST A. L., KURMAN R. J., SCULLY R. E. & POSKANZER D. C. (1972) Clear cell carcinoma of genital tract in young females. *New England J. Med.*, **287**, 1259.

[78] CONSTANTINIDIS K. (1977) Asbestos exposure—its related disorders. *Brit. J. clin. Pract.*, **31**, 89.

[79] FARBER E. (1973) Carcinogenesis—cellular evolution as a unifying thread. *Cancer Res.*, **33**, 2537.

[80] MITELMAN F., MARK J., LEVAN G. & LEVAN A. (1972) Tumor etiology and chromosome pattern. *Science*, **176**, 1340.

[81] SAMTER M. & BEERS R. F. (1967) Concerning the nature of intolerance to aspirin. *J. Allergy*, **40**, 281.

CHAPTER 6

Living Agents Which Cause Disease

These may be either cells of the body itself or parasitic and hostile foreign organisms. Injury by cells of the body itself will first be considered.

INJURY BY CELLS OF THE BODY ITSELF

The body's own cells can injure by the following mechanisms:

1. Deprivation of nutriments.
2. Liberation of harmful substances.
3. Mediation of harmful immune responses.

Deprivation of nutriments by cells of the body

Abolition of pulmonary absorption by cellular proliferation

Occlusion of pulmonary alveoli by fibrosis is a potent cause of hypoxia in both silicosis (p. 145) and asbestosis (p. 183). Similarly, exudates, which fill alveoli of the lung in lobar pneumonia and in pulmonary tuberculosis (p. 241), impede absorption of oxygen and produce severe hypoxia; this may be a terminal event in these diseases.

Occlusion of blood vessels as a result of cellular disorder

Chronic proliferation of cells in arterial intima and intercellular accumulation of their products, whether collagen fibres or lipid deposits, are potent causes of vascular occlusion in atherosclerosis and result in severe and lethal ischaemic damage to heart and brain.

Aggregation of platelets, which are themselves cellular fragments, is also an important contributor to occlusive vascular disease. This aggregation may be increased by local hypoxia which can increase concentration of ADP. ADP can cause rapid aggregation of platelets [1]. This effect is associated with spectacular alteration in the shape of the platelets which simultaneously change from discs to spheres.

Injury of platelets with liberation of thromboplastin followed by diffuse intravascular coagulation is a dreaded event in septicaemia due to Gram-negative bacteria (p. 231). This can result in very severe ischaemic injury to brain and kidney.

Disorders of cells in the walls of blood vessels and of platelets within the blood are thus most important causes of ischaemic injury.

Liberation of harmful substances by cells of the body

Substances which exert harmful effects on cells and tissues may be formed and liberated by cells of the body itself. Many of these substances are normal products of cellular metabolism and only when metabolism is accelerated, retarded or diverted are these substances formed in harmful concentration. In other instances cellular damage liberates intracellular constituents which exert harmful effects when they emerge in excess into the extracellular environment.

Glucose

In severe diabetes glucose fails to enter various cells and its metabolism is retarded (p. 96). As glucose still continues to be liberated into the blood by hepatic and intestinal cells, this retardation of utilisation of glucose causes intense hyperglycaemia, and the blood plasma and extracellular fluid become hypertonic. Affected patients may then become stuporous and lapse into coma. This condition is called hyperosmolar coma and is probably caused by neuronal dehydration [2]. Thus glucose, which is one of the most important cerebral nutriments, can, in excess, cause profound malfunction of cerebral cells.

Vaso-active mediators of inflammation

Acute inflammation is itself injurious when it results in prolonged vascular stasis or profuse local exudates. The latter are particularly harmful in the pleura or pericardium or when they produce extensive epidermal vesication.

Vaso-active substances *formed by the tissues themselves* enhance and prolong the harmful phenomena of acute inflammation, even when the latter are initiated by external physical or chemical agents. These endogenous substances cause vasodilation and increase in vascular permeability as well as contraction of bronchial smooth muscle. The effect of such mediators in promoting leakage of plasma is confined to the venules, where these substances stimulate separation of endothelial cells with formation of gaps at intercellular junctions. These vaso-active mediators include:

1. *Histamine*, stored in granules of mast cells, liberated when the granules are ejected from the cells as an immediate sequel to trauma, thermal injury, exposure to UVL and type 1 allergic reactions (p. 203). The liberated histamine can cause vasodilation, oedema and bronchospasm.

2. *5-Hydroxytryptamine*. This vaso-active amine is present in mast cells of rats and mice, in which animals it exerts similar action to that of histamine in man and guinea-pigs.

3. *Kinins*. These are vaso-active peptides formed by fission from globulins of the plasma. These peptides may be produced by action of proteases liberated

from necrotic polymorphs in the intense inflammation produced by pyogenic bacterial infection.

4. *Prostaglandins*. These local hormones are long chain fatty acids, some of which are highly active vasodilators. They are probably formed by cell damage which may activate phospholipase A in cell membranes; this results in hydrolysis of phospholipids so as to liberate polyenoic acids, such as arachidonic acid, which are then converted to prostaglandins. Prostaglandins are present in

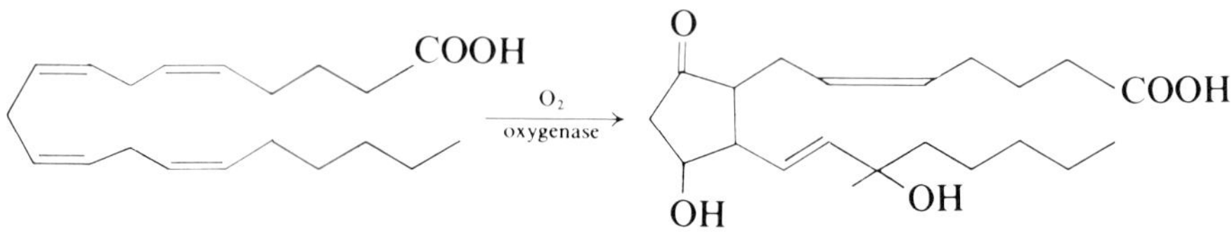

arachidonic acid　　　　prostaglandin PGE_2

inflammatory exudates of burnt tissues and blister fluid. They are also found in perfusates of human skin swollen by cell mediated allergic reactions, produced by sensitization to Ni or chromates [3]. Prostaglandins thus probably contribute greatly to the erythema and oedema initiated by burns and by delayed hypersensitivity (p. 214). Prostaglandins are also formed by the cells of medullary carcinoma of the thyroid and carcinoid tumours of the intestine and may be responsible for attacks of intense flushing produced by these tumours. Carcinoid tumours of the intestine can also form 5-hydroxytryptamine which exerts a similar effect.

Potassium

The normal concentration of $K^+(K^+)$ inside cells is about 30 times as great as that in extracellular fluid and plasma. Release of intracellular K^+ from damaged cells may therefore be highly injurious to other cells by exposing their external surfaces to abnormally high (K^+) or high $(K^+)/(Na^+)$. Injurious effects of this change will now be considered.

Drowning by fresh water. Inhalation of fresh water is much more rapidly lethal than inhalation of salt water; the former may produce sudden death from ventricular fibrillation, while the latter more slowly causes asphyxia. When *fresh* water partly fills the lungs, it is very rapidly absorbed into the lungs by osmosis into the plasma; this dilution of plasma by water results in intravascular haemolysis. (Na^+) therefore falls by dilution, and (K^+) rises as a result of release of K^+ from the lysed red cells. When the ratio $(K^+)/(Na^+)$ reaches the cardiotoxic level, the ventricular muscle commences to fibrillate and arterial blood pressure falls to zero (4, 5]. Thus K^+ released from the lysed red cells become a highly lethal agent.

Traumatic injury. After prolonged compression of human limbs by crush injury many of the muscle fibres are severely injured by ischaemia, so that K^+ leak out of the dying cells when circulation is re-established. Similarly (K^+) in plasma of animals rises after release of tourniquets applied for 2 h. Moreover, after this release of tourniquets, the toxicity of K^+ to mice is magnified eight-fold; the injection of such toxic doses of K^+ to animals after release from tourniquets is followed by heart failure and death within a few minutes [6]. This effect of tissue injury in enhancing the toxicity of K^+ is probably determined by simultaneous fall in (Na^+) owing to leakage of Na^+ and Cl^- from the plasma into the damaged tissue. In this way (K^+)/(Na^+) in plasma rises to a greater extent than by an equal increase in (K^+) produced by injection of K^+ into uninjured animals. The consequential rise in (K^+)/(Na^+) of plasma probably results in cardiac arrest or ventricular fibrillation.

Ischaemic injury of brain. Under anaerobic conditions K^+ rapidly inhibit anaerobic glycolysis of cerebral cortex (Fig. 6.1). K^+ are probably liberated from hypoxic neurones and also from extravasated red cells, which infiltrate nervous tissue after cerebral haemorrhage and infarction. These liberated K^+ ions may cause additional injury to the hypoxic neurones by inhibiting anaerobic glycolysis and so depriving the cells of their last remaining source of energy (p. 92). Locally liberated K^+ may thus aggravate neuronal injury initiated by ischaemia.

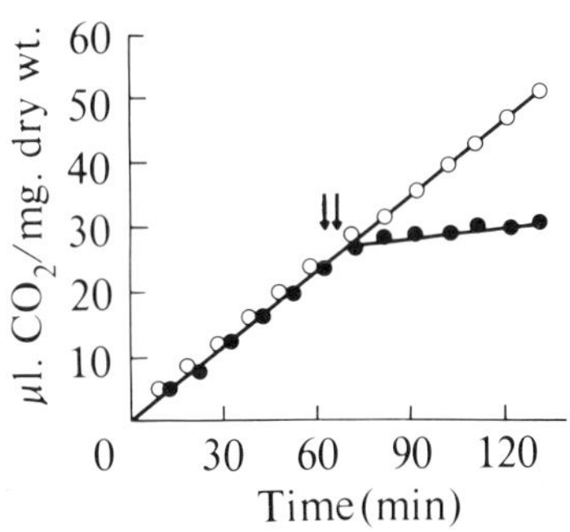

FIG. 6.1 Inhibition of anaerobic glycolysis of slices of rabbit cerebral cortex by K^+. Both series of points record normal anaerobic glycolysis in two parallel experiments up to the period between the arrows. Then K^+ were added, increasing final concentration of K^+ by 50 mmol/litre in the experiment marked •—•—•; in the experiment marked ○—○—○ no K^+ added. Dixon K. C. (1949) *J. Physiol.*, **110**, 87.

Burns. The liberation of K^+ from lysed red cells after exposure of the body to blasts from hot air or scalding fluids causes intense hyperkalaemia (p. 121); this ionic change may be followed by cardiac arrest and sudden death.

Acute renal failure. with anuria or oliguria, may annul the excretion of K^+ and is therefore followed by a rise of (K^+) in plasma; this may also result in lethal cardiac arrest.

K^+, which are such a universal necessity for the intracellular milieu, may thus exert gravely harmful effects when they accumulate excessively on the outer surface of cell membranes.

Myoglobin

Following ischaemic necrosis of limbs due to crush injuries myoglobin, as well as K^+, leaks out of the dying muscle fibres. In some of the patients, who survive the effects of immediate hyperkalaemia and immediate heart failure, the urine later becomes scanty and dilute and also contains myoglobin detectable by spectroscope [7]. Some of these patients recover after developing a diuresis, but in others oliguria or anuria persists and is followed by fatal uraemia. In the kidneys of the latter patients granules of pigment (probably acid haematin) are visible in the renal tubules; these precipitates, which are probably formed from myoglobin, may initiate anuria by obstructing renal secretion.

Abnormal haemoglobins

Variant types of haemoglobin may be so defective in structure and function that the molecules harm the red cells which contain them. Red cells with HbS instead of HbA have a severely shortened life span and may become so viscous that they cause vascular occlusion; the harmful action of some abnormal forms of Hb is considered with other inherited defects in Chapter 2.

Harmful precursors of haem: porphyria

Accumulation of porphyrins and their precursors can be highly injurious. Excessive formation of δ-aminolaevulinic acid (ALA) and porphobilinogen (PBG) in *acute intermittent porphyria* is closely related to the attacks of mania, pain and vomiting occurring in this disease (p. 167); these attacks are indeed precipitated and exacerbated by barbiturates which induce formation of ALA-synthase and thus increase formation of ALA and PBG (see Fig. 5.10, p. 168).

In other forms of hereditary porphyria enzymes, which catalyse later stages in the formation of haem. are deficient; tetrapyrrole porphyrinogens or protoporphyrin then accumulate and become harmful in excess.

Thus in *porphyria variegata*, which affects 1 in 250 Afrikaners, intermediary porphyrinogens accumulate and some of these are oxidised to porphyrins; these tetrapyrroles are deposited as pigmented granules in liver, erythropoietic cells and skin. Hepatic deposition can eventually lead to cirrhosis. The skin containing these pigments becomes photosensitised which can lead to necrosis and severe scarring in parts of the skin exposed to light. The porphyrins formed as by-products by diversion in metabolism of porphyrinogens can thus be extremely harmful. In porphyria variegata attacks of pain and vomiting may also occur; these crises probably result from feed-back acceleration in formation of ALA due to interruption in synthesis of haem as in acute intermittent porphyria (see Fig. 5.10).

In *protoporphyria* the normal metabolite protoporphyrin IX accumulates in excess and similarly exerts harmful effects. This inherited disease is determined by deficiency of the enzyme ferrochelatase, normally present in liver and erythroid cells. This enzyme catalyses the conversion of protoporphyrin IX to haem by chelation with Fe^{++}:

$$\text{protoporphyrin IX} \xrightarrow[\text{ferrochelatase}]{Fe^{++}} \text{haem}$$

In protoporphyria, therefore, this reaction is retarded; the concentration of protoporphyrin in red cells and plasma rises, and protoporphyrin enters the skin in excess and produces harmful photosensitisation. Exposure of the skin of these patients to sunlight is followed by an intense itch and a stinging sensation with later oedema and erythema. This photodermatitis is produced by light of a narrow spectral band near the ultraviolet (wave length about 400 nm), which is of the same wave length as that of maximum absorption by porphyrins [8]. The liver is blackened by deposits of protoporphyrin in hepatocytes and macrophages; this deposition may be followed by cirrhosis, and gallstones composed of protoporphyrin are also sometimes produced. This accumulation of protoporphyrin is primarily determined by retardation of its removal, but its rate of formation may also be augmented by feedback mechanism caused by deficient formation of haem (p. 168).

Bilirubin

The harmful action of bilirubin illustrates the toxic potentialities of a normal metabolite when formed in gross excess. This happens in children with *haemolytic disease of the newborn*, if they survive antenatal life and so are removed from their mother's capacity to eliminate excessive bilirubin. The red cells of these newborn children continue to be haemolysed by adsorbed maternal antibodies (p. 206), but the bilirubin formed from the released Hb cannot be removed, as the neonatal hepatic cells are deficient in glucuronyl transferase and therefore cannot excrete excessive bilirubin. As well as being severely anaemic these children then become grossly jaundiced as the concentration of bilirubin in their plasma reaches extremely high levels (e.g. 300 μmol/l). This bilirubin, which is held in loose combination with albumen, passes freely from the plasma through the poorly developed blood-brain barrier of newborn infants. On entering the brain this bilirubin then stains various nuclei in the grey matter a deep yellow (*kernicterus*, nuclear jaundice). The zones most usually coloured are the subthalamic and medullary nuclei, the globus pallidus and patchy areas in the cerebral cortex. In these zones many of the neurones are necrotic and shrivelled and are intensely coloured by adsorbed bilirubin.

Neuronal damage in haemolytic disease of the newborn is probably, at least in part, caused by toxic action of bilirubin, since similar shrunken yellow neurones are found in kittens after injection of bilirubin-albumen [9]. In baby rabbits, however, the cerebral neurones can only be coloured by injected bilirubin, if the brain is first injured by hypoxia which may also cause injury [10]. In human haemolytic disease of the newborn the neurones may thus first be damaged by hypoxia and subsequently be coloured selectively by bilirubin. If these jaundiced children survive they commonly suffer from involuntary movements (choreoathetosis), due to loss of neurones in corpus striatum, and also from nerve deafness [11]; fortunately exchange transfusion at birth greatly diminishes this risk.

In children affected by the *Crigler-Najjar syndrome* similar neonatal jaundice is prominent; in those who die soon after birth the grey nuclei of the brain are intensely stained by bilirubin, while those who survive suffer from severe mental defect. In this disease inherited lack of glucuronyl transferase in liver cells is responsible for accumulation of bilirubin in the blood, but there is *no* haemolysis *nor* anaemia. This indicates that excess of bilirubin *alone*, without anoxia, can enter cerebral neurones of the newborn and cause necrosis as well as staining by absorption of this toxic pigment.

Monosodium urate: gout

The formation of excessive amounts of monosodium urate (MSU) is the basic determinant of gout. This disorder arises either as a result of inherited metabolic disease (primary gout), or when cell nuclei are excessively destroyed as in leukaemia or in patients treated by cytotoxic drugs (secondary gout). Gout seldom affects women, though they may transmit the inherited metabolic form. The clinical disability commences with acute arthritis affecting single joints and then slowly progresses to chronic articular disease.

Acute gout is characterised by sudden attacks of arthritis and fever. The metatarsophalangeal joint of the big toe is often first affected. The diseased joints become inflamed and swollen by an exudate containing numerous polymorphs and microcrystals of MSU.

In chronic gout hard nodules called tophi are formed in the subcutaneous tissue and also around or within joints *previously* affected by acute gout. White tophaceous masses are also deposited on articular cartilages so as to coat the opposing surfaces with paint-like material. The cartilages later become eroded and severe chronic arthritis follows. Tophi consist of connective tissue in which are embedded crystals of MSU along with 'foreign body' giant cells.

Metabolic defect. The deposition of MSU in gout depends on acceleration in formation of uric acid. By feeding uric acid labelled with ^{15}N an estimate can be made of the 'uric acid pool' in the body; in gouty patients this pool is increased from three-to ten-fold. Moreover ^{15}N-glycine is converted to uric acid in this metabolic pool more rapidly in patients with primary gout than in healthy persons. The increase in the uric acid pool is reflected by a rise in concentration of uric acid in the plasma. This persistent hyperuricaemia may ultimately produce renal deposits of MSU followed by renal failure.

Uric acid is formed in the body by (1) synthesis from glycine and glutamine, and (2) catabolism of nucleic acids. An abbreviated summary of these metabolic routes is given in Fig. 6.2; this shows how formation of MSU results from accumulation of precursors of uric acid (xanthine, hypoxanthine, guanine) irrespective of whether they are formed by (1) or (2).

In secondary gout accumulation of these precursors clearly arises from increased destruction of nuclei followed by catabolism of nucleoprotein and

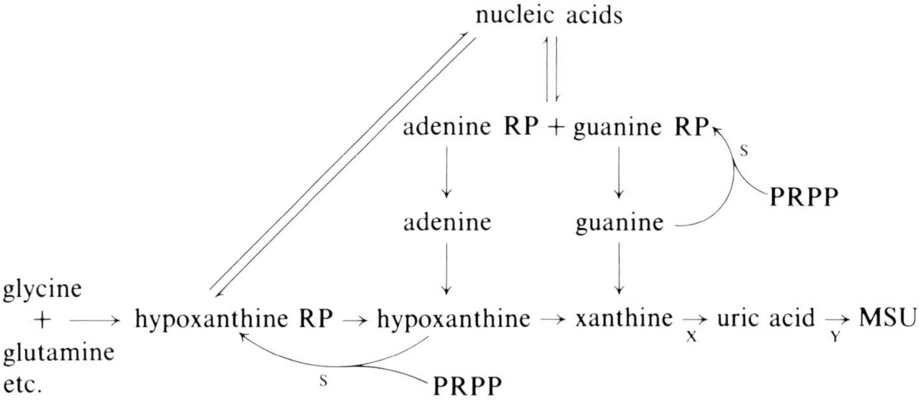

FIG. 6.2 Precursors of uric acid and monosodium urate in gout. In gout, reactions X and Y are accelerated; this probably results from a metabolic aberration which causes accumulation of precursors of uric acid, e.g. xanthine, hypoxanthine and guanine. There is some evidence that inherited deficiency in phosphoribosyl transferases responsible for salvage pathways S is the immediate determinant of accumulation of these precursors of uric acid.

MSU	monosodium urate
hypoxanthine RP	hypoxanthine ribose phosphate
adenine RP	adenine ribose phosphate
guanine RP	guanine ribose phosphate
PRPP	5-phosphoribosyl-l-pyrophosphate
S	salvage pathways

hydrolysis of nucleotides, so that hypoxanthine, guanine and xanthine are formed in excess (Fig. 6.2).

In primary gout, however, the mechanism of accumulation of the purine precursors is not so clear, it may depend on inherited defect in the synthesis of nucleotides from free purines. In many cells free purines are converted into nucleotides (e.g. hypoxanthine-ribose-phosphate, guanine-ribose-phosphate) by intracellular *phosphribosyl transferases*; these enzymes catalyse reactions S in Fig. 6.2, and thus prevent needless loss of free purines capable of participating in the synthesis of nucleic acids. These reactions are called 'salvage pathways', and they normally tend to *retard* the formation of uric acid by removing its *immediate* precursors. Deficiency of these enzymes would accelerate formation of uric acid. There is evidence that hereditary deficiency of such enzymic transferases is responsible for excessive accumulation of uric acid in some patients suffering from inherited primary gout.

Crystallisation of monosodium urate. This is the immediate cause of injury in gout. Aspirates from joints affected by acute gout contain enormous numbers of microcrystals of MSU many of which are enclosed within polymorphs [12]. The site of crystallisation of MSU in articular cartilage and around joints may be related to the abundance of chondroitin sulphate in these regions [13]. The solubility of MSU in water is greatly diminished in the presence of increasing concentrations of chondroitin sulphate. Thus, MSU, formed where there is a high concentration of chondroitin sulphate, may be excluded from solution in local intercellular water already occupied by intertwining proteoglycan chains. The *steric exclusion* of MSU may induce crystallisation in remaining pockets of water which become supersaturated. This explanation would only account for the localised crystallisation of MSU in and around joints, *provided* MSU is formed at this site.

Mechanism of damage by crystalline MSU. Microcrystals of MSU, injected as a *suspension* into unaffected joints of gouty or of normal people, produce an acute inflammatory exudate similar to that of gout; *solutions* of MSU do not produce this effect [12]. Subcutaneous injection of suspensions of MSU produce a similar exudate. Crystals of MSU are therefore clearly responsible for causing acute gout. Phagocytosis of MSU by polymorphs is extremely rapid and is followed within a few minutes by release of an active chemotactic factor which attracts

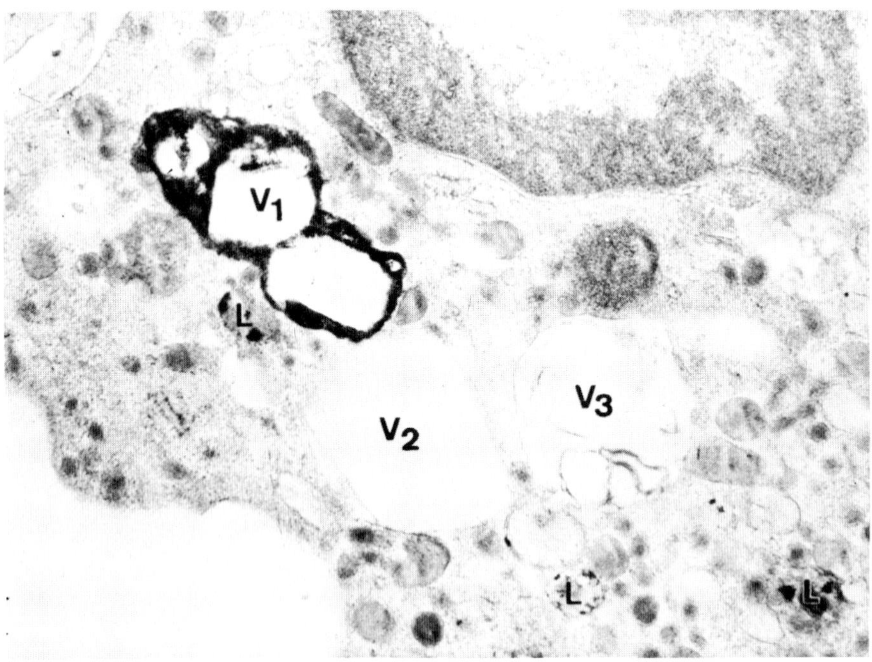

FIG. 6.3 Crystalline MSU within a polymorph; 15 min after commencement of phagocytosis of MSU, the cell was fixed and treated by cytochemical method for acid phosphatase and then examined by EM. Cytoplasmic vacuoles V_2 and V_3 show crystal spaces from which MSU has been extracted. V_1 marks similar spaces which are clearly outlined by heavy deposits of lead phosphate indicating site of lysosomal acid-phosphatase activity and the merging of lysosome with vacuoles containing MSU to form phagolysosomes. Part of nucleus seen in upper right quadrant of field. ×20 000. Courtesy of Professor T. R. Shirahama & Professor A. S. Cohen. *Amer. J. Path.* (1974), **76**, 501.

more polymorphs. Intra-articular injection into either men or dogs of MSU crystals (10–15 μm in length) excites an exudate of polymorphs [14], but this synovitis produced in canine joints by injection of MSU crystals is abolished after induction of leucopenia by pre-treatment with vinblastine [15]. This indicates that gouty arthritis is dependent on the phagocytosis of MSU by polymorphs and thus no longer occurs in their absence.

Observations by EM on polymorphs after phagocytosis of microcrystals of MSU show that the crystals are first enclosed in cytoplasmic vacuoles (phagosomes), which then merge with lysosomes to form phagolysosomes [16]. Fig. 6.3 shows (by EM) a polymorph which has rapidly engulfed microcrystals of MSU. Some of the microcrystals are enclosed in simple vacuolar phagosomes, while others are in phagosomes which have coalesced with lysosomes (forming phagolysosomes) and are therefore enveloped by a layer of material rich in lysosomal acid-phosphatase; this is detectable histochemically as an electron-opaque product of enzyme activity (Fig. 6.3). Soon the phagolysosomes become ruptured by contact with the crystals. The internal surface of the cell membrane is then injured either by direct contact with MSU microcrystals or by lysosomal proteases.

This toxic action of MSU microcrystals after phagocytosis by polymorphs is thus probably first exerted on the inner surface of the membranes of phagolysosomes by a process similar to that effected by hydrated silica (p. 146). Both MSU and hydrated silica can lyse human red cells and free lysosomes as well as artificially made phospholipid vesicles [17]. This lysis is inhibited by agents (such as urea) which prevent hydrogen bonding. Crystalline MSU probably contains orientated –OH groups capable of hydrogen bonding to the arrayed oxygen atoms of membrane phospholipids or peptides (Fig. 6.4). The

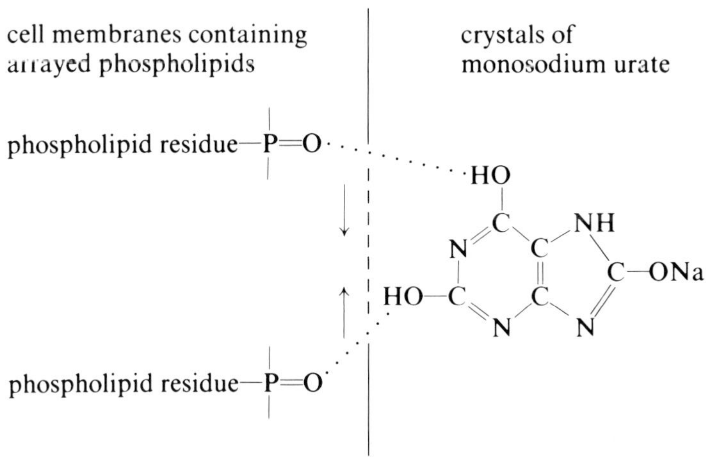

FIG. 6.4 Possible mechanism of injury to cell membranes by crystalling monosodium urate. Adduction of MSU microcrystals by hydrogen bonding to O atoms in phospholipids (or peptides) of cell membranes may lead to disarray followed by lysis.

uniform spacing of these groups in microcrystalline MSU thus accounts for its toxic effects which are not possessed by MSU in solution. This adduction may cause stresses in the membrane followed by rupture of the phagolysosomes with liberation of uncovered MSU microcrystals and of lysosomal enzymes into the cytoplasm; either or both of these agents may then lyse the cell membrane with later release of both MSU and lysosomal enzymes from the damaged cells. These enzymes cause extensive damage to the surrounding tissue and promote acute inflammation. Liberation of endogenous pyrogens (p. 232) from the lysed polymorphs may produce the coincident attacks of fever which are typical of acute gout.

The extreme rarity of gout in women may be due to two factors: (1) the concentration of urate in the plasma of women is lower than in men, thus preventing saturation being reached, and (2) oestrins may exert a protective effect on lysosomal membranes in polyporphs and so diminish harmful action of crystalline MSU [17].

Microcrystalline MSU is thus a highly noxious agent elaborated by the cells of the body themselves. Its power to produce disease depends on its phagocytosis by polymorphs followed by their death and lysis as well as on the damaging effect of the lysosomal enzymes released into the tissues from the lysed phagocytic cells. Gout thus results from the excessive production of a normal metabolic product, which is only toxic when deposited in microcrystalline form; the location of the lesions is probably determined by a macromolecular environment rich in proteoglycans which incites this crystallisation.

Mediation of harmful immune mechanisms

Lymphocytes, and cells derived from them, cause disease by generating harmful immune reactions on re-encounter with antigenic substances to which they have previously become sensitised; this they do in two principal ways:

1. By developing into clones of cells which form soluble antibodies (immunoglobulins); these bind specifically with the original antigen to cause harmful effects which follow rapidly within minutes or hours. This is called *humoral* or *immediate hypersensitivity*.
2. By developing into clones of cells with receptors on their surface, which bind specifically with the original antigen on re-encounter, and then themselves cause harmful effects usually within a few days. This is called *cell-mediated* or *delayed hypersensitivity*.

The antigens which evoke harmful hypersensitivity have three sources:

1. *Foreign substances*. Platinum salts or pollen can cause humoral hypersensitivity, while dinitrochlorobenzene or tubercle bacilli can stimulate cell-mediated hypersensitivity; the harmful antigenic action of hostile organisms and their products is considered later (p. 234).
2. *Fetus*. Fetal red cells, such as those containing surface antigen D, may enter the mother during labour and evoke the formation of maternal antibodies,

which may later cause haemolytic disease in the children of subsequent pregnancies, if their red cells also carry D antigen (p. 206).

3. *Cells of the body itself.* Self made antigens may also induce formation of antibodies which then react with the antigens to produce harmful effects (autoimmune disease). This kind of reaction probably accounts for the formation of harmful immune complexes both in systemic lupus erythematosus (p. 209) and in rheumatoid arthritis (p. 208). Moreover in Graves' disease an antibody is present in the blood which binds specifically to receptors in thyroid cells and stimulates them to secrete excessive amounts of thyroid hormones; it is likely that this antibody is formed in response to release of an antigen originating from these same cells.

Humoral or immediate hypersensitivity

This depends on the formation of specific immunoglobulin antibodies by individual clones of plasma cells derived from B-lymphocytes and developed in response to initial encounter with an individual antigen. These antibodies react specifically with the same antigens on re-encounter by three kinds of mechanism called respectively types 1, 2 and 3 allergic reactions [18].

Type 1 (mast cell generated) allergic reactions

In this kind of reaction antigen present in solution combines with antibody already adsorbed on the surface of mast cells. As a result the mast cell granules are discharged and the histamine contained in them is liberated to produce vasodilation of post-capillary venules and bronchiolar spasm.

Foreign substances such as Pt salts, penicillin, grass pollen or fungal spores excite this kind of allergy. Pt salts probably first form complexes with protein which are the initial antigens. But pollens and fungal products may contain macromolecules which are complete antigens in themselves. The antibodies to these substances, which are generally bivalent IgE, become attached by their Fc portions to the surface of mast cells (Fig. 6.5a, p. 204). On re-exposure to the same foreign antigen, either through the skin or by inhalation, the antigen becomes interlinked with bivalent antibody previously attached to the surface of mast cells in the tissues (Fig. 6.5b). This interlinkage produces a change both in the cell membrane and in the granules within the mast cells; the granules swell, become less dense and some of them emerge through the cell membrane, although others remain behind as empty cavities communicating with the extracellular space [19]. During these changes the granules lose their metachromatic staining due to heparin while histamine and 5-hydroxy tryptamine are released at the same time. These vasoactive amines then cause vasodilation and contraction of smooth muscle and thus produce urticaria, acute rhinitis or bronchospasm respectively when released in skin, nasal mucosa or bronchioles.

The interlinkage of *bivalent* antibody on the surface of the sensitised mast cells by this interaction with antigen (Fig. 6.5b) initiates the process of degranulation. Indeed, if univalent antibody is attached to the mast cells instead of bivalent antibody, discharge of granules on exposure to antigen does not occur.

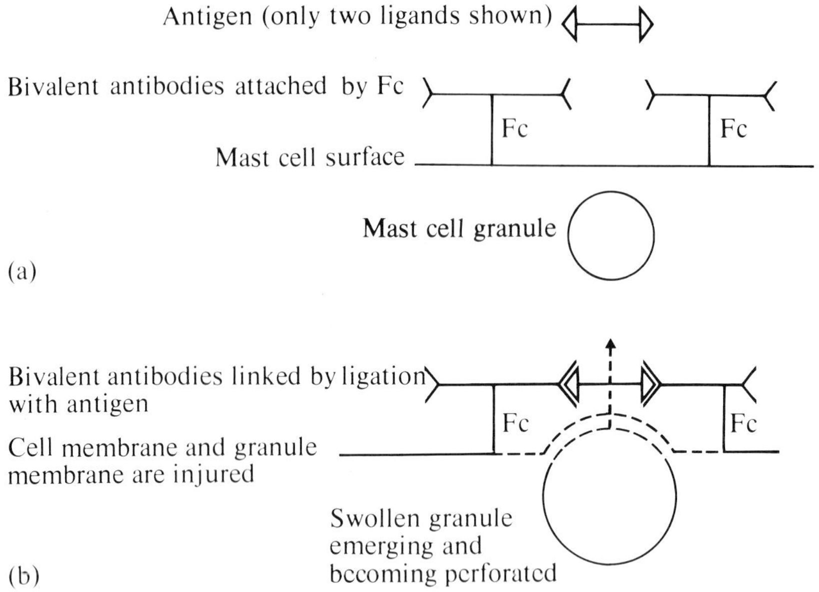

FIG. 6.5 Injury to mast cell membrane by type 1 allergic reaction.
a. Shows mast cell surface sensitized by adsorbed antibody before reaction with antigen.
b. Shows cell surface injured by reaction of antigen with antibody adsorbed on cell surface. The mast cell granules swell and their surface is also injured and some of them are ejected from the damaged cell. Although the contents of the granules are largely expelled from the cell many of their swollen envelopes remain within the cell remnant after rupture and discharge [19].

Wherever antigen can come in contact with bivalent antibody already attached to surface of mast cells this reaction of discharge of granules occurs rapidly (usually within a few minutes). Accessible tissues in man subject to these reactions include:

1. Skin, where urticaria is produced by Pt salts or penicillin.
2. Upper respiratory tract, where allergic rhinitis may follow inhalation of fungal spores and hyphae.
3. Bronchioles, where allergic asthma with bronchiolar spasm results from similar allergy to horse hair, house mites or fungal products.

In many of these sensitised patients a prick by a fine needle into the skin through a drop of fluid containing the specific antigen is followed within 15 min by development of an urticarial weal as a result of liberation of vasoactive amines from sensitised mast cells [20].

More widespread degranulation of sensitised mast cells can occur in man, with disastrous consequences, following injection of antitoxins containing horse serum proteins into patients sensitised by previous injection of these antigens possibly many years before. This may result in anaphylactic shock in which serious bronchospasm and vasomotor failure follow extensive release of vasoactive amines. Fortunately man is not so readily sensitised as some animals, such as guinea-pigs, and this generalised anaphylaxis is rare.

The tendency to form IgE antibodies, which attach to mast cells and thus generate type 1 allergy, is inherited. Persons with this tendency are said to be atopic and often develop multiple sensitivity to a variety of antigens such as house mites, foods and pollens.

Type 2 (cytotoxic) allergic reactions

In these reactions antigens, which are generally component parts of the cell surface, combine with antibodies present in the extracellular fluid. This ligation of antibody produces invisible alteration in the cell membrane which may lead to injury or lysis of the cell. Results of such cytotoxic reactions which contribute to human illness include:

Effects of mismatched blood transfusion. Following these errors antigen A or B on donor erythrocytes may ligate respectively with anti-A or anti-B antibody in plasma of recipient. The antibody-coated red cells are then rapidly sequestered by the liver, as was shown by injecting small amounts of incompatible red cells labelled by ^{51}Cr; this was followed almost immediately by radioactive emission detectable over the liver where the foreign red cells are trapped by the hepatic macrophages. This capture is effected by (*a*) *opsonic adherence*, in which the antibody, initially bound to antigen on the red cell surface, links through attachment sites on its Fc portion to special receptors on the macrophages, or (*b*) *complement-dependent immune adherence* in which the C_3 component of complement is first adsorbed on bound antibody and is then similarly linked to other receptors on the macrophages. The macrophages then engulf the trapped antibody-coated red cells and lyse them internally. This lysis is extremely rapid and soon the products of disintegrated Hb, such as globin and bilirubin, escape from the macrophages and appear in the blood.

As well as this intraphagocytic lysis of donor red cells in the liver, intravascular lysis also follows mismatched transfusions owing to action of the complete 'complement cascade' (p. 291) on the antibody-coated red cells. This results in the appearance of Hb in the plasma and also sometimes in the urine. In some cases also the consequences of mismatched transfusion are further aggravated by intravascular agglutination of donor red cells by anti-A or anti-B antibodies.

Massive transfusion of incompatible blood is almost immediately followed by rigors with flushing and dyspnoea succeeded by renal failure and sometimes terminal coma. The initial symptoms may depend on the action of histamine-like substances released from the lysed cells; but clumping of donor red cells probably also contributes to renal and cerebral ischaemia. In patients who survive these initial hazards lysis results in jaundice and persistent anaemia with failure to replace the depleted red cells.

Haemolytic disease of newborn and hydrops fetalis. This defect, which can cause intense hyperbilirubinaemia (p. 197) in the newborn child, is a consequence of damage by cytotoxic antibodies. When a child with antigen D on its red cells is born to a D-negative mother, fetal red cells bearing antigen D may pass into the maternal circulation during the third stage of labour. This D antigen can then sensitise the mother so that she synthesises anti-D antibody thereafter. The anti-D antibody can later cross the placenta during subsequent pregnancies and ligate with D antigen on red cells of a D-positive fetus conceived by the same mother. This ligation is followed rapidly by sequestration of antibody-coated red cells, which become attached to macrophages in the spleen and monocytes in the blood by opsonic adherence with subsequent phagocytosis and intracellular lysis; monocytes containing these ingested red cells are conspicuous in peripheral blood. The severe anaemia produced by this phagocytosis and lysis leads to hypoxia with increase in vascular permeability and intense oedema of the fetal tissues (hydrops fetalis) terminating in abortion or stillbirth. If the child survives till term, then continued haemolysis *after* birth can produce intense hyperbilirubinaemia followed by kernicterus and cerebral injury (p. 197); this does not happen *before* birth, since in prenatal life bilirubin formed by haemolysis within the fetus is removed by the maternal circulation.

Multiple sclerosis. Lytic action of specific antibody together with complement is probably concerned in the destruction of myelin in mutiple sclerosis (MS). In this disease plaques of demyelination develop in the white matter of brain and spinal cord and produce spastic paralysis and loss of sensation. These effects are often temporary at first but they may recur and be followed by progressive or permanent disability. In the plaques of demyelination at first the myelin sheaths alone are affected but later the axons also disintegrate. In the serum of these patients a specific MS type of antibody appears, which, in the presence of complement, causes the destruction of myelinated nerve fibres and oligodendrocytes in cultures of neonatal rat myelin [21]. Moreover some of the myelin sheaths of nerve fibres in the plaques are coated with human IgG and complement detectable by staining with fluorescent antibodies. This binding of antibody and complement to the myelin may thus indicate the site of damage in oligodendroglial cell membranes which initiates this serious disorder of myelinated fibres. There is, however, evidence (p. 392) that loss of protein from the myelin sheath may precede this binding of immunoglobulin.

Type 3 (immune complex) allergic reactions

The antigen in solution and the antibody also in solution interact to form complexes. When antigen is present in excess, these complexes are initially *soluble* but finally become deposited as minute micellar particles in or around small blood vessels generally in skin, lymph nodes, joints and renal glomeruli. When antibody is in excess, large insoluble complexes are formed which rapidly precipitate near the point of reaction as can happen in the lungs after intrapulmonary inhalation of antigenic particles by sensitised persons; this kind of effect may produce severe dyspnoea ('farmer's lung') which develops about 6 h after exposure to mouldy hay containing antigenic fungal products.

These immune complexes, composed of antigen conjoined to antibody, soon adsorb complement at their site of deposition. Then the consecutive reactions of the complement-cascade, along with its amplifying enzymic mechanisms, occur on the surface of the complexes [22, 23]. As a result of participation of C_3 and C_5 components of complement active peptides of low molecular weight (C_3a and C_5a respectively) are liberated. These peptide fragments are largely responsible for the tissue damage caused by deposition of immune complexes, although changes in the residual protein of complement are concerned in the further lytic action of complement adsorbed on cells (p. 291). The peptide fragments exert two principal harmful effects:

1. *Anaphylatoxic action.* This releases vasoactive amines from neighbouring mast cells; as a result vasodilation, oedema and bronchospasm may ensue.
2. *Chemotaxis.* This attracts neutrophil granulocytes. These cells then disintegrate and release their lysosomal enzymes and endogenous pyrogens; the former rapidly injure adjacent tissues, while the latter may cause fever (p. 232).

Precipitation of immune complexes also causes aggregation of platelets which may reinforce effect of (1) above by additional release of vasoactive amines. Diseases in which tissue damage depends on the formation of immune complexes include:

Serum sickness. In this disorder fever, generalised urticaria, swelling of lymph nodes and glomerulonephritis with oliguria and oedema develop 1–2 weeks after first injection of xenogeneic serum or more rapidly after subsequent injection. The formation of immune complexes followed by ligation of complement (C) is largely responsible for these effects; indeed the absorption of C is reflected by a rapid fall in concentration of C in the blood during the course of the disease.

The location of the lesions with swelling and inflammation is apparently determined by the site of deposition of complexes, as around the lymph nodes where much antibody is formed. Initially the antigen is present in gross excess so that soluble complexes of low MW circulate in the blood and are finally filtered out and form deposits in the walls of small vessels of skin, joints and renal glomeruli. In the glomerular capillaries the complexes readily pass through fenestrae in the specialised endothelial cells and thus rapidly reach the basement membrane (BM) where they are arrested and form deposits which fix C. Both IgG and C can be detected by immunofluorescence of the deposits formed on the BM, which are also visible (by EM) as irregular 'lumpy' particles. The peptide fragments, liberated from activated C, then cause inflammation, swelling and accumulation of neutrophils. The neutrophils and proliferated endothelial cells add to the swelling which may induce glomerular ischaemia and renal failure. Finally disruption of the neutrophils causes local tissue damage, owing to escape of their lysosomal hydrolases, as well as fever due to liberation of endogenous pyrogens (p. 232). These effects may occur wherever the immune complexes are deposited.

Injection of foreign serum into persons previously sensitised by the same antigen may also produce acute degranulation of antibody-coated mast cells with immediate bronchospasm and shock (p. 204) before the onset of more usual effects resulting from deposition of immune complexes.

Rheumatoid arthritis (*RA*). Deposition of immune complexes plays a prominent part in pathogenesis of RA. This disease, which most commonly occurs in women between 20 and 40, is characterised by arthritis, formation of subcutaneous nodules, anaemia and bouts of fever. In affected joints the synovial membrane is oedematous with pulpy masses of granulation tissue infiltrated by neutrophils, plasma cells and monocytes. The joints are swollen by excessive synovial fluid which is turbid with enormous numbers of neutrophils (Fig. 6.6a). Later the granulation tissue erodes the articular cartilages and ankylosis may ensue. The serum usually contains high concentration of a specific IgM called 'rheumatoid factor' which can agglutinate latex particles coated with denatured IgG. The neutrophils in the synovial fluid contain spherical cytoplasmic inclusions formed by aggregates of IgM, IgG and complement (C); the cells containing these immune complexes are called RA cells [24]. In some of these neutrophils the nuclear lobes are conspicuously

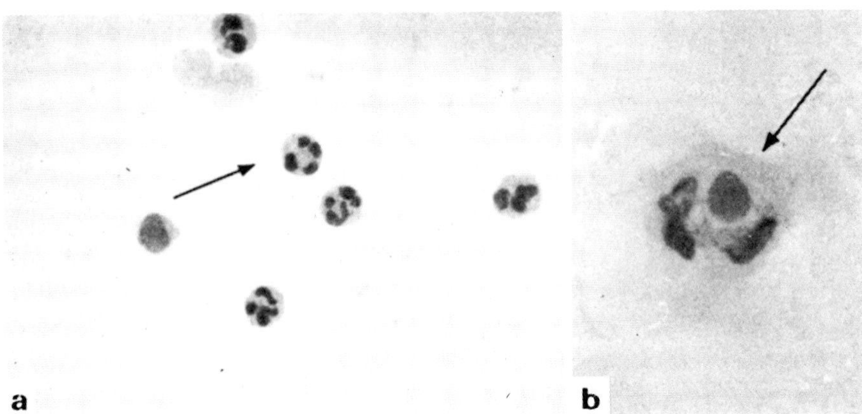

FIG. 6.6 Synovial fluid rich in neutrophil granulocytes from joints affected by rheumatoid arthritis.

a. Numerous neutrophils with multilobed nuclei; cell indicated by arrow shows peripheral displacement of nuclear chromatin. Haematoxylin eosin-azure II. ×400.

b. Neutrophil with marked peripheral displacement of nucler lobes and a central inclusion of tannophilic protein. Feulgen-oxidised tannin-azo method. ×1100. Courtesy of Professor T. Malinin, Dr T. J. Pekin & Professor N. J. Zvaifler. *Amer. J. clin. Path.* (1967), **47**, 203.

displaced towards the periphery of the cells (Fig. 6.6a, b). This displacement is caused by central deposition of protein [25] which forms clearly outlined inclusions coloured by the oxidised tannin-azo method for protein (Fig. 6.6b). These inclusions doubtless correspond to aggregates of immunoglobulin and C detectable by immunofluorescence in RA cells. IgM 'rheumatoid factor' is also present in inclusions within neutrophils and in perisynovial plasma cells, while intercellular deposits containing both IgG and C are present in swollen synovial tissue and in the subcutaneous nodules of patients with RA.

Probably RA is initiated by the formation of 'rheumatoid factor' in synovial plasma cells as an antibody to *altered* IgG. This antibody may then react with its antigen to form immune complexes, which are precipitated in the synovial membranes, where they fix C and then liberate potent chemotactic substances. Immense numbers of neutrophils then enter the synovial fluid; indeed, C_3 component of C, which is known to generate chemotactic peptides, is detectable in the inclusions within the polymorphs [26]. Probably about 300×10^6 neutrophils enter an affected knee joint daily [27]. As these cells degenerate their lysosomal enzymes and leucocytic pyrogens are set free. The enzymes include collagenase as well as neutral proteases capable of hydrolysing the peptidoglycans of cartilage. These enzymes may thus be responsible for severe tissue damage with erosion of cartilage and bone which is such an injurious event in the disease, while release of leucocytic pyrogens may account for characteristic bouts of fever. Fig. 6.7 (pp. 210, 211) shows by sequential radiographs the progressive erosion of cartilage and bone in the metacarpophalangeal joints of a patient with RA. The loss of articular cartilage is revealed by disappearance of radio-translucent gaps between the bones, while the erosion of bone is seen by loss of density in both metatarsals and phalanges.

Deposition of immune complexes followed by adsorption of C with chemotaxis of leucocytes and release of their harmful enzymes thus appear to be dominant events in causing RA, but the mechanism by which the initial antigen is generated, possibly by alteration of IgG, is obscure.

Systemic lupus erythematosus (*SLE*) is another illness in which deposition of immune complexes is a paramount event. This disorder of connective tissue produces symmetrical rashes, fibrinous arthritis and pericarditis, myalgia with bouts of fever, and frequently oedema and proteinuria due to glomerulonephritis. In affected regions the basement membranes (BM) of blood vessels are thickened, while fibrinoid material is deposited in synovial membranes of joints and in cardiac and pleural connective tissue. In these fibrinoid lesions and in zones of necrosis in lymph nodes characteristic spherical bodies rich in DNA and containing immunoglobulin are deposited (see below).

SLE is probably determined by immune complex reactions between antigenic constituents of human nuclei and antinuclear antibodies (ANA) followed by adsorption and activation of complement (C) adsorbed on the complexes. In the kidney of patients with SLE there is clear evidence of deposition of immune complexes. The glomerular BM is thickened and on both sides of it granular deposits may be visible. These deposits contain:

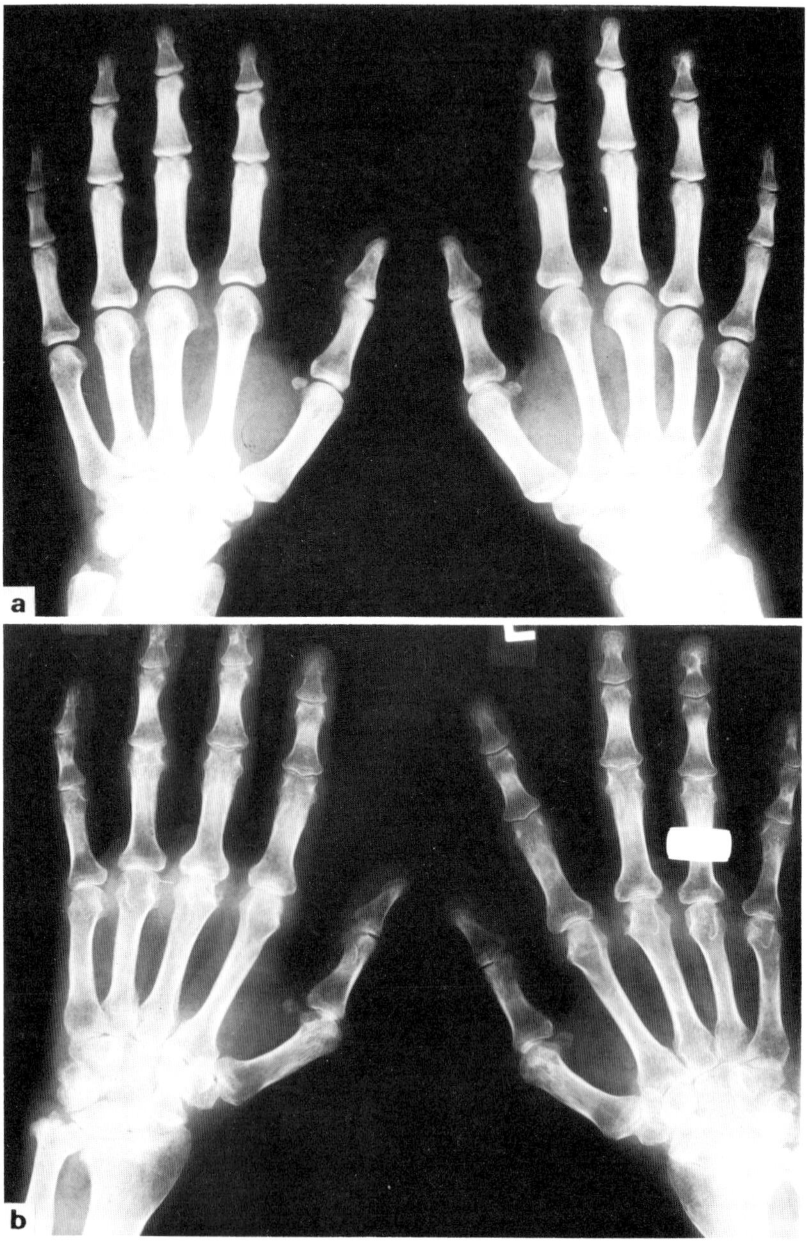

FIG. 6.7 Rheumatoid arthritis. Successive stages in erosion of cartilage and bone around metacarpophalangeal joints.

a. Radiotranslucent gaps between heads of metacarpals and phalanges demonstrate intact articular cartilages; only slight loss of osseous density.

b. Erosion of cartilage has eliminated these radiotranslucent gaps in joints; considerable loss of density both in metacarpal heads and phalanges due to erosion of bone.

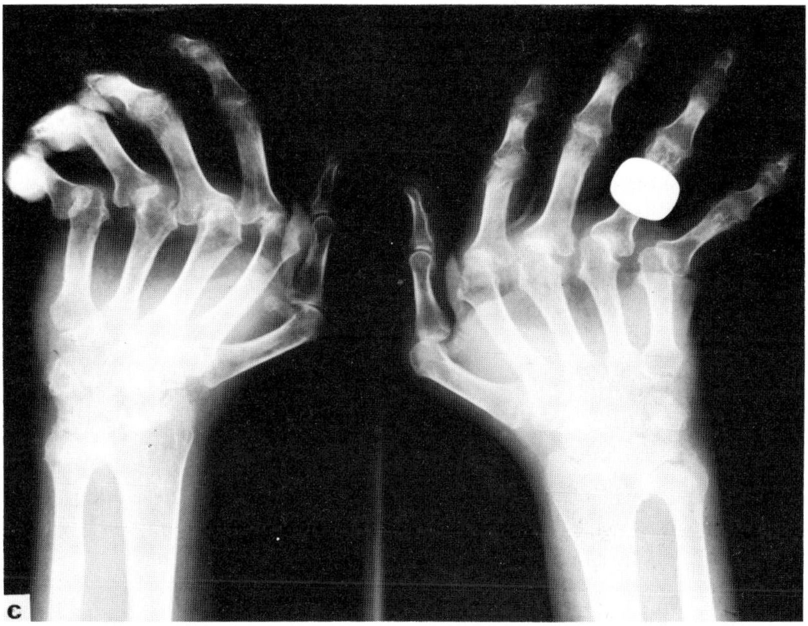

FIG. 6.7 cont.
c. Further osseous erosion and more severe deformity. Courtesy of Dr A. K. Dixon.

1. DNA stainable by the Feulgen method and also by fluorescent antibody to native DNA.
2. Immunoglobulins including antibodies to specific nuclear antigens (such as DNA).
3. Components of C detectable by immunofluorescence [26].

Moreover, the concentration of C in the serum of patients with SLE is abnormally low especially when there is concomitant renal disease. The immune complexes deposited in the kidney absorb C and this probably leads to local inflammation, chemotaxis of neutrophils, endothelial swelling and mesangial proliferation often terminating in glomerular ischaemia and renal failure.

Deposits containing immunoglobulins are also found in undamaged skin of many patients with SLE. These aggregates are detectable by treatment of sections with fluorescent anti-human globulins and are visible along the dermo-epidermal BM [28]. This *lupus band test* is positive in the majority of patients with lupus nephritis and in nearly all patients with a low level of serum C. Moreover the globulins present in these deposits include IgG, IgM, IgA and C_3, and are generally of the same classes as those found in renal lesions of the same patient [29]. Probably these deposits are also immune complexes which precipitate on the dermo-epidermal BM in the same way as similar complexes are filtered out on the glomerular BM.

Antinuclear antibodies (ANA) are generally present in the serum of patients with SLE. ANA can be detected by adsorption on nuclei in sections of rat liver followed by specific ligation of fluorescent anti-human immunoglobulins to the adsorbed ANA. These antibodies belong principally to the IgG class and some of them ligate with nucleoprotein or with DNA itself. They also include the *LE factor* which exerts a remarkable homogenising effect on nuclei by reacting with their nucleoprotein. When neutrophils or lymphocytes from normal blood (or from blood of SLE patients) are exposed to LE factor (from a patient's serum) *in vitro*, the nuclei of the older white cells swell and become homogeneous and are then extruded from the cells. The LE factor can only enter the older white cells or those that have been damaged artificially, as by shaking with glass ballotini. Within 5 sec of contact with LE factor, the nuclei swell and their lobes fuse [30]; the nuclei are then expelled from the cells. The resultant spherical and homogeneous nuclear remnants are called *LE bodies*; they are faintly basophilic and Feulgen-positive, owing to presence of DNA, and they also contain immunoglobulin adsorbed from the LE factor [31]. On further incubation with blood the LE bodies are taken up by phagocytes which are then seen (in blood

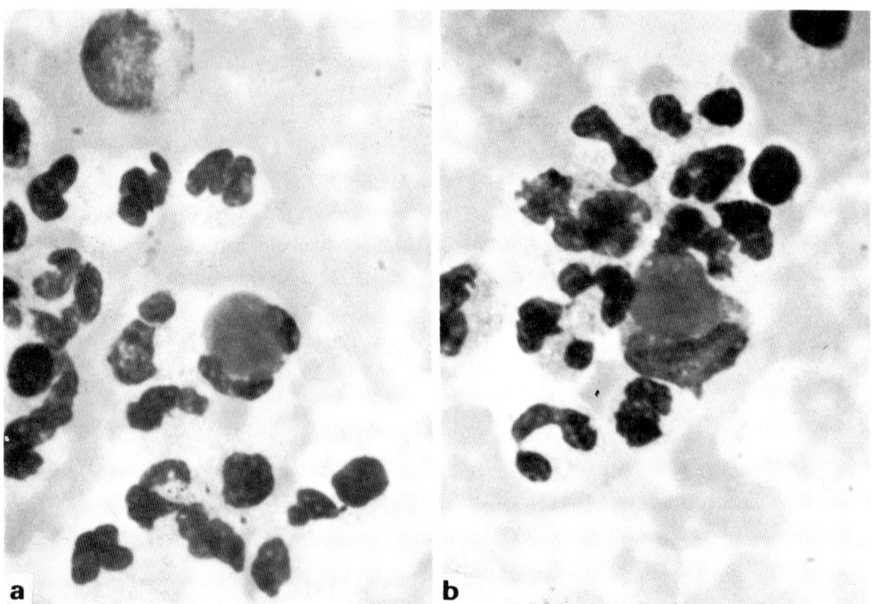

FIG. 6.8 LE cells after phagocytosis of spherical nuclear remnants (LE bodies); from a preparation of human leucocytes incubated with serum from a patient with SLE. ×910.

a. Neutrophil with dense nuclear lobes attached to periphery of enclosed spherical LE body.

b. Macrophage also enclosing a spherical LE body.

films) enclosing these swollen nuclear remnants. These phagocytes are called *LE cells* and include both neutrophils (Fig. 6.8a) and macrophages (Fig. 6.8b).

The formation of LE cells thus involves two sequential stages:

1. Action of LE factor on nuclei; in this stage Ig detectable by fluorescent antibody is adsorbed by nuclei which are swollen, homogenised and extruded from the cells to form LE bodies.

2. LE bodies are taken up by phagocytes to form LE cells; this process requires the presence of complement [31]. Indeed this second stage depends on the chemotactic attraction of C components activated by adsorption on immune complexes.

This swelling and homogenisation of nuclei and expulsion of nuclear remnants probably also occurs in the tissues of patients with SLE. Within the lesions in cardiac connective tissue, lymph nodes, synovial membranes and renal glomeruli, masses of Feulgen-positive basophilic material are frequently visible. These granular masses are strongly coloured by alum-haematoxylin and are called 'haematoxylin bodies'; they are probably formed by action of LE factor on the nuclei of older cells in these patients, and their presence indicates previous action of soluble antinuclear antibodies on nuclear antigens.

How far this action of antinuclear antibodies is directly concerned with causing the principal lesions of SLE is uncertain. Transfusion of plasma from patients containing LE factor does not transmit overt disease to recipients. Moreover LE factor exerts the same antinuclear action on normal neutrophils as on those from patients with SLE. Also antinuclear antibodies show no toxic effects on healthy intact cells in culture [26]. The lesion therefore cannot result from direct toxic effect of autoantibodies on nuclei of *healthy* cells.

However there is cogent evidence (see above) that renal lesions in SLE are related to location of immune complexes between ANA and nuclear constituents along with adsorption and activation of C, and it seems likely that degenerative and fibrinoid changes in other tissues are similarly excited. The antigens which initiate this allergic reaction appear to be DNA and other nuclear constituents. DNA and also antibodies to DNA are present in serum of patients with SLE [32, 33], while immunoglobulins are found adsorbed on some of the nuclei in zones of dermal and renal inflammation in SLE [26].

Antigenic change in nuclear DNA (or loss of tolerance to it) may be initiated by various agents such as drugs, viral infection or even by ultraviolet light (UVL). Indeed UVL can cause antigenic change in DNA of epidermal nuclei (p. 129). It is thus significant that erythematous lesions in the skin in SLE appear on exposed parts of the body and are exacerbated by UVL. Adsorption by nuclei of a specific antibody to altered DNA may thus be a crucial event in extending nuclear damage and release of additional nuclear antigens which then evoke further autoimmune sensitisation. Thus a wider and less specific assortment of ANA is evolved. This amplification in the synthesis of ANA then heralds more extensive deposition of immune complexes with activation of C in kidney, skin, joints and other tissues which ultimately causes widespread and severe injury in this remarkable nuclear malady.

Cell-mediated or delayed hypersensitivity

This involves formation of specific clones of sensitised thymus-derived lymphocytes (T-lymphocytes), which are developed in response to an encounter with an individual antigen. These cells carry on their surface specific receptors, which ligate with the same antigen on re-encounter, so as to produce a reaction of swelling, induration and erythema at site of contact within 1–2 days. This state of reactivity is called cell-mediated hypersensitivity (CMH); it becomes established after a latent period generally of 1–3 weeks following first exposure to the antigen.

Antigens which initiate CMH

These include:

1. Micromolecules such as Ni, $HgCl_2$, picryl chloride, 4-phenylenediamine and 2,4-dinitro-1-chlorobenzene (DNCB), which are probably absorbed through skin and then chelated to tissue proteins before becoming fully antigenic.
2. Macromolecular complexes, such as the protein (tuberculin) and lipids of the tubercle bacillus, which together act as a complete antigen and thus induce CMH caused by tuberculous infection; CMH arising in this way is a common sequel to chronic bacterial infection (p. 236).

Some substances, which induce CMH *after* a latent period, are also directly irritant and rapidly produce non-allergic lesions at higher concentration even in *unsensitised* patients. Thus $HgCl_2$ in 1–3 per cent aqueous solution is directly irritant to human skin (whether sensitised or unsensitised). But, after sensitisation by previous exposure, reapplication of $HgCl_2$ in 0.1 per cent solution or less produces typical delayed reaction of CMH [34].

Access of an antigen to reactive cells: contact dermatitis

Exposure of the skin by mere *contact* with an antigen which is readily absorbed (such as DNCB or 4-phenylenediamine) establishes CMH within 7–14 days. Thereafter re-exposure to the same antigen causes an allergic reaction within 48 h. This consists of swelling, induration and erythema of the skin, due to vasodilation and *infiltration* of the dermis with lymphocytes and monocytes. The epidermis becomes oedematous and this may be followed by blistering and necrosis resulting in severe vesicular dermatitis; the condition is called *contact dermatitis* (CD). Common substances in the human environment, which act in this way, include the chemicals mentioned above and also hair dyes and mascara cosmetics as well as nickel-plated watches and suspender belts.

The antigens which initiate contact dermatitis are taken up in the epidermis and dermis by *dendritic* cells; these are specialised macrophages with long processes and are called Langerhans cells. After preliminary sensitisation the reapplication of antigens (such as $HgCl_2$ or DNCB) is followed within 3–5 h by movement of Langerhans cells into close apposition with lymphocytes [34, 35]. This apposition, however, does not occur in lesions caused by primary irritants. Antigens labelled with electron-dense ferritin are seen by EM to be picked up in the skin by Langerhans cells, which transport the labelled antigens to lymphocytes both in the skin and related lymph nodes [36]. In this way the antigens are probably transported from the epidermis to T-lymphocytes both in the initial process of sensitisation and in the subsequent allergic reaction which rapidly follows re-exposure to the same antigen.

Antigenic constituents of invasive pathogens such as the tubercle bacillus reach T-cells by transport within phagocytic macrophages, in which the bacilli disintegrate. In this way the T-cells become sensitised and produce harmful CMH which contributes greatly to the pathogenicity of these bacteria (p. 239).

Effects of antigens on sensitised cells: consequences of CMH

The consequences of ligation of antigen to specific receptors on sensitised T-lymphocytes (T-cells) are numerous and include:

1. *Direct mitogenic action* (*clonal expansion*). This increases the number of sensitised T-cells; these cells contribute to swelling and induration in cell-mediated allergic reactions including both CD and the tuberculin reaction (Fig. 6.9, p. 216).

2. *Liberation of lymphokines.* The antigen also stimulates the specifically sensitised T-cells to liberate highly active soluble substances called lymphokines [37], which:

a. Exert mitogenic action on both sensitised and unsensitised T-cells (indirect clonal expansion); this further increases local swelling and induration in both CD and in reaction to tuberculin, and causes lymphocytic infiltration in tuberculosis.

b. In low concentration stimulate mitosis of macrophages and activate their lysosomes to produce 'angry macrophages' which are effective in killing ingested bacteria (Fig. 6.9). This results in cell-mediated immunity (CMI).

c. In higher concentration attract macrophages and alter their surface so that they are immobilised and cohere together and even fuse to form giant cells. These coherent and fused cells may then die and disintegrate into caseous debris. These effects are responsible for the formation of groups of coherent epithelioid cells and giant cells in tuberculous exudates (see Fig. 6.14), and also contribute significantly to the highly necrotising action of the tubercle bacillus (see Fig. 6.14c and Fig. 7.33).

d. Cause swelling and separation of capillary endothelial cells and thus initiate the prolonged inflammation of CD and other forms of CMH; this severe inflammatory stasis may lead to ischaemic necrosis. Prostaglandins, which are formed in CD (p. 194) also contribute to the prolonged inflammation.

3. *Aggressor action as 'killer' cells.* After sensitisation by antigen T-cells can develop aggressive power and transform into 'killer' (cytotoxic) cells which then attach themselves to 'target' cells bearing the *same* antigen on their surface. This attachment damages the surface membrane and is followed by the death of the

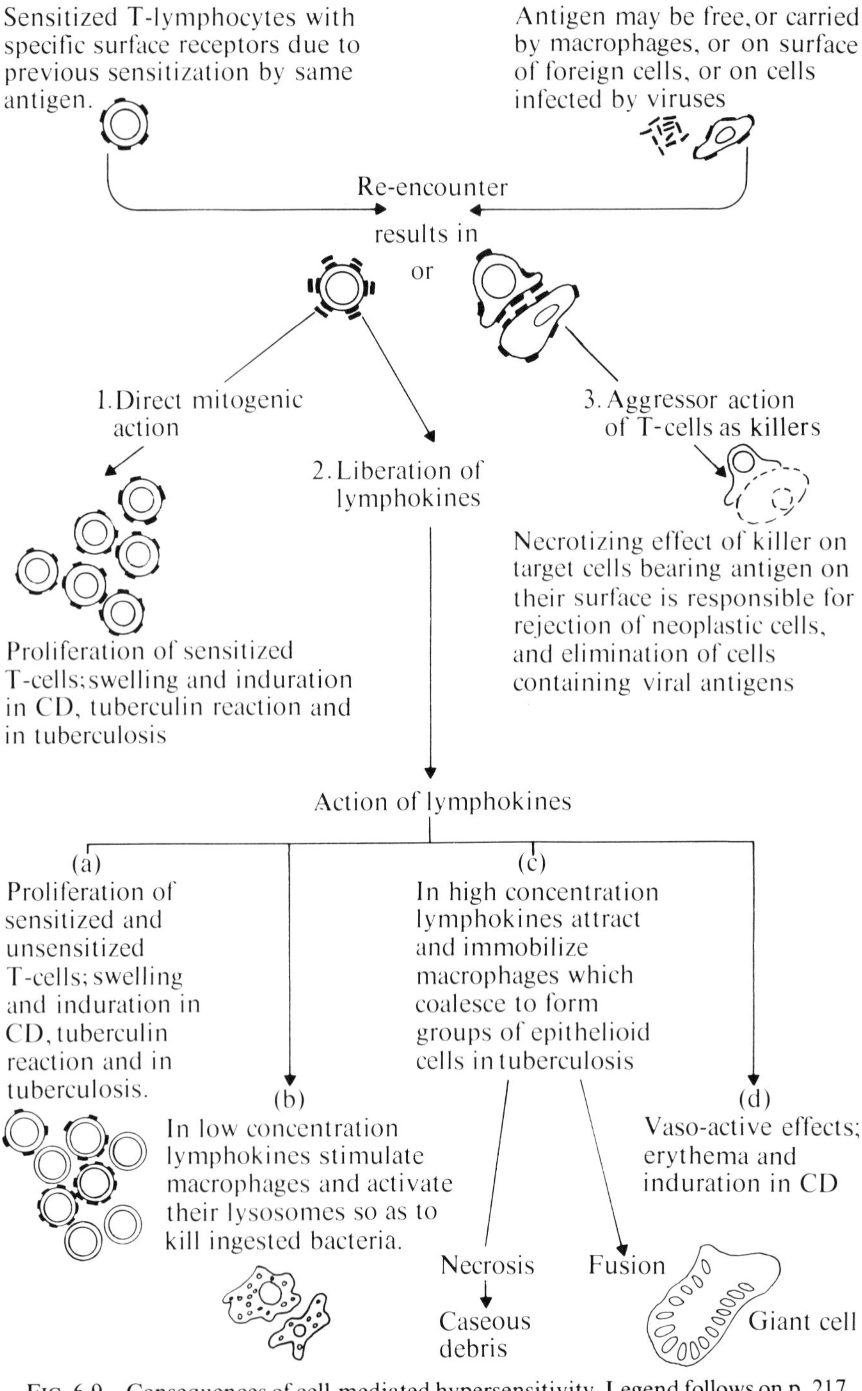

FIG. 6.9 Consequences of cell-mediated hypersensitivity. Legend follows on p. 217 opposite.

'target cell'. The contact of killer to target is extremely close and involves intercellular communication between the two, which can be revealed by passage of a fluorescent dye from one partner to another in this kiss of death [38]. The necrotising action of killer on target is probably an important factor in killing transplanted allogeneic cells in the rejection of allografts (Fig. 6.9). Similarly lymphocytes obtained from patients with squamous carcinoma can kill the cells of the same cancer grown in tissue culture after excision; the lymphocytes firmly adhere to the cancer cells, which then round up and become amorphous [39]. The lymphocytes of these patients thus probably become sensitised and transformed by contact with the antigens of the carcinoma. This action may be highly effective in preventing the spread of neoplasm. Also cytotoxic T-cells sensitised by viral antigens can kill cells freshly infected by the same virus; this elimination of infected cells before the virus is fully formed is probably a major determinant of recovery and immunity in viral infection (p. 270).

Fig. 6.9 summarises (in a diagram) the various consequences of re-encounter of antigen with specifically sensitised T-cells.

INJURY BY HOSTILE FOREIGN ORGANISMS

This discussion will be limited to the action of pathogenic microorganisms.

Pathogenicity is the power to cause disease; this depends on two principal characteristics—toxigenicity and invasiveness. Toxigenicity is the capacity to form harmful substances, while invasiveness is the power to grow, divide and spread in the tissues and cells of the body.

Pathogenic microbes (pathogens) are in general toxigenic, or invasive, or both. Indeed these hostile microbes show a gradation in the relative magnitude

---

FIG. 6.9 Consequences of cell-mediated hypersensitivity. Re-encounter of sensitised T-lymphocytes (T-cells) with sensitising antigen (which may be free in solution or on surface of foreign or virus-infected cells) results in:

1. Direct mitogenic action on T-cells.
2. Liberation of lymphokines from T-cells which give rise to further effects a, b, c and d.
3. Aggressor action of T-cells which can kill foreign or virus-infected cells bearing the specific antigen on their surface.

unsensitised T-cell 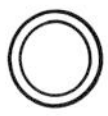

sensitised T-cell with specific surface receptors 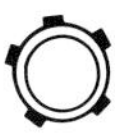

antigenic molecules (which ligate specifically to these receptors) -

these antigenic molecules may be free in solution 

or may be attached to surface of a foreign or virus-infected cell 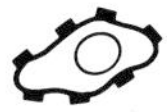

of these two characteristics. At one end of the scale there is extreme toxigenicity with very little or no invasiveness, as for instance *Clostridium botulinum*, which does not invade the body but produces one of the most lethal of all toxins. Some pathogens show both properties, such as *Streptococcus pyogenes*, which is toxigenic in causing scarlet fever, but highly invasive and also toxigenic when producing septicaemia. At the other end of the scale little or no toxigenicity may be displayed but extreme invasiveness is prominent; this is so with *Treponema pallidum* which, in causing syphilis, can penetrate and invade mucous membranes and the placenta, and can also spread throughout the body, but yet forms no known toxin.

One might fairly ask how a microbe can injure cells, if it forms no toxins at all; indeed most visitors are not poisonous hooligans. Yet, in the case of cells, the invader may interfere with their nutrition, or liberate harmful substances from them, or as a xenogeneic alien, the invader may exert harmful antigenic action. Thus invasiveness alone may be sufficient as an initial determinant which actually causes disease because of consequential effects, which occur after infection is established.

We shall consider four principal mechanisms by which hostile microorganisms injure the cells of the body so as to produce disease:

1. Deprivation of nutriments.
2. Formation and liberation of harmful substances; which may be:
   (a) Exotoxins formed by microbial metabolism.
   (b) Endotoxins liberated from disintegrating microbes.
   (c) Endogenous poisons liberated from injured cells of the body, as a result of microbial activity.
3. Harmful antigenic action.
4. Intracellular growth.

More than one of these mechanisms may contribute to injurious effects of disease produced by one and the same pathogen; thus the varied injury resulting from infection by *Mycobacterium tuberculosis* illustrates these four mechanisms. Moreover in some diseases caused by microbial pathogens the mechanism of injury is undetermined.

Deprivation of nutriments by hostile organisms

The activity of pathogenic microbes may interfere with absorption of oxygen by the lungs and its transport by the blood.

Thus the 'false membrane' produced in the larynx by infection with *Corynebacterium diphtheriae* (p. 223) can obstruct the narrow air entry in children with diphtheria and so cause death by asphyxia. Inflammatory exudate formed in the lungs in lobar pneumonia and pulmonary tuberculosis also interferes with absorption of O_2. In prenatal congenital syphilis the pulmonary alveoli become occupied by fibrous tissue and exudate, so that the lungs become white and solidified (*pneumonia alba*); the newborn child can never inhale air, and dies from asphyxia immediately after birth.

Hostile microbes can also produce profound cellular injury by interrupting the supply of blood. Thus blood vessels may become occluded by red cells parasitised by *Plasmodium falciparum* with disastrous consequences to the brain or the heart in malignant tertian malaria (p. 247).

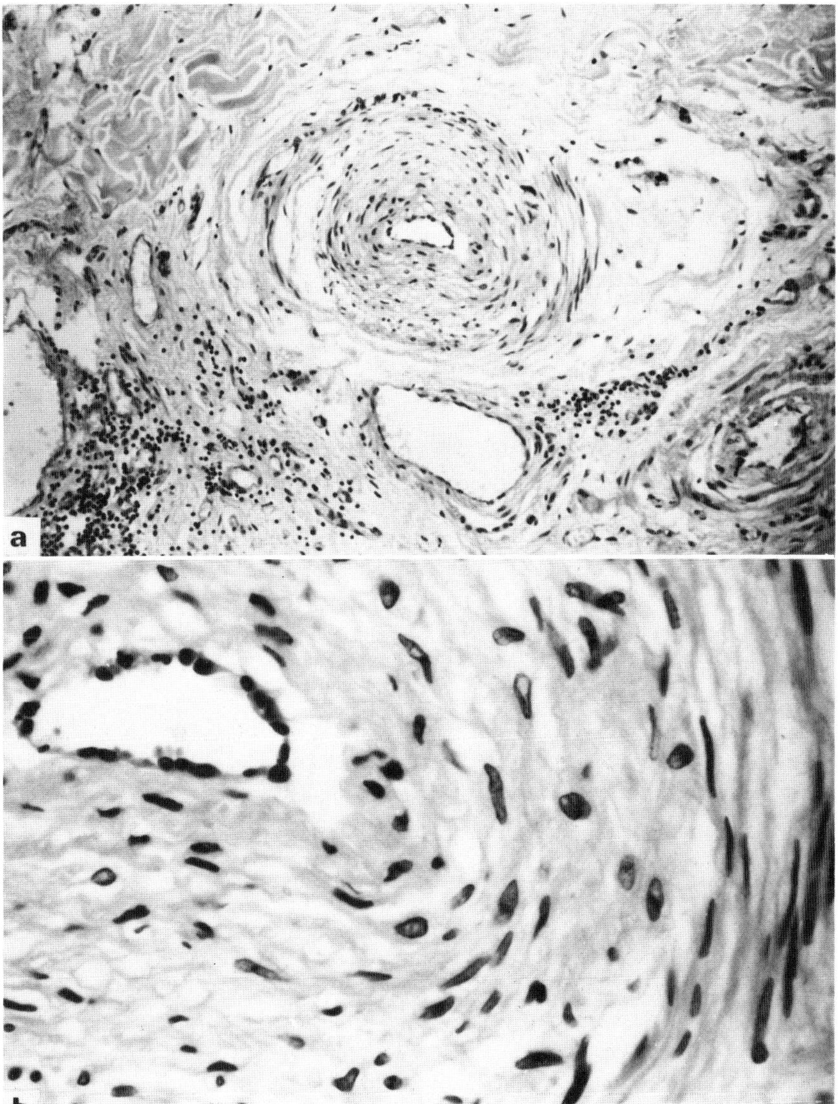

FIG. 6.10 Aortic syphilis. Partial occlusion of an arteriole in the adventitia by syphilitic endarteritis obliterans; intense proliferation of intimal connective tissue.
a. ×130.
b. ×510.

Inflammatory stasis caused by bacterial infection can also result in ischaemic injury. This stasis is particularly harmful when the infecting organisms produce exotoxins capable of injuring the capillary endothelium and thus increasing vascular permeability. Such action by the exotoxins of *Clostridium oedematiens* and *Bacillus anthracis* contribute respectively to the necrotising inflammation occurring in gas gangrene of muscle and in cutaneous anthrax. Occlusion of blood vessels may also result from septic emboli which become detached from thrombi formed on mural endocardium by bacterial infection during subacute bacterial endocarditis or generalised bacterial septicaemia.

By stimulating cellular proliferation some pathogenic bacteria can cause narrowing of blood vessels and so interrupt cellular nutrition. This thickening of arterioles with narrowing of their lumina (endarteritis obliterans) is a prominent feature of tertiary and late syphilis, and may cause ischaemic injury of the surrounding tissue. In aortic syphilis such narrowing affects the arterioles of the adventitia and may thus restrict nutrition of the media; this defect may cause destruction of elastic tissue in the aortic media along with dilatation of the aortic wall, which is responsible for both formation of aneurysms and incompetence of the aortic valve. Fig. 6.10 shows an arteriole in aortic adventitia which is in this way severely narrowed by syphilitic endarteritis.

Intense cellular proliferation and mutual coherence of macrophages, in exudates excited by *Mycobacterium tuberculosis* (p. 244), may also deprive these cells of nutriments and so contribute to the devastating caseous necrosis which is so typical of tuberculous infection. Compressed mononuclear cells in exudates may similarly become necrotic in the lesions of typhoid fever (p. 229).

Formation of toxic substances by bacteria: exotoxins

Exotoxins are intensely harmful proteins formed and excreted by pathogenic bacteria in the course of their metabolism. Many exotoxins are the dominant agents by which organisms of high pathogenicity cause specific diseases. They either directly affect cell function or behaviour without first causing any visible injury to the cell, or they kill the cell and so stop its function. The action of some exotoxins which primarily affect cellular function or behaviour will be considered first.

Clostridium botulinum

This anaerobic pathogen produces an exotoxin which is one of the most powerful of all known poisons; 1 mg of the pure protein (MW 60 000D) could kill 200×10^6 mice. Formed in infected meat or vegetables under anaerobic conditions the toxin is consumed in food. The organism itself is entirely non-invasive. The toxin is absorbed from the bowel, then enters the blood and is finally adsorbed at the fine unmyelinated terminals of cholinergic fibres in muscle and spinal cord preventing the release of acetyl choline [40, 41]. In the disease botulism there is early paralysis of eye muscles with diplopia and ptosis. Later there is more general muscular paresis and death is due to the effect of the toxin in paralysing the muscles of respiration and deglutition.

Clostridium tetani

This anaerobe also forms and releases an intensely poisonous protein: 1 mg could kill 10×10^6 mice. This toxin is formed when the spores of *Cl. tetani* germinate in the anaerobic tissue of necrotic wounds.

The toxin is specifically adsorbed by the axonal terminals of nerve fibres. This happens very readily when wounded striated muscle becomes infected; the toxin then passes up the axons of motoneurones to reach the spinal cord. This mode of transit was demonstrated by injecting toxin labeled with ^{125}I into muscles of rats or mice and then crushing the nerves supplying the muscles a few hours afterwards; the toxin labelled by ^{125}I then accumulated inside the axons *distal* to the crush where it became detectable by autoradiography [42]; this showed that the toxin can rapidly move up the nerves to the spinal cord by *retrograde axonal transport*. Similarly labeled toxin was located 7–14 h after injection into muscles by EM-autoradiography within the corresponding perikarya and dendrites of motoneurones in the ventral horn grey matter of spinal cord [43]. The glial elements and dorsal horn grey matter were unlabeled, but much of the labeled toxin also appeared in synaptic terminals afferent to the motoneurones. This work provided evidence of transsynaptic migration of tetanus toxin in spinal cord and motoneurones.

This adsorption of toxin probably prevents liberation of inhibitory transmitters such as glycine and γ-aminobutyrate from the presynaptic terminals with annulment of spinal inhibition, so that the excitatory function of motoneurones becomes hyperactive.

Homogenised nervous tissue specifically removes tetanus toxin from solution, but other tissues fail to do so (Wassermann-Takaki phenomenon). Apparently the toxic group is directly bound since toxoid is not similarly adsorbed. This ligation to nervous tissue is probably due to binding of the toxin to a sialidase-labile disialosyl ganglioside which acts as a membrane receptor for the toxin [44].

In clinical tetanus the toxin adsorbed at motor terminals passes by retrograde intra-axonal transport along the nerve fibres innervating the infected muscle and finally reaches the synapses of the corresponding motor cell bodies in the spinal cord, where inhibitory impulses are suppressed; this may first excite the muscles of the injured region alone so as to give preliminary *local tetanus*. Transsynaptic spread of the toxin in spinal grey matter can then cause more general suppression of central inhibition with widespread magnification of reflex motor activity; this induces intense convulsive spasms affecting many groups of muscles characteristic of *generalised tetanus*. Death is usually due to spasm of respiratory muscles.

Vibrio cholerae

The causative organism of cholera grows and multiplies in enormous numbers within the lumen of the small intestine; there it forms and excretes a heat labile toxic protein (MW 84 000D). This substance, which is called cholera toxin (CT), exerts a remarkable effect in stimulating enterocytes of the small intestine to secrete large volumes of isotonic fluid, resulting in serious loss of water and electrolytes from the body. If this is not replaced the patient shrivels owing to dehydration produced by the efflux of many litres of water a day. CT stimulates the active secretion of Cl^- and water through isolated pieces of ileal mucosa; $3^1,5^1$-cyclic AMP exerts the same action. Moreover CT increases the activity of adenyl cyclase in homogenates and membrane preparations of the mucosal cells. The toxic effects of CT are thus believed to depend on its power to activate adenylcyclase in the mucosal enterocytes [45]. These membranes bind CT with avidity and this ligation is effected through sialidase-stable monosialosyl ganglioside receptors on the enterocyte surface [44]. After binding, CT activates adenylcyclase so that cyclic AMP is formed; this rapidly increases the secretory action of the cells and finally may kill the patient by devasting depletion of fluid. The introduction of CT into an isolated loop of intestine rapidly increases the mucosal activity of adenylcyclase and also the flow of fluid into the loop [46]; boiled toxin is inactive. CT does not kill mucosal cells and exerts its harmful effects entirely by stimulating their activity.

Enteropathogenic strains of *Escherichia coli*, which cause infantile gastroenteritis, also produce enterotoxins with action on the intestinal mucosa similar to that of CT. This may result in extreme fluid loss resembling that of cholera. These toxins like CT probably activate adenylcyclase. By this mechanism cell-free culture filtrates from these strains of *E.coli*, and also CT, are able to induce formation of ketosteroids by adrenocortical cells in culture, and simultaneously they can make the cells round up and separate from each other. These effects may all be caused by activation of adenylcyclase [47].

Another hostile enteropathogen which is apparently one of the most common causes of human enteritis is the microaerophilic vibrio *Campylobacter* (καμπύλος, curved). This vibrio, now that its requirements in culture and its capacity to pass through millipore filters are recognised, is frequently isolated from patients with diarrhoea [48]. Infection may be transmitted to man from poultry. *C.jejuni* and *C.coli* produce severe diarrhoea along with intense abdominal pain, fever and headache; the ileum becomes acutely inflamed and oedematous, while the mesenteric lymph nodes are enlarged. It is uncertain whether *Campylobacter* causes its harmful action by means of an exotoxin, akin to that of *V.cholerae*, or invades the enteric mucosa like *Shigella dysenteriae* (p. 244).

Other exotoxins exert their principal pathogenic effects by killing cells. This necrotising action may be preceded by interruption in function or it may involve visible structural damage from the start. Bacteria which secrete necrotising exotoxins include the following.

Corynebacterium diphtheriae

This highly toxigenic pathogen is only locally invasive and produces all its clinical effects by the action of an extremely powerful exotoxin which it forms and excretes.

When *C. diphtheriae* grows in the throat its toxin is liberated and first kills the mucosal cells. These dead cells, together with the fibrin formed by the intense concomitant inflammatory reaction, produce a greyish yellow exudate called the 'false membrane' which may cover extensive zones of the pharyngeal and laryngeal mucosa. In children the laryngeal 'membrane' can occlude the larynx and produce asphyxia. The membrane provides an ideal culture medium for *C. diphtheriae*, which then multiplies and produces more exotoxin; a vicious cycle then develops. Absorption of the toxin is followed by fatty deposition and necrosis in heart muscle with cardiac failure and arrest. The toxin also causes demyelination of peripheral nerves accompanied by paralysis. Splitting and fragmentation of myelin lamellae precede the destruction of myelin; the axons of the nerves are often unharmed although the degenerating myelin retracts from the nodes, and the Schwann cells and myelin disintegrate [49–51].

The exotoxin, as secreted by *C. diphtheriae*, is a single polypeptide chain (MW 62 000D) with two disulphide bridges. This substance diffuses into the body and causes injury by its uniquely necrotising effect on the cells which absorb it. The exotoxin is extremely lethal to susceptible animals such as man and guinea-pig for whom the lethal dose of the pure polypeptide may be as low as 10^{-1} μg/kg. But the cytocidal effect, which depends on enzymic action of a portion of the peptide absorbed by the cell, may be exerted by even lower concentrations of the toxic fragment (see below).

The toxin blocks the incorporation of amino acids into protein in mammalian cells. This inhibition of protein synthesis by the toxin was first demonstrated in human Hela cells in culture [52]; the cells round up, become granular and finally disintegrate, leaving shreds of cytoplasm round apparently intact nuclei. At a concentration of 10^{-8} M the toxin arrests the incorporation of amino acids into mammalian cells. The complete toxin is inactive in inhibiting protein synthesis in cell extracts, but it alone can *enter* intact cells. The incorporation of amino acids into peptides in cell extracts is, on the other hand, powerfully inhibited by a fragment made from the toxin within the cell (activated toxin). This effect is due to inactivation of elongation factor 2 (EF2 or transferase II), one of the highly soluble enzymes necessary for transferring amino acids from aminoacyl-t-RNA to the elongating peptide chain on the ribosome during synthesis of peptides [53, 54].

This inactivation of EF2 is an enzymic process catalysed by the activated toxin in which an ADP-ribosyl group is transferred from nicotinamide adenine dinucleotide (NAD^+) to EF2 so as to form an *inactive* addition compound ADP-ribosyl-EF2.

$$NAD^+ + EF2 \rightleftharpoons \text{ADP-ribosyl-EF2} + \text{nicotinamide} + H^+$$

By this mechanism the activated toxin abolishes the activity of EF2 and interrupts the elongation of peptide chains. Protein synthesis is thus arrested and cellular death follows.

The exotoxin secreted by *C. diphtheriae* is a polypeptide (62 000D). It can be split into fragments A (24 000D) and B (38 000D). A without B cannot injure whole animals or intact cells. Fragment A alone can inhibit synthesis of protein in *cell free extracts* by catalysing inactivation of translocation (elongation) factor EF2. But the complex with both factors is necessary for intoxication of *whole cells* or animals. It is thought that fragment B is required for attachment of the whole molecule of the toxin to the cell membrane, where fragment A is split off and enters the cell. A single molecule of fragment A is sufficient to convert all the EF2 within the cell into its inactive ADP-ribosyl derivative [55, 55a].

The power of the toxin of *C. diphtheriae* to exert this profound inhibition on protein synthesis doubtless accounts for its necrotising effects on pharyngeal epithelial cells and cardiac muscle fibres. Moreover the highly specific fission and fragmentation of myelin lamellae followed by demyelination and necrosis of Schwann cells (p. 223), which occur in diphtheritic neuropathy, may also depend on the action of the toxin in abolishing the supply of protein essential for maintaining myelin lamellae. Lack of protein needed for membrane structure and semipermeability may similarly induce swelling of hepatic and renal cells which is a conspicuous effect after injection of rabbits with *sublethal* doses of diphtheria toxin [56].

Pathogenicity of the exotoxin for different species of animal apparently varies with capacity of fragment B of toxin to bind to their individual cellular receptors; without this ligation the toxic fragment A cannot enter the cells. This difference in ligation to cell surfaces probably explains why the whole toxin is about 1000 times more lethal (per unit of body weight) to man and guinea-pigs than to rats and mice.

Virulence of C. diphtheriae. C. diphtheriae only forms its exotoxin when lysogenised by a temperate phage; this provides the genetic code for synthesis of the singularly damaging A–B peptide. Strains not infected by this phage are *avirulent*. Virulence is clearly advantageous to the toxigenic strains of *C. diphtheriae*, as it enables them to produce a highly fertile pharyngeal exudate in which colonial growth occurs at an enhanced rate.

Other *bipartite peptides* similar to the toxin of *C. diphtheriae* are now known. In these peptides, as in diphtheria toxin, fragment A is a toxic enzyme. This can *only* enter cells when fragment B ligates to receptors on the cell membrane; then fragment A passes through the membrane. These A–B toxins include the exotoxin of *Pseudomonas aeruginosa*, which so harmfully infects burns, and also the toxic peptide ricin of castor oil seeds [57]. Ricin has apparently been used by injection as an offensive weapon.

Clostridium welchii (*and gas gangrene*)

Clostridium welchii is the prime pathogen responsible for gas gangrene. In this disease clostridia and anaerobic streptococci grow in the anaerobic medium formed *in vivo* by traumatised infected muscle, where necrotic tissue is sufficiently anoxic to enable clostridial spores to germinate. In these conditions the clostridia form and liberate various exotoxins which cause highly injurious effects. Exotoxins elaborated by *Cl. welchii* kill the adjoining muscle fibres, while its carbohydrases ferment the muscle glycogen to produce bubbles of gas in the infected muscle; hence the name gas gangrene. Finally proteases formed by other clostridia convert the dead muscle into a greenish black deliquescent mass.

Death of the muscle fibres in gas gangrene is mainly caused by the α-toxin of *Cl. welchii*; this is a phospholipase C, which splits lecithin into diglyceride and phosphoryl choline [58].

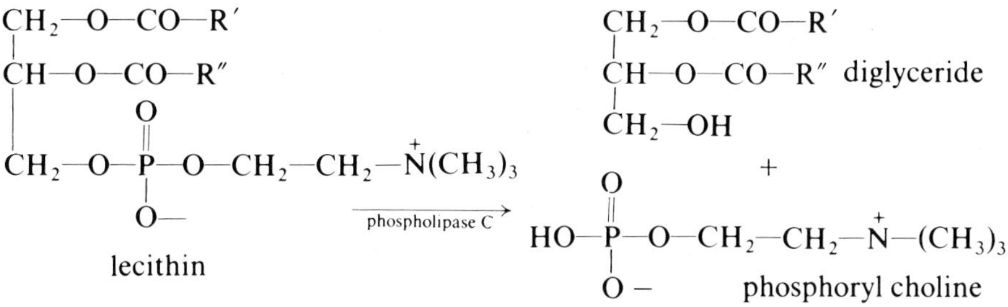

This action decomposes phospholipids in cell membranes and mitochondria and lyses red blood cells [59]. The α-toxin thus directly disrupts the laminar micelles of cell membranes and so kills the muscle fibres. It also causes fatty change by destroying solubilising phospholipids and by forming hydrophobic diglycerides (p. 371); thus the dying muscle may contain visible fat [60].

Other exotoxins secreted by *Cl. welchii* include the κ-toxin. This is a collagenase which dissolves collagen fibres and probably produces the pronounced softening of striated muscle that occurs in gas gangrene; the softened muscle becomes pulpy and can be smeared out on a plate. This destruction of collagen accounts for the rapid spread of gas gangrene as a progressive fulminating infection throughout whole groups of muscles. Glycogenase is also formed; this enzyme breaks down muscle glycogen to glucose, which is then fermented to form bubbles of gas beneath the sarcolemma of affected fibres. Release of this captive gas makes the dying muscle crepitant on palpation.

Besides *C. welchii* other clostridia can cause or contribute to production of gas gangrene. Thus the highly pathogenic *Cl. oedematiens* elaborates several exotoxins; it forms an α-toxin which causes intense inflammatory oedema by injuring capillary endothelial cells, and a β-toxin which has lecithinase activity and lyses red cells. Moreover the final liquefaction and blackening of the dead muscle in gas gangrene results from the action of proteolytic enzymes secreted by saprophytic anaerobes such as *Cl. histolyticum* and *Cl. sporogenes* which also colonise the dying tissue.

As well as suffering from these severe local lesions, patients with gas gangrene may become desperately ill with pallor, fall in blood pressure and feeble irregular pulse, and then pass terminally into delirium or coma. Although the action of clostridial exotoxins adequately accounts for the local condition of gas gangrene, the mechanism of these general symptoms is obscure. Perhaps the final lethal effects are caused by substances liberated from dying muscle tissue by lecithinase activity on an extensive scale [61].

Streptococcus pyogenes

Exotoxins formed by *Str. pyogenes* contribute considerably to its pathogenicity.

But these substances are not sufficiently powerful in terms of MLD (or lethal molar concentration) for localised infection to be a threat of imminent death as in diphtheria. Indeed *localised* streptococcal tonsillitis, although causing a high fever, is seldom if ever a mortal illness unless complicated by spread of infection or other consequential disease like glomerulonephritis or rheumatic fever (pp. 234, 235).

However *Str. pyogenes* possesses a specific antigenic protein on its surface which exists in many different antigenic types. This M substance enables the streptococcus to attach to the pharyngeal mucosa and also to resist phagocytosis unless the specific antibody to this particular antigen becomes available. The M substance thus determines much of the invasive power of *Str. pyogenes*. Invasion may then result in spreading cellulitis or lymphangitis culminating in septicaemia. Invasion is of course aided by simultaneous liberation of exotoxins, two of which are highly lethal to phagocytes. In this way an invasive bacterium, which does not form the most powerful exotoxins, can, because of power to spread, induce just as deadly effects as less invasive pathogens which produce toxins of extreme lethal potency.

Another way by which *Str. pyogenes* can cause mortal infection is by colonisation of very extensive surfaces from where exotoxins in large quantities diffuse into the body as a whole. Thus, after extensive vesiculation of the epidermis by burns or variola virus, highly lethal cutaneous infection by *Str. pyogenes* may ensue.

Exotoxins formed by *Str. pyogenes* thus become of extreme importance because of its invasive powers. Some of these exotoxins will now be considered.

Erythrogenic toxin is a highly active protein produced by many strains of *Str. pyogenes* infected by a specific temperate phage. First infection with one of these strains which usually cause tonsillitis is followed by fever together with an erythematous rash. The patient is then said to suffer from scarlet fever. This rash is due to intense dermal vasodilation which results from action of this erythrogenic toxin even in very low concentrations. This toxin is a potent stimulator of humoral immunity, and, since the toxin only occurs in one form, subsequent streptococcal infection cannot produce recurrence of the rash. However owing to multiplicity of types of the M antigen repeated infections by *Str. pyogenes* can occur, although 'scarlet fever' is only suffered once. Unfortunately spreading infection without the erythematous rash is just as likely to produce lethal effects.

Streptolysin O and *streptolysin S* haemolyse red cells and also cause severe cellular injury. Streptolysin O produces cardiac arrest when perfused even in low concentration into isolated hearts; this loss of cardiac contractility is irreversible. Streptolysin O also kills neutrophil polymorphs and macrophages with great rapidity. The action of streptolysin O on living neutrophils was studied by motion pictures taken with phase contrast microscopy [62]. The first change is rapid and extensive lysis of the cytoplasmic granules, which are in fact lysosomes covered by vesicular lipid membranes. The lysosomes explode and are replaced momentarily by clear spaces which rapidly disappear. Then long filamentous processes protrude from the surface of the cell membrane. The cell rounds up and finally the nuclear lobes swell and fuse to form a homogeneous spherical mass. Apparently this explosive disappearance of the lysosomes by the action of streptolysin O involves rupture of their membranes and liberation of their hydrolases, including actively proteolytic cathepsin, into the cytoplasm. Intracellular enzymic fission then changes the cell membrane so that the dying cell rounds up into a sphere and also causes globation and homogenisation of the nucleus. Thus cellular armaments so useful in digesting bacteria within phagolysosomes are diverted into self-destructive backfire. This sequence of changes terminating in cell death is completed with 5 min of exposure of neutrophils to streptolysin O. Streptolysin S has similar effects, but these begin after a latent period of 30 min. The harmful action of these exotoxins, including the cardiotoxicity of streptolysin O, probably play an important part in illness caused by streptococcal infection.

Bacterial endotoxins: pyrogens and fever

The endotoxins are structural components of bacterial walls which are released by pathogenic bacteria inside the host where they exert toxic effects. Although these substances, when extracted from organisms grown *in vitro*, are harmful to animals on injection, their minimum lethal dose is large in comparison with that of exotoxins. Toxic concentrations of these substances can only be reached inside the body by disintegration of relatively large numbers of the infecting pathogens, which are essentially invasive and able to grow massively within the tissues. Some of the harmful effects of endotoxins are indirect and depend on their power to liberate endogenous poisons from the cells around them or on their capacity to cause allergic reactions.

Harmful action of Gram-negative bacteria

The virulence of Gram-negative pathogenic bacteria primarily depends on extreme invasiveness due to their power to resist phagocytosis and bactericidal activity of phagocytic cells. However the endotoxins released from these organisms, on disintegration within the tissues, also contribute to the harmful effects of invasive infection.

Gram-negative bacteria possess a well developed and complex external cell calyx which is responsible for much of their pathogenic activity. Indeed the harmful effects of *Salmonella typhi* and other species are largely dependent on components of the superficial glycocalyx which envelops these organisms and protects their plasma membrane.

The glycocalyx of *Salmonella* is largely composed of lipoglycosaminoglycans (LGAGs) which have toxic properties. These endotoxins can be extracted from the surface of the bacterial cells. The antigenic specificity of LGAG in each species of *Salmonella* depends on the monosaccharide units in the outer glycosaminoglycan (GAG) covering of the complex LGAG. The solution of extracted endotoxin of *S. typhi* is precipitated by the specific O-antibody and a similarly precipitable O-antigen is present in the blood of patients with typhoid fever. The extracted endotoxins are lethal on injection into animals and also produce foci of necrosis in bone marrow and liver. Injection of smaller amounts cause fever both in animals and man; this pyrogenic effect develops after a latent period following injection (see below) and progressively declines and disappears after repeated injection (tolerance).

Further analysis of the LGAG in the enveloping glycocalyx of *Salmonella* and other Gram-negative pathogens shows that this complex contains several biologically active components which occur in successive zonal layers from without inwards [63, 64]. These zones are as follows:

1. Superficial GAG containing O-antigen, on which the invasive power of each *Salmonella* mainly depends.
2. Deeper GAG containing R-antigen, which is common to all species of *Salmonella* but differs among other genera.
3. Glycolipid containing both 2-keto-3-deoxyoctonic acid (KDO) and lipid-A. The latter is composed of a pair of glucosamine residues esterified with fatty acids which include β-hydroxymyristic acid. This glycolipid is both toxic and pyrogenic.

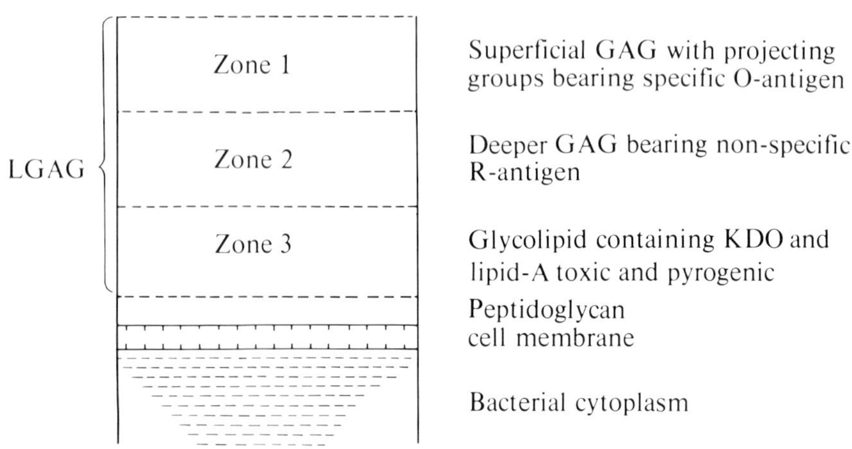

FIG. 6.11 Diagram of endotoxic envelope (glycocalyx) of *Salmonellae* and other Gram-negative bacteria. The glycocalyx is composed of lipoglycosaminoglycan (LGAG) arranged in three zonal layers.
GAG glycosaminoglycan.
KDO 2-keto-3-deoxyoctonic acid.

Fig. 6.11 shows diagrammatically these three zones of the LGAG which envelops the bacterial surface and also a still deeper layer of peptidoglycan which intervenes between the LGAG and the cell membrane.

Infection by S. typhi. This pathogen is much more invasive in man than other species of Salmonella and it also produces a more lethal disease accompanied by prolonged fever and stupor (typhoid fever). *S. typhi* penetrates the intestinal epithelium, spreads by lymphatics and blood and ultimately infects the reticuoendothelial system of the whole body; it excites an exudate of macrophages in which it grows. These infected cells then aggregate and die to produce necrotic foci in bone marrow, spleen and liver (Fig. 6.12a, p. 230). Masses of necrotic macrophages also appear in lymphoid tissue of intestinal submucosa (Fig. 6.12b) and in the sinuses of lymph nodes (Fig. 6.12c).

The invasiveness and virulence of *S. typhi* largely depend on its specific glycosaminoglycan (GAG) containing the O-antigen. This GAG is part of the superficial zone 1 of the bacterial calyx (see Fig. 6.11); the projecting chains of GAG, containing the O-antigenic determinants, probably protrude from the bacterial surface where they can react with O-antibody and complement at a *distance* from the inner parts of the bacterial cell wall. Thus the usual lytic and opsonic potentialities of antibody and complement are needlessly expended far from the zone where their activity can mediate bacteriolysis or phagocytosis. In the case of *S. typhi* the even more superficial GAG of the Vi-antigen may further add to this protective bacterial envelope. The GAGs of the endotoxic complex are thus dominant factors in virulence.

Apart from determining invasiveness of *S. typhi* the extent to which the endotoxin is responsible for the pathogenesis of typhoid fever is uncertain. The lipid-A component of the endotoxin is apparently essential for its pyrogenic activity, while lipid-A and KDO are both toxic [63]. Moreover the fatty acids in lipid-A can injure cell membranes [64] and so cause necrosis; this glycolipid also produces spectacular coagulation of proteins from white cells of Limulus, which thus serve as a delicate indicator of the presence of endotoxin.

Hyperplasia of reticuloendothelial cells is a most conspicuous feature of typhoid fever and induces swelling of lymph nodes and of intestinal lymphoid follicles along with aggregation of massed Kupffer cells in the liver. These macrophages may become coherent and immobilized as a reaction to cell-mediated hypersensitivity (p. 215), and then later become necrotic. Whether the necrosis is due to lack of nutriments among the compressed cells or to lethal action of endotoxin is unknown; but the dying macrophages in lymph nodes may well be casualties of endotoxic action as they appear to be entirely uncompressed (Fig. 6.12c).

Necrosis of macrophages in the intestinal submucosa (Fig. 6.12b) is succeeded by mucosal ulceration ('typhoid ulcers') and this is followed by haemorrhage into the bowel or perforation into the peritoneum. In patients dying of typhoid fever the distal small intestine and caecum are thus commonly filled with clotted blood.

The intense stupor of typhoid fever has not been adequately explained, but may be due to action of endotoxin on cerebral cells, or else the endotoxin may act on the pituitary to release opioid peptide hormones (encephalins) which then induce stupor by direct effect on the brain. The prolonged fever produced by *S. typhi* in man is probably *not* caused by the endotoxin, since repeated injection of the endotoxin soon ceases to exert a pyrogenic effect. Possibly the pyrogenic effects of immune complexes may be responsible for continued fever (p. 232).

The characteristic leucopenia of typhoid fever may partly be due to the

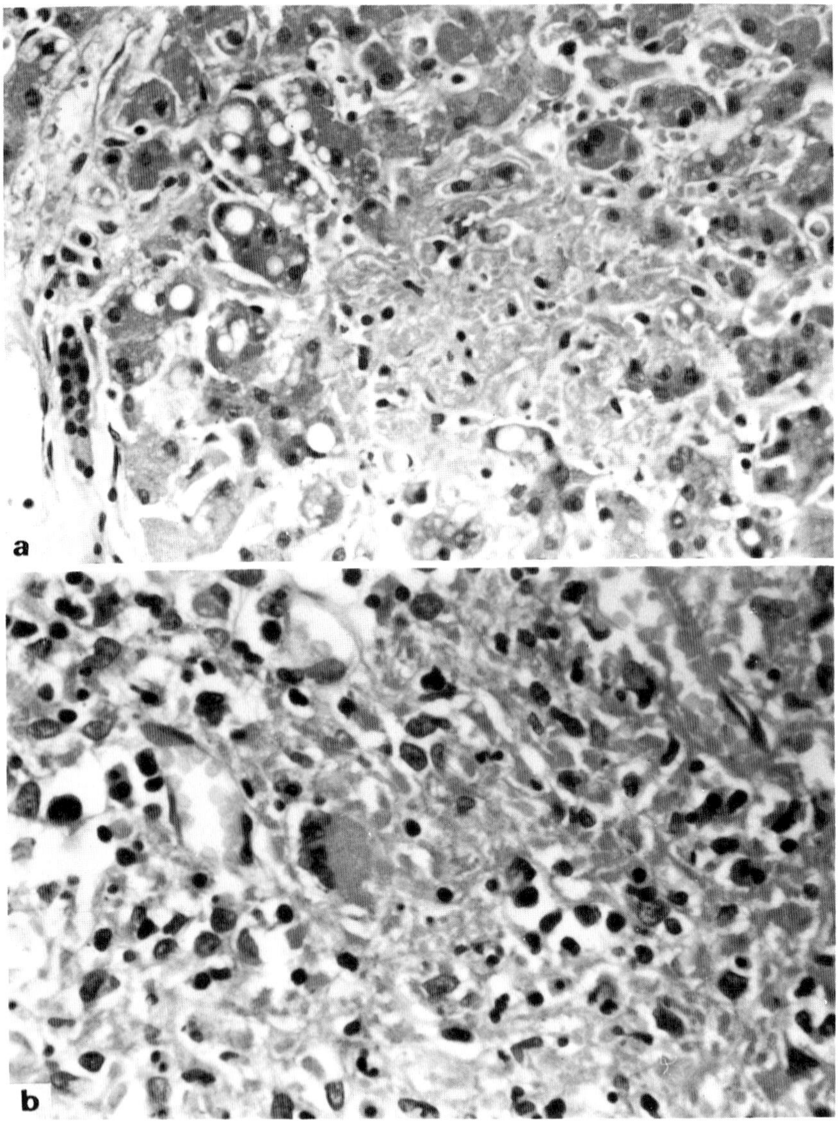

FIG. 6.12 Aggregation and necrosis of macrophages in typhoid fever.
a. Necrotic focus composed of aggregated macrophages in a liver lobule. Fat droplets in hepatocytes × 330.
b. Aggregate of necrotic macrophages in an intestinal lymphoid follicle. × 330.

injurious effect of endotoxin on neutrophils or their precursors. But leucopenia may also result from suppression of myelopoiesis in bone marrow as a sequel of reticuloendothelial hyperplasia, as well as from sequestration of neutrophils owing to their absorption by immune complexes (p. 232).

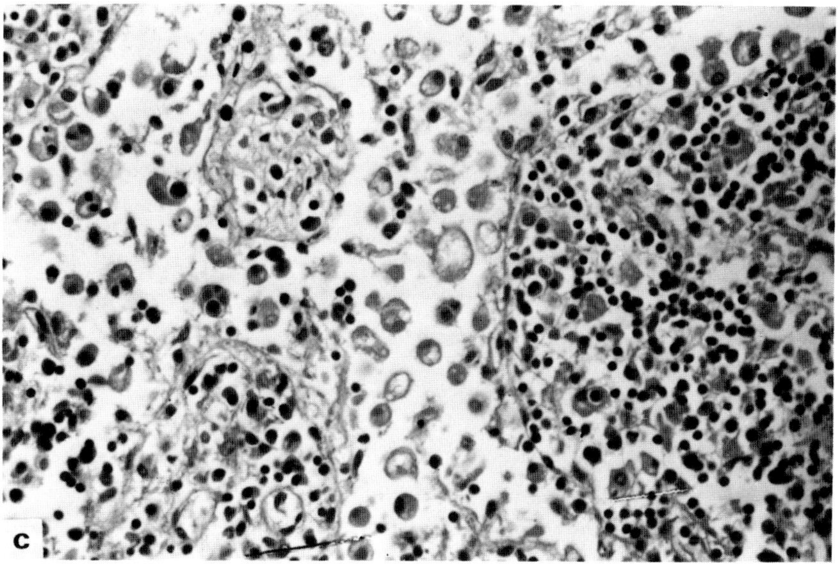

FIG. 6.12 cont.
c. Dilated sinuses in a lymph node containing necrotic macrophages. General hyperplasia of reticuloendothelial cells. × 330.

Bacteriogenic and endotoxic shock

Other Gram-negative bacteria such as *Escherichia coli* also liberate endotoxins when they disintegrate. *E. coli* is usually only locally invasive and is a common cause of chronic infection of the urinary tract; some of its strains (p. 222) can also secrete an exotoxin with enterotoxic activity and thus cause infantile diarrhoea. But, after intestinal trauma or urogenital operations, *E. coli* may enter the blood *en masse* and produce septicaemia associated with severe shock and ischaemic injury to various organs.

This bacteriogenic shock usually has a sudden onset with rigors followed by fever, hypotension and vasoconstriction. These effects are probably caused by liberation of endotoxins during the course of septicaemia. The endotoxins also injure vascular endothelium as well as the surface of platelets and leucocytes. This is followed by release of thromboplastin with widespread formation of fibrin to produce disseminated intravascular coagulation (DIC). Both DIC and the loss of fluid through damaged endothelium combine to produce ischaemia which may affect many organs and result in confusion and coma, respiratory distress, or acute renal failure [65]. Gram-negative anaerobes which are normal colonists of the large bowel, such as *Bacteroides fragilis*, may also cause septicaemia and bacteriogenic shock following surgery of the large intestine.

Severe shock and general vasodilation occur in septicaemic plague; these effects are probably caused by the endotoxin of Yersinia pestis which acts directly on vascular endothelium to increase permeability.

Endotoxins of Gram-negative bacteria may also be formed by contamination of distilled water in which these organisms may multiply. Even though the distilled water is subsequently sterilised before being used for making up solutions for intravenous infusion, intense rigors and bouts of fever follow their use owing to the presence of heat-stable endotoxins.

Shock with DIC can also occur in septicaemia produced by some Gram-positive organisms such as *Staphylococcus pyogenes*. This invasive pathogen forms an α-toxin, which causes constriction of venules, and coagulase which clots fibrinogen; these bacterial products may be active in promoting DIC [64].

Endogenous pyrogens and fever following infection

Saline extracts of neutrophil leucocytes contain a rapidly acting pyrogen which causes fever by direct effect on the cerebral heat regulating centre [66]. This *endogenous* pyrogen, because of its direct effect on the brain, acts even more readily on intracarotid than on intravenous injection. Endogenous pyrogen extracted from rabbit neutrophils is a highly labile protein which in amounts as low as 1–2 μg can produce fever in rabbits [67]. Unlike endotoxin-pyrogens, endogenous pyrogen extracted from polymorphs continues to act on repeated injection and does not induce tolerance. Moreover the pyrogenic action of endotoxins is in part indirect by causing release of endogenous pyrogen from neutrophils [68]. But endotoxin-pyrogens can also (like endogenous pyrogen) exert a direct effect on the subthalamic thermoregulatory centre [64].

Endogenous pyrogens are formed and released by neutrophils during phagocytosis of bacteria and also when neutrophils aggregate around immune complexes [69]. During acute infection by bacteria and viruses both bacterial and viral antigens are liberated and react with specific antibodies to produce complexes which absorb complement and then attract neutrophils (p. 207). This effect is probably a major cause of fever occurring during infection both by bacteria and viruses. The fever of serum sickness may arise in the same way (p. 208). In the course of extensive infection by a highly invasive pathogen, such as *S. typhi*, the liberation of bacterial antigens may be substantial and prolonged; this may lead to continuous formation of immune complexes over several weeks with resultant sequestration of neutrophils followed by release of their endogenous pyrogen with continued fever.

Fever has several harmful effects, especially if high or long lasting. Thus high temperature produced by pneumonia, typhoid or relapsing fever may reach levels that cause delirium and coma by direct action on cerebral cells (p. 121). Prolonged fever by increasing metabolic rate may summate with anorexia to produce severe wasting of tissues and eventual heart failure.

Toxic action of spirochaetes: Jarisch–Herxheimer reaction

Although no known toxins have been extracted from *Treponema pallidum*, harmful substances are probably formed when it disintegrates in the body and these may contribute to the injurious effects of syphilitic infection.

Treatment of patients with early syphilis by penicillin is followed in over 50 per cent of cases by attacks of acute illness which is called the Jarisch–

Herxheimer reaction (JHR). This involves fever, malaise, headache, sweating and exacerbation of signs of the disease, such as skin rash in secondary syphilis. Similar reactions occurred when arsphenamines were formely used as the method of treatment. JHR occurs in nearly every patient in whom treatment with penicillin is started in seropositive (late) primary and early secondary syphilis, when large numbers of treponemata are probably destroyed with great rapidity.

Liberation of a toxic substance from the dying treponemata probably causes this reaction, but the nature of the supposed endotoxin is unknown. However, possibly the mechanism is *indirect* and results from an immune complex reaction in which an antigen is suddenly released by death of numerous treponemata and then forms complexes (p. 234) with antibody already in the tissues. Indeed the dermal lesions of secondary syphilis, which are temporarily exacerbated by JHR, simultaneously become infiltrated with neutrophils. This may be the result of chemotactic attraction to immune complexes; in any case the release of endogenous pyrogen from the attracted neutrophils probably contributes to fever in JHR.

Spectacular acute reaction also follows destruction within the tissues of another invasive spirochaete, namely *Borrelia recurrentis*, which causes louse-born relapsing fever. In this disease treatment with tetracyclin or penicillin may be followed by rise of temperature, rigors and sudden death from heart failure [70]. The heart muscle shows intercellular oedema and diffuse histiocyte infiltration. This lethal effect of treatment may result from release of large amounts of a toxic component from the dying spirochaetes. In relapsing fever intensity of infection is so great that spirochaetes are usually visible in the blood. Thus treatment by bactericidal drugs may suddenly liberate a toxic substance in high concentration, which then causes lethal effects.

Toxic action of entamoeba histolytica

This highly injurious protozoon, which is the causal organism of amoebic dysentery, kills human cells by a unique lethal mechanism. *Entamoeba histolytica* colonises the submucosa of the colon where it produces destructive ulceration with rectal outflow of blood-streaked slime. The entamoeba engulfs and destroys red cells and neutrophils; it also dissolves the cells and tissues around it, so that in sections each parasite appears to be encircled by a clear halo.

Observations by phase contrast [71] and by EM [72, 73] on human neutrophils *in vitro* and on cultures of Hela cells have done much to reveal the toxic mechanism of this necrotising pathogen. Initially neutrophils move towards the amoebae which appear to exert chemotactic attraction. The neutrophils then put out pseudopodia towards the amoeba. As soon as contact is established the neutrophils are trapped and adhere to the parasites until killed. Within 2 min of contact the neutrophils lose their motility and round up into spheres; their cytoplasmic granules disappear, their nuclear lobes fuse and finally the nuclear outline fades. This death by touch is complete within 10 min and is followed by phagocytosis of the remnant of the neutrophil by the entamoeba.

This effect is seen by EM to depend on injection by a trigger mechanism of fluid from an enlarged lysosomal vesicle of the entamoeba into the neutrophil, followed by sudden loss of the osmiophilic cell membrane of the neutrophil. Probably amoebic lysosomal hydrolases rapidly destroy the cell membrane and granules of the neutrophil; the cell remnant is then engulfed by the amoeba as it terminates this spectacular act of murder followed by cannibalism.

E. histolytica causes similar contact-dependent lysis of other mammalian cells. Non-pathogenic *E. coli* is also attractive to human neutrophils, but, unlike *E. histolytica*, exerts no toxic effect on them.

Harmful antigenic action of microorganisms

Invasive pathogenic microbes can introduce foreign antigenic substances into the body or antigenic microbial products can enter by inhalation. These antigens may then evoke harmful immune responses which thus become dominant factors in disease.

Another possibility is that invasive pathogenic microbes can disintegrate cells and tissues within the body and thereby liberate substances which are harmfully antigenic in themselves. Mechanisms of this kind have been suggested as possible determinants of diseases such as rheumatoid arthritis (p. 209) and SLE (p. 213) in which antigen/antibody interactions of unknown origin appear to play a prominent part. A similar mechanism, may also be actuated by the highly invasive *Treponema pallidum* which in causing syphilitic infection simultaneously excites intense formation of immunoglobulins.

Microbial antigens excite harmful hypersensitivity in four principal ways, types 1, 2 and 3 allergic reactions [18], depending on interaction of antigens with humoral antibodies, and cell-mediated reaction of antigens with sensitised T-cells (Fig. 6.9). These four types of injury involve:

1. Mast cell-generated allergy in which antibody to microbial antigen becomes bound to mast cells and then reacts harmfully with the antigen on re-encounter (p. 204); asthma and allergic rhinitis, caused by sensitisation to house mites or to fungi such as *Aspergillus fumigatus*, arise in this way.
2. Induction or formation of antibodies which cross-react with human tissue to give cytotoxic effects. Antibody formed in this way to microbial antigens of *Streptococcus pyogenes* may account for injury and inflammation of joints and heart muscle in rheumatic fever, which is a common sequel to repeated streptococcal infection of the pharynx. Antibodies to other streptococcal antigens, such as anti-streptolysin O, are constantly present in the blood in rheumatic fever.
3. Formation of antibody which reacts with microbial antigen to produce harmful immune complexes. This kind of mechanism is probably responsible (p. 232) for some of the harmful effects of endotoxins and also plays a prominent role (see below) in producing lesions both in kidney and the skin.
4. Sensitisation of T-lymphocytes, which react harmfully with the microbial antigen on re-encounter, and thus produce the injurious effects of cell-mediated hypersensitivity (p. 239). This kind of reaction has great importance in lesions initiated by mycobacterial and viral antigens.

Microbial antigens may thus excite harmful immune responses in several ways. In some diseases which are probably initiated by microbial antigens, such as rheumatic fever (see above), the actual pathogenic mechanism is obscure. But in other disorders, especially those in which microbial antigens generate harmful immune complexes or cell-mediated hypersensitivity, the sequential events are much clearer.

Immune complexes caused by microbial antigens: acute glomerulonephritis
The renal glomeruli have the power to retain immune complexes formed between microbial antigens and their antibodies; these precipitated complexes can then induce development of serious glomerular lesions.

Acute post-streptococcal glomerulonephritis occurs as a sequel to infection by *Str. pyogenes* and commonly arises about two weeks after the start of streptococcal pharyngitis in children. The onset is sudden with fever, oliguria and oedema. This disease is probably initiated by reaction between excess of streptococcal M antigen with antibody, when the latter begins to be formed. In this way small complexes, typical of antigen excess, are produced which penetrate the fenestrae in glomerular capillaries but are filtered out on the basement membrane (BM).

In post-streptococcal glomerulonephritis these complexes usually appear as lumpy granules containing IgG and complement (C) which are deposited on the outer side of the BM. As in other immune-complex reactions (p. 207) the precipitated complex absorbs C which results in two principal effects:

1. Liberation of vasoactive amines and production of oedema.
2. Attraction of neutrophils, which cause further swelling and other injury.

The local oedema and infiltration by neutrophils produce glomerular ischaemia. This results in oliguria as well as damage to the glomerular BM which enables proteins to leak into the glomerular filtrate and urine. In consequence hypoproteinaemia and generalised oedema develop. Further injury to the glomeruli is caused by release of lysosomal enzymes from the attracted neutrophils, while escape of their endogenous pyrogens accounts for fever. Although recovery occurs in most patients, oliguria may progress to acute renal failure or chronic glomerular lesions may persist.

This post-streptococcal glomerulonephritis, depending on interaction between streptococcal antigen and its specific antigen, only follows infection by a few types of *Str. pyogenes*, notably type 12. For this reason recurrence of post-streptococcal glomerulohephritis is very uncommon.

Glomerulonephritis due to a similar immune-complex reaction initiated by a foreign microbial antigen also may follow infection by *Plasmodium malariae*. In this disease antigen derived from the malarial parasites can be detected in the glomerular deposits.

Immune complexes caused by microbial antigens: lesions in the skin
The sudden liberation of large amounts of antigenic material from an invasive pathogen can cause spectacular effects in the skin if antibodies are already

present in large amounts in blood and tissues. This happens in about 50 per cent of patients with *lepromatous leprosy* when treatment with sulphones is started. Although cell-mediated immunity is deficient in lepromatous leprosy, antibodies to mycobacterial antigens are present in the serum. Treatment of these patients with sulphones may kill myriads of mycobacteria with release of antigens in excess into the blood. This treatment is frequently followed by transient appearance of crops of erythematous nodules in the skin. This effect is due to the formation of immune complexes containing mycobacterial antigen, immunoglobulin and complement. These complexes are deposited in the skin and this is followed by attraction of neutrophils, intense erythema and nodular swelling (erythema nodosum), and also fever due to liberation of pyrogens.

Similar erythema nodosum may occur after streptococcal infection. This is probably also caused by dermal deposition of immune complexes derived from streptococcal antigens and their antibodies.

The skin, like the kidney, thus filters out immune complexes, and so also becomes a target for lesions produced by the noxious effects of microbial antigens when ligated to their specific antibodies.

Cell-mediated hypersensitivity (CMH) to microbial antigens

CMH exerts a dominant effect in causing the mild and chronic lesions of *tuberculoid leprosy*. In this disease scanty infection of the dermis with *Mycobacterium leprae* slowly produces dermal plaques of thickening with erythematous edges; these chronic localised lesions are caused by infiltration with lymphocytes and macrophages (epithelioid cells) with formation of giant cells, resulting from reaction of sensitised T-cells with myobacterial antigen. This dermal infiltration is harmful by its effect in compressing cutaneous nerve fibres which ultimately degenerate to produce anaesthetic zones. The skin in these areas later becomes further damaged by trauma or burns owing to absence of sensation. In tuberculoid leprosy cell-mediated immunity due to activated macrophages is so efficient that infective bacilli are mostly destroyed and, in contrast to lepromatous leprosy, scarcely any mycobacteria can be found in the lesions.

CMH is also evoked by antigens of *M. tuberculosis*. Indeed the effects of the reaction of these antigens with sensitised T-cells play such a crucial part in the course of human tuberculosis that they will be considered in the next section along with other factors which affect the outcome of this highly lethal infection.

Pathogenic action of tubercle bacillus

The injurious effects of this most necrotising of all human parasites are related both directly and indirectly to harmful components of the bacilli; these components may be directly toxic, they may exert harmful antigenic action and they may promote intracellular growth of the invading bacilli (Fig. 6.13). Moreover the antigenic effects of bacillary components mediated by lymphokines induce the formation of an abundant avascular exudate, in which necrosis readily occurs both from lack of nutriments and from the toxic action of substances, such as proteases, released from dying cells.

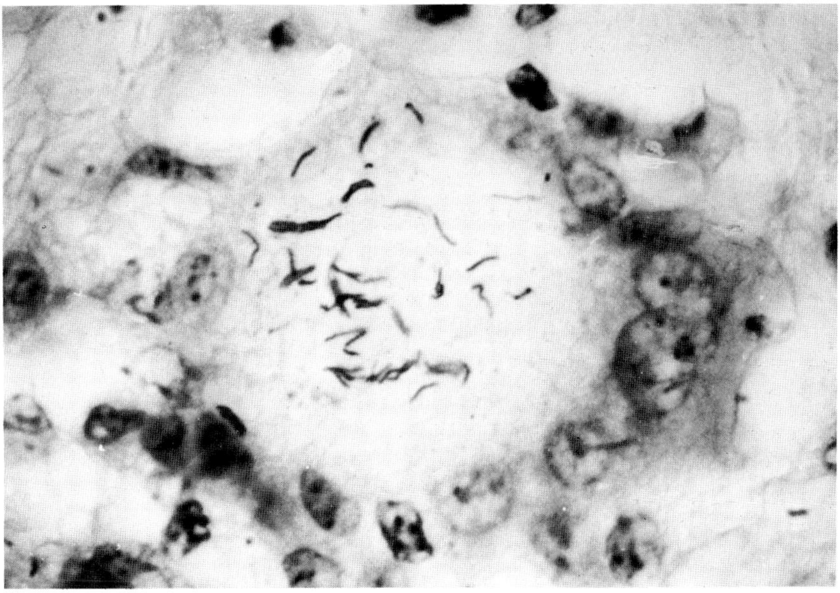

FIG. 6.13 Intracellular growth of *Mycobacterium tuberculosis* within a multinucleate tuberculous giant cell. From an enlarged lymph node in a giraffe which died of generalised tuberculosis caused by infection with human tubercle bacillus. Numerous rod-shaped mycobacteria (stained deep crimson) visible in centre of the cell. Ziehl-Neelsen stain. × 1300. Specimen by courtesy of Professor G. A. Gresham.

Fig. 6.13 shows a multinucleate giant cell in a tuberculous exudate. This cell contains tubercle bacilli growing within it. The capacity for intracellular growth probably adds to the other harmful attributes of the bacilli. These features of tuberculous infection will now be considered.

Harmful components

Both human and bovine strains of tubercle bacilli cause tuberculosis in man; both these organisms will be referred to as *Mycobacterium tuberculosis.* Two components of these mycobacteria are paramount in determining their pathogenicity and antigenicity; these are (a) lipids of the bacterial cell walls, and (b) proteins of the cytoplasm.

Lipids of cell walls

The cell envelope is exceptionally rich in lipids which have remarkable biological properties and enable the bacilli to resist the major defences of the body and grow within cells and between them.

The lipids include (1) waxes, (2) glycolipids, and (3) phospholipids. The fatty acids of the waxes and glycolipids are branched β-hydroxyacids called mycolic acids [74]; they contain about 60 C atoms and are substituted in α-position by a second long fatty acid chain

$$\ldots CH_2{-}CHOH{-}\underset{\displaystyle C_{24}H_{49}}{\underset{|}{CH}}{-}COOH$$

mycolic acid

Mycolic acids are acid-fast when stained with hot basic dyes. The presence of free mycolic acid along with waxes may determine the tenacity of tubercle bacilli to basic dyes which makes them both 'acid-fast' and 'alcohol-fast'.

The general hyrophobic nature of the waxes may be a dominant factor in invasiveness and resistance to phagocytes. However certain specific lipids of the cell wall may contribute to pathogenicity in more definite ways. These specific lipids are:

1. Wax D, which contains mycolic acid and a glycopeptide. It is a unique adjuvant to tuberculin; together they compose the antigen which evokes both sensitivity to tuberculin and to the whole tubercle bacillus.
2. Glycolipid 6, 6^1-dimycolyltrehalose. This is extractable from surface of virulent strains, in which the bacilli grow in serpentine cords, and is sometimes called the cord factor; it is toxic to mice (LD_{50} 10μg), and it resembles virulent tubercle bacilli in its capacity to inhibit the migration of neutrophils. When dissolved in oil and inhaled by mice this glycolipid induces pulmonary granuloma.
3. Fatty acids, obtained from the bacterial phospholipids, which, on injection into guinea pigs, cause accumulation of mononuclear cells and giant cells followed by necrosis.

Protein of cytoplasm (tuberculin)

This is a soluble protein extractable from disintegrated tubercle bacilli. The native protein contains two moieties distinguishable by electrophoretic mobility. The release of this protein from dead tubercle bacilli within the body is a major factor in the necrotising action of tuberculous infection (see below).

Antigenic action of tuberculin and of tubercle bacilli

Tuberculin acts specifically on thymus-derived lymphocytes (T-cells) of sensitised animals to give the response of cell-mediated hypersensitivity (p. 215). But tuberculin by itself cannot *initiate* this sensitisation of T-cells. The sensitisation, however, can be effected by:

1. Infection with live tubercle bacilli (including BCG).
2. Injection of dead tubercle bacilli.
3. Injection of tuberculin along with wax D; this wax exerts a potent adjuvant effect which takes part in the development of cell-mediated hypersensitivity (sensitisation) during natural infection by tubercle bacilli. Wax D makes the protein (tuberculin) a complete antigen, so that together they can induce the

formation of sensitised cells, which thereafter will react specifically with tuberculin by itself. Similar cooperative action of wax D and tuberculin is believed to cause sensitisation to tuberculin during the course of tuberculous infection (see below).

Tuberculin alone, however, can cause intense reaction on encounter with senstitised T-cells. Thus although harmless to uninfected animals tuberculin injected into guinea pigs during the course of tuberculous infection causes, within 1–2 days, intense swelling of lesions and infiltration with lymphocytes. Similarly in man intradermal injection of tuberculin produces no reaction in previously uninfected persons, but in those who have previously been infected, swelling and infiltration with lymphocytes occurs around the point of infection within two days owing to CMH.

Antigenic effects during tuberculous infection

During infection of man or animals by tubercle bacilli exposure of T-lymphocytes to tuberculin along with wax D, released from the bacilli, induces cell-mediated hypersensitivity (CMH); this involves development of clones of specifically sensitised cells. When these cells re-encounter tuberculin, also released from invasive tubercle bacilli, either during first infection or re-infection, the cells proliferate and display the reaction of CMH outlined on p. 215 and in Fig. 6.9. The most significant of these reactions, which has crucial effects in tuberculosis, is the liberation of non-specific lymphokines from the sensitised T-cells on contact with tuberculin.

These lymphokines then:

a. Stimulate mitosis of lymphocytes which proliferate around foci of tuberculous infection.

b. In *low* concentration stimulates mitosis of macrophages and activate their lysosomes which become more effective in killing bacteria; this effect is paramount in arresting spread of infection and shows that cell-mediated immunity (CMI) is a consequence of CMH (p. 215).

c. In *higher* concentration similarly induce proliferation of macrophages but also alter their surface so that they are immobilised and cohere into ovoid masses or follicles (Fig. 6.14a, p. 240). These coherent macrophages are called 'epithelioid' cells. Some of the epitheloid cells fuse to form giant cells and they also die and disintegrate into caseous debris (Fig. 6.14b). This latter effect significantly contributes to the necrotising action of tuberculin in severe infection.

d. Exert vasoactive effects resulting in oedema and inflammatory stasis and may lead to ischaemic necrosis.

Tuberculous lesions and course of tuberculosis in man

Tuberculous lesions thus contain follicles of epithelioid cells (Fig. 6.14a) surrounded by infiltrating lymphocytes. The production of these follicles depends largely on the action of lymphokines liberated from sensitised T-cells by contact with tuberculin formed by the mycobacteria. The lipids of the

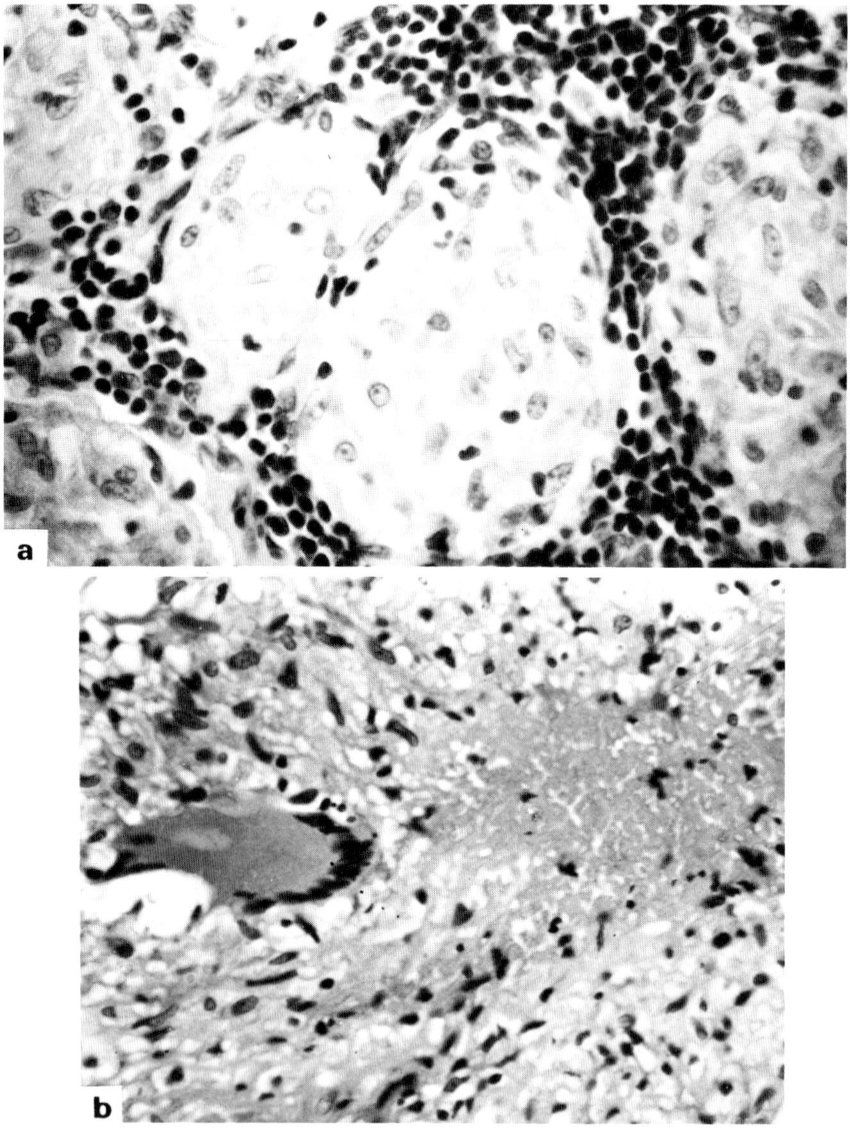

FIG. 6.14 Lymph node from a child with tuberculous lymphadenitis.
a. Macrophages aggregated into ovoid masses (follicles) of contiguous 'epithelioid' cells. × 330.
b. Fusion of epithelioid cells to form a giant cell at left of field; complete disintegration of epithelioid cells into caseous debris at right of field. × 410.

mycobacteria also attract macrophages and thus contribute to this effect. As infection extends daughter follicles appear around the initial follicles so as to produce visible whitish foci called tubercles (Fig. 6.14c). This process is often

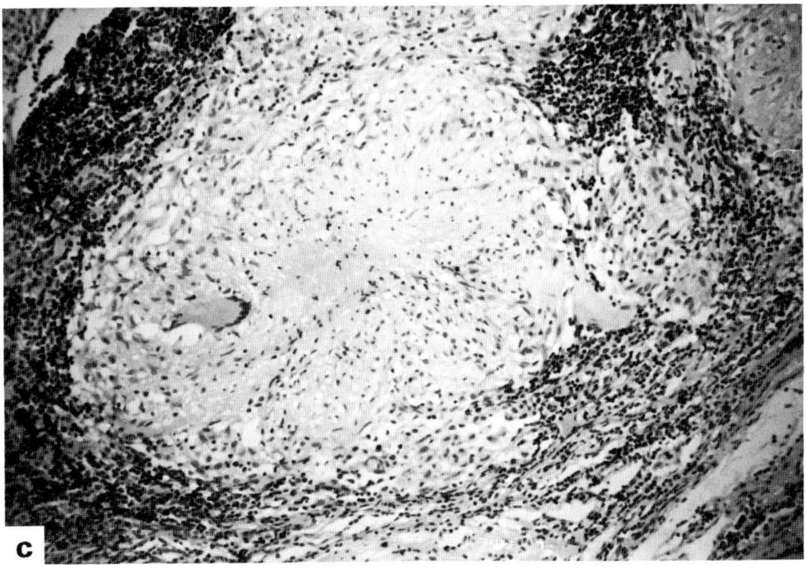

FIG. 6.14 cont.
c. Coalescence of follicles and daughter follicles to produce a visible tubercle. ×130.

accompanied by the most devastating caseous necrosis (p. 7) in which cellular tissue is replaced by cheese-like debris (Fig. 6.14b).

In human tuberculosis there is a continuous conflict between healing on the one hand and spread to progressive disease on the other.

Activation of macrophages as a result of (b) above (p. 239), which enables them to kill tubercle bacilli, is a prime requirement for healing. This activation depends on CMH evoked by tuberculin in low concentration; in these circumstances liberation of tuberculin is beneficial (Fig. 6.15a, p. 242).

On the other hand, the sudden release of large amounts of tuberculin, owing to rapid proliferation of tubercle bacilli, causes extensive necrosis of macrophages by mechanisms (c) and (d) above. This may herald transition to acutely progressive disease such as tuberculous bronchopneumonia; under these conditions tuberculin exerts a harmful action (Fig. 6.15b).

Two other factors may hasten a lethal outcome:

1. Rupture of an infected pulmonary focus into a bronchiole (Fig. 6.16, p. 243); this provides immediate access of oxygen which enables the aerobic mycobacteria to flourish and multiply.

2. Macrophages may develop intense proteolytic power by increase in activity of cathepsin in their lysosomes; this activation follows phagocytosis of necrotic material rich in protein [75]. The release of these activated proteases may then liquefy the lesion or else promote rupture of a bronchiole. Liquefaction,

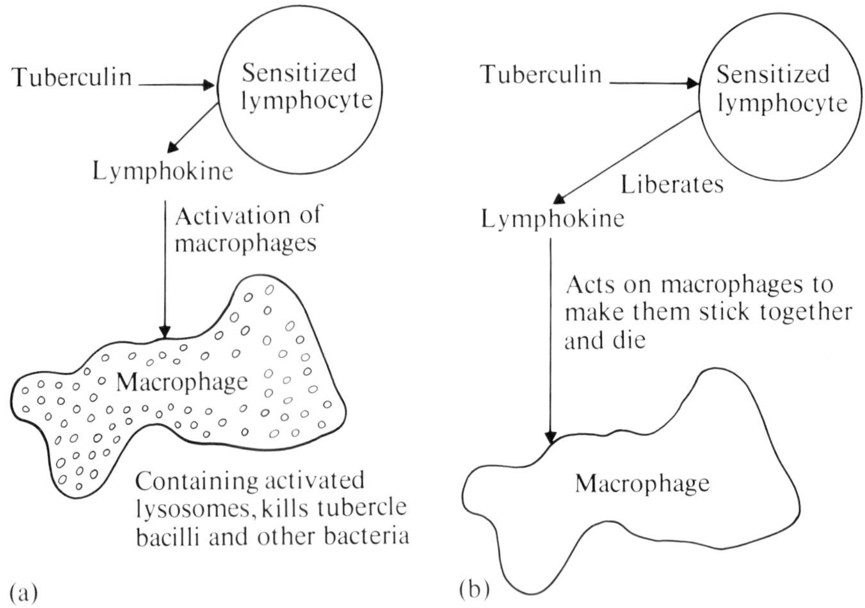

FIG. 6.15a Beneficial action of tuberculin. Sensitized lymphocytes on contact with tuberculin in small amounts liberate lymphokines in low concentration; these stimulate macrophages to divide and form activated lysosomes which kill tubercle bacilli.

FIG. 6.15b Harmful action of tuberculin. Sensitised lymphocytes on contact with tuberculin in large amounts liberate lymphokines in high concentration; these stimulate macrophages to divide and then make them cohere together and die, without killing tubercle bacilli. In pulmonary tuberculosis this results in filling of alveoli with necrotic macrophages followed by fibrosis and progessive loss of respiratory function.

by disseminating mycobacteria, is one of the most adverse events in the pathogenesis of human tuberculosis [76].

Invasiveness and intraphagocytic growth

The lipid envelope of tubercle bacilli repels neutrophils and attracts macrophages; the bacilli are then ingested by macrophages and divide within them. Fig. 6.13 shows intracellular tubercle bacilli which have grown within a giant cell formed by the fusion of macrophages.

The lipids of the bacterial envelope appear to be essential for this intracellular survival which so greatly enhances the power of the bacilli to spread in the body and cause extensive disease. The survival of virulent bacilli in cultured macrophages probably depends on their power to prevent lysosomes from fusing with phagosomes in which the bacilli are first enclosed after phagocytosis [77]. This inhibition of fusion to form phagolysosomes precludes the exposure of intracellular mycobacteria to lysosomal hydrolases and thus enables the bacilli

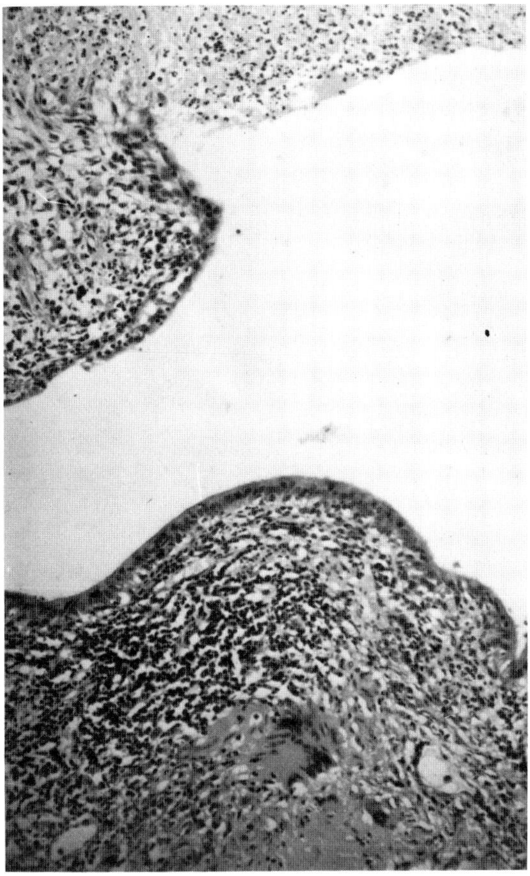

FIG. 6.16 Pulmonary tuberculosis: erosion of a bronchiole. In the lower part of the figure epithelioid cells and a large giant cell are seen enveloped by lymphocytes; this part of the lesion is still covered by intact bronchial epithelium. But in the upper part of the figure the bronchial epithelium is eroded and infected granulation tissue is exposed directly to air. Consequent multiplication of tubercle bacilli then may produce disastrous effects. × 130.

to survive and kill. This inhibitory effect on fusion may be determined by the nature of the surface lipids.

Virulent tubercle bacilli cause degeneration of macrophages in culture; avirulent strains do not [78]. The difference may be due to direct necrotising action of virulent strains owing to the presence of cord factor or other toxic lipids on their surface.

Summary of pathogenic mechanisms in tuberculosis

In summary therefore the singularly harmful effects of infection by *M. tuberculosis* depend on:

1. Necrosis of epithelioid cells as a result of their immobilisation and cohesion to form avascular aggregates (p. 239).

2. Ischaemic injury in the lesions owing to extreme pressure of exudate and inflammatory stasis (p. 239).

3. Directly harmful action of dimycolyltrehalose and other lipids of bacillary envelope.

4. Power of bacilli to kill epithelioid cells by intracellular growth (p. 242), which may also be related to bacterial lipids.

Of these factors (1) and (2) are the outcome of cell-mediated hypersensitivity to tuberculin, while (3) and (4) depend on directly noxious properties of the bacteria themselves.

All these four factors contribute and combine to make the tubercle bacillus one of the most lethal and necrotising parasites alike of animals and of man.

The capacity to produce disease by intracellular growth is possessed by many other hostile microorganisms besides the tubercle bacillus: further examples of cell injury caused by intracellular infective agents will now be considered.

Intracellular growth: bacteria

Some pathogenic bacteria can survive and grow in epithelial cells, such as colonic epithelium, or in phagocytes including both macrophages and polymorphs. Some examples of disease produced by such intracellular growth will be considered.

Intraepithelial growth

To enter epithelial cells bacteria may possess special powers of adherence or attachment. Thus *Shigella dysenteriae* becomes specifically attached to colonic epithelial cells and then penetrates their membranes. Within the cells *S. dysenteriae* multiplies and elaborates an exotoxin (enterotoxin); this exotoxin causes hypersecretion of the colonic mucosa and also exerts cerebral neurotoxic effects. The latter consist of convulsions simulating meningitis in severely affected children, as well as drowsiness and stupor in adults. Infection by *Shigella* also produces necrosis and severe ulceration of the colonic mucosa along with passage of blood and slime *per rectum*; the excreted mucopus contains numerous neutrophils. This necrosis of the mucosa may be due to the action of endotoxin liberated by *Shigella* growing within the epithelial cells. Necrosis and ulceration of the colon also occurs in dysentery produced by *S. flexneri*, which forms an endotoxin similar to that of *S. dysenteriae*, but does not form an exotoxin. Intracellular growth of these organisms is probably a prime determinant in their necrotising effects.

Other pathogenic bacteria, which can attach to epithelial cells and grow within them, include *Streptococcus pyogenes* (pharynx) and *Neisseria gonorrhoeae* (urethra). The attachment of *N. gonorrhoeae* to urogenital epithelium is aided by pili on the surface of the coccus which make it adhere to urothelial cells.

Intraphagocytic growth

Profuse multiplication of several kinds of pathogenic bacteria occurs in phagocytic cells and this intraphagocytic growth not only increases invasiveness and spread, but may also determine the principal lesions of disease.

Phagocytosis of non-pathogenic bacteria commences by endocytosis of the organisms by invagination of the cell surface of the phagocytes, so that the bacteria become enclosed in membrane-covered cytoplasmic vacuoles called phagosomes. Inside neutrophil leucocytes these phagosomes fuse rapidly with leucocytic granules which then disappear [79]. After this fusion lysosomal enzymes, including lysozyme which disintegrates bacterial glycosaminoglycans, digest the bacterial cell walls. The naked bacteria then swell by osmosis and burst. This bacteriolysis together with degranulation of neutrophils occurs in sequential stages [80]:

1. Within 30 sec after ingestion of bacteria by the neutrophils the phagocytic vacuoles coalesce with small 'specific' granules which contain alkaline phosphatase and lysozyme.
2. The phagocytic vacuoles then fuse with larger 'azurophil' granules which contain typical lysosomal enzymes such as acid phosphatase.
3. Bacteriolysis then follows.

One of the most immediate sequels to contact with foreign bacteria is increase in respiratory oxidation of glucose to CO_2 by the phagocytic neutrophils. This change is detectable within 30 sec, even before any change in the granules can be discerned [81].

Pathogenic bacteria may however elude this process in two ways: *either* their surface repels the phagocytes (unless previously opsonised by antibody) *or* they have the power to survive inside the phagocyte without injury by lysosomal enzymes.

Neisseria gonorrhoeae and *N. meningitidis* multiply inside neutrophils so that their cytoplasm may become stuffed with Gram-negative diplococci (Fig. 6.17, p. 246). The mechanism of intraphagocytic survival is unknown but proteases secreted by the cocci may interfere with lysosomal activity. Eventually the infected neutrophils are killed and the cocci are liberated and can then cause further infection. Possibly endotoxins liberated by the cocci are responsible for necrosis and the intense pyogenic inflammation. The injurious lesions of both gonorrhoea and meningococcal meningitis are initiated by this intense inflammation and exudation of netrophils; this process is substantially enhanced by the power of the pathogenic diplococci to proliferate within the phagocytic neutrophils.

Mycobacterium tuberculosis, although lethal and repulsive to neutrophils, can attract and survive in macrophages by precluding the fusion of lysosomes with phagosomes containing the bacilli (p. 242) and can then cause extensive necrosis of the infected macrophages; when the macrophages are activated by cell-mediated immunity (CMI) due to CMH (p. 215), the fusion of lysosomes with phagosomes is resumed and the ingested bacilli are killed.

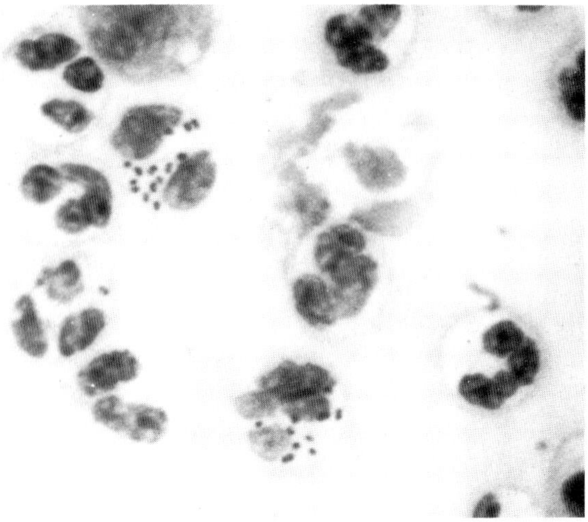

FIG. 6.17 *Neisseria gonorrhoeae* inside neutrophils. This Gram-negative diplococcus can grow and divide within the phagocytes. The cocci are seen as pairs elongated in the plane of fission. Gram stain. × 1300.

M. leprae can multiply in enormous numbers within macrophages in patients with the lepromatous form of leprosy, in which CMI is deficient. In contrast, when CMI is effective, macrophages become activated and kill intracellular *M. leprae* as happens in tuberculoid leprosy (p.236). When CMI is depressed, especially in undernourished patients, *M. leprae* can grow in macrophages and survive in them for years. A more pathogenic organism, such as *M. tuberculosis*, rapidly kills infected macrophages unless they are protected by CMI, but the relatively bland leprosy bacilli and the phagocytes can survive together in symbiosis.

Intracellular pathogenic protozoa

Their harmful effects on man are illustrated by a brief account of some pathogenic mechanisms displayed by *Plasmodium* and *Leishmania*.

Plasmodium and malaria

After introduction to man by the bite of an anopheline mosquito the malarial sporozoite multiples by several cycles of extraerythrocytic schizogony within the liver cells. Although the liver cells are ruptured on emergence of merozoites after each cycle of schizogony, this phase of infection produces no signs of disease.

Subsequently merozoites penetrate erythrocytes by creating depressions on the red cell surface which are then invaginated into the cell. This process, as revealed by EM, is initiated by adherence of the merozoite to the surface of the red cell. This attachment is mediated by filaments which project from the surface coat of the merozoite [81a]. These filaments adhere to specific receptors on red cell surface. When this contact is made at site of the *apical prominence* situated at one pole of the merozoite, then invasion follows. Proteins released from organelles in the apical prominence may alter the red cell surface which becomes pliable and invaginates to form a cup-like depression. The merozoite rapidly passes into this depression possibly impelled by suction [81a]. This depression then expands to form the so-called *parasitophorous vacuole* which becomes detached internally from the red cell membrane and encloses the merozoite.

This whole sequence of events occurs in less than 1 minute. Thus the invading merozoite, without breaking the red cell membrane, becomes enclosed in an intracellular vacuole where it spends its intraerythrocytic life and where it also absorbs nutriments from the cell [81b]. The formation of malarial pigment from Hb, however occurs *within* the parasite, where chunks of Hb can be seen initially. The globin is then utilized while the haem is converted to black malarial pigment. After schizogony, which forms 8–24 daughter merozoites from each schizont, the red cells are ruptured and the multiplied merozoites are liberated.

The mechanism of rupture and emergence of merozoites from the red cell is undetermined. Reduced glutathione (GSH) decreases in the red cell during infection. This loss of SH groups may damage the red cell membrane and produce haemolysis as in deficiency of glucose-6-phosphate dehydrogenase (p. 29); in this case disarray in the membrane may result from lack of the stabilising effect of GSH. Another possibility is that sudden rise in osmolality within the parasitophorous vacuole initiates swelling and rupture of the red cell. The red cell is seen to swell and within a few seconds the merozoites are released into the plasma through an aperture in the red cell membrane.

As each batch of infected red cells is synchronously ruptured throughout the body the patient suffers an attack of rigors followed by intense fever. Whether pyrogens released from the products of ruptured red cells or from the plasmodia are responsible for these bouts of shivering and fever is unknown. The fever terminates with drenching sweats and the patient then becomes afebrile until a new cycle of schizogony is completed and merozoites again emerge following rupture of the red cells to produce a fresh attack.

The liberated merozoites enter previously uninfected red cells during the attacks of shivering and are then visible within the red cells as young trophozoites ('ring forms'). In the case of *P. falciparum* these are very fine 'hair rings' often showing two or three thickened dots of chromatin (Fig. 6.18, p. 248) which give the rings a jewelled appearance. The growing trophozoites then may undergo schizogony or become gametocytes.

The formation of schizonts by *P. falciparum*, which causes malignant tertian malaria, exerts a singularly harmful effect not produced by the other species of *Plasmodium*. The schizonts of *P. falciparum* occur mainly in capillaries of internal organs such as brain, heart or small intestine. These schizonts make the infected red cells sticky so that they adhere together and to the capillary endothelium and so occlude the capillaries of internal organs. This may have

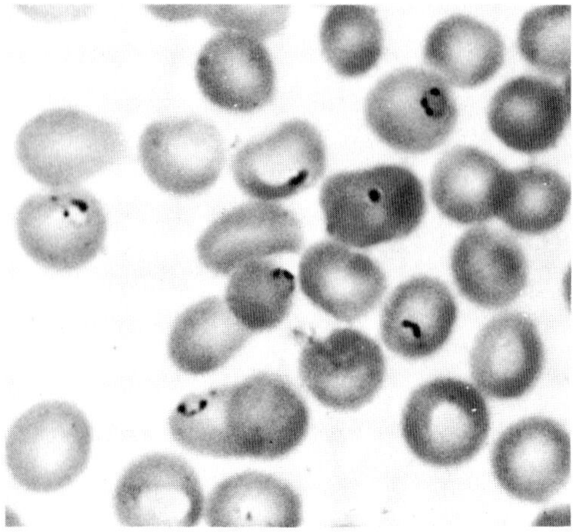

FIG. 6.18 Young trophozoites of *Plasmodium falciparum* within human red cells. These parasites are in the form of 'hair rings' with small beads of chromatin. Leishman's stain. ×1300.

disastrous effects on the brain and myocardium. Fig. 6.19 shows a cerebral capillary occluded by schizonts of *P. falciparum*; each schizont is seen splitting into merozoites. This occlusion of cerebral capillaries is responsible for the terminal coma of cerebral malaria. The cerebral capillaries become filled with enormous numbers of schizonts containing malarial pigment which gives the brain a slaty grey appearance.

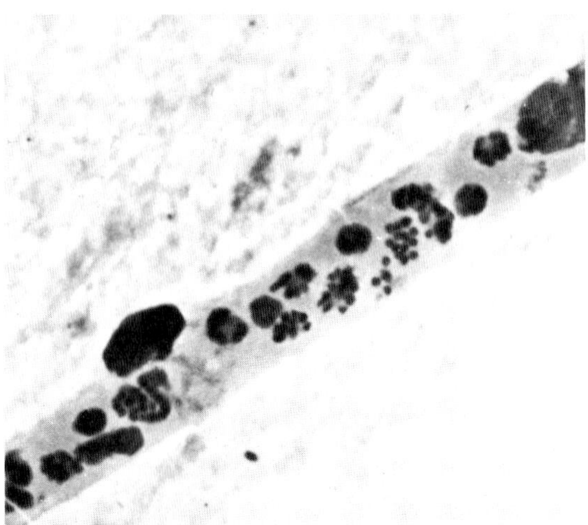

FIG. 6.19 Cerebral malaria; brain film. Schizonts of *Plasmodium falciparum* each splitting into merozoites are seen occluding a cerebral capillary. Leishman's stain. ×1300.

Leishmania

This highly pathogenic protozoon produces disease by its ability to grow inside phagocytic cells. It is transmitted to man by the bite of infected sandflies which contain the flagellate leptomonad form of the parasite.

Once inside human or other mammalian tissue the flagellate leptomonad is transformed to the leishmanial form (amastigote) which has no flagellum. This form consists of minute spheroids (2 μm in diameter) which are called amastigotes or Leishman–Donovan bodies (LDBs); each contains a spherical nucleus and a rod-shaped kinetoplast, which is coloured deep purple by Romanovski stains.

LDBs have a remarkable capacity for intracellular life within reticuloendothelial cells; in fact they parasitise macrophages, which are usually the archkillers of parasites. Within macrophages LDBs divide once in 24 h and eventually fill the grossly enlarged phagocytes with up to a hundred parasites.

Different species and strains of *Leishmania*, although morphologically identical, produce different clinical lesions. Thus *L. donovani* can invade macrophages throughout the whole reticuloendothelial system including bone marrow, spleen and liver to produce generalised or 'visceral' leishmaniasis, while *L. tropica* infects macrophages in the skin alone and causes localised or dermal leishmaniasis.

Infection by *L. donovani* can produce a severe febrile illness called kala-azar which results in progressive wasting and severe anaemia. The liver is enlarged and the spleen may become enormous owing to multiplication of swollen reticuloendothelial cells filled with amastigotes. In patients with this non-healing form of visceral leishmaniasis no reaction of cell-mediated hypersensitivity follows intradermal injection of an extract of *Leishmania*; and cell-mediated immunity appears to be absent. The resultant proliferation of parasites probably stimulates humoral immunity along with intense hyperglobulinaemia. The latter can be detected by adding a drop of aqueous formaldehyde to the patient's serum: within a few minutes the serum becomes opaque and sets into a solid gel ('formol-gel' test). Other persons, however, infected by *L. donovani* develop cell-mediated immunity and then show little or no clinical signs of disease except for epithelioid cell granulomata detectable by liver biopsy [82].

Infection by *L. tropica*, on the other hand, is confined to the skin, where dermal accumulation of infected giant macrophages along with lymphocytes causes swelling and ulceration ('oriental sore') at the site of entry of the parasite. This lesion exudes sticky pus containing giant macrophages stuffed with the amastigotes (LDBs) as well as numerous lymphocytes (Fig. 6.20, p. 250).

The type of dermal leishmaniasis which occurs in rural middle East and on Mediterranean islands is caused by the strain *L. tropica major*. Infection by this strain results in ulceration and intense inflammation usually followed by rapid healing [83]. In this type of infection cell-mediated immunity is rapidly developed as shown by the numerous lymphocytes in the exudate and the appearance of a reaction of cell-mediated hypersensitivity after intradermal injection of an extract of the amastigotes. The initial lesion may however produce unsightly scarring although followed by permanent immunity. For this

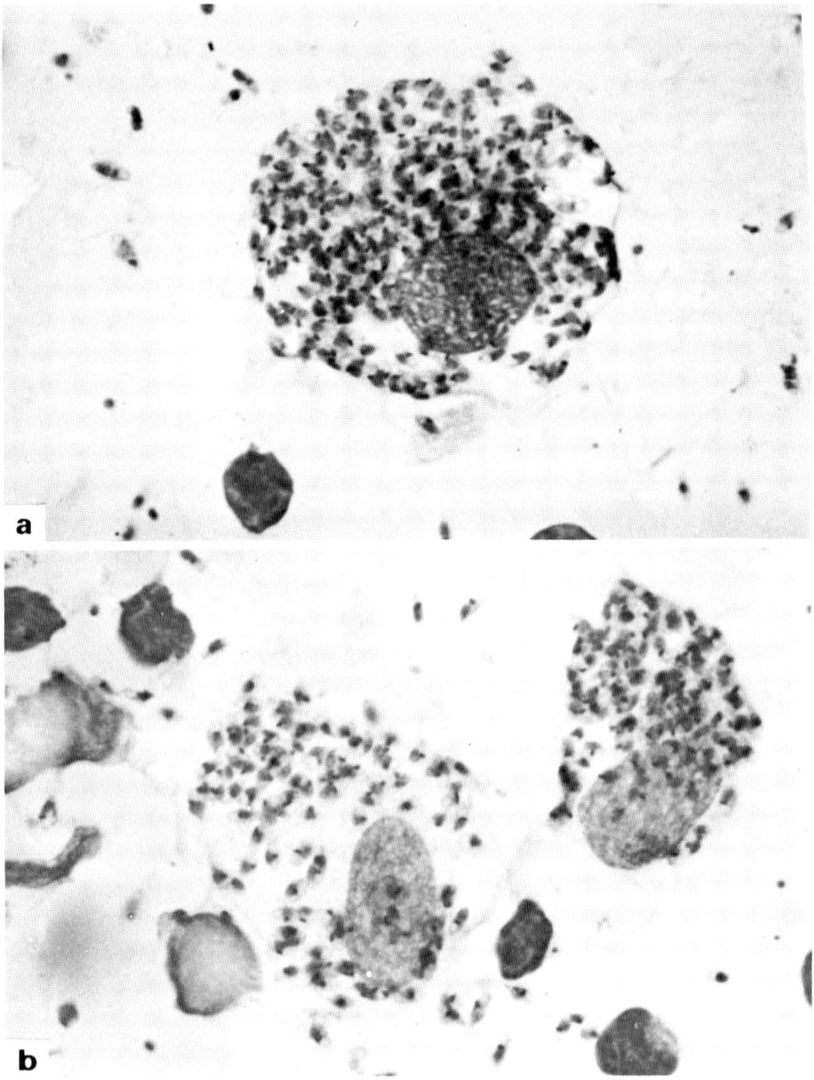

FIG. 6.20 Film from cutaneous sore caused by *Leishmania tropica*: giant macrophages stuffed with amastigotes (LDBs). Each parasite contains an ovoid nucleus and a rod-shaped darkly stained kinetoplast. Leishman's stain. × 1300.
a. Large macrophage with many intracellular LDBs.
b. Two macrophages with intracellular LDBs and some lymphocytes.

reason ladies in Iraq were sometimes inoculated with material from one of these lesions, which was introduced at a site of minimal cosmetic importance; this secured life-long immunity for the remainder of their skin from infection by *L. tropica major* as well as other strains. These other strains of *L. tropica*, occurring in Ethiopia and among urban communities in middle East, may fail

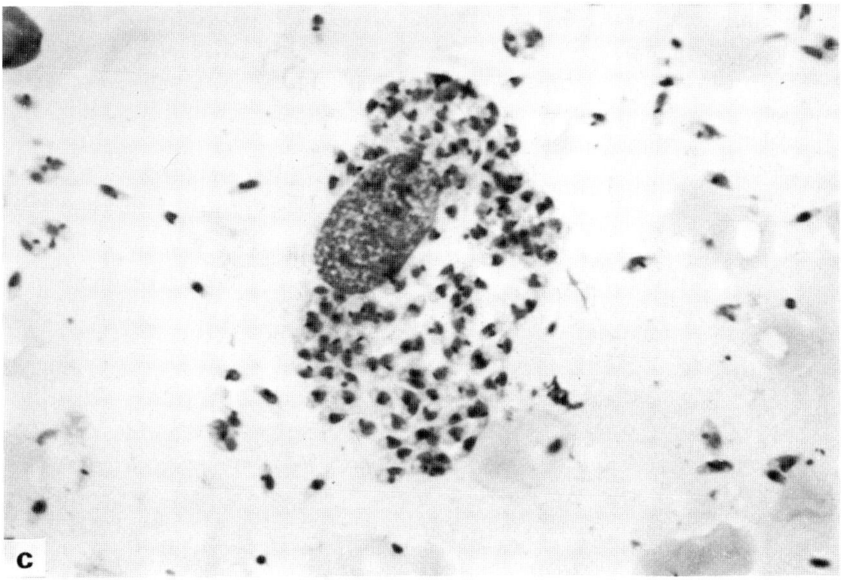

FIG. 6.20 cont.
c. Macrophage with intracellular LDBs and also extracellular LDBs; nucleus and kinetoplast clearly visible in nearly every parasite.

to induce cell-mediated immunity and tend to produce dermal lesions which are slow to heal and may spread or recur.

Leishmania is thus a successful and hostile intracellular parasite. It causes disease by:

1. Promoting accumulation of infected giant macrophages (Fig. 6.20).
2. Inducing intense cell-mediated hypersensitivity.

Intracellular growth: rickettsiae

Rickettsia prowazekii, the causative organism of epidemic typhus, grows and multiplies in endothelial cells of capillaries, especially those of the skin and the brain. The infected cells swell and proliferate and thrombi form on their surfaces. The capillaries therefore become occluded and the surrrounding tissues are injured by ischaemia and are also swollen by an exudate of macrophages; in the skin these changes are associated with a maculopapular rash. In the brain characteristic nodules of microglial mononuclear cells coalesce around the occluded capillaries to produce typhus 'nodules'. Cerebral ischaemia resulting from capillary occlusion probably accounts for the profound stupor and confusion which are so typical of typhus fever.

Intracellular growth: viruses

Intracellular replication of viruses is a potent initiator of cellular injury, although the mechanism of this damage, which is here our prime concern, is still largely undetermined.

Viruses replicate in some cells with little harmful action while in others the same virus may produce devastating injury. Thus poliovirus, on entry to the human body, normally multiplies without ill effect in gastrointestinal lymphoid tissue, but occasionally it penetrates spinomedullary neurones where viral replication is followed by necrosis, and this may result in respiratory paralysis and death.

Similar differences are observed in cells infected in culture. Thus paramyxovirus SV5, a common and harmless colonist of monkey kidney, multiplies in cultured monkey kidney cells with no cytopathic effects; the same virus profoundly alters baby hamster kidney cells in culture by making them fuse together to form multinucleate giant cells which subsequently degenerate [84].

These examples show how fine is the balance between harmless intracellular existence of viral visitors and their assumption of the noxious characteristics of a Trojan horse.

Entry of viruses into cells

Entry is probably initiated by attachment of virus to receptors on cell membranes. Vaccinia virus thus becomes attached to L cells in culture by adhesion to the cell surface [85]; the virus is then absorbed by endocytosis.

Influenza virus is initially adsorbed on cilia and microvilli of tracheal epithelium as shown by EM observations on tracheal tissue grown in organ culture [86, 87]; the junction appears to be effected between haemagglutinin spikes on the viral surface and neuraminic acid groups in the cellular glycocalyx of the tracheal cilia. Influenza virus also possesses enzyme neuraminidase on its surface which enables it to detach from cells it cannot enter and then be free to attach to other cells. The entry of virus is an active process; the virus induces formation of vacuoles immediately inside the cell membrane into which the viral particles become embedded and so enter the cell.

Location of lesions caused by viruses

In some illnesses produced by viruses the principal lesions appear in the initially infected cells.

Such initial infection in the ciliated epithelium of the bronchial mucosa and nasopharynx accounts for the most conspicuous lesions produced by influenza viruses and rhinoviruses. Influenza viruses cause necrosis of the bronchial epithelium, while the rhinoviruses (of common colds) produce degeneration of nasopharyngeal mucosal cells in organ cultures [88]. The illness produced by these viruses depends on this epithelial damage and subsequent mucopurulent inflammation.

Changes produced in the initially infected cells also result in the more localised condition of human warts. In forming a wart this papovavirus may infect only one epidermal cell which then divides to produce a clone of transformed cells. These cells behave abnormally and aggregate into a slowly growing mass of contiguous cells uncontrolled by the polarising action of their

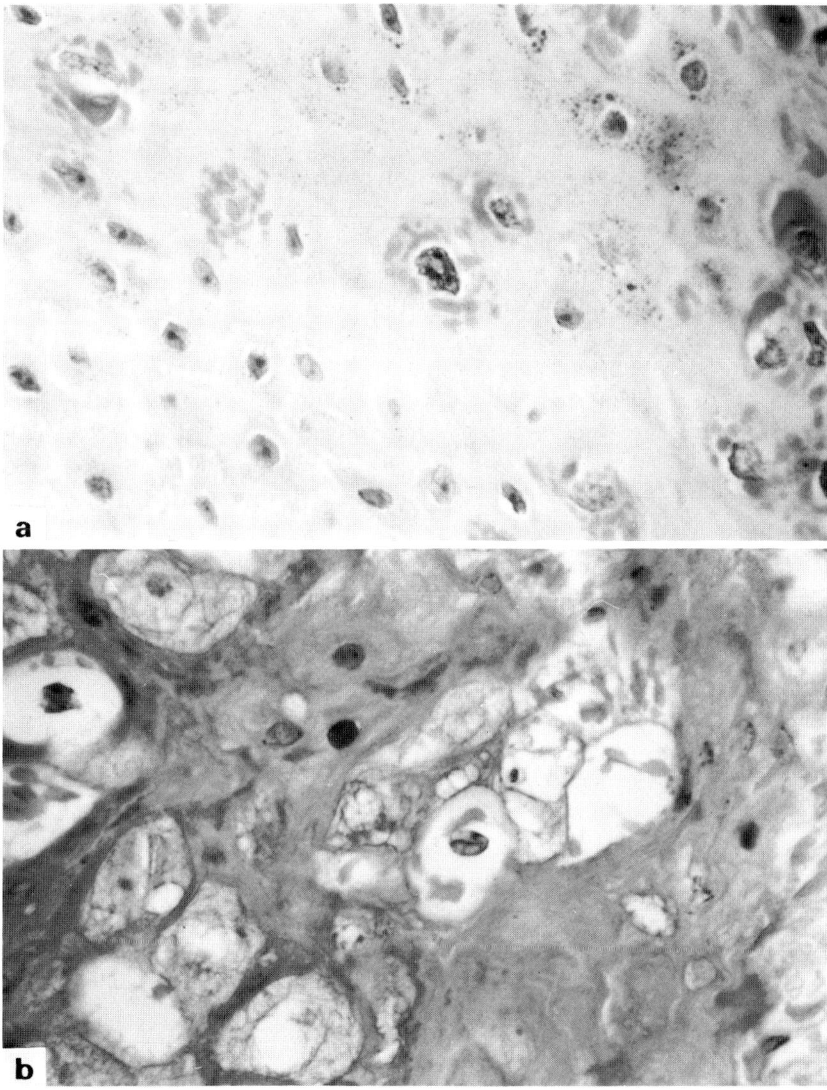

FIG. 6.21 Human wart. ×510. The neoplastic epithelium includes:
a. Enlarged epidermal cells with eosinophilic cytoplasmic inclusions around the nuclei.
b. Swollen (ballooned) cells, some also containing eosinophilic cytoplasmic inclusions.

neighbours. The cells in these small benign papillomata enlarge and some of them contain extensive cytoplasmic inclusions (Fig. 6.21a) composed of abnormal keratohyalin [89]; other cells become intensely swollen with ballooning degeneration (Fig. 6.21b). Ultimately the transformed cells are discarded, as

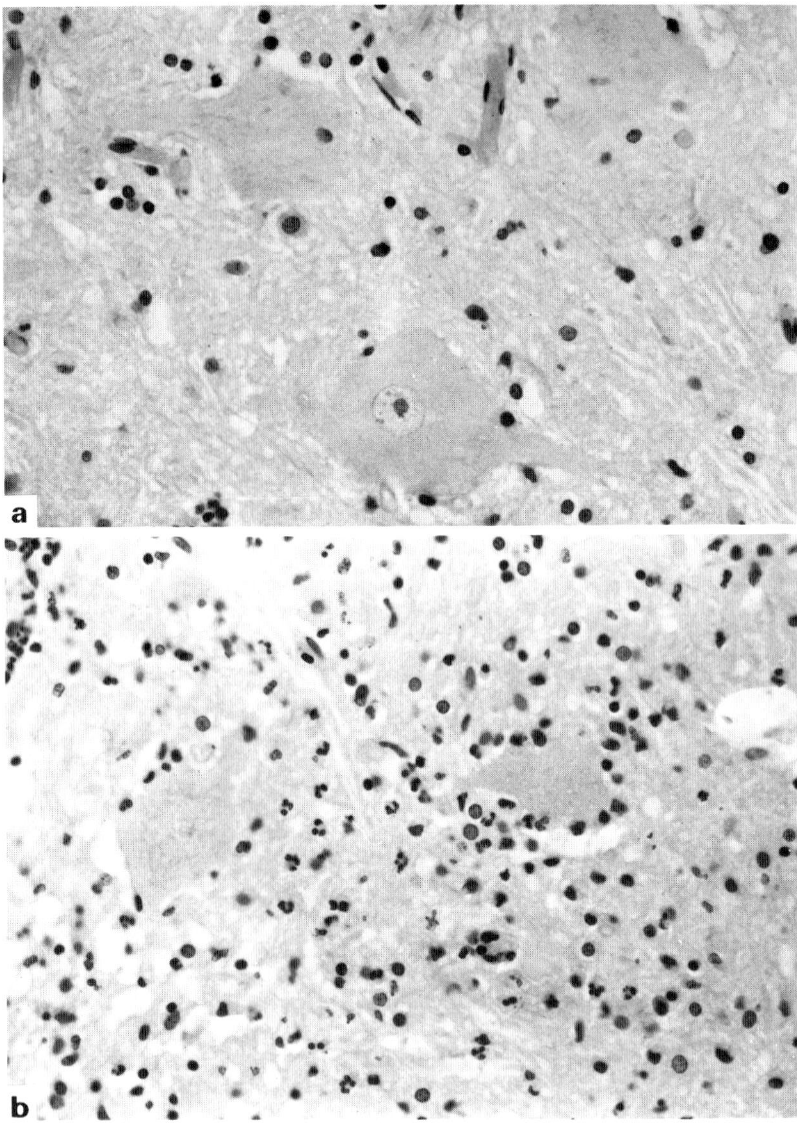

FIG. 6.22 Acute paralytic poliomyelitis: spinal cord grey matter. × 330.
a. Loss of Nissl substance from anterior horn cells; neuronal nuclei visible.
b. Necrotic neuronal cell bodies; perineuronal infiltration by neutrophils and monocytes.

they become more completely keratinised, but continuation of the process may occur through infection of neighbouring cells.

Invasive viruses on entering the body may never reach an organ where they injure cells and only occasionally penetrate cells where viral growth is actively

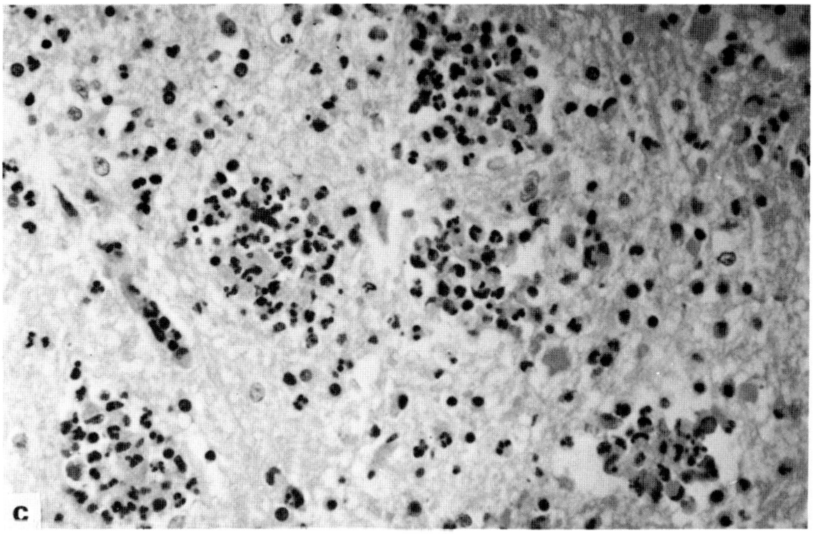

FIG. 6.22 cont.
c. Dead neurones consumed by aggregates of phagocytic cells (neuronophagia).

harmful. The most prominent signs of disease then depend on injury to these distant target cells, and only develop if the infection spreads to the organ where these susceptible cells are situated.

Thus poliovirus usually produces a harmless infection of the gastrointestinal lymphoid tissue followed by development of immunity; in some patients the virus spreads further by the blood and may cause fever and sore throat. But in an even smaller proportion of persons infected the virus then enters the central nervous system giving headache, backache, neck stiffness with recurrence of fever (pre-paralytic phase) followed by a variable degree of muscular paralysis due to replication of the virus within spinomedullary motor neurones (paralytic phase). Extensive intraneuronal replication has disastrous consequences and produces crippling loss of motor power or lethal paralysis of respiration and deglutition. Paralysis is accompanied by conspicuous loss of Nissl substance in spinal and medullary motor neurones (Fig. 6.22a; see Fig. 1.3a, p. 3) followed by devastating necrosis as the cytoplasm shrivels and becomes granular (Fig. 6.22b); the dead neurones are then surrounded by phagocytes which finally consume them entirely (neuronophagia, Fig. 6.22c). In lethal infection these changes are most prominent in the grey matter of motor nuclei in spinal anterior horns and medulla, which is intensely infiltrated with neutrophils and macrophages (Fig. 6.22b,c). This inflammatory exudate is a reaction to the products of the disintegrating neuronal cell bodies and is mainly confined to the grey matter; this originally gave rise to the term poliomyelitis (πολιός), grey).

Neuronal necrosis in paralytic poliomyelitis is greatly extended by physical exertion in the pre-paralytic phase of the disease; this suggests that excessive activity of the lower motor neurones increases the harmful effects of viral replication. Another adverse factor in promoting severe disease is preceding tonsillectomy which increases the risk of bulbar poliomyelitis with extensive necrosis of medullary neurones.

Infection by some viruses however is almost always followed by spread to susceptible target cells and is thus often accompanied by severe disease. Such spread with serious consequences usually occurs when a non-immune person is infected by the highly invasive smallpox virus (variola). The virus enters the body by infecting cells in the respiratory tract without overt injury. The virus then spreads by blood stream to other organs where it multiplies again without destructive effects. This replication is followed by more intense secondary viraemia which results in general infection of groups of epidermal cells which are the principal target for severe damage. The virus replicates in the epidermal cells which swell and die; this results in formation of macules which quickly become papules and vesicles and are surrounded by zones of acute inflammation in the dermis. Neutrophils then enter the vesicles to form pustules (Fig. 6.23). The encircling inflammation and local necrosis are enhanced by secondary infection with pyogenic cocci, while damage to the subjacent dermis results later in severe scarring and disfigurement. Similar focal epithelial lesions occur in the pharynx, larynx and oesophagus. Death in smallpox usually results from this secondary infection of lesions in skin and respiratory tract, although the

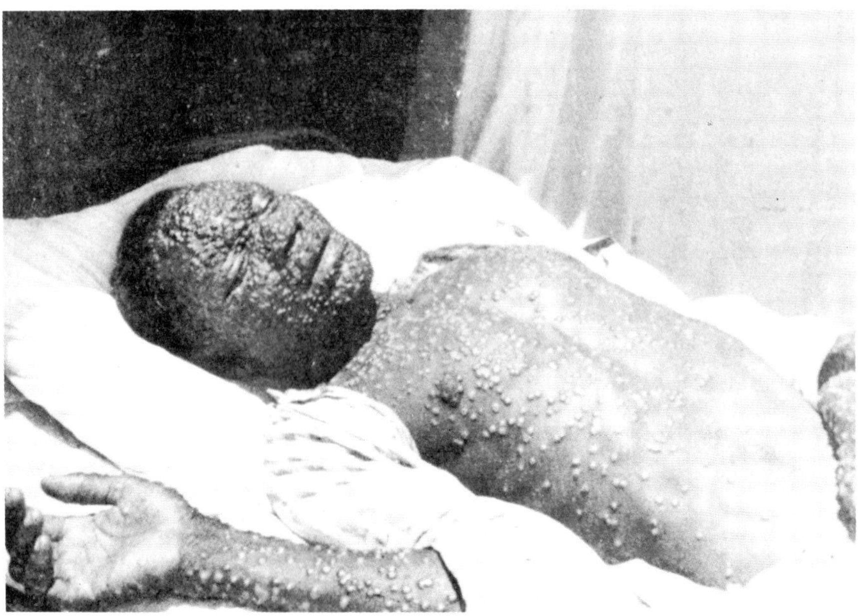

FIG. 6.23. Pustular lesions of smallpox on ninth day of illness; confluent pustules on face. Courtesy of Professor A. J. Rhodes & Professor C. E. Van Rooyen. Reproduced from *Textbook of Virology* (1962) Williams & Wilkins, Baltimore.

toxic effects of liberation of large amounts of virus into the blood may account for early death with haemorrhagic rashes produced before appearance of the epidermal vesicles.

Different tissues may thus greatly differ in their susceptibility to damage by one and the same virus. This phenomenon is strikingly illustrated by the effects of infection with rubella virus; this usually produces overt lesions in the skin with mild fever and transient rash (German measles), possibly caused by immune complex reaction between viral antigen and antibody. But, in pregnancy, spread of the virus across the placenta can infect the embryo and cause crippling maldevelopment of fetal heart, eyes or inner ear followed by congenital heart disease, blindness or deafness.

Injury induced by intracellular viral growth

Although pathogenic viruses can cause latent infection, their intracellular growth frequently induces conspicuous visible alteration and injury both to cells in culture and within the body in disease.

Cytopathic effects produced by viruses on cells in culture include:

1. Contraction into spherical necrotic remnants with pyknotic nuclei (poliovirus, vaccinia).
2. Coalescence to form multinuclear syncytia (respiratory syncytial virus, measles and herpesvirus).
3. Formation of cytoplasmic inclusion bodies (measles, vaccinia and variola).
4. Formation of nuclear inclusion bodies (measles, herpesvirus and cytomegalovirus).
5. Changes in cell membranes of infected cells so that they adsorb foreign red cells (parainfluenza virus 1).
6. Transformation to neoplastic cells (polyoma virus and SV40).

Similarly when viruses replicate within cells of the body in disease they also cause prominent visible changes; these include:

1. Swelling and vacuolation (vaccinia, Fig. 6.24 and see Fig. 1.2, p. 3). This aqueous swelling accounts for the epidermal lesions produced by vaccinia and variola viruses and also by herpes simplex and herpes zoster viruses (see Fig. 6.32).
2. Loss of Nissl substance from motor neurones (poliovirus, see Fig. 1.3a and Fig. 6.22a).
3. Formation of syncytial cells, such as multinucleate Warthin–Finkeldey giant cells in lymph nodes and nasal secretion in measles and coherent groups of epidermal cells within cutaneous vesicles in herpes zoster (see Fig. 6.32).
4. Formation of cytoplasmic inclusion bodies (vaccinia, Fig. 6.25 and 6.26; variola; rabies, Fig. 6.27 and 6.28).
5. Formation of nuclear inclusion bodies (cytomegalovirus, Fig. 6.29; herpes simplex; herpes zoster, see Fig. 6.32).

These changes may be followed by the most devastating necrosis, as can happen in the epidermis infected by smallpox or vaccinia (Fig. 6.23 and 6.24),

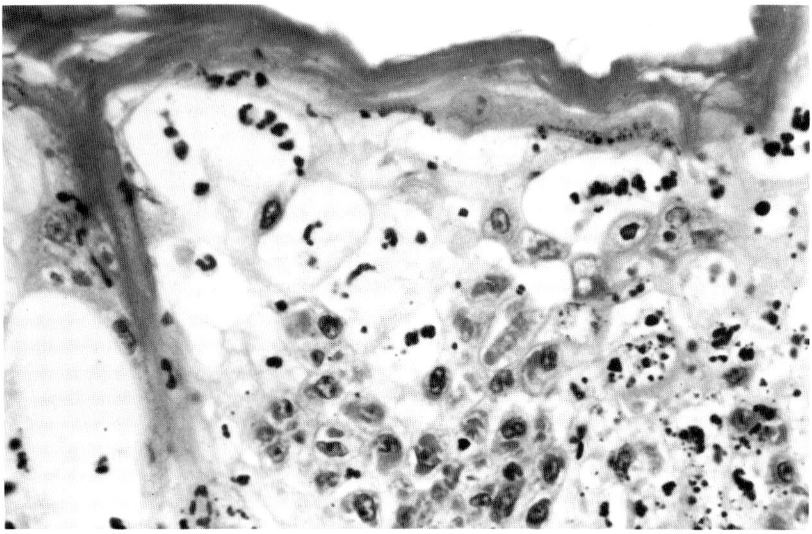

FIG. 6.24 Lesion caused by vaccinia virus in epidermis of newborn rabbit. Conspicuous cellular swelling with ballooning degeneration and infiltration with polymorphs. In lower part of the figure cytoplasmic inclusion bodies are visible in the epidermal cells. ×510.

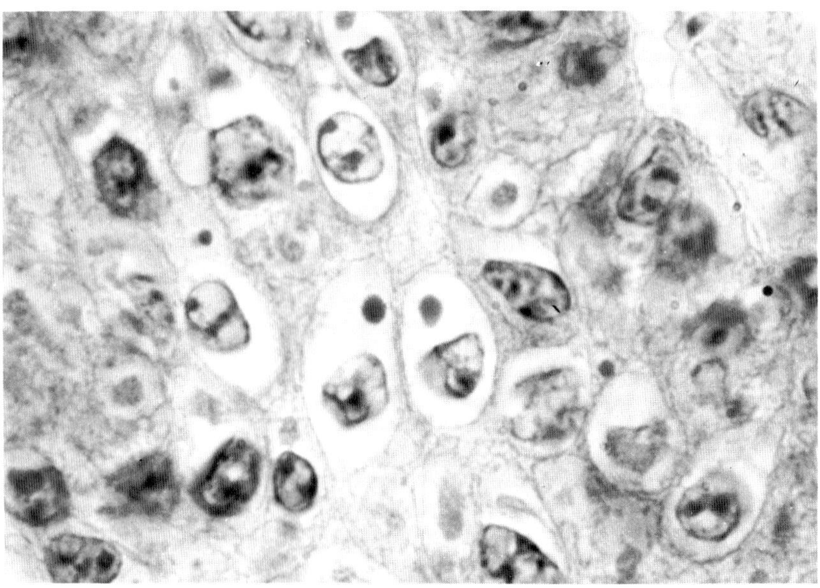

FIG. 6.25 Vaccinial lesion in rabbit epidermis (same as in Fig. 6.24). Swollen epidermal cells containing cytoplasmic inclusion bodies. ×1300.

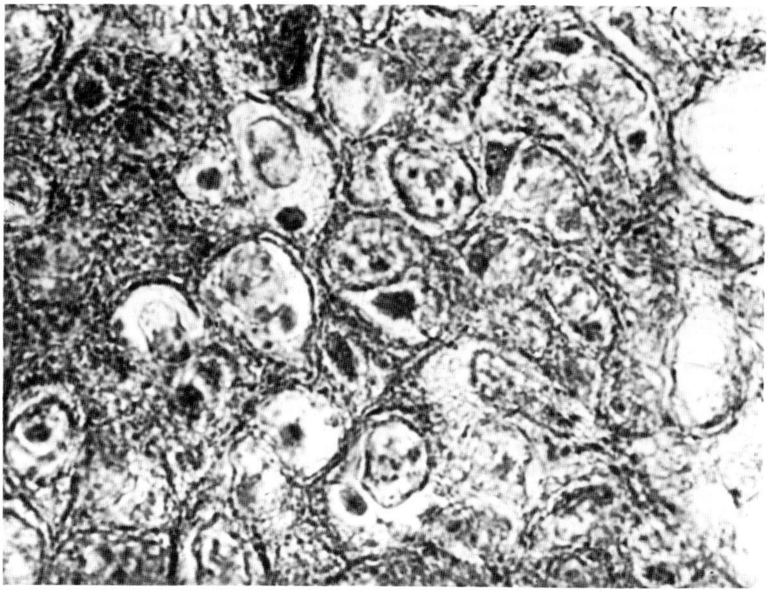

FIG. 6.26 Vaccinial lesion in rabbit epidermis (same as in Fig. 6.24). Epidermal cells contain cytoplasmic inclusion bodies stained by oxidised tannin-azo method for protein. ×1140. Dixon K. C. (1959), *Amer. J. Path.*, **35**, 249.

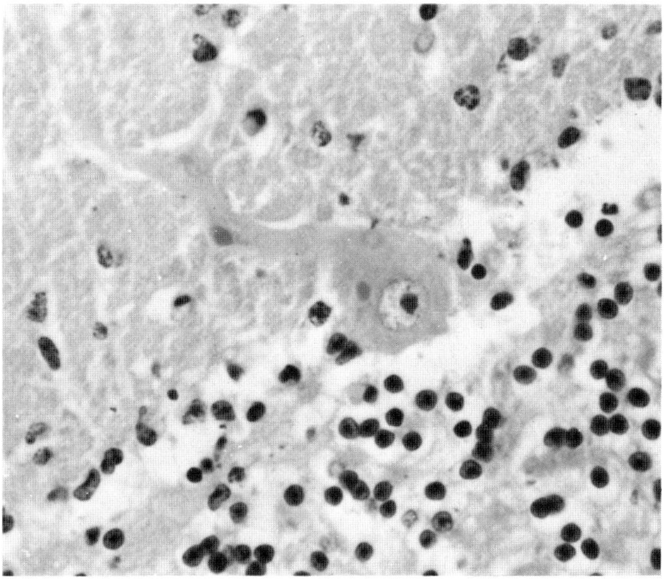

FIG. 6.27. Cerebellar cortex from sheep infected with rabies 'street' virus. Negri bodies in perikaryon and in apical dendrite of a Purkinje cell; these cytoplasmic inclusion bodies contrast strongly with the much more basophilic neuronal nucleolus. ×510.

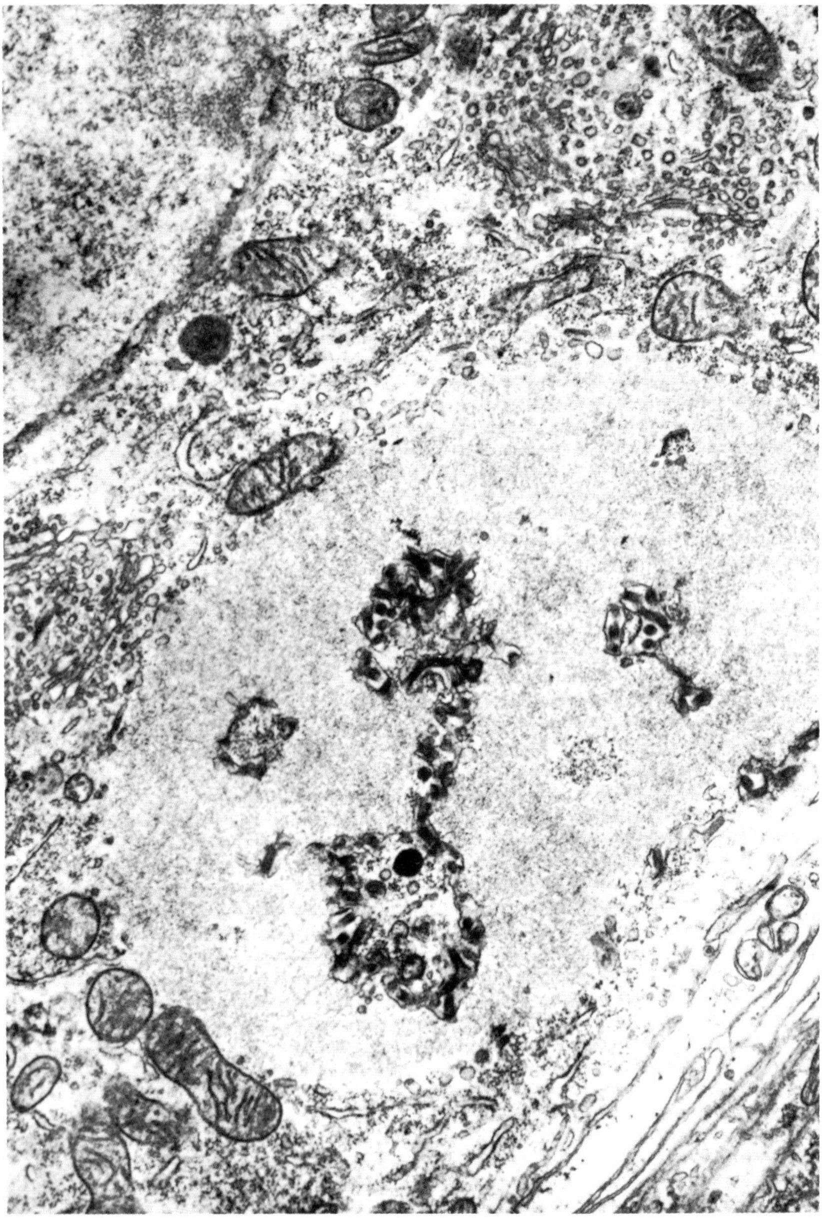

FIG. 6.28 Negri body in cytoplasm of a neurone in hippocampal cortex of mouse infected with rabies 'street' virus. The Negri body contains a fine homogeneous fibrous matrix in which several 'inner bodies' are embedded; these consist of swollen vesicles of endoplasmic reticulum in which are seen virions of rabies virus. Mitochondria are visible in cytoplasm around Negri body, EM. × 19 200. Courtesy of Professor S. Matsumoto. *Advances in Virus Research* (1970), **16**, 257.

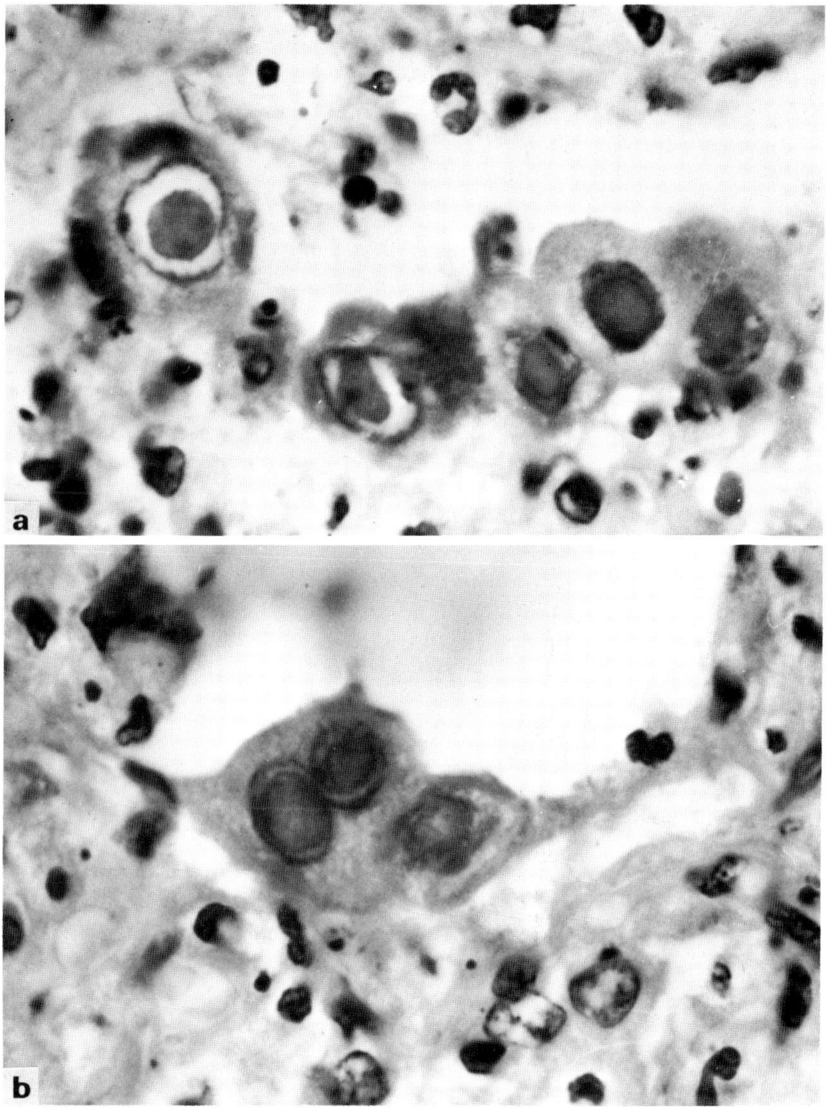

FIG. 6.29 Type A nuclear inclusion bodies due to infection of alveolar cells of human lung by cytomegalovirus from a patient who had been treated by immunosuppressive drugs which enabled opportunist infection to become established. × 1300.

a. Enlarged alveolar cells containing type A nuclear inclusions: a clear halo separates these hyaline inclusions from the nuclear membranes.

b Fusion of three alveolar cells containing nuclear inclusions to form a giant cell.

and in spinomedullary motor neurones in poliomyleitis (Fig. 6.22b). Even in the absence of necrosis cell function may substantially be altered; thus infection by smallpox or by vaccinia virus causes intense cellular hyperplasia before the onset of necrosis (see Fig. 1.2 and 6.33a), while oncogenic viruses can induce neoplastic transformation, as in human warts (see Fig. 6.21), without severe necrotising effects. Similarly excitement followed by coma, without neuronal necrosis, occurs in rabies caused by 'street virus' (p. 264).

Neoplasia caused by viruses

Human warts (see above) are caused by a DNA virus of the papova group. How far other kinds of human neoplasia are caused by viruses is uncertain. There is some evidence that carcinoma of the cervix is related to previous infection by herpes virus hominis type 2 and that another virus of the herpes group (the Epstein–Barr virus) may be concerned with causing Burkitt's lymphoma. Recently particles with the appearance of a retrovirus were observed in cell lines grown from patients with acute monocytic leukaemia [90].

Papova viruses, such as the polyoma virus, can produce malignant tumours in mice and hamsters. Retroviruses also cause leukaemia in animals; retroviruses are enveloped RNA viruses which replicate by means of reverse transcriptase. Bittner's mouse mammary tumour virus is a retrovirus which is transmitted by maternal milk and causes mammary carcinoma in female mice and also in male mice after treatment with female sex hormones (p. 183). Another retrovirus is responsible for murine leukaemia. This agent (discovered by Gross in 1951) is present in the tissues of some strains of mice and is transmitted in a latent form from mother to offspring, which may later develop leukaemia and lymphoma if the virus becomes activated by an external stimulus such as radiation; this virus buds from cell membranes in the form of central nucleoids surrounded by membranes derived from the cell surface (see Fig. 9.22, p. 474). Erythromyeloblastosis of birds as well as Rous chicken sarcoma are also caused by similar RNA viruses.

Viral replication

Visible damage of cells by viruses is usually accompanied by viral replication and synthesis, which are revealed by:

1. Multiplication of infective particles in terms of plaque-forming units, each of which produces a visible plaque of degeneration among cultured cells *in vitro* or a separate pock lesion on chick embryo membranes.
2. Formation of 'matrices' (inclusion bodies) in cytoplasm or nuclei of infected cells where individual virions become visible by EM, e.g. vaccinia and rabies in cytoplasm [91, 92] (Fig. 6.28) and herpes zoster and cytomegalovirus in nucleus [93] (Fig. 6.30).
3. Appearance and accumulation of viral antigens detectable by immunofluorescence, e.g. influenza, rabies [92, 94].

Viral inclusion bodies

Inclusion bodies visible by LM are prominent features of many cells infected by viruses. Inclusions are usually formed in zones of viral replication and

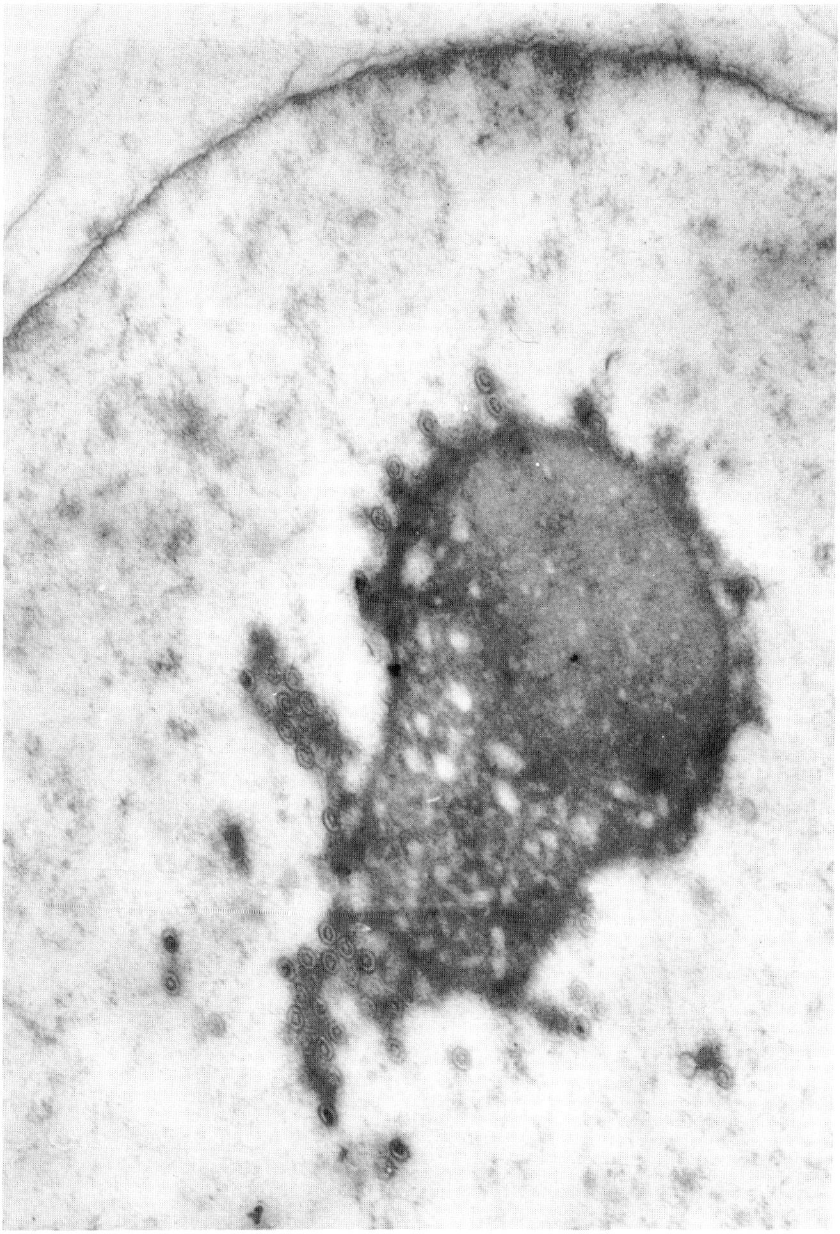

FIG. 6.30 Intranuclear formation of virions of cytomegalovirus in cultures of human lung fibroblasts. Dense delimited nuclear inclusion (factory matrix) from which virions are emerging; nuclear membrane visible at top of field. EM ×40 000. Courtesy of Dr P. Becker, Professor J. L. Melnick & Dr H. D. Mayor. From *Exp. molec. Path.* (1965), **4**, 11.

correspond to 'matrices' or dense zones visible by EM where the virions (elementary bodies) of the virus are assembled. Within the matrices virus-coded proteins are formed which constitute the polymerases necessary for replication, transcription and translation of the macromolecules of the formed virions. These 'factory' sites are then visible by LM as inclusion bodies and by EM as fibrillar matrices from which the formed virions emerge (Fig. 6.28 and 6.30). In some cases however inclusions are merely aggregates of protein which are indirect results of injury produced by viral infection but are not directly related to the sites of viral assembly. Inclusion bodies are situated either in the cytoplasm or in the nucleus.

Cytoplasmic inclusion bodies. infection by pox virus produces spheroidal eosinophilic masses in the cytoplasm of epidermal cells. These dense zones sometimes enlarge and fuse to fill most of the cytoplasm. Fig. 6.25 (p. 258) shows spheroidal inclusion bodies in swollen cells of rabbit epidermis infected by vaccinia virus. In Fig. 6.26 (p. 259) epidermal cells from the same vaccinial lesion are stained by the oxidised tannin azo method for protein; the inclusions are seen to contain a high concentration of tannophilic protein [95].

Inclusion bodies produced by vaccinia virus enclose within them virions (elementary bodies) of the virus, which are visible by EM and are elaborated within the protein matrix of the inclusion body [96]. The envelopes of the virions and also their nucleocapsids are assembled within these dense matrices or factory zones.

In rabies of man or animals, caused by naturally occurring 'street' virus, large inclusion (Negri) bodies visible by LM appear in the cytoplasm of cerebral neurones; Fig. 6.27 (p. 259) shows inclusions in a Purkinje cell of sheep cerebellum as seen by LM. Fig. 6.28 (p. 260) shows by EM an inclusion body in a neurone of hippocampal cortex of a mouse infected by 'street' virus; the inclusion bodies seen by EM consist of faintly fibrillar matrices enclosing in places some swollen vesicles of ER into which project budding virions of the rabies virus. These vesicles with budding virions probably correspond to basic particles visible within some of the Negri bodies seen by LM.

Negri bodies are not present in the neurones of animals with rabies caused by brain-adapted 'fixed' virus. But smaller dense zones are visible by EM in neurones infected by 'fixed' virus; these dense zones are similar in consistency to the larger matrices visible after infection by 'street' virus. Matsumoto [92] suggested that the 'fixed' virus injures cells so severely that full development of the large matrix (Negri body) cannot occur before necrosis arrests further viral growth. Infection by 'street' virus, on the other hand, although producing mania terminating in coma and death, usually does not produce neuronal necrosis; therefore large inclusion bodies composed of viral 'factory' protein have time to develop. Antigenic proteins of rabies virus stainable by immunofluorescence extend through much of the cytoplasm of infected neurones irrespective of whether introduced by 'street' or 'fixed' virus.

Cytoplasmic inclusions thus commonly appear in factory sites of viral replication and assembly. But in some instances viral infection induces denaturation and aggregation of cell protein not involved in viral assembly. Thus deposits of altered eosinophilic keratohyalin appear in the cytoplasm (Fig. 6.21a, p. 253) of epidermal cells in human warts produced by a papova (DNA) virus, which itself replicates in the nucleus. Similarly, degeneration of the cytoplasm of liver cells injured by yellow fever virus can produce large aggregates of denatured protein (Councilman bodies) which retract from the remainder of the cell (p. 292).

Nuclear inclusion bodies. Infection by viruses of the herpes group, including cytomegalovirus, herpes simplex and herpes zoster, commonly produces type A nuclear inclusion bodies both in cells in culture and *in vivo*. These bodies are large hyaline masses of protein which occupy most of the nucleus except for a clear peripheral halo separating them from the nuclear membrane (Fig. 6.29 and 6.32). This group of viruses are enveloped DNA viruses which replicate in the nucleus (see below); the inclusions visible by LM are in fact situated where 'factory' sites with developing virions are seen by EM.

Figs. 6.29a and 6.29b (p. 261) show (by LM) type A nuclear inclusions caused by cytomegalovirus in alveolar cells of the lung from a patient treated by immunosuppressive drugs; this immunosuppression had enabled opportunistic infection of the lungs by cytomegalovirus to become established. Some of the infected alveolar cells are visible as giant cells with one or more nuclei enclosing large hyaline inclusions. These nuclear inclusions seen by LM indicate the sites of 'factory' zones in which the virions of cytomegalovirus are elaborated [93]. Fig. 6.30 shows (by EM) an inclusion within the nucleus of an embryonic lung fibroblast infected in culture by cytomegalovirus; this inclusion is mainly composed of a dense matrix (factory site) from which formed virions are emerging. Fig. 6.31 shows groups of virions of cytomegalovirus formed in a more diffuse intranuclear matrix of a similarly infected embryonic fibroblast. Type A nuclear inclusion bodies induced by intranuclear viral replication are also present in cells infected by herpes zoster virus (Fig. 6.32, p. 269).

Infection of cells by measles virus causes the appearance of both type A intranuclear inclusions as well as inclusions in the cytoplasm. This enveloped RNA virus replicates in both cytoplasm and in nucleus, and the inclusions visible by LM correspond with viral 'factory' zones visible by EM. In human measles these intranuclear inclusions are present in oral epithelial cells in Koplik spots in the mouth, which develop about 3 days before the onset of the rash. In children with defective CMI (p. 267) measles virus can spread rapidly in pulmonary tissue to produce 'giant cell pneumonia' characterised by development of large polykaryocytes containing both cytoplasmic and type A intranuclear inclusions.

Type B nuclear inclusions are minute eosinophilic particles not surrounded by halos, which are visible in some cells infected by viruses. They are seen for instance in the nuclei of spinal anterior horn cells infected by poliovirus; as this virus replicates in the cytoplasm and not in the nucleus, these intranuclear inclusions are probably not directly related to viral replication.

Viral inclusion bodies are generally eosinophilic owing to the presence of

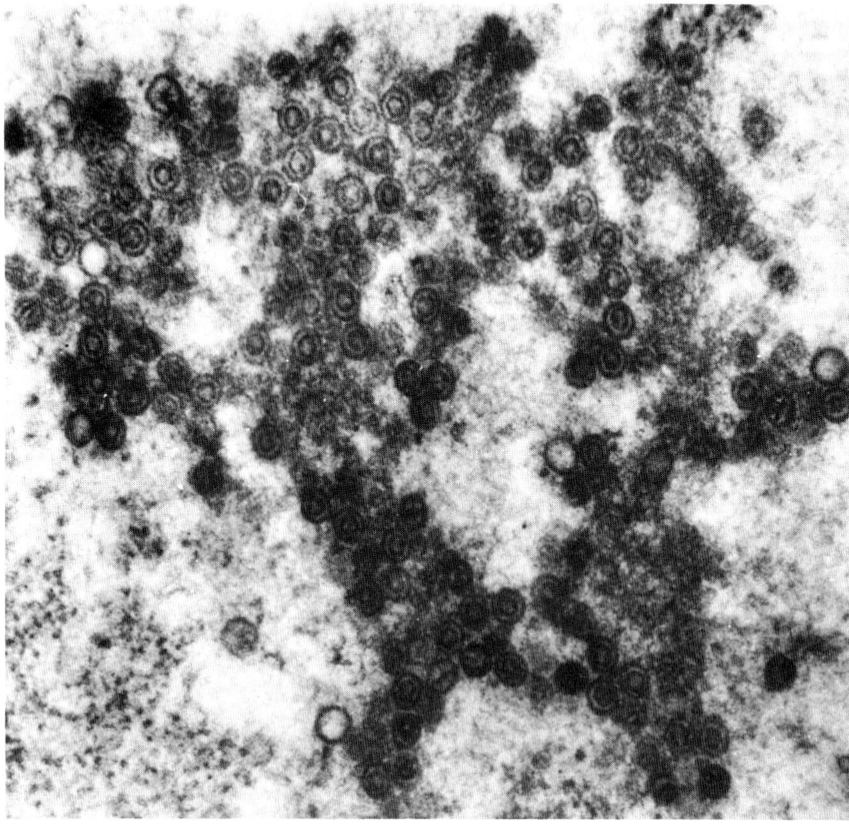

FIG. 6.31 Same tissue as Fig. 6.30 showing groups of virions of cytomegalovirus in a more diffuse intranuclear matrix. EM ×36 000. Courtesy of Dr. P. Becker, Professor J. L. Melnick & Dr H. D. Mayor. From *Exp. molec. Path.* (1965), **4**, 11.

anionophilic protein; but degrees of eosinophilia and basophilia depend greatly on pH of stains and other conditions of staining. DNA, stainable by the Feulgen method, is detectable in inclusions related to 'factory' sites for DNA viruses during the process of replication. DNA may disappear from these zones after emergence and discharge of the virions from the site of their formation. Thus the large type A intranuclear inclusions produced by herpes simplex virus in chick embryonic membranes [97, 98] and in Hela cells [99] at first contain Feulgen-positive DNA; but this is later lost from the degenerating nuclei.

Mechanism of necrosis and other cytopathic effects

Why viral replication is so necrotising only to some cells in which viruses multiply is obscure. Perhaps in these cases the formation of viral nucleic acids or proteins can exhaust the supply of available nucleotides or amino acids necessary for synthesis of the cell's own macromolecules. However, cytopathic effects usually arise more rapidly than could be effected by such deprivation. Moreover rapidly induced cytopathic effects, such as rounding of cells in culture caused by vaccinia virus, are prevented by inhibition of synthesis of viral protein by puromycin or cycloheximide, but on removal of the inhibitors the synthesis of viral protein is resumed and rounding of the cells begins almost immediately and is complete in one hour [100, 101]. Proteins formed by the virus thus appear to determine the cytopathic effects.

Other viral components may also contribute to changes in the infected cells. Thus a substance synthesised in cells infected by herpes virus may account for its typical power to induce the formation of syncytia; this syncytium-forming activity develops in cell cultures infected by herpes virus even before the appearance of infectious virus and is thought to be caused by a lipoprotein toxin [102]. The formation of syncytia also contributes to necrosis as the nutrition of these gigantic cells may easily become defective.

Viruses can thus cause injury by elaborating toxic substances. This view is substantiated by the recent discovery of a remarkable toxic protein formed by frog virus 3 (FV3) which is lethal to tadpoles. This amphibian DNA virus can only grow in mammalian cells at low temperatures. But the viral particles, although unable to replicate at 37°, can even at this temperature cause rapid inhibition of synthesis of both RNA and DNA in mammalian and chick embryonic cells in culture, and also produce margination of nuclear chromatin in the affected cells. These effects are due to the action of a structural protein which can be extracted from the viral particles and which binds avidly to DNA [103–105]. These observations imply that some toxic proteins formed by viruses can inactivate the principal biological activities of DNA and so may contribute substantially to the pathogenesis of viral disease.

Another cause of injury by viruses may be release of lysosomal enzymes and dissemination of these hydrolases through the cytoplasm of infected cells. Thus in cultured chick embryo cells infected by fowl plague virus lysosomal acid phosphatase becomes liberated from the disrupted lysosomes [106, 107]. Moreover an *early* change produced by poliovirus grown in human epithelial cells is the appearance of β-glucuronidase (another lysosomal hydrolase) *free* in the cytoplasm [108]; this appears to be the result of damage associated with the synthesis of viral proteins. Cytoplasmic dissemination of the hydrolase is then *followed* by leakage of the protein out of the cells. This suggests that viral proteins may induce release of lysosomal enzymes which in turn injure the plasma membrane with concomitant leakage of protein from the dying cells.

The necrotising effects of viral infection may thus depend on the formation of toxic proteins by viruses or also on the release of harmful enzymes by disruption of lysosomes. Indeed the toxic action of viral proteins may in some cases be exerted by damage to lysosomal membranes followed by release of lysosomal enzymes which are then responsible for further irreversible injury and discharge of virions through damaged cell membranes.

Another factor which may contribute to death of cells infected by viruses is cell-mediated immunity (CMI); death of infected cells, damaged by cytotoxic T-cells sentsitized by CMH (p. 217), may then become a major event in termination of viral infection. Moreover the necrotising effects of some viruses, such as hepatitis B, may largely depend on this elimination of the infected cells by CMI. When this process is exceptionally extensive the patient (with hepatitis B) may die from massive hepatic necrosis with acute yellow atrophy (p. 269).

Persistence in latent state

Following some viral diseases, although the acute infection terminates in the normal way as a result of CMI, intracellular virus may persist in a latent state and subsequently become reactivated. Such latent virus commonly persists in the cell bodies of sensory neurones. Possibly the permanence of neurones and their incapacity to divide enables dormant virus to survive within them.

Thus after recovery from chickenpox in childhood the varicella-zoster virus disappears from the healed lesions in the skin, but the infection may spread from the epidermis to reach spinal or trigeminal ganglion cells which harbour the virus in a latent state for many years or for life. The dormant virus may be reactivated in older people or in patients with Hodgkin's disease possibly owing to decline or suppression of CMI. The reactivated virus replicates in the ganglion cells and then passes down the sensory fibres so as to infect epidermal cells in skin area (dermatome) supplied by the corresponding nerve. The first sign of illness is deep seated intense pain vaguely referred to the same skin area in which crops of vesicles then develop. This disease is called shingles or *herpes zoster*.

The cutaneous lesions in shingles are produced by swelling and rupture of groups of epidermal cells in which this reactivated virus replicates. These swollen zones then form epidermal vesicles, around which are visible enlarged cells containing eosinophilic type A nuclear inclusions (Fig. 6.32). Similar inclusions also develop in the nuclei of neuronal cell bodies and satellite cells in the sensory ganglia of the same dermatomes corresponding to the affected cutaneous zones. The ganglionic cells also become swollen and intraganglionic foci of necrosis and haemorrhage may develop. This swelling and haemorrhage exert pressure on the nerve fibres within the ganglia which accounts for the intense pain of shingles. By EM viral particles are visible in the nuclei both of epidermal cells in the vesicles and of neuronal cell bodies of the affected ganglia, while the virus can be cultured from the epidermal vesicles [109, 110]. Sometimes the epidermal vesicular infection spread extensively in the skin to produce gerneralised herpes zoster; this tends to occur in patients with Hodgkin's disease, probably owing to extreme depression of CMI.

The virus of herpes simplex can similarly persist in a dormant state in sensory ganglia. This virus usually first infects children causing vesicular stomatitis. After healing the virus disappears from the mouth but may pass up sensory nerves to infect ganglion cells in the trigeminal ganglia. Reactivation of virus later in life by colds or other febrile illnesses enables the virus to spread down nerves and produce vesicular sores ('cold sores') in skin areas around mouth and nostrils which are supplied by nerves from the same ganglia.

Hepatitis B virus can also cause prolonged latent infection. This DNA virus persists in liver cells and in plasma of both apparently healthy carriers and also

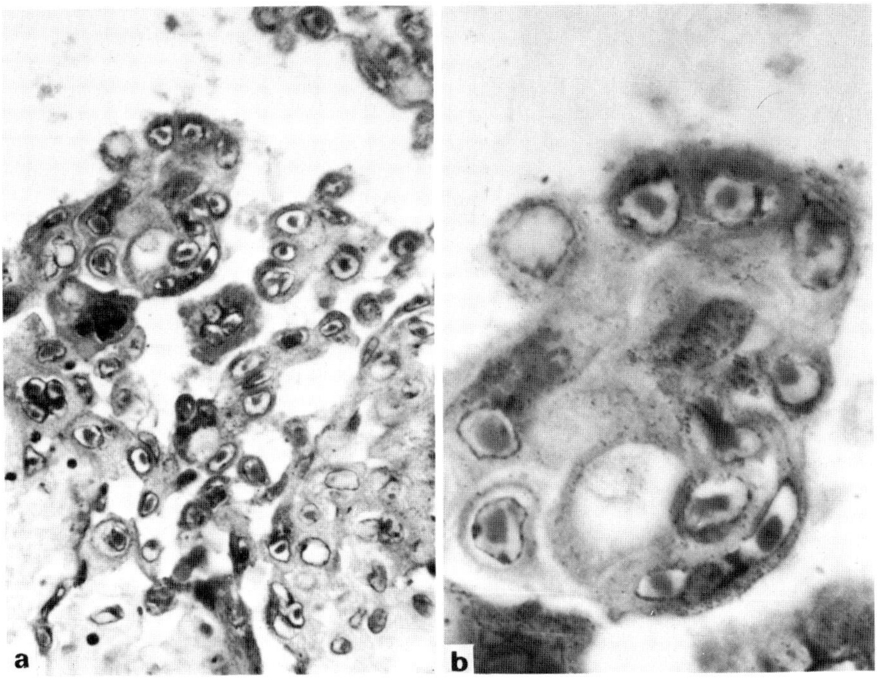

FIG. 6.32 Epidermal herpeszoster in a patient (with Hodgkins' disease), who developed generalised herpes zoster/varicella with vesicular lesions over face and trunk caused by zoster/varicella virus.

a. Epidermal vesicle surrounded by enlarged epidermal cells with type A intranuclear inclusions: these cells are coalescing to form syncytia. ×400.

b. Same field, showing cell fusion. ×1000.

of patients with chronic hepatic disease. In both cases hepatitis B virus surface antigen (HBsAg, Australia antigen) is detectable in the plasma. Infection usually occurs by transfusion of blood from carriers to previously uninfected persons. Infection also follows exposure to infected blood from use of contaminated syringes or needles, or even by entry of virus by cutaneous abrasions or inhalation. One of three possibilities [111] may then ensue:

1. Acute centrilobular hepatic necrosis with fever and jaundice along with rapid elimination of virus-infected cells by *fully effective CMI*. This is usually followed by complete recovery without any persistence of virus, though sometimes extensive hepatic necrosis may terminate rapidly in hepatic coma and death (p. 449).

2. Imperfect elimination of virus-infected hepatic cells when *CMI is less effective*. This may result in asynchronous piecemeal necrosis with successive sporadic infection of other hepatocytes, producing chronic hepatitis with progressive scarring (cirrhosis, p. 376) and portal obstruction; hepatic encephalopathy may ultimately follow (p. 449).

3. Little or no necrosis of the infected hepatic cells, when *CMI fails to be evoked*. This happens in healthy carriers whose hepatocytes contain large cytoplasmic inclusions rich in HBsAg detectable by immunofluorescence [112]. These infected cells occur in cords or clusters in the hepatic lobules; their cytoplasm (seen by direct transmission microscopy) is eosinophilic and finely granular with the appearance of 'ground glass'. In the absence of CMI the infected cells are not killed and many of them persist indefinitely. Such persistence of infection by hepatitis B virus may be a determinant of hepatocellular carcinoma [114].

Hepatitis A virus, on the other hand, does not lead to latent or persistent infection, nor does it cause chronic liver disease [113]. This RNA virus, which is the commonest cause of acute hepatitis with jaundice, can be isolated from faeces in the early acute phase of the disease. Infection is not transmitted by blood transfusion, but by the faeco-oral route.

Latent infection of a more extreme type occurs with some of the tumour viruses, which only produce overt disease if activated by additional stimuli; thus viruses of murine leukaemia are transmitted from mother to offspring among certain strains of mice without any pathogenic action unless activated by another injurious agent such as exposure to X-rays (p. 473).

Termination of infection

In viral diseases the development of cell-mediated immunity (CMI) is usually a principal factor in terminating infection (p. 217 and Fig. 6.9). CMI results in killing of infected cells before viral replication can take place. The presence of viral antigen on the cell surface can attract either specific killer cells (T-lymphocytes) or lymphokine-stimulated macrophages, which eliminate the infected cells so that viral growth is arrested. In this way the lesions of smallpox cease to enlarge and the solitary pustule of vaccination heals and shrivels.

In some persons CMI is defective and this power to eliminate virus-infected cells does not develop. This happens in patients with hereditary thymic aplasia, irrespective of whether or not this is accompanied by inherited defect in synthesis of immunoglobulins. In these children measles virus causes acute spreading infection among bronchopulmonary cells with formation of multinucleate giant cells—'giant cell pneumonia' (p. 265). This defect of CMI may also be specially harmful after vaccination; thus, instead of terminating in a limited pustule with healing, the vaccinial lesion continues to enlarge as the vaccinia virus spreads to neighbouring epidermal cells which in their turn swell and die. The virus shed from such an enlarged lesion then infects other areas of the body to produce multiple expanding vaccinial sores with extensive epidermal necrosis in skin (Fig. 6.33) and mucous membranes; this highly lethal condition is called generalised vaccinia or *vaccinia gangrenosa*.

Unknown pathogenic mechanisms

Some pathogenic micro-organisms which produce severe cellular injury form no known toxin and do not appear to interfere with nutrition, nor penetrate cells.

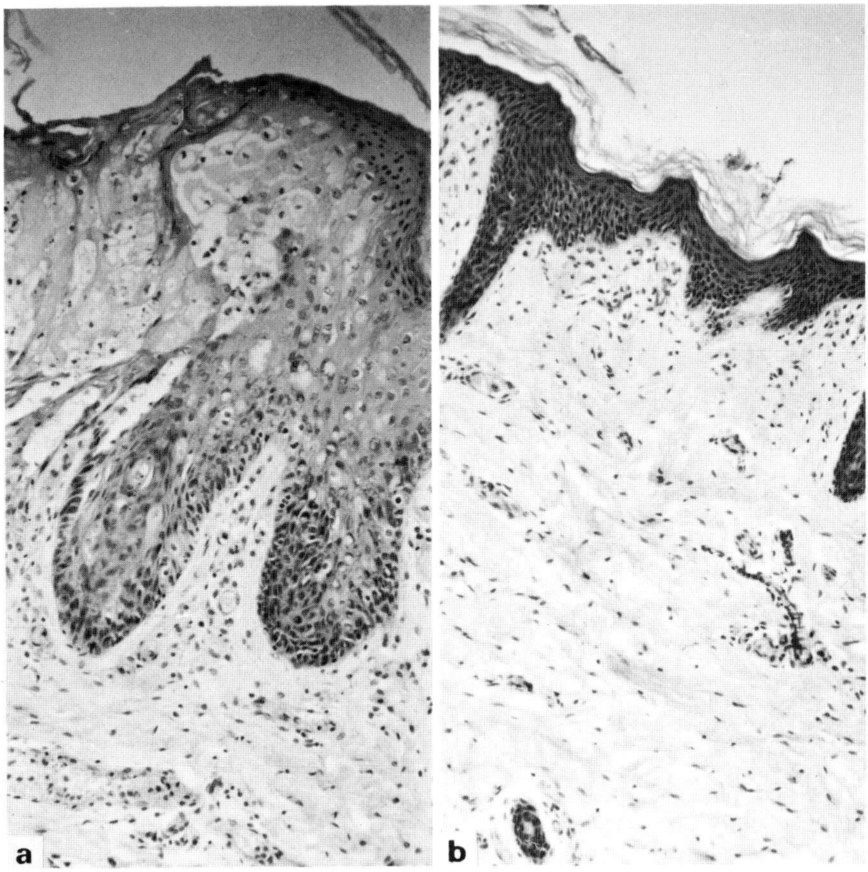

FIG. 6.33 Vaccinia gangrenosa in a child aged 7 months. Insidious development and progression of epidermal contact lesions, probably owing to defective CMI, following vaccination (on the forearm) 5 months earlier.

a. Contact lesion of inguinal skin; hyperplasia and enlargement of epidermal cells followed by ballooning degeneration, necrosis and intraepidermal vesiculation. × 130.

b. Adjacent unaffected epidermis for comparison. × 130.

Thus *Leptospira icterohaemorrhagiae*, which causes human leptospiral jaundice (Weil's disease), produces hepatic necrosis with jaundice and haemorrhages into the skin, as well as necrosis of cardiac and striated muscle together with fever and intense muscle pain; yet the mechanism underlying these severe lesions is unknown. This organism harmlessly colonises the renal tubules of rats. Human infection is acquired by contact with water contaminated by rat urine (as in sewers); *L. icterohaemorrhagiae* then penetrates the human skin and produces this highly injurious infection of man by some specific mechanism which leaves the rat unharmed.

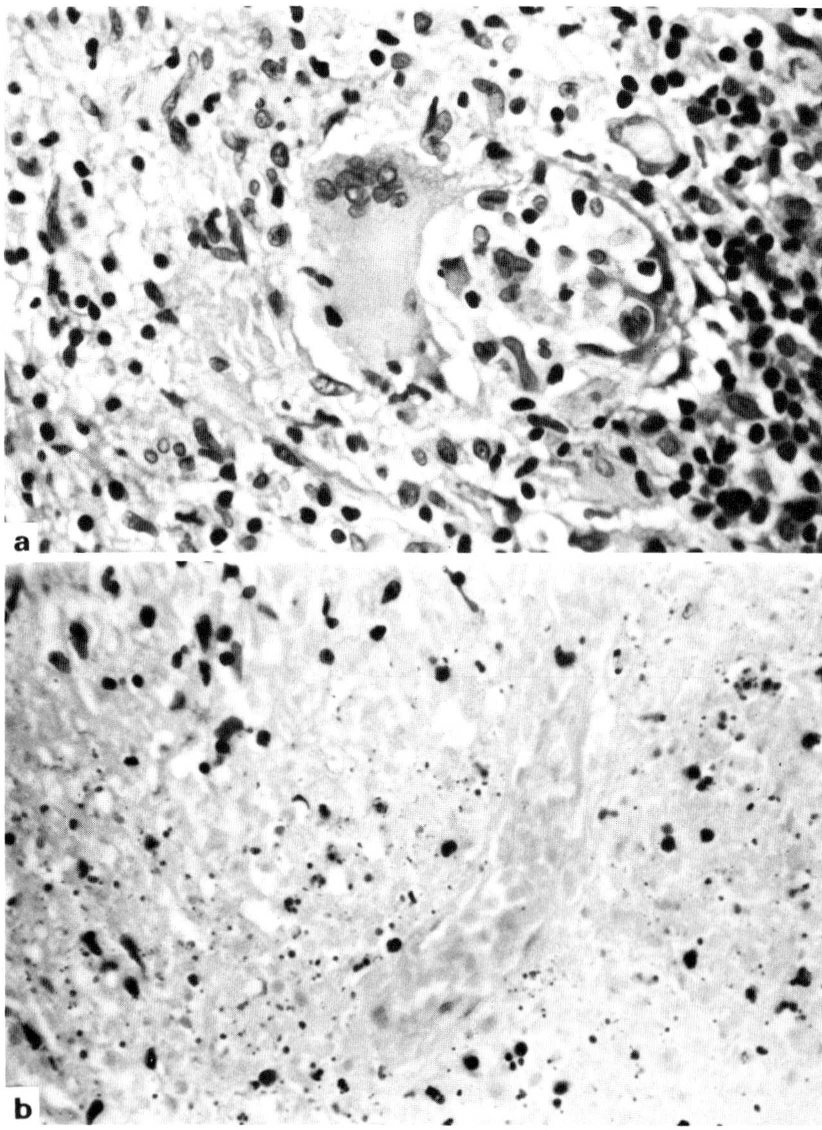

FIG. 6.34 Gumma of testis. Around a central focus of necrosis is a peripheral zone containing epithelioid cells and occasional giant cells along with granulation tissue composed of small blood vessels surrounded by lymphocytes. ×510.

a. Peripheral zone showing giant cell, epithelioid cells and lymphocytes.

b. Necrotic focus in centre of gumma showing pyknosis, karyorrhexis and karyolysis of nuceli, but in which outlines of some cells and a blood vessel persist.

Similarly the mechanism of many injurious effects produced by *Treponema pallidum* are undetermined. In tertiary syphilis *diffuse lesions*, composed of granulation tissue infiltrated by plasma cells and lymphocytes along with fibrosis, are the usual sequels to prolonged infection. But for some unknown reason epithelioid cells and giant cells occasionally appear (Fig. 6.34a) and parts of the lesions become necrotic. Such a zone of necrosis is called a gumma; this is a rubbery mass of dead tissue in which cellular structure is destroyed, but in which the outlines of blood vessels and of some cells and fibres persist (Fig. 6.34b). Gummatous necrosis occurs typically in testis, liver and lung and also in the facial bones and nasal cartilages where it may produce mutilating disfigurement. Possibly this accumulation of mononuclear cells coupled with necrosis may be related to cell-mediated hypersensitivity as in tuberculosis, but there is no evidence of any treponemal antigen akin to tuberculin which might incite or contribute to this necrotising hypersensitivity.

Prolonged syphilitic infection also produces devastating damage to the central nervous system in *general paralysis of the insane* (GPI). In this disease deterioration of personality with loss of memory, disorientation and confusion are followed by apoplectiform and epileptiform attacks terminating in paresis and dementia. The neurones of the cerebral cortex atrophy and disintegrate; the dendritic and axonal arborisations of the neurones are gradually replaced by proliferating microglial cells and the brain gyri become shrivelled by loss of neuronal substance. Usually masses of *Treponema pallidum* are visible in parts of the cerebral cortex (Fig. 6.35). Possibly toxins released by these abundant

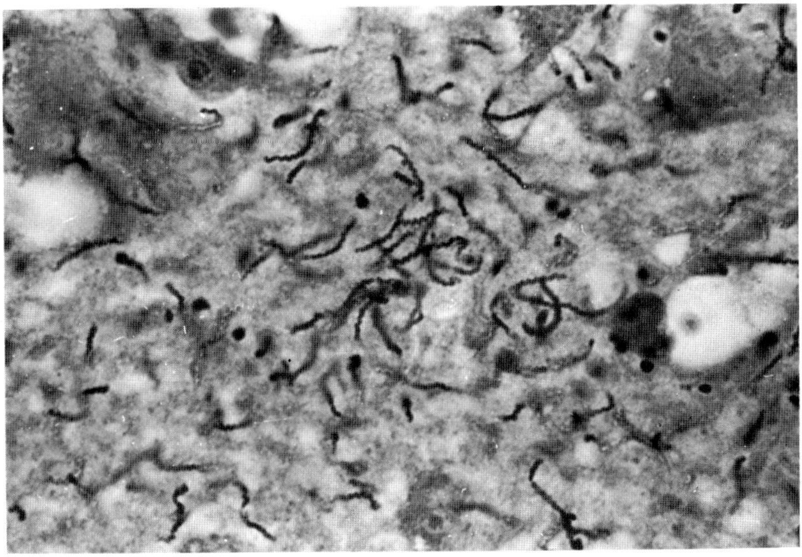

FIG. 6.35 Brain from a patient with GPI; swarms of *Treponema pallidum* between neuronal elements. Levaditi's silver impregnation. × 1300. Courtesy of Professor P. O. Yates.

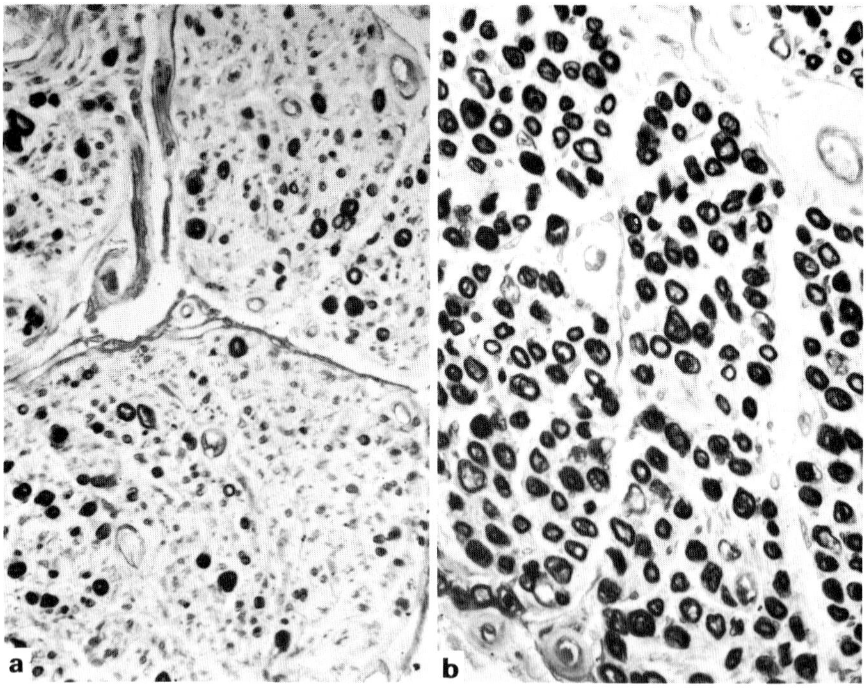

FIG. 6.36 Spinal nerve roots, from a patient with severe tabes dorsalis, stained by Weigert-Pal method for myelin. ×265.

a. Posterior roots: shrinkage and loss of fibres, also loss of myelin.

b. Anterior roots at same level: unaffected. Specimen by courtesy of Dr B. M. Herbertson.

spirochaetes are responsible for some of the more transient early symptoms, while syphilitic endarteritis affecting the smaller arterioles (p. 220) may cause ischaemic injury with permanent neuronal loss. Thus the activity of myriads of spirochaetes almost certainly initiates this crippling cerebral disintegration, but the actual steps in its pathogenesis are undetermined.

Another outcome of prolonged syphilitic infection, with even more uncertain mechanism, is *tabes dorsalis*. This disorder involves highly damaging degeneration of the sensory fibres entering the spinal cord from the posterior root ganglia; ultimately the posterior columns of spinal white matter become shrivelled and wasted (L. *tabes*, wasting) owing to loss of most of their myelinated fibres. The concomitant loss of proprioception as well as of sensation eventually produces most incapacitating disability with extreme incoordination of movement. Fig. 6.36a and 6.37a show the loss of myelin from the posterior roots and posteromedial tracts respectively in the spinal cord of a patient with severe tabes dorsalis: Fig. 6.36b and 6.37b show, for comparison, the corresponding anterior roots and anteromedial tracts which are seen to be completely unharmed. The mechanism for this highly discriminating degeneration affecting a single functional group of myelinated fibres is obscure. No

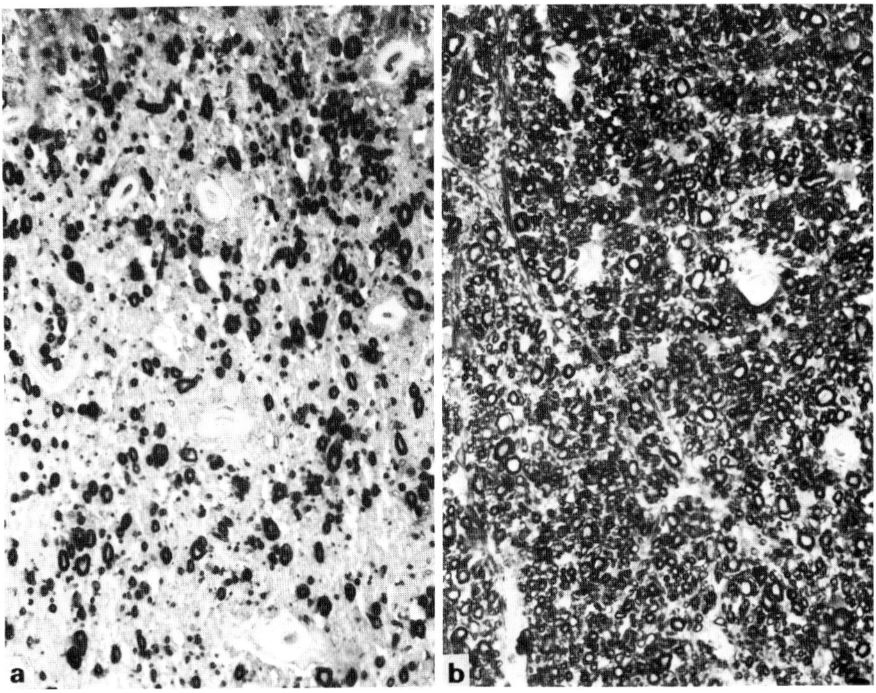

FIG. 6.37 Spinal tracts from patient with severe tabes dorsalis; same section as Fig. 6.36. ×265.
a. Posteromedial tract: shrinkage and loss of fibres, also loss of myelin.
b. Anteromedial tract: unaffected.

swarms of massed spirochaetes are detectable as in GPI, nor is there consistent evidence of any other pathogenic mechanism. The selective loss of myelin appears to originate in the radicular nerves entering the spinal cord from the posterior root ganglia. Is the origin of this selective and highly injurious degeneration ischaemic, toxic or allergic? It is well to remember that in spite of continuous and progressive advance in knowledge we are still ignorant of many of the basic mechanisms of cellular disorder.

Trace science then with modesty thy guide
First strip off all her equipage of pride
Alexander Pope

REFERENCES

[1] BORN G. V. (1971) Functional physiology of platelets. In *Human Blood Coagulation, Haemostasis and Thrombosis*, p. 168, ed. by R. Biggs. Blackwell Scientific Publications, Oxford.
[2] FULOP M., ROSENBLATT A., KREITZER S. M. & GERSTENHABER B. (1975) Hyperosmolar nature of diabetic coma. *Diabetes*, **24**, 594.

[3] GREAVES M. W., SONDERGAARD J. & GIBSON W. McD. (1971) Recovery of prostaglandins E & F in human cutaneous inflammation. *Brit. med. J.*, **2**, 258.
[4] GORDON A. S., RAYMON F. & IVY A. C. (1954) Drowning phenomena in various species. *Fed. Proc.*, **13**, 58.
[5] DONALD K. W. (1955) Drowning. *Brit. med. J.*, **2**, 155.
[6] TABOR H. & ROSENTHAL S. M. (1945) Effects of potassium administration, of sodium loss and fluid loss in tourniquet shock. *Publ. Hlth. Rep.* (*NIH*), **60**, 373 and 401.
[7] BYWATERS E. L., DELORY G. F., RIMINGTON C. & SMILES J. (1941) Myohaemoglobin in the urine of air raid casualties with crushing injury. *Biochem. J.*, **35**, 1165.
[8] MEYER U. A. & SCHMID R. (1978) In *The Metabolic Basis of Inherited Diseases*, 4th Ed., p. 1166, ed. by J. B. Stanbury, J. B. Wyngaarden & D. S. Fredrickson. McGraw-Hill, New York.
[9] ROZDILSKY B. & OLSZEWSKI J. (1961) Experimental study of the toxicity of bilirubin in newborn animals. *J. Neuropath.*, **20**, 193.
[10] CHEN H.-C., LIEN I.-N. & LU T.-C. (1965) Kernicterus in newborn rabbits. *Amer. J. Path.*, **46**, 331.
[11] TIZARD B. M. (1980) Cerebral palsies. The Croonian lecture 1978. *J. roy. Coll. Phycns. Lond.*, **14**, 72.
[12] SEEGMILLER J. E., HOWELL R. R. & MALAWISTA S. E. (1962) The inflammatory reaction to sodium urate. *J. Amer. med. Ass.*, **180**, 469.
[13] LAURENT T. C. (1964) Solubility of sodium urate in the presence of chondroitin-4-sulphate. *Nature*, **202**, 1334.
[14] FAIRES J. S. & McCarty D. J. (1962) Acute arthritis in man and dog after intrasynovial injection of sodium urate crystals. *Lancet*, **2**, 682.
[15] PHELPS P. & MCCARTY D. J. (1966) Crystal-induced inflammation in canine joints. II. Importance of polymorphonuclear leucocytes. *J. exp. Med.*, **124**, 115.
[16] SHIRAHAMA T. & COHEN A. S. (1974) Ultrastructural evidence for leakage of lysosomal contents after phagocytosis of monosodium urate crystals. A mechanism of gouty inflammation. *Amer. J. Path.*, **76**, 501.
[17] WEISSMANN G. & RITA G. A. (1972) Molecular basis of gouty inflammation: interaction of monosodium urate crystals and lysosomes and liposomes. *Nature, new Biol.*, **240**, 167.
[18] COOMBS R. R. A. & GELL P. G. (1975) In *Clinical Aspects of Immunology*, 3rd Ed., p. 761, ed. by P. G. Gell, R. R. A. Coombs & P. J. Lachmann. Blackwell Scientific Publications, Oxford.
[19] LAWSON D., FEWTRELL C., GOMBERTS B. & RAFF M. C. (1975) Anti-immunoglobulin induced histamine secretion by rat peritoneal mast cells studied by immunoferritin electron microscopy. *J. exp. Med.*, **142**, 391.
[20] PEPYS J. (1975) Skin testing (for allergic reactions). *Brit. J. Hosp. Med.*, **14**, 412.
[21] LUMSDEN C. E. (1971) The immunogenesis of the multiple sclerosis plaque. *Brain Res.*, **28**, 365.
[22] LINDQUIST R. (1975) in *Immunology*, p. 33, ed. by B. A. Thomas. Upjohn, Kalamazo, Michigan.
[23] ROITT I. M. (1980) *Essential Immunology*, 4th Ed., p. 161. Blackwell Scientific Publications, Oxford.
[24] HOLLANDER J. L., MCCARTY D. J., ASTORGA G. & CASTRO-MURILLO D. J. (1965) Studies on the pathogenesis of rheumatoid joint inflammation: I The 'R.A. cell' and a working hypothesis. *Ann. intern. Med.* **62**, 271.
[25] MALININ T. I., PEKIN T. J. & ZVAIFLER N. J. (1967) Cytology of synovial fluid in rheumatoid arthritis. *Amer. J. clin. Path.*, **47**, 203.
[26] VAUGHAN J. H. (1972) Infectious and immunologic considerations in rheumatic diseases. In *Arthritis and Allied Conditions*, 8th Ed., p. 248, ed. by J. L. Hollander & D. J. McCarty. Lea & Febiger, Philadelphia.
[27] ZVAIFLER N. J. (1972) Pathogenetic mechanism in rheumatoid arthritis. In *Arthritis*

and Allied Conditions, 8th Ed., p. 302, ed. by J. L. Hollander & D. J. McCarty. Lea & Febiger, Philadelphia.

[28] KAY D. M. & TUFFANELLI D. L. (1969) Immunofluorescent techniques in clinical diagnosis of cutaneous disease. *Ann. intern. Med.*, **71**, 753.

[29] GILLIAM J. N., CHEATUM D. E., HURD E. R., STASINY P. & ZIFF M. (1974) Immunoglobulins in clinically uninvolved skin in SLE. *J. clin. Invest.*, **53**, 1434.

[30] RIFKIND R. A. & GODMAN G. C. (1957) Phase contrast & interferometric microscopy of the LE cell phenomenon. *J. exp. Med.*, **106**, 607.

[31] FRIOU G. J. (1972) The LE cell phenomenon and antinuclear antibodies. In *Arthritis and Allied Conditions*, 8th Ed., p. 172, ed. by J. L. Hollander & D. J. McCarty. Lea & Febiger, Philadelphia.

[32] TAN E. M., Schur P. H. & KUNKEL H. G. (1965) DNA in serum of patients with SLE. *J. clin. Invest.*, **44**, 1104.

[33] HUGHES G. V. R. (1971) Significance of anti-DNA antibodies in SLE. *Lancet*, **2**, 861.

[34] SILBERBERG I. (1971) Ultrastructural studies of Langerhans cells in contact sensitive and primary irritant reactions to mercuric chloride. *Clin. Res.*, **19**, 715.

[35] SILBERBERG I., BARR R. L. & ROSENTHAL S. A. (1974) The role of Langherhans cells in contact allergy. *Acta derm.- venereol. (Stock.)*, **54**, 321.

[36] SILBERBERG-SINAKIN I., THORBECK G. J., BAER R. L., ROSENTHAL S. A. & BEREZOWSKY V. (1976) Antigen-bearing Langerhans cells in skin, dermal lymphatics and lymph nodes. *Cell Imm.*, **25**, 137.

[37] DUMONDE D. C., WOLSTENCROFT R. A., PANAYI G. S., MATTHEW M., MORLEY J. & HOWSON W. T. (1969) Lymphokines: non-antibody mediators of cellular immunity generated by lymphocytic activation. *Nature*, **224**, 38.

[38] SEILIN D., WALLACH D. F. H. & FISCHER H. (1971) Intercellular communication in cell-mediated cytotoxicity (fluorescein transfer between target cells and sensitised lymphocytes). *Europ. J. Immunol.*, **1**, 453.

[39] NAIRN R. C., NIND A. P. P., GULI E. P. G., MULLER H. K., ROLLAND J. M. & MINTY C. C. J. (1971) Specific immune response in human skin carcinoma. *Brit. med. J.*, **4**, 701.

[40] AMBACHE N. (1948) Peripheral action of botulinum toxin. *Nature*, **161**, 482.

[41] BURGEN A. S. V., DICKENS F. & ZATMAN L. J. (1949) The action of botulinum toxin on the neuromuscular junction. *J. Physiol.*, **109**, 10.

[42] PRICE D. L., GRIFFIN J., YOUNG A., PECK K. & STOCKS A. (1975) Tetanus toxin: direct evidence for retrograde intra-axonal transport. *Science*, **188**, 945.

[43] SCHWAB M. E. & THOENEN H. (1976) EM evidence for transsynaptic migration of tetanus toxin in spinal cord and motoneurons: an autoradiographic and morphometric study. *Brain Res.*, **105**, 213.

[44] VAN HEYNINGEN W. E. (1974) Gangliosides as membrane receptors for tetanus toxin, cholera toxin and serotonin. *Nature*, **249**, 415.

[45] KIMBERG D. V., FIELD M., JOHNSON J., HENDERSON A. & GERSHON E. (1971) Stimulation of intestinal mucosal adenylcyclase by cholera enterotoxin and prostaglandins. *J. clin. Invest.*, **50**, 1218.

[46] SHARP G. W. G. & HYNIE S. (1971) Stimulation of intestinal adenylcyclase by cholera toxin. *Nature*, **229**, 266.

[47] DONTA S. T., MOON H. W. WHIPP S. C. (1974) Detection of heat labile *E. coli* enterotoxin with use of adrenal cells in culture. *Science*, **183**, 334.

[48] SKIRROW M. B. (1977) Campylobacter enteritis. *Brit. med. J.*, **2**, 9.

[49] WEBSTER H. DE F., SPIRO D., WAKSMAN B. & ADAMS R. D. (1961) Phase and EM studies of experimental demyelination. II Schwann cell changes in guinea pig sciatic nerves during experimental diphtheritic neuritis. *J. Neuropath.*, **20**, 5.

[50] CAVANAGH J. B. & JACOBS J. M. (1964) Some quantitative aspects of diphtheritic neuropathy. *Brit. J. exp. Path.*, **45**, 309.

[51] WELLER R. O. (1965) Diphtheritic neuropathy in the chicken, an EM study. *J. Path. Bact.*, **89**, 591.

[52] STRAUSS N. & HENDEE E. D. (1959) The effect of diphtheria toxin on the metabolism of Hela cells. *J. exp. Med.*, **109**, 145.

[53] COLLIER R. J. (1967) Effect of diphtheria toxin on protein synthesis: inactivation of one of the transfer factors. *J. molec. Biol.*, **25**, 83.

[54] GILL D. M., PAPPENHEIMER A. M., BROWN R. & KURNICK J. T. (1969) Studies on the mode of action of diphtheria toxin. VII Toxin-stimulated hydrolysis of nicotinamide adenine dinucleotide in mammalian cell extracts. *J. exp. Med.*, **129**, 1.

[55] GILL D. M. & PAPPENHEIMER A. M. (1971) Structure-activity relationships of diphtheria toxin. *J. biol. Chem.*, **246**, 1492.

[55a] YAMAIZUMI M., MEKADA E., UCHIDA T. & OKADA Y. (1978) One molecule of diphtheria toxin fragment A introduced into a cell can kill the cell. *Cell*, **15**, 245.

[56] POPJAK G. (1948) The mechanism of parenchymatous degeneration produced by diphtheria toxin. *J. Path. Bact.*, **60**, 75.

[57] GILL D. M. (1978) Toxic peptides that cross cell membranes. In *Bacterial Toxins and Cell Membranes*, p. 291, ed. by J. Jeljaszewicz & T. Wadstrom. Academic Press, London.

[58] MACFARLANE M. G. & KNIGHT J. G. (1941) The biochemistry of bacterial toxins. I. The lecithinase action of *Clostridium welchii* toxins. *Biochem. J.*, **35**, 884.

[59] MACFARLANE M. G. & DATTA N. (1954) Observations on the immunology and biochemical properties of liver mitochondria with reference to the action of *Clostridium welchii* toxin. *Brit. J. exp. Path.*, **35**, 191.

[60] MACFARLANE R. G. & MACLENNAN J. D. (1945) The toxaemia of gas gangrene. *Lancet*, **2**, 328.

[61] MACLENNAN J. D. & MACFARLANE R. G. (1945) Toxin and antitoxin studies on gas gangrene in man. *Lancet*, **2**, 301.

[62] HIRSCH J. G., BERNHEIMER A. W. & WEISSMANN G. (1963) Motion picture study of the toxic action of streptolysins on leucocytes. *J. exp. Med.*, **118**, 223.

[63] WORK E. (1971) Chemistry of bacterial pyrogens. In *Pyrogens and Fever*, p. 23, ed. by G. E. W. Wosterholm & J. Birch. Churchill Livingstone, Edinburgh.

[64] WARDLE N. (1979) Bacteraemic and endotoxic shock. *Brit. J. Hosp. Med.*, **213**, 223.

[65] PRESTON F. E. (1979) Haematological problems associated with shock. *Brit. J. Hosp. Med.*, **213**, 232.

[66] BENNET I. L. & BEESON P. B. (1953) Studies in pathogenesis of fever. *J. exp. Med.*, **98**, 477 and 492.

[67] MURPHY P. A., CHESNEY P. J. & WOOD W. B. (1971) Purification of an endogenous pyrogen. In *Pyrogens and Fever*, p. 59, ed. by G. E. W. Wosterholm & J. Birch. Churchill Livingstone, Edinburgh.

[68] ATKINS E. & WOOD W. B. (1955) Studies on pathogenesis of fever: I. The presence of transferable pyrogen in the blood stream following the injection of typhoid vaccine. *J. exp. Med.*, **101**, 519. II. Identification of an endogenous pyrogen in the blood stream following the injection of typhoid vaccine. *J. exp. Med.*, **102**, 499.

[69] ATKINS E. & BODEL P. T. (1971) Role of leucocytes in fever. In *Pyrogens and Fever*, p. 81, ed. by G. E. Wosterholm & J. Birch. Churchill Livingstone, Edinburgh.

[70] JUDGE D. M., SAMUEL I., PERINE P. L. & VICKOTIC D. (1974) Louse-borne relapsing fever in man. *Arch. Path.*, **97**, 136.

[71] JARUMLINTA R. & KRODOLFER F. (1964) The toxic effects of *Entamoeba histolytica* on leucocytes. *Ann. trop. Med. Parasit.*, **58**, 375.

[72] EATON R. D. P., MEEROVITCH E. & COSTERTON J. W. (1969) A surface active lysosome in *Entamoeba histolytica*. *Trans. roy. Soc. trop. Med. & Parasitol.*, **63**, 678.

[73] EATON R. D. P., MEEROVITCH E. & COSTERTON J. W. (1970) The functional morphology of pathogenicity of *Entamoeba histolytica*. *Ann. Trop. Med. Parasit.*, **64**, 299.

[74] GOREN M. B. (1972) Mycobacterial lipids: selected topics. *Bact. Rev.*, **36**, 33.
[75] ROJAS-ESPINOSA O., DANNEBERG A. M., STEINBERGER L. A. & TSUDA T. (1974) The role of cathepsin D in the pathogenesis of tuberculosis. *Amer. J. Path.*, **74**, 1.
[76] DANNEBERG A. M. (1968) Cellular hypersensitivity and cellular immunity in the pathogenesis of tuberculosis. *Bact. Rev.*, **32**, 85.
[77] ARMSTRONG J. A. & HART P. d'A. (1971) Response of cultured macrophages to *Mycobacterium tuberculosis* with observations on fusion of lysosomes with phagosomes. *J. exp. Med.*, **134**, 713.
[78] FONG J., SCHNEIDER P. & ELBERG S. S. (1957) Studies on tubercle bacillus–monocyte relationship. II Induction of monocyte degeneration by bacteria and culture filtrate: specificity of serum and monocyte effects on resistance to degeneration. *J. exp. Med.*, **105**, 25.
[79] HIRSCH J. G. (1962) Cinematographic observations on granule lysis in polymorphonuclear leucocytes with continuing locomotion of cells. *J. exp. Med.*, **116**, 827.
[80] BAINTON D. F. (1973) Sequential degranulation of the two types of polymorphonuclear leucocyte granules during phagocytosis of micro-organisms. *J. cell Biol.*, **58**, 249.
[81] ZATTI M., ROSSI F. & MENEGHELLI V. (1965) Morphologic and metabolic concomitants of phagocytosis in polymorphonuclear leucocytes. *J. Microscopie*, **4**, 95.
[81a] BANNISTER L. (1977) Invasion of red cells by Plasmodium. *Symposia brit. Soc. Parasitol.*, **15**, 27
[81b] NEWTON B. A. (1972) Protozoal pathogenicity. In *Microbial Pathogenicity in Man and Animals*, p. 269. Eds H. Smith & J. H. Pearce, Cambridge University Press, Cambridge.
[82] HUTT M. S. R. & SPENCER H. (1978) Tropical diseases in Britain. In *Recent Advances in Pathology 10*, p. 311, ed. by P. P. Anthony & N. Woolf. Churchill Livingstone, Edinburgh.
[83] BRYCESON A. D. M. (1974) Mechanisms of disease in leishmaniasis. In *Pathogenic Processes in Parasitic Infections*, p. 85, ed. by A. E. R. Taylor & R. Muller. Blackwell, Oxford.
[84] HOLMES K. W. & CHOPPIN P. W. (1966) On the role of the response of cell membrane in determining virus virulence. *J. exp. Med.*, **124**, 501.
[85] DALES S. (1962) An EM study of the early association between two mammalian viruses and their hosts. *J. cell Biol.*, **13**, 303.
[86] DOURMASHKIN R. R. & TYRRELL D. A. J. (1970) Attachment of two myxoviruses to ciliated epithelial cells. *J. gen. Virol.*, **9**, 77.
[87] TYRRELL D. A. J. (1977) The entry of viruses into cells. *Parasite Invasion*, Symposia of the British Society of Parasitology 15, p. 83, ed. by A. E. R. Taylor & R. Muller. Blackwell, Oxford.
[88] HOORNE B. & TYRRELL D. A. J. (1965) On the growth of newer respiratory viruses in organ culture. *Brit, J. exp. Path.*, **46**, 109.
[89] NASEMAN T. (1977) *Viral Diseases of Skin, Mucous Membranes and Genitals*, p. 140 (translated by P. J. Frosch). Theme, Stuttgart.
[90] KARPAS A., WREGHITT T. & NAGINGTON J. (1978) Transformation of normal bone marrow cells by a leukaemic cell line associated with presumptive new human virus. *Lancet*, **2**, 1016.
[91] DALES S. & SIMINOVITCH L. (1961) The development of vaccinia virus in Earle's strain cells as examined by EM. *J. biophys. biochem. Cytol.*, **10**, 475.
[92] MATSUMOTO S. (1970) Rabies virus. *Advanc. Virus Res.*, **16**, 257.
[93] BECKER P. B., MELNICK J. L. & MAYOR H. D. (1965) A morphologic comparison between the development stages of herpes zoster and human cytomegalovirus. *Exp. molec. Path.*, **4**, 11.
[94] NIVEN J. S., ARMSTRONG J. A., BALFOUR B. M., KLEMPERER H. G. & TYRRELL D. A. J. (1962) Cellular changes accompanying growth of influenza virus in bovine cell cultures. *J. Path. bact.*, **84**, 1.

[95] DIXON K. C. (1959) Protein in vaccinial lesions revealed by oxidised tannin-azo (OTA) method. *Amer. J. Path.*, **35**, 249.

[96] DALES S. (1971) in *Cell Membranes: Biological and Pathological Aspects.*, p. 131, ed. by G. W. RICHTER & D. G. Scarpelli. Williams & Wilkins, Baltimore.

[97] CROUSE H. V., CORIELL L. L., BLANK H. & SCOTT T. F. McN. (1950) Cytochemical studies on the intranuclear inclusions of herpes simplex. *J. Immunol.*, **65**, 119.

[98] WOLMAN M. & BEHAR A. J. (1952) Cytochemical evidence for the nature of herpes simplex inclusion bodies. *J. infect. Dis.*, **91**, 63.

[99] WILDY P., SMITH C., NEWTON A. A. & DENDY P. (1961) Quantitative cytological studies on Hela cells infected with herpes virus. *Virology.* **15**, 486.

[100] BABLANIAN R. (1968) The prevention of early vaccinia-virus-induced cytopathic effects by inhibition of protein synthesis. *J. gen. Virol.*, **3**, 51.

[101] BABLANIAN R. (1970) Studies on the mechanism of vaccinia virus cytopathic effects. *J. gen. Virol.*, **6**, 221.

[102] TOKUMARU T. (1968) The nature of toxins of herpes simplex virus: I Syncytial giant cell producing components in tissue culture. *Arch. ges. Virusforsch.*, **24**, 104.

[103] GUIR J., BRAUNWALD J. & KIRN A. (1971) Inhibition of host-specific DNA and RNA synthesis in K B cells following infection by frog virus – 3. *J. gen. Virol.*, **12**, 293.

[104] AUBERTIN A. M., TRAVO C. & KIRN A. (1976) Proteins solubilised from frog virus – 3 particles: effect on transcription. *J. Virol.*, **18**, 34.

[105] KELLY D. C. (1975) Frog virus replication: EM observations on the sequence of infection in chick embryo fibroblasts. *J. gen. Virol.*, **26**, 71.

[106] ALLISON A. C. & MALLUCCI L. (1965) Histochemical studies of lysosomal enzymes in virus-infected cells. *J. exp. Med.*, **121**, 463.

[107] ALLISON A. C. (1967) Lysosomes in virus infected cells. *Perspect. Virol.*, **5**, 29.

[108] BLACKMAN K. E. & BUBEL H. C. (1969) Poliovirus-induced cellular injury. *J. gen. Virol.*, **4**, 203.

[109] ESIRI M. E. & TOMLINSON A. H. (1972) Herpes zoster: demonstration of virus in trigeminal nerve and ganglion by immunofluorescence and EM. *J. neurol. Sci.*, **15**, 35.

[110] GHATAK N. R. & ZIMMERMANN H. M. (1973) Spinal ganglion in herpes zoster. *Arch. Path.*, **95**, 411.

[111] SCHEUER P. J. (1978) In *Recent Advances in Histopathology 10*, p. 180, ed. by P. P. Anthony & N. Woolf. Churchill Livingstone, Edinburgh.

[112] HADZIYANNIS S., GERBER M. A., VISSOULIS C. & POPPER H. (1973) Cytoplasmic hepatitis B antigen in 'ground-glass' hepatocytes of carriers. *Arch. Path.*, **96**, 327.

[113] ZUCKERMAN A. I. (1981) Acute viral hepatitis. *J. roy. Coll. Phycns. Lond.*, **15**, 88.

[114] BEASLEY R. P., HWANG L-Y., LIN C-C. & CHIEN C-S. (1981) Hepatocellular carcinoma and hepatitis B virus. *Lancet,* **2**, 1129.

PART II

Nature of Cellular Disorder in Disease

In the following chapters some of the principal kinds of cellular defect which occur in disease will be considered.

Disorders of cells consist of abnormalities in composition, conformation and arrangement of their constituent molecules determined by the mechanisms considered in the previous chapters. Some of these abnormalities involve such profound lesions of macromolecular assembly as to produce changes visible by naked eye, LM or EM. These changes in addition to concomitant alterations in cellular metabolism and behaviour are responsible for the symptoms and signs of disease. Other cellular abnormalities may only affect structure at molecular level and cause no visible alteration in the immediately affected cells. Such changes become perceptible only when they also produce such severe aberration in metabolism, behaviour or growth as to cause overt disease. Disease has thus suggested the existence of underlying molecular derangements which might otherwise never have been unmasked or detected.

With these principles in mind three types of cellular defect are considered, realising that many derangements involve events in more than one of the descriptive compartments, and that each type may be attended by the others in its wake.

The three kinds of defect are:

1. Disintegration of the visible macromolecular fabric of the cell.
2. Intracellular aggregation or deposition.
3. Invisible derangement of metabolism, behaviour and growth.

CHAPTER 7

Disintegration of the Macromolecular Fabric of the Cell

MECHANISM OF DISINTEGRATION

Disintegration of the visible cell fabric depends on two kinds of process, macromolecular disarray and chemical fission. These two processes may succeed each other or may occur simultaneously.

Macromolecular disarray

This consists of disorientation of aligned macromolecules with disruption of cell membranes sometimes accompanied by denaturation of protein. This is a physico-chemical phenomenon which can arise by:

1. *Direct* action of adverse physical conditions (e.g. trauma, heat, cold) or of noxious substances (e.g. SiO_2, monosodium urate).
2. *Indirectly* through cessation of exergonic reactions necessary for stabilising or maintaining orientated macromolecules (e.g. inhibition of respiratory oxidation).

Chemical fission

Lesions of this kind consist of chemical decomposition of macromolecules into smaller units of low molecular weight, and commonly arise from derangement in the normal equilibrium between anabolism and catabolism. Loss of essential macromolecules can thus result by retardation of anabolism or by acceleration of catabolism.

Retardation of anabolism

Anabolism of macromolecules normally replaces their continuous loss by catabolism in active cells. If this compensation by anabolic synthesis is arrested and catabolism continues, the resultant net loss of essential macromolecules can result in necrosis.

Thus, when transcription of RNA is abolished by actinomycin (p. 157), RNA is still consumed and necrosis occurs because this RNA is not replaced.

Similarly, when elongation of peptide chains in translation and synthesis of protein is specifically eliminated by action of the exotoxin of *Corynebacterium diphtheriae* (p. 223), loss of protein without replacement is followed by devastating necrosis.

Anabolism may also slowly be interrupted by lack of nutriments which normally provide essential units for synthesis of the cell fabric; thus starvation can cause shrivelling of myocardial fibres with terminal cardiac arrest (p. 46).

Acceleration of catabolism

In some remarkable instances chemical fission initiates the process of cellular disintegration. Thus the exotoxin of *Clostridium welchii* is a phospholipase/C (p. 225), which probably kills the fibres of skeletal muscle by initial fission of aligned phospholipids in their cell membranes; this toxin also hydrolyses the phospholipids of isolated mitochondria. Similarly the first stage in the lysis of polymorphs and colonic mucosal cells by *Entamoeba histolytica* in amoebic dysentery (p. 234) probably depends on rapid hydrolysis of lipids in cell membranes by hydrolases discharged through a trigger mechanism from the lysosomes of this singularly aggressive protozoon.

Catabolic reactions can also occur as a *sequel* to macromolecular disarray, which may increase accessibility of enzymes previously separated from their substrates by membranous barriers, or may activate enzymes by exposure of initially occluded reactive sites.

Thus in silicosis (p. 146) and in gout (p. 201) initial hydrogen bonding of SiO_2 and MSU respectively to membranes of phagolysosomes is followed by membrane injury and liberation of lysosomal hydrolases which are ultimately responsible for extensive tissue damage by splitting proteins and lipids. Similarly in acute inflammation (p. 194) initial damage may consist of activation of membrane-bound phospholipase A followed by fission of phospholipids leading to formation of prostaglandins. Moreover ligation of antibodies in the presence of complement to antigens in the surface membrane of cells may initiate a sequential chain of activation and attachment of pre-enzymic components of complement which finally results in splitting of phospholipids in cell membrane to cause increase in permeability followed by swelling and lysis (p. 291).

In all these examples disarray of cell membranes is responsible for initiating chemical fission by enzymic action.

In the living cell many of the disruptive enzymes are thus locked away inside organelles such as lysosomes. Also the free water necessary for hydrolysis may not be available in uninjured cells. Structural injury of the fabric may accordingly accelerate catabolism, not only by making hydrolytic enzymes more accessible, but also by permitting ingress of water necessary for hydrolytic fission. Indeed, osmotic entry of water may promote a vicious cycle of catabolism and aqueous swelling; the extreme swelling and disintegration which occurs in the ballooning degeneration of epidermis in smallpox and vaccinia (Fig. 7.1) may arise in this way. The ballooned cells contain little protein stainable by cytochemical methods, probably because of hydrolytic fission in the swollen cells (p. 341).

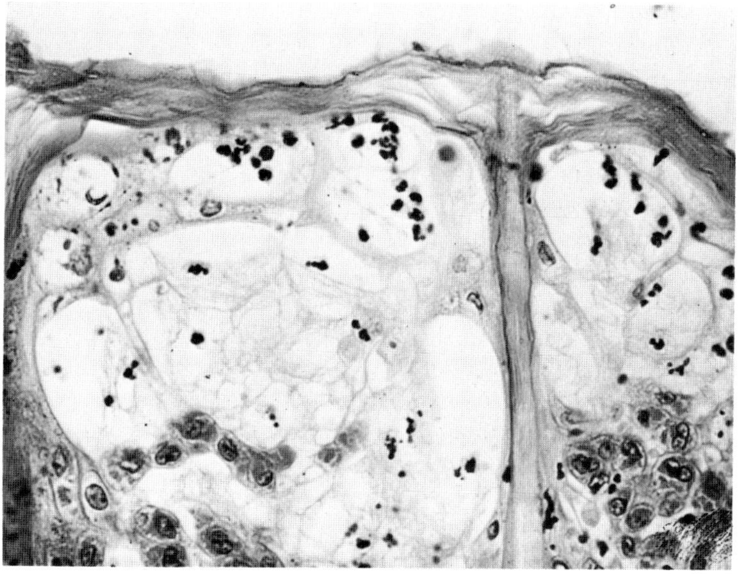

FIG. 7.1 Extreme swelling and disintegration of epidermal cells in skin of newborn rabbit infected by vaccinia virus. This ballooning degeneration is visible in the upper epidermis where some of the vacuolated cells are invaded by neutrophils. The lower epidermal cells are less swollen and contain cytoplasmic inclusion bodies. × 420. Dixon K. C. (1959) *Amer. J. Path.*, **35**, 249.

Although changes in the cytoplasm and nucleus occur simultaneously, in this chapter cytoplasmic disintegration will for convenience be considered first, followed by nuclear disintegration. Cellular disintegration will be discussed from four principal aspects:

1. Cytoplasmic disintegration.
2. Nuclear disintegration.
3. Reversible injury and death.
4. Fate of the remnants in dead and dying cells.

CYTOPLASMIC DISINTEGRATION

This involves changes in various parts of the cell which may occur simultaneously or in succession or as isolated events:

1. Injury to cell membranes; this may be followed by swelling, lysis, fusion, fission or shrinkage.
2. Chromatolysis and loss of cytoplasmic basophilia.
3. Mitochondrial disintegration.
4. Changes in other cytoplasmic constituents.

Injury to cell membranes

Minor invisible changes to cell membranes may only be detectable by changes in *cellular behaviour*. Thus the surface of polymorphs and vascular endothelial cells become sticky during acute inflammation, while invisible adsorption of exotoxins of *Clostridium botulinum* and of *Clostridium tetani* by cell membranes of neurones can abolish release of neurotransmitters (p. 221) and thus produce profound neuronal malfunction causing botulism and tetanus respectively. Invisible alteration in molecular structure in glycocalyx or cell membranes may similarly account for defective cohesion of epidermal cells in psoriasis (p. 327) and also for the invasive behaviour of neoplastic cells (p. 461).

Conformational changes in the molecular assembly of the cell membrane probably occur rapidly as a result of trauma. Thus myelin sheaths of nerves retract from the nodes of Ranvier with great rapidity after crush injury (p. 110). This kind of change may also occur in other cell membranes but is only visible in myelin sheaths where the effect is magnified by multiplicity of cell membranes packed in parallel; the synchronous contraction of these contiguous laminae is then clearly visible by LM.

More serious injury to cell membranes usually increases permeability. This either causes swelling of the cell with watery fluid (*aqueous swelling*) that may lead to lysis or, if so severe as to make the cell completely permeable, may be followed by shrinkage.

Aqueous swelling

The irreversibly injured membrane of dead cells is fully permeable. But cell injury may initially increase the permeability of membranes without making them fully permeable. Then water may be drawn into the cells by osmosis and the cells become swollen. The cell membrane is believed to contain orientated phospholipid bilayers which occur in a liquid-crystalline state [1]; this arrangement would enable swelling of the cell towards a spherical state to occur without increase in surface area, but further enlargement might even develop with increase in surface, if the surface received additional fluid lipid from membranes of internal organelles.

This aqueous swelling of injured cells may be accompanied by the formation of vacuoles in the cell sap or blebs which develop beneath the surface. Cellular swelling may also involve formation of vesicles in the cisternae of endoplasmic reticulum and enlargement of mitochondria which change from sausage-shaped tubules into spheres. In irreversibly injured cells when the cell membrane can itself no longer act as an osmotic barrier so as to cause swelling of the whole cell, swelling of internal organelles may even still develop (p. 302).

Examples of aqueous swelling are illustrated in Fig. 7.1, 7.2 and 7.3. Fig. 7.1 shows grossly distended epidermal cells in the skin of a baby rabbit infected with vaccinia virus; the extreme expansion of injured cells by aqueous fluid is called ballooning degeneration. Fig. 7.2 and 7.3 respectively, show (by EM) aqueous intracytoplasmic vacuolation and formation of swollen blebs in the surface membrane of ischaemic hepatocytes 15 min after clamping the pedicle to a liver lobe [2]; these changes are early phases in aqueous swelling.

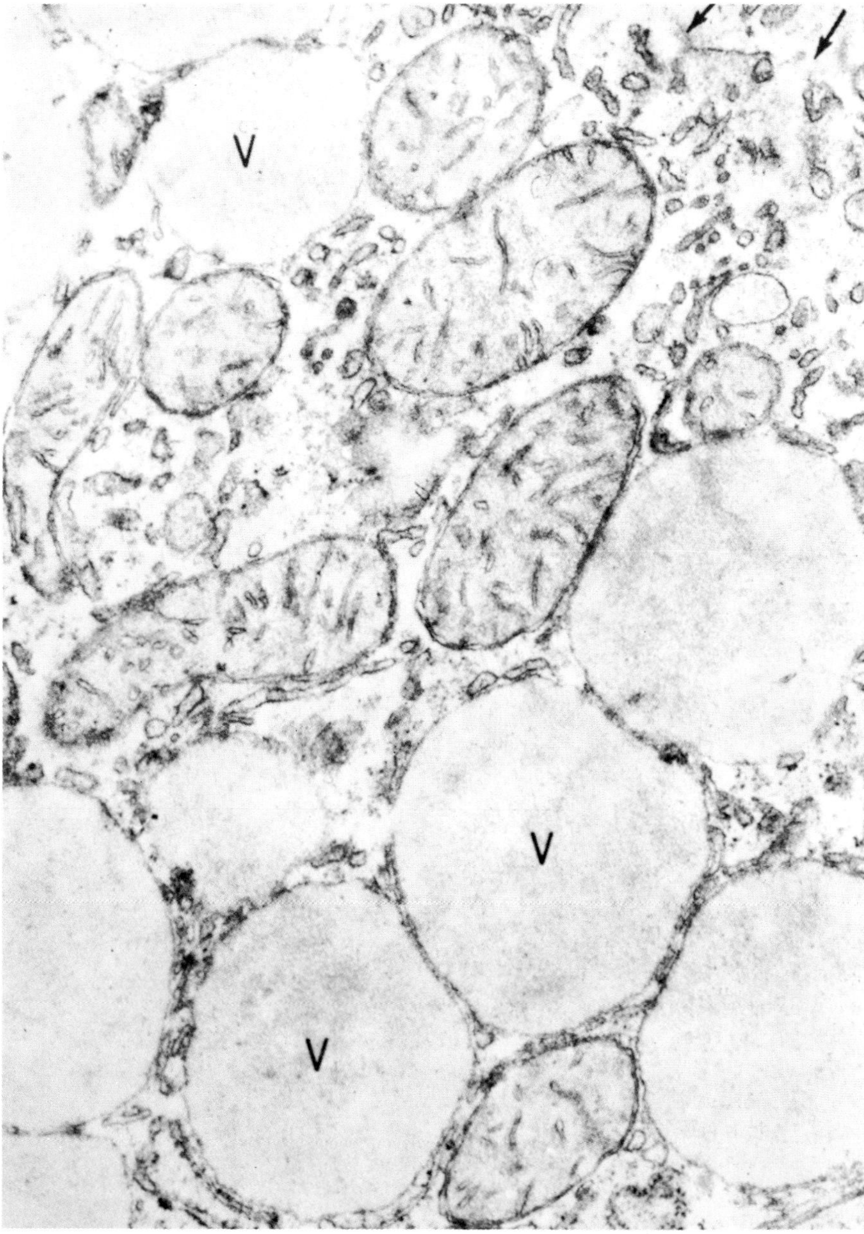

FIG. 7.2 Aqueous swelling near sinusoidal border of rat hepatocyte after 15 min ischaemia. Numerous vacuoles (V) and focal interruptions of plasma membrane (arrows). EM ×30 000. Courtesy of Dr Maria Bassi & Professor A. Bernelli-Zazzera. Reproduced from *Exp. molec. Path.* (1964) **3**, 332.

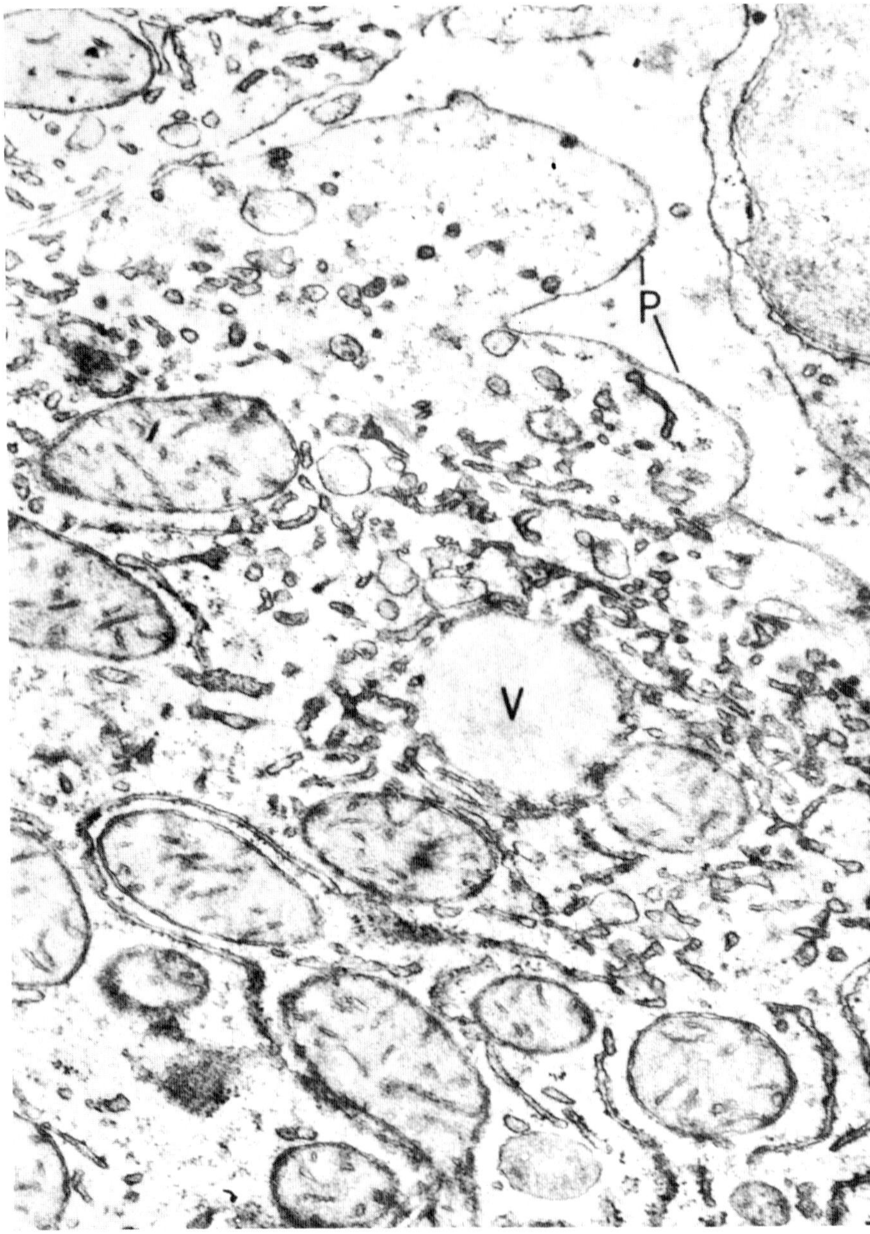

FIG. 7.3 Aqueous swelling in sinusoidal region of rat hepatocyte after 15 min ischaemia. Microvilli on cell surface have disappeared and two large blebs (P) are visible on plasma membrane; a small vacuole (V) is also visible. EM ×28 000. Courtesy of Dr Maria Bassi & Professor A. Bernelli-Zazzera. Reproduced from *Exp. molec. Path.* (1964) **3**, 332.

Mechanism of aqueous swelling

The internal osmotic pressure (OP) of healthy cells is equal to that of the external fluid [3] but, after injury to the cell, the internal OP may exceed the external OP for two reasons:

1. Injury may result in net catabolism of macromolecules, e.g. proteins, nucleic acid and glycogen and also of smaller molecules like ATP and CrP and hexose esters. This net catabolism increases the concentration of solutes [4]; the internal OP then rises and water is drawn into the cell.
2. Healthy cell membranes exclude Na^+ and Cl^-. These extracellular ions may be actively extruded by a sodium pump, which is propelled by energy provided by catabolism of ATP, or the membrane itself directly excludes these ions so long as its structure is maintained by exergonic reactions. Thus when ATP is no longer formed or when the membrane is directly damaged, the membrane is changed and Na^+ and Cl^- can enter the cells. These ions then no longer contribute to the external OP which therefore falls to a lower level than the internal OP; water is thus drawn into the cells which become swollen.

Both these mechanisms probably contribute to swelling of cells deprived of O_2. Thus hypoxia initially inhibits formation of ATP and results in net fission of ATP (Fig. 3.13, p. 85) along with rise in intracellular concentration of solutes with increase of internal OP; this effect is magnified by simultaneous interference with synthesis of macromolecules in absence of ATP, which results in uncompensated catabolism and further rise of concentration of solutes within the cell. Moreover lack of ATP in anoxia also makes the cell membrane more permeable to external Na^+ and Cl^- and hence effectively lowers external OP which causes additional osmotic swelling.

This latter effect may be ascribed to intake of previously isotonic saline which can penetrate the injured cell membrane [5–7]. Although K^+ may simultaneously escape from injured cells, the loss of K^+ from cells damaged by metabolic depression is not so great as the entry of Na^+ [5, 6]. Retention of K^+ may depend on ligation to anionic groups of intracellular proteins. These intracellular proteins still exert full colloid OP provided that the initial damage is not great enough to permit proteins to penetrate the cell membranes.

The internal OP which is primarily dependent on osmotic action of intracellular macromolecules may thus be fully maintained in the injured cells so long as they remain impermeable to colloids; the external OP which so much depends on Na^+ and Cl^- falls rapidly, once the damaged membranes become fully permeable to crystalloids. The osmotic action of intracellular colloids then become a key factor in aqueous swelling.

The dependence of aqueous swelling on osmosis means that swelling only occurs when the cell membranes retain their semipermeable nature. But if they are so severely injured as to become fully permeable, osmosis and aqueous swelling are precluded. Human cells in dead bodies usually show neither swelling nor vacuolation, because ischaemic injury *post mortem* disintegrates the cell membranes before swelling can occur (see Figs 1.7 and 1.8, pp. 10, 11).

Indeed when cells are *killed* in disease shrinkage is a more usual phenomenon than swelling (p. 292).

Agents which injure cell membrane may also damage the membranes of its organelles, and then cause rise of OP inside saccules of ER and mitochondria. Thus OP within these organelles may exceed that of the cytoplasm, when the cytoplasmic concentration of solutes becomes diluted by entry of water. Thus swelling of vesicles of ER and mitochondria may follow aqueous swelling of the cell as a whole, and may occur or continue when the cell membrane is so grossly damaged as to be incapable of osmotic swelling.

The action of CCl_4, in causing intense aqueous swelling of midzonal cells and necrosis of centrilobular cells in hepatic lobules, probably depends on lipoperoxidation of membrane phospholipids by a toxic intermediary formed from CCl_4 by microsomal oxygenase (p. 164). This effect is most severe in the centrilobular zones, where this enzyme is most abundant, and declines progressively towards the periphery of the lobules. Many of the centrilobular cells die without swelling (see Fig. 7.14b). But, where the membranes are injured without disintegration, water may be drawn into the cells by osmosis to produce aqueous swelling, which thus occurs principally in the midzonal cells (see Fig. 7.14b). On the other hand the peripheral cells which lack oxygenating enzymes are initially unaffected (see Fig. 5.7).

Aqueous swelling of hepatic cells in animals poisoned by CCl_4 commences in the cisternae of ER, while the mitochondria become swollen later [8, 9]. Ultimately the midzonal cells enlarge into spongiose saccules filled by vacuoles covered by tenuous films of cytoplasm (Fig. 7.4). This extreme effect is probably

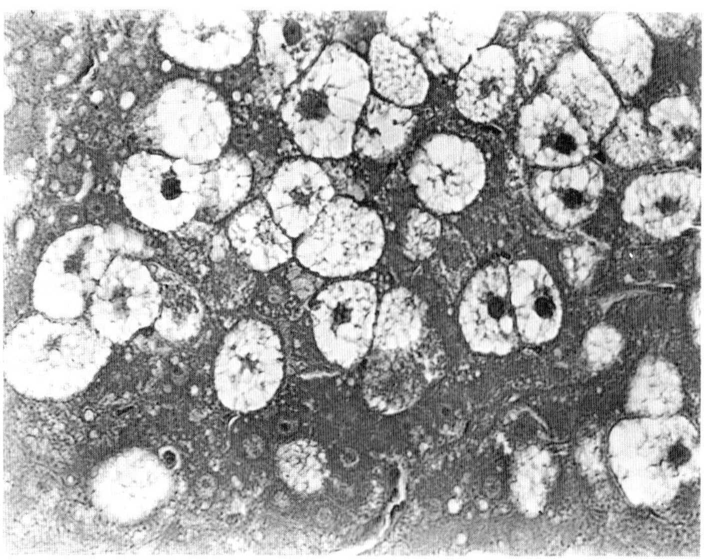

FIG. 7.4 Aqueous swelling in midzonal hepatocytes of rat one day after injection of CCl_4 0.75 ml/100 g bodyweight. Intensely swollen hydropic cells filled by vacuoles covered by tenuous films of cytoplasm. Coupled tetrazonium method for protein. ×420.

a terminal sequel to continued osmotic swelling of the injured organelles after the external cell membrane has become completely permeable.

Aqueous swelling of neuronal cell bodies which develops after section of axons is discussed on p. 112.

Lysis

When the plasma membrane of injured cells disintegrates sufficiently for large molecules to escape, then cellular lysis is said to have occurred. When red cells are lysed, their haemoglobin escapes and enters the external medium and so serves as a visible indicator of lysis. Uncoloured large molecules such as enzymes are also liberated from lysed cells; thus esterases and phosphatases emerge from polymorphs lysed by saponin, and cathepsin may leak out of macrophages in tuberculosis (p. 241), while aminotransferases and other enzymes are released from dying myocardial fibres killed by ischaemia (p. 300).

Intravascular lysis of antibody-coated red cells can occur following mismatched transfusion (p. 205) in addition to the more usual intraphagocytic lysis. This direct lysis involves the complete complement cascade with absorption of components C_8 and C_9 on the antibody-coated cell membranes in addition to the initially absorbed components C_1–C_7 of complement. The terminal absorption of C_8 and C_9 is accompanied by development of permeable zones in the cell membrane through which Na^+, Cl^- and H_2O then enter by osmosis to cause swelling. This swelling finally produces rents in the swollen membrane which are large enough to permit the escape of macromolecules including Hb; this is the ultimate and essential process of lysis. This terminal osmotic swelling followed by rending can, however, be prevented by immersing the red cells in serum albumen which cannot enter through the permeable zones in the membrane and thus maintains the effective external OP [10]. The final stage of lysis can thus be precluded, although initial latent damage has occurred.

During the sequential binding and activation of components of C some of the complex $C_5C_6C_7$ is activated but remains free in extracellular fluid where it binds with other cells and activates them by contagion [11]; the latter cells then ligate C_8 and C_9 and themselves become lysed. This process of *reactive lysis* magnifies the lytic effects of C.

Along with the terminal effects exerted by the complement cascade, which result in development of permeable zones in the antibody-coated cell membrane, lesions detectable by EM also become visible. These lesions appear as dark holes (10 μm in diameter) penetrated by electron-dense ‘negative’ stain and surrounded by electron-translucent rims [12]. The question arises whether these holes (or pits) correspond to the functional zones of increased permeability which initiate lysis. However Lachmann *et al.* [13, 14] showed that artificially made vesicles (liposomes), which are composed of dispersed phospholipids, develop lesions with similar appearance by EM, on treatment with activated complexes of $C_5C_6C_7$, *provided* C_8 and C_9 are added; at the same time permeable zones are formed in the membranes of the liposomes as shown by release of previously incorporated crystalloidal markers, such as chromate. These important observations therefore indicate that the permeable zones, which develop in cell membranes during lysis by C, do in fact correspond with the structural lesions (visible by EM) imprinted simultaneously on the lipids of the cell surface.

Lysis of antibody-coated red cells by the components of complement thus involves two principal stages:

1. The sequential adsorption of components of complement terminating in development of permeable zones in the cell membrane which freely admit entry of Na^+, Cl^- and H_2O but not of macromolecules.
2. Osmotic entry of water with swelling followed by rending of the cell membrane and liberation of macromolecules.

This two-staged process of lysis of antibody-coated red cells by complement probably contributes to lysis following mismatched transfusions and also to haemolytic anaemia caused by SLE (p. 205).

Lysis by freezing probably also follows two sequential stages. First the formation of ice crystals generates eutectic mixtures of hypertonic saline which produce latent lesions in the cell membrane. The latter only result in actual disintegration of the membrane on thawing and re-exposure to isotonic saline (p. 124). Other agents, such as heat, may lyse cells by immediate disintegration of their membranes by disarray of lipids or removal of bound water (p. 119).

Fusion, fission, shrinkage and separation

Injury or change in conformation of cell membrane can so alter its physical properties that cells cohere together and fuse into syncytia, or, on the other hand, split into membrane-bound fragments.

Thus lymphokines liberated from sensitised T-lymphocytes on contact with tuberculin are probably responsible for the fusion (p. 239) of epithelioid cells in tuberculous exudates to form giant cells (see Fig. 6.14b, c). Infection by viruses of measles and herpes zoster can also make cells fuse into syncytia (see Fig. 6.32).

Fission into membrane-bound fragments follows action of heat on red cells (see Fig. 4.11, p. 120) and also occurs in the removal of redundant cells during embryonic development. The latter process, which has been called *apoptosis* (ἀπό, away from; πτῶσις, falling), also occurs in atrophic liver lobes of rats made partially ischaemic by ligation of branches of the portal vein [15, 16]. This apoptosis involves a sequence of cellular separation succeeded by shrinkage of the separated cells, which then split into condensed membrane-bound fragments containing crowded organelles. In the liver these fragments are then ingested by macrophages or hepatocytes in which they are seen as eosinophilic cytoplasmic inclusions. The Councilman bodies visible in the cytoplasm of hepatocytes in yellow fever (p. 265) probably arise in this way.

Shrinkage of dead and dying cells is a common sequel to severe injury of cell membranes. Separation of shrunken cells from each other is often conspicuous among centrilobular hepatocytes killed by general ischaemia of heart failure (see Fig. 1.6, p. 8), while rapid dissociation of dying hepatic cells is characteristic of fatal leptospiral jaundice. Dissociation of hepatic and renal cells is also a prominent concomitant of post mortem change (see Figs 1.7 and 1.8, pp. 10, 11).

Injury to the surface membrane of cells and their organelles is thus responsible for conspicuous changes such as swelling, vacuolation, lysis, fission and fusion. Two of the commonest initial determinants of these changes are (a) hypoxia and ischaemia, and (b) infection by pathogenic microbes. Examples of injury due to these causes will now be considered.

Ischaemic and hypoxic injury to cell membranes: liver

Although hepatic cells are only irreversibly injured after their circulation is interrupted for more than 1 hour (p. 79), changes in the permeability of their cell membrane occur within 15–20 min of circulatory arrest. Thus when starved rats are killed by asphyxia watery vacuoles appear within 20 min in the liver cells (p. 80), provided the animals are not bled between death and dissection. Large aqueous vacuoles also appear in human liver cells after death from acute haemorrhage of asphyxia [17]. Similar vacuoles become visible (by EM) after exposing starved rats to coal gas [18]. These vacuoles apparently develop by gross enlargement of minute aqueous droplets which are continuously formed in hepatic cells by pinocytosis from the exterior. The vacuoles can in fact be labelled by electron-opaque thorotrast injected a few minutes before exposure to coal gas; the thorotrast is then absorbed into the cells along with the aqueous microdroplets. These observations support the view that hypoxia is responsible for osmotic absorption of water, which results in aqueous swelling of the cell as a whole or of vacuoles or organelles within it.

After occlusion of blood supply to hepatic cells *in vivo* for 15 min (p. 79) spectacular changes become visible by EM in the cell membranes along the sinusoidal borders of the hepatocytes [2]; the microvilli projecting from the cell surface disappear while blebs and discontinuities appear in the plasma membrane and vacuoles covered by membranes are formed in the cytoplasm (Figs 7.2 and 7.3).

Alterations produced by hypoxia in the surface membranes of hepatic cells probably also account for change in behaviour of ischaemic liver tissue on compression. Thus when fresh liver of rats is rolled into films by steel rollers almost all the cells are burst (Fig. 7.5a) but when liver is first incubated for 1–2 hr at 37° *in vitro* and then rolled into films numerous entire cells are visible (Fig. 7.5b, p. 294). Softening or loss of microvilli in the cell membranes may thus permit entire cells to be rolled out into films without rupture [19, 20].

The surface membranes of liver cells of animals observed by EM are also strikingly altered after incubation *in vitro* at 37°; within 0.5 h blebs and large gaps appear in the membranes along the sinusoidal borders of the cells, while microvilli are lost and mitochondria become swollen [21]. Observations of this kind show that a profound change occurs in the cell membranes of the dying

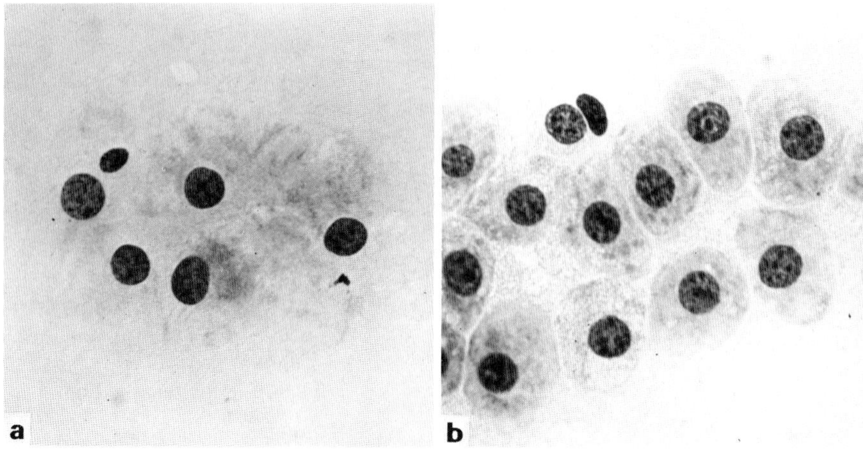

FIG. 7.5 Films of rat hepatocytes rolled by steel rollers, fixed in ethanol and stained H & E. ×650.
a. Film of fresh liver rolled within 3 min of death by cardiotomy: all cells ruptured, nuclei intact.
b. Film made from liver incubated 1 h at 38° post mortem: large numbers of entire cells, nuclei intact. Dixon K. C. (1964) *Brit. J. exp. Path.*, **45**, 481.

cells, but they do not establish that portions of the plasma membrane are eliminated or become ruptured by ischaemia. Such rupture and disappearance of membranes visible by EM along the sinusoidal border of hepatocytes may be an artefact produced by section in which fragile, weakened membranes are disintegrated by the trauma of microtomy. However the existence of such visible alterations proves that the macromolecular conformation of the cell membrane has become profoundly modified. It is notable, however, that this change is only detectable on the unsupported sinusoidal border and the membranes of contiguous hepatic cells appear undamaged.

Ischaemia for longer periods injures the membranes of ER and mitochondria as well as the surface membrane of hepatic cells [2]. The laminar compartments of ER then become fragmented into rounded vesicles and the mitochondria swell from sausage-shaped into rounded vesicles. The damage to mitochondria is further accentuated if the supply of blood is restored after an initial period of ischaemia; eccentric blebs covered by single membranes then emerge from some of the swollen mitochondria (Fig. 7.6) [22]. This more severe injury to the mitochondrial membranes may depend on free availability of water for hydrolytic catabolism of phospholipids in the membranes as well as for entry of water by osmosis. This kind of lesion emphasises the importance of reflow of blood in increasing visible damage to membranes after temporary arrest of circulation.

Ischaemic injury to cell membranes: mycocardium

Cardiac muscle is irreversibly injured by ischaemia lasting more than 30 min.

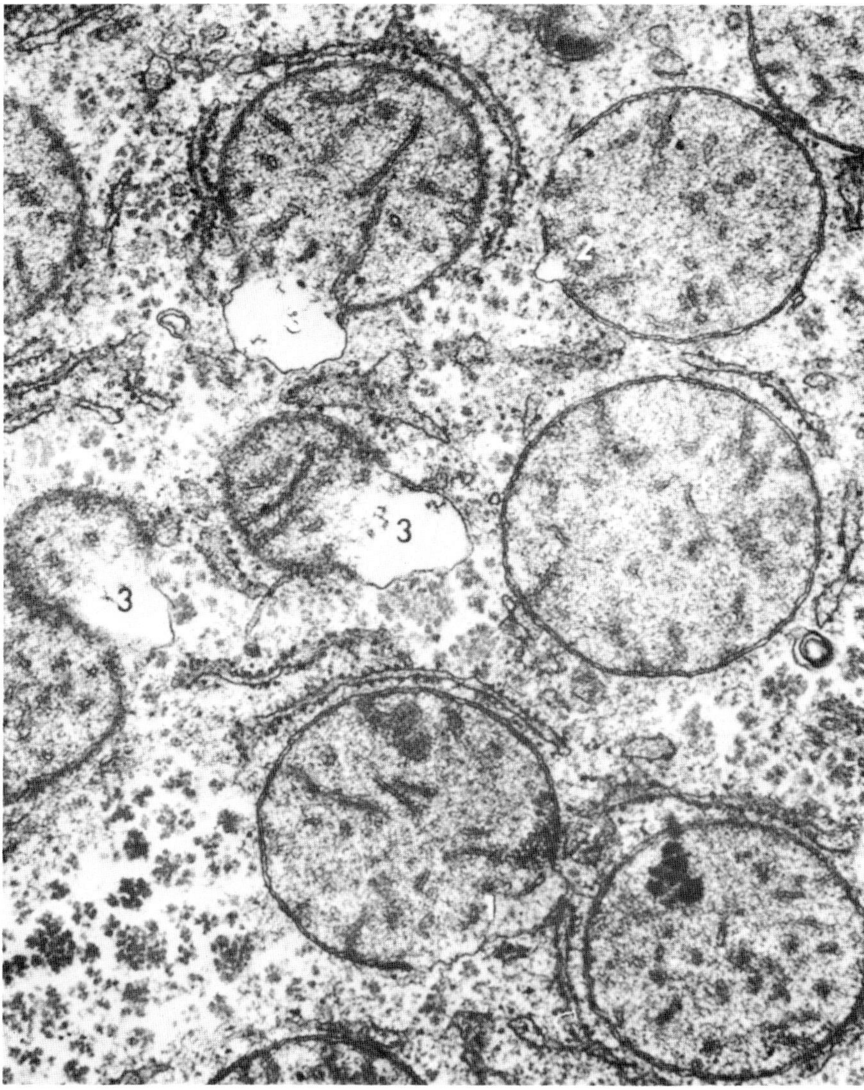

FIG. 7.6 Rat hepatocyte after 15 min ischaemia followed by 15 min normal circulation. Gross swelling of mitochondria and formation of mitochondrial blebs. EM ×34 000 (approx). Courtesy of Dr F. Cajone, Dr G. Ragnotti, Professor A. Bernelli-Zazzera & Dr Maria Bassi. Reproduced from *Exp. molec. Path.* (1971) **14**, 392.

Spaces visible by EM appear within the fibrils of ischaemic myocardial fibres within 5 min of occlusion of branches of the left coronary artery of rabbits [23]; these spaces probably represent aqueous vacuoles which form in the hypoxic fibres.

Temporary ischaemia produces particularly conspicuous lesions in myocardial fibres when followed by re-entry of flowing blood [24]. Thus necrosis with only moderate swelling of mycocardial fibres of left ventricle follows occlusion for 40 min of circumflex branch of left coronary artery in dogs, if the tissue is fixed *immediately* after the period of ischaemia. But, if reflow of blood is permitted for 2–20 min *before* the cells are fixed, then large vacuoles appear in the cytoplasm and the cells become grossly swollen, while the cell membranes are lifted away from the myofibrils to produce spectacular subsarcolemmal blebs (Fig. 7.7, 7.8 and 7.9). In addition to the explosive cell swelling during brief periods of reflow the myofibrils develop prominent bands of contraction (Fig. 7.7) and the mitochondria become intensely swollen (Fig. 7.7 and 7.9) but *no* significant changes occur in the lysosomes.

Thus myocardial fibres killed by ischaemia rapidly become distended by fluid after re-access of flowing blood. Discontinuities also appear in the sarcolemma

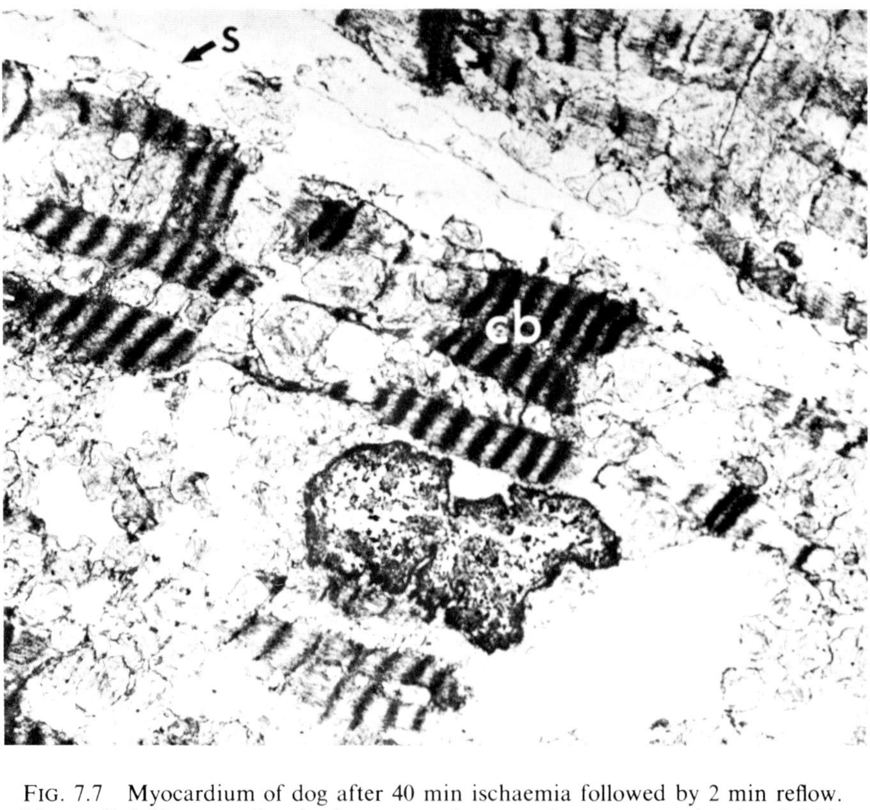

FIG. 7.7 Myocardium of dog after 40 min ischaemia followed by 2 min reflow. Myocardial fibres swollen by large vacuoles, prominent contraction band (cb), lifting of sarcolemma (s) away from rest of cell, swelling of mitochondria and clumping with margination of nuclear chromatin. EM ×6000. Courtesy of Dr. R. A. Kloner, Dr E. Ganote, Dr D. A. Whalen and Professor R. B. Jennings. Reproduced from *Amer. J. Path.* (1964) **74**, 399.

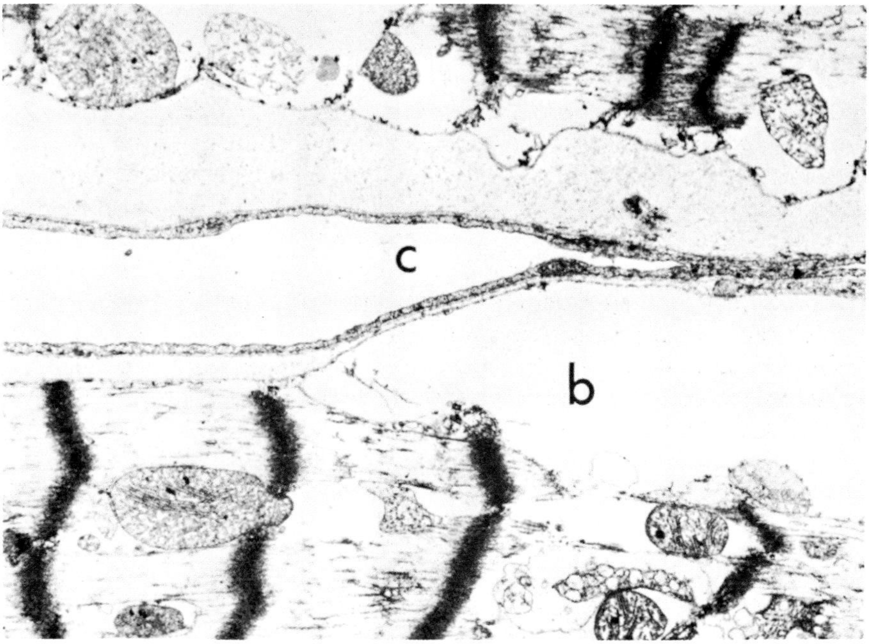

FIG. 7.8 Myocardium of dog after 40 min ischaemia followed by 10 min reflow. Large subsarcolemmal bleb (b) compressing a capillary (c), intracellular oedema of myocardial fibres with mitochondrial swelling. EM ×9600. Courtesy of Dr. R. A. Kloner, Dr E. Ganote, Dr D. A. Whalen and Professor R. B. Jennings. Reproduced from *Amer. J. Path.* (1974) **74**, 399.

of some of these injured fibres (Fig. 7.9, p. 298). These lesions may be caused by artefact during section, or by trauma to these weakened fibres in the still beating heart (p. 294). But the presence of such points of weakening and rupture implies that ischaemia produces membrane disarray, and this may herald lysis with later escape of enzymic macromolecules through the injured sarcolemma (p. 300).

These observations thus emphasise the importance of latent injury produced by ischaemia which only becomes fully apparent on re-access of flowing blood. The existence of such latent damage also explains why changes in human heart muscle from patients who temporarily survive ischaemic accidents are more prominent than after complete cardiac arrest accompanied by sudden death.

Deformation of ischaemic myocardial fibres

At the margins of zones of ischaemic necrosis in human heart muscle conspicuously wavy deformed fibres may intervene between necrotic and unaffected myocardium [25]. This transition is shown in Fig. 7.10 (pp. 299, 300). Between the frankly necrotic fibres of a myocardial infarct (Fig. 7.10a) and the unaffected fibres in surrounding myocardium (Fig. 7.10c), wavy fibres (Fig.

7.10b) are visible in the intervening marginal zone. These filiform wavy fibres are usually arranged in parallel as multiple serpentine groups (Fig. 7.10b).

The mechanism of formation of wavy fibres probably depends on exposure to incomplete anoxia. These marginal fibres at the border of necrotic zones apparently receive enough O_2 to stay alive; possibly they are so hypoxic that they are paralysed and are then stretched into attenuated filiform shapes by contraction of surrounding active muscle. This plasticity may depend on retention of sufficient ATP to prevent excessive interaction of myosin and actin as may occur in the completely anoxic fibres, which then are converted into rigid and inextensible necrotic remnants. Another possibility is that hypoxia, not severe enough to cause necrosis, makes the cell membranes of the hypoxic fibres initially more *fluid* so that they become deformed and stretched by contractions of adjacent active fibres. The deformation of the wavy fibres may thus be a consequence of limited ischaemic damage to the cell membranes of fibres in this marginal zone of incomplete anoxia.

Recent observations, however, suggest that wavy fibres are present in about half the human hearts examined *post mortem* whether 'normal' or infarcted [26].

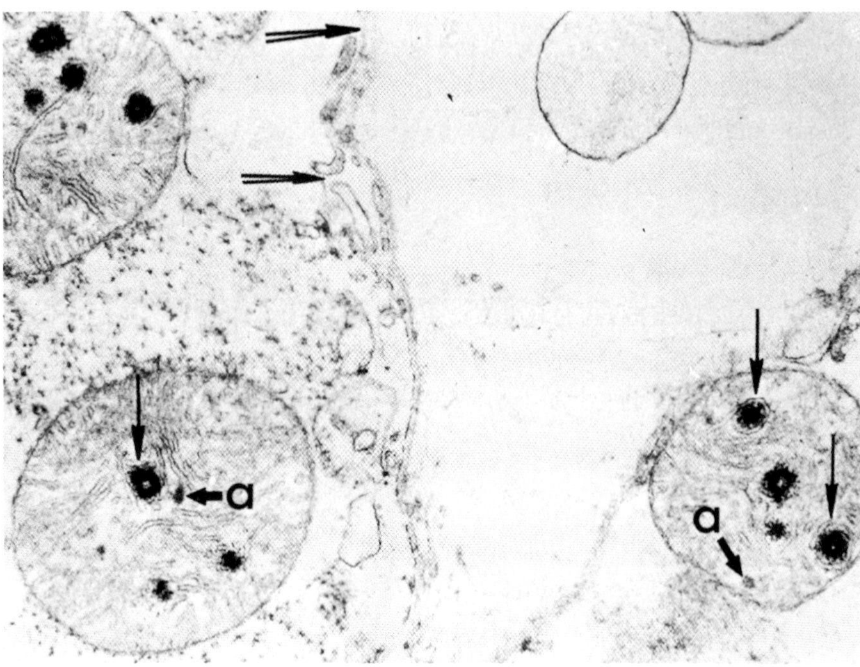

FIG. 7.9 Myocardium of dog after 40 min ischaemia followed by 20 min reflow. Large vacuolar spaces in myocardial fibres with breaks in sarcolemmal membrane (double arrows); swollen mitochondria contain dense bodies (a). EM ×28 900. Courtesy of Dr. R. A. Kloner, Dr E. Ganote, Dr D. A. Whalen and Professor R. B. Jennings. Reproduced from *Amer. J. path.* (1974) **74**, 399.

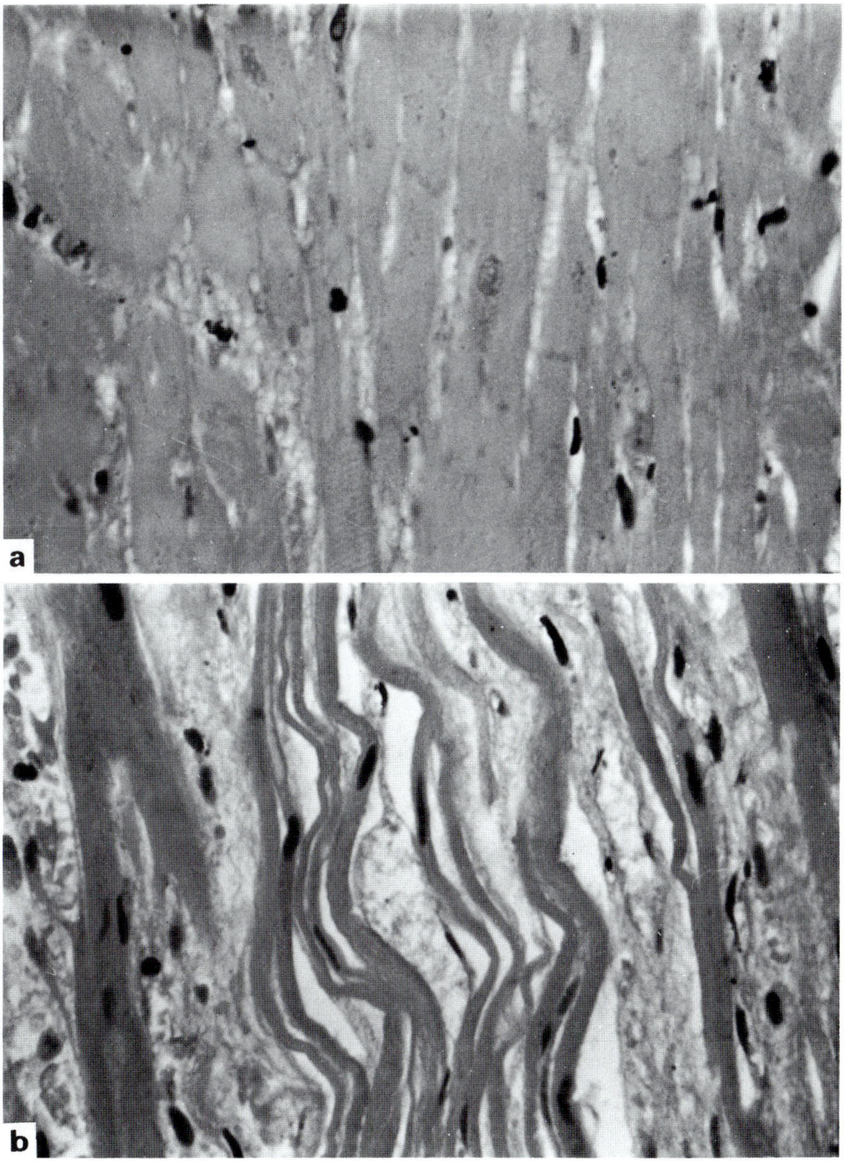

FIG. 7.10 Human myocardium showing deformation and stretching of myocardial fibres adjacent to an infarct resulting from coronary occlusion 6 days before death. H & E. ×510.

a. Necrotic fibres within the infarct; karyolysis of myocardial nuclei, pyknosis of nuclei of connective tissue.

b. Wavy fibres immediately adjacent to infarct showing deformation and stretching.

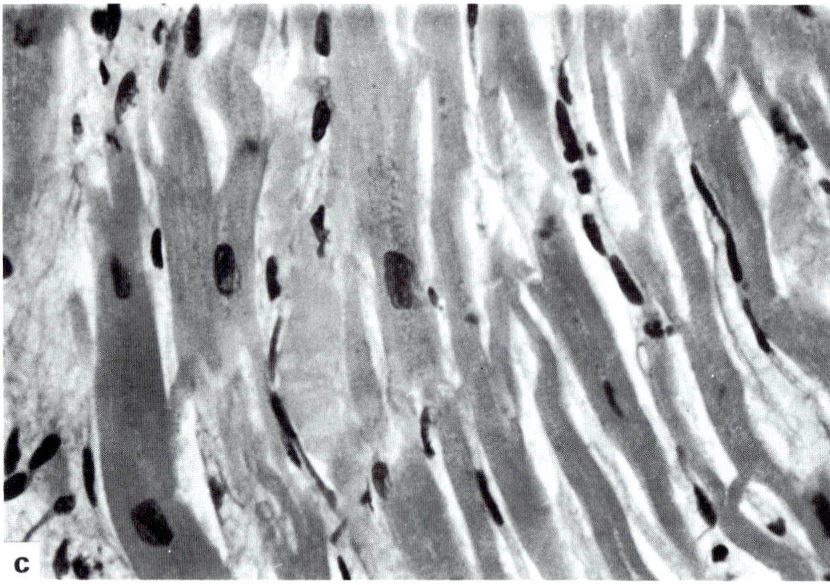

FIG. 7.10 cont.
c. Unaffected myocardium external to the infarct.

If undulations are formed by stretching of hypoxic fibres or of their membranes owing to continued contraction of their neighbours, there is no reason why such an agonal phenomenon should be confined to the vicinity of previous infarction. Indeed waviness may merely be a terminal state assumed by some fibres that become paralysed and are then deformed by the activity of neighbours, which maintain contractility for a longer period up to the time of final cardiac arrest. Wavy fibres may thus be of common occurrence in dying heart muscle.

Release of enzymes from ischaemic myocardium

Lysis or rupture of the sarcolemma of hypoxic myocardial fibres is responsible for the sudden release of cardiac enzymes into the blood after infarction of the heart. Myocardial enzymes which then appear in the blood plasma include creatine kinase (CK), lactic dehydrogenase (LDH) and aspartate aminotransferase (ASA).

Of these enzymes CK leaks out first following the onset of precordial pain due to acute cardiac ischaemia. Activity of CK begins to rise within 3–6 h after the onset of ischaemia and reaches a peak of 7- to 12-fold of the normal upper limit 18–24 h later. Liberation of LDH and ASA then follows. Increase in the concentration of these enzymes in plasma thus provides valuable confirmation of diagnosis of cardiac infarction.

Along with the release of myocardial enzymes from the dying fibres into the blood, loss of enzymes also is detectable in the fibres themselves; thus conspicuous diminution in the activity of succinic dehydrogenase [27] and of cytochrome oxidase [28] is found in myocardial cells after ischaemic necrosis. Both the liberation of enzymes into the blood and their loss from the dying fibres emphasise the increase in permeability of their cell membranes, which no longer restrict the free passage of macromolecules. Indeed plasma albumen and globulin detectable by specific fluorescent antibodies enter necrotic myocardial cells of dogs after ligation of the anterior descending branch of left coronary artery [29]. Thus the membranes of the necrotic myocardium become so permeable as to permit the transit of macromolecules in either direction.

Ischaemic and hypoxic injury to cell membranes: neurones

Ischaemia very rapidly alters the surface membrane of cerebral neurones. At first reversible osmotic swelling of the whole neurone occurs but soon the cell membrane becomes permanently disorganised and cell swelling ceases; however, osmotic swelling of internal organelles still continues in these irreversibly injured neurones.

Arrest of circulation to the brain in rabbits is followed after a latent period of about 3 min by rapid rise in electrical resistance of the tissue coupled with increase in volume of the apical dendrites of pyramidal cells in the cerebral cortex. These changes are accompanied by entry of Cl^- and water into the cell bodies and their apical dendrites [30, 31]. Arrest of circulation causes similar swelling and entry of Cl^- into the apical dendrites of Purkinje cells of the cerebellum and the adjacent glial fibres of Bergmann [32].

Temporary occlusion of the aorta in rabbits or cats for 15min produces *reversible* swelling and vacuolation of the spinal anterior horn cells [33–35]. Longer periods of aortic occlusion result in irreversible damage to the spinal anterior horn cells. Thus, following temporary ischaemia lasting for 1 h, minute vacuoles become visible in the cell bodies 1 h later, but the cells themselves do not enlarge; the cells then become grossly vacuolated and shrink into necrotic remnants within 1–2 days [34]. Similar microvacuolation develops following ischaemic and hypoxic injury to cerebral pyramidal cells both in man and animals [36–39]. This change is the earliest visible alteration in cerebral neurones after irreversible injury by hypoxia which may be induced by deprivation of O_2 for only a few min. (p. 87). These vacuolated neurones later shrink into homogeneous necrotic remnants.

Observations by LM and EM on cerebral neurones of rats and monkeys, made hypoxic by exposure to N_2, show that this microvacuolation is mainly due to swelling of mitochondria [39]. Moreover these vacuoles develop rapidly and become visible in cerebral neurones of animals killed by perfusion-fixation after hypoxia lasting 15 min. The vacuoles later become indistinct and the irreversibly injured neurones finally become shrivelled.

Neuronal swelling produced by ischaemia depends on osmotic entry of water into hypoxic cells and can only occur if the injured neurones retain semipermeable envelopes. But longer periods of hypoxia may result in such complete disintegration of arrayed lipids that the cell membranes become fully permeable; osmotic swelling of the cell as a whole is then arrested.

After such disorganisation of the cell membrane, however, mitochondria and other internal organelles may temporarily remain semipermeable. Therefore swelling by osmosis of membrane-covered organelles *within* the cell continues (p. 290) even when the cell membrane is so severely injured as to prevent swelling of the whole cell. Thus, localised vacuolation *inside* neurones without cellular enlargement is a characteristic of irreversibly damaged cells [40]. Microvacuolation of irreversibly injured neurones probably results from osmotic swelling of mitochondria within the dying cells.

Much larger vacuolar spaces may be formed in disintegrating ischaemic cerebral cortex (Fig. 7.11b, c); these probably arise by coalescence and fusion of smaller vacuoles produced by hypoxic injury in both glial and neuronal processes (p. 303). This cerebral swelling in ischaemic disease is considered in the next section.

Cerebral swelling in ischaemic disease

When patients develop coma and apnoea as a result of temporary cardiac arrest or cerebral vascular accidents and are kept alive for 24 h or more by artificial respiration, the brain is found to be soft, visibly swollen and darkened by congestion and is usually increased in weight. This condition is called 'respirator brain' and it is accompanied by necrosis, lysis and loss of neurones in cerebral and cerebellar cortex [41]. In this 'brain death' the cerebral circulation is probably permanently and progressively interrupted.

The morphological characteristics of similar 'brain death' were examined in the brain of animals made ischaemic for 20 min by inflation of balloons placed in the epidural space [42]. Following this temporary compression the animals remain comatose and do not recover spontaneous respiration but their cardiac activity continues provided oxygenation is maintained by respirator. The brain of cats and baboons kept 'alive' in this way becomes swollen and, after 6 h or more, examination by EM reveals cerebral oedema along with complete obstruction of capillaries. The capillaries are occluded by compression from swollen astrocytes as well as by swelling of the capillary endothelial cells, which form intravascular blebs visible by EM. As well as the astrocytes, the oligodendrocytes and the cytoplasmic processes of the neuropil become swollen and filled with vacuoles. Later the glial cells develop more extreme swelling and contain large and apparently empty spaces, while the neurones shrivel and their membranous components disappear.

Cerebral swelling with increase in water content also develops in the brain of rats after exposure to anoxic ischaemia (by the Levine technique, p. 67) for periods of about 1 h [43]; this change commences after 4 h and attains a maximum in about 1 day. Possibly incomplete ischaemia can initially produce a latent change in membranes of cerebral cells which is afterwards followed by prolonged osmotic swelling.

Vacuolation or fenestration can also develop in ischaemic zones of cerebral cortex in patients with spontaneous respiration, who die in coma following cerebral haemorrhage or vascular occlusion [40, 44, 45].

The nature of this vacuolation is illustrated in Figs 7.11a and 7.11b, which

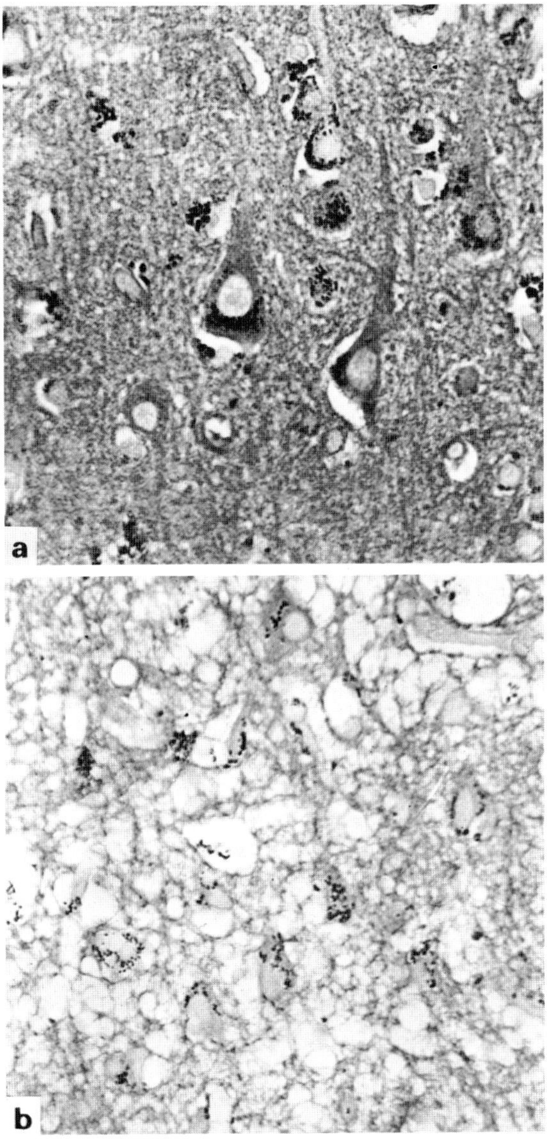

FIG. 7.11 Intensely vacuolated human cerebral cortex stained by paraldehyde-fuchsin after pre-treatment with $KMnO_4$. ×420.

This method probably colours lipoprotein membranes and it also stains granules of lipofuscin present in neuronal cell-bodies, thus enabling them clearly to be recognised even in grossly vacuolated cerebral cortex.

a. *Unaffected right* parietal cortex.

b. *Vacuolated left* parietal cortex contralateral to that shown in (a), from a hypertensive patient who died in coma 3 days after haemorrhage into *left* cerebral hemisphere; the cell processes of the interpyramidal grey matter have disintegrated into vacuolar spaces bounded by the remnants of cell membranes; pyramidal cell bodies containing granules of lipofuscin are clearly discernible.

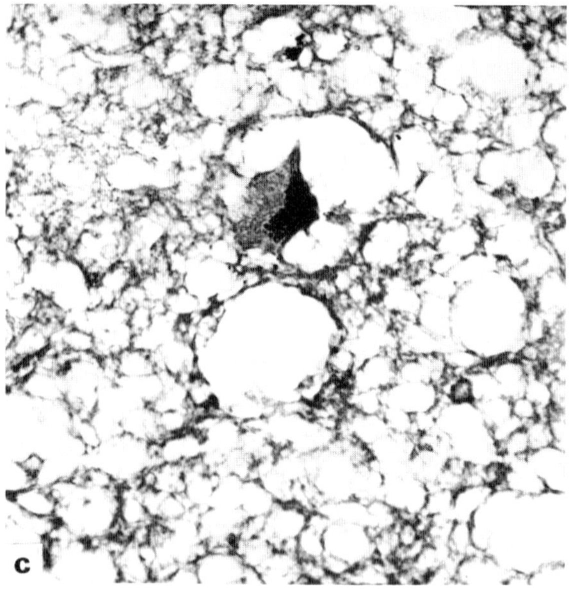

FIG. 7.11 cont.
c. Extreme vacuolation and disintegration of *left* precentral cortex of a patient who died in coma 2 days after occlusion of *left* middle cerebral artery. The interpyramidal grey matter consists of coalescent vacuolar remnants of cell processes; a shrivelled cell body of a large pyramidal neurone with prominent granules of lipofuscin is still visible. Dixon K. C. (1955) *J. Path. Bact.*, **69**, 251.

show respectively *unaffected right* parietal cortex and *ischaemic left* parietal cortex from a patient who died in coma 3 days after haemorrhage into the white matter of the left cerebral hemisphere accompanied by extensive ischaemic injury in the left cerebral cortex. The left parietal cortex is grossly disorganised (Fig. 7.11b); although the pyramidal cell bodies are still discernible, the interpyramidal grey matter consists of swollen vacuolated remnants of neuronal and glial processes bounded by lipoprotein membranes. Fig. 7.11c shows even more intense vacuolation with swelling in necrotic left precentral cortex from a patient who died in coma 2 days after occlusion of the left middle cerebral artery; the interpyramidal grey matter has disintegrated into swollen cystic spaces bounded by membranous remnants, although a large pyramidal cell body with darkly stained granules of lipofuscin is still visible.

Thus ischaemic injury to the brain can cause osmotic swelling in neuronal and glial processes with formation of large empty vacuoles. This swelling coupled with fusion of vacuoles and autolysis may produce these large clear spaces enclosed by remnants of distended membranes which gives a fenestrated appearance to the interpyramidal grey matter (Fig. 7.11b, c).

These changes can only occur if the injured cell membranes are at first semipermeable so that water can be absorbed by osmosis. But when ischaemia is so rapid in onset and so severe as to make the membranes completely permeable before absorption of water can occur through the immense area of damaged surfaces, then swelling and autolysis are precluded (p. 289). For this reason neither swelling nor vacuolation is conspicuous in the cerebral cells of dead bodies kept in refrigerators *post mortem*. Also in cerebral infarcts, when necrosis is rapid, these large vacuoles may not be formed, although other features of irreparable cellular damage are present (p. 337).

Retinal 'cotton wool' spots

These discoid lesions are caused by temporary swelling of neuronal processes as a result of partial ischaemia.

Cotton wool spots are whitish slightly raised discs 0.1–1 mm in diameter, situated in the nerve fibre layer of the retina. Most commonly these lesions occur in hypertensive patients and develop rapidly within 24 h of an attack of increased blood pressure. They also appear when retinal vessels are occluded by microthrombi, as in subacute bacterial endocarditis or by fat emboli following fractures. Similar whitish zones of swelling form rapidly in the retina of animals after intracarotid injection of glass microspheres [46]. Cotton wool spots also appear in the retina of diabetics; these lesions are more greyish and their onset is slower. In hypertensive patients cotton wool spots generally disappear within a few months, but in diabetes resolution is slower.

The prime determinant of these discoid swellings is focal arrest of circulation in the retinal vessels in the affected zones. When retina, removed *post mortem*, is perfused with Indian ink, the capillaries within the cotton wool spots are not injected or are injected incompletely, although the surrounding capillaries are fully perfused [47]. The microcirculation in the cotton wool spots is thus obstructed and the capillaries appear to be closed. In hypertension this interruption of microcirculation probably results from sudden closure of arterioles already partly occluded by intramural hyaline, while in diabetes localised thickening of basement membranes both in capillaries and precapillary arterioles may result in more gradual closure.

In an illuminating study of cotton wool spots in man and animals Ashton established that these lesions are composed of localised fusiform swellings of the axons of retinal ganglion cells as they traverse the nerve fibre layer of the retina (Fig. 7.12, p. 306). This axonal swelling develops with great rapidity after embolisation of the retina in animals with glass microspheres injected into the carotid artery. Fig. 7.13 (p. 307) shows by EM these intensely swollen axons along with adjacent normal fibres in the retina of a pig 1 h after intracarotid injection of glass micropsheres [46]. Later these swollen axonal vesicles become filled with proliferated mitochondria; this probably accounts for the whitish appearance of the swollen zones.

The axonal swelling which produces cotton wool spots is a consequence of *partial* ischaemia. *Complete* retinal ischaemia which follows occlusion of the central retinal artery produces necrosis of ganglion cells followed by degeneration of the axons. But the axons in cotton well spots are not killed immediately, and

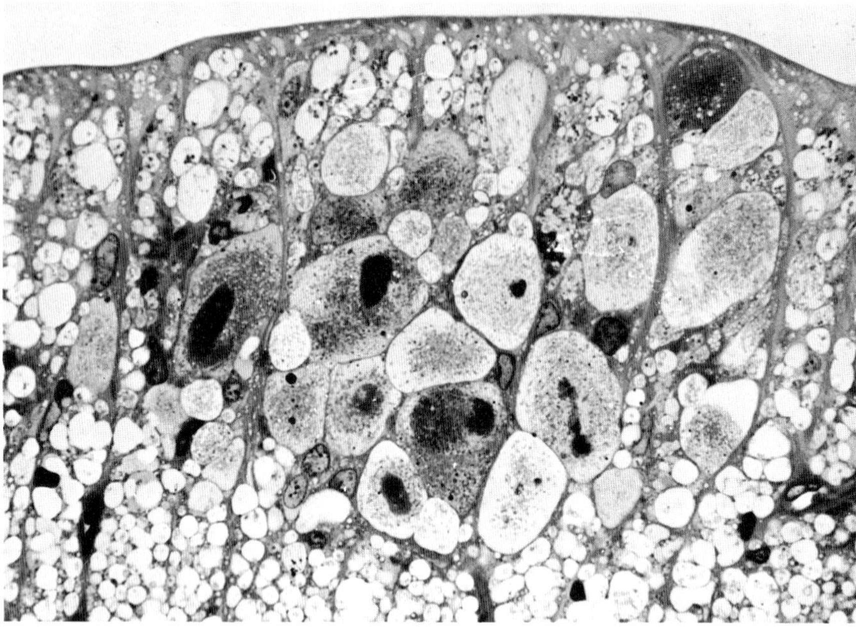

FIG. 7.12 Nerve fibre layer of retina from a hypertensive monkey showing a group of grossly swollen axons which compose a cotton wool spot; these contrast with surrounding unaffected axons. Some of the swollen axons contain central inclusions. Fixed with OsO_4, stained toluidine blue. × 550. Courtesy of Professor N. Ashton. Reproduced from *Brit. med. Bull.* (1970) **26**, 143.

their external membranes remain semipermeable and so permit osmotic absorption of water along with swelling.

This swelling probably depends on a unique feature in the structure of retinal axons, which are *unmyelinated* as they emerge from the ganglion cells and traverse the nerve fibre layer; they only acquire myelin sheaths on entering the optic nerve at the optic disc. In unmyelinated fibres the propagation of impulses requires spread of depolarisation and activity over the entire axonal surface and thus lacks the economy of energy derived from *saltatory* conduction in myelinated fibres. This exceptionally high axonal activity causes rapid consumption of ATP by the axonal membranes as well as rapid depletion of ATP within the axons, when its restoration after activity is retarded by ischaemic hypoxia (p. 91). Depletion and fission of ATP within the axons result in fall of external osmotic pressure and rise of internal osmotic pressure (p. 289), which together promote aqueous swelling of the axons so long as their membranes remain semipermeable.

The formation of cotton wool spots may thus be determined by hypoxic osmotic swelling of the naked retinal axons.

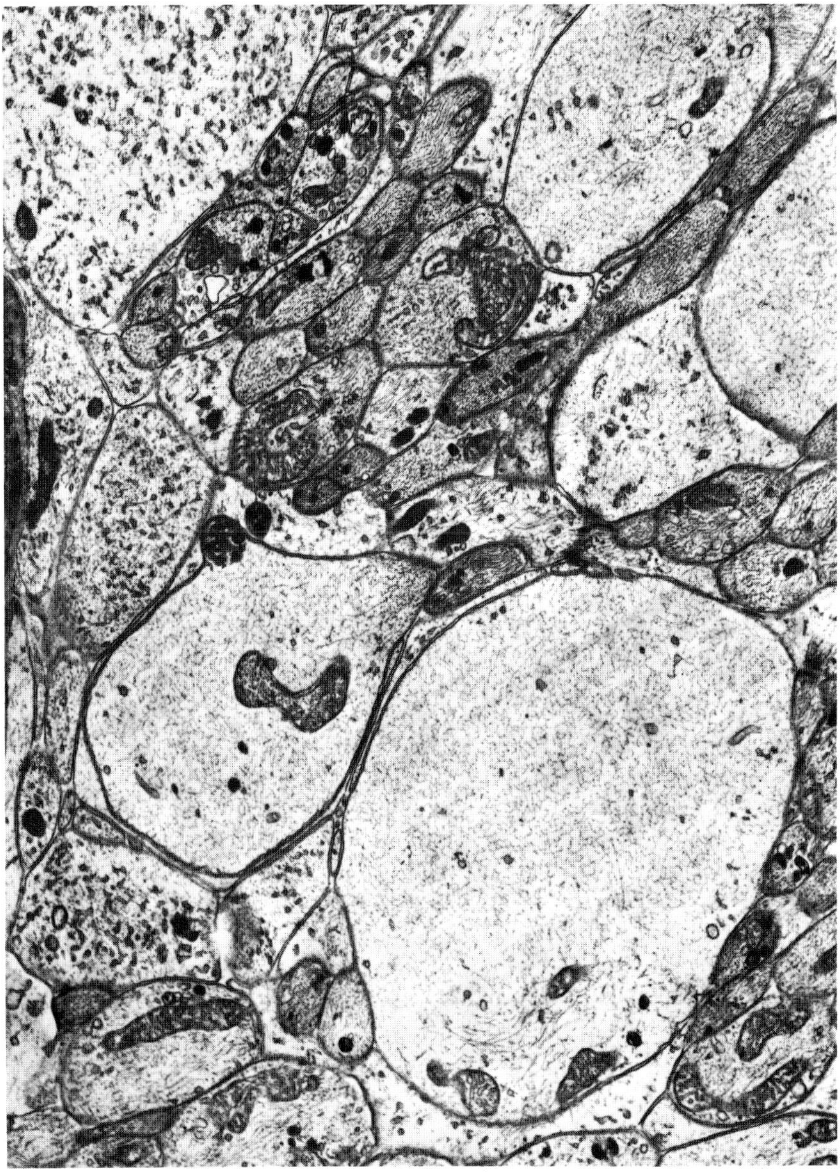

FIG. 7.13 Early stage in formation of a retinal cotton wool spot. Nerve fibre layer of pig retina 1 h after embolization with glass microspheres. Some axons are grossly swollen but others are unaffected. EM ×1200. Courtesy of Professor N. Ashton. Reproduced from *Brit. med. Bull.* (1964) **26**, 143.

Injury to cell membranes by pathogenic microbes

Hostile bacteria, protozoa and viruses can cause serious lesions by their effects on cell membranes. These are chiefly produced by effects of exotoxins and of intracellular growth.

Some exotoxins exert dramatic lytic action. Thus the α-toxin of *Clostridium welchii* hydrolyses phospholipids in cell membranes and so kills the muscle fibres in gas gangrene (p. 225). Staphylococcal leucocidin makes the surface of polymorphs so permeable that K^+ and also intracellular granules escape through the damaged cell membrane. Streptolysin O first bursts lysosomes of polymorphs, which then round up and die, while filamentous processes emerge from the cell membrane; probably initial release of lysosomal enzymes is responsible for the other changes (p. 227). *Entamoeba histolytica* also rapidly kills polymorphs, probably by discharging a membrane splitting enzyme (p. 234).

Other exotoxins, such as those of *Cl. botulinum* and *Vibrio cholerae*, combine with receptors on the cell surface membrane and thus seriously alter cellular function (p. 222), but produce no visible damage to the cells.

Infection by *Mycobacterium tuberculosis* is responsible for cohesion of macrophages to form follicles of epithelioid cells and the fusion of epithelioid cells to form giant cells (see Fig. 6.14). These effects are probably consequences of changes in surface membranes of macrophages actuated by lymphokines liberated from previously sensitised T-lymphocytes on contact with tuberculin (p. 239). This cohesion and fusion of macrophages in tuberculosis may be followed by devastating caseous necrosis.

Viral infection exerts profound effects on cell membranes. Some viruses are released by rapid lysis of the cells in which they have replicated. Thus poliovirus kills MK and Hela cells in culture and makes their membranes fully permeable; the lysed cells then shrivel and disintegrate. Probably similar change occurs in anterior horn cells of human spinal cord which also shrivel when killed by poliovirus, although later consumed by phagocytes (p. 255).

Other viruses, which are released slowly, *abduct* a portion of the cell membrane into their outer envelope. Into this part of the cell membrane myxoviruses insert some of their own component protein; then this portion of the cell membrane buds out enclosing the internally adherent nucleocapsid so as to form a separate infective particle, while the cell membrane is chemically changed by insertion of viral protein.

Changes caused by viruses in the surface of infected cells are responsible for coalescence to form syncytia both in culture and in the body in disease (e.g. measles and herpes zoster; p. 269 and Fig. 6.32). Moreover tumour viruses also profoundly alter surface of infected cells and thus induce neoplastic behaviour (p. 465).

Some viruses such as those of the pox group initially cause cell enlargement which is followed by intense aqueous swelling. Probably the cell membrane and the membranes of organelles become more permeable so that water enters by osmosis and this is followed by autolysis (p. 284), which promotes further osmotic swelling; in this way ballooning degeneration develops, which is such a prominent feature of epidermal cells infected by viruses of variola and vaccinia (Fig. 7.1) and also by the papova virus of human warts (see Fig. 6.21b). This kind of lesion can only occur if injury to membranes is not severe enough to preclude osmotic swelling.

Infection by viruses also indirectly injures cell membranes by evoking cell-mediated immunity against the membranes of infected cells bearing the viral antigen. Thus chronic active hepatitis caused by hepatitis B virus (p. 269) induces lymphocytic infiltration at margins of liver lobules followed by piecemeal disappearance of contiguous hepatocytes (p. 376). This destruction of hepatocytes may be actuated by apoptosis (p. 292); in this process the liver cells bud and split up into cell fragments which are then phagocytosed by adjacent hepatocytes and macrophages [48]. This fission of virus-infected cells following contact with sensitised T-lymphocytes (killer cells) may in fact be a general mechanism (see Fig. 6.9) by which target cells bearing a specific antigen are killed by cell-mediated hypersensitivity [48]; simultaneous liberation of lymphokines from these sensitised T-cells may also be responsible for fibrogenesis leading to cirrhosis, which is such an adverse consequence of chronic active hepatitis (p. 376).

Chromatolysis and loss of cytoplasmic basophilia

Chromatolysis means disintegration or loss of cytoplasmic aggregates of basophilic material, which are so prominent in cells capable of intensely active

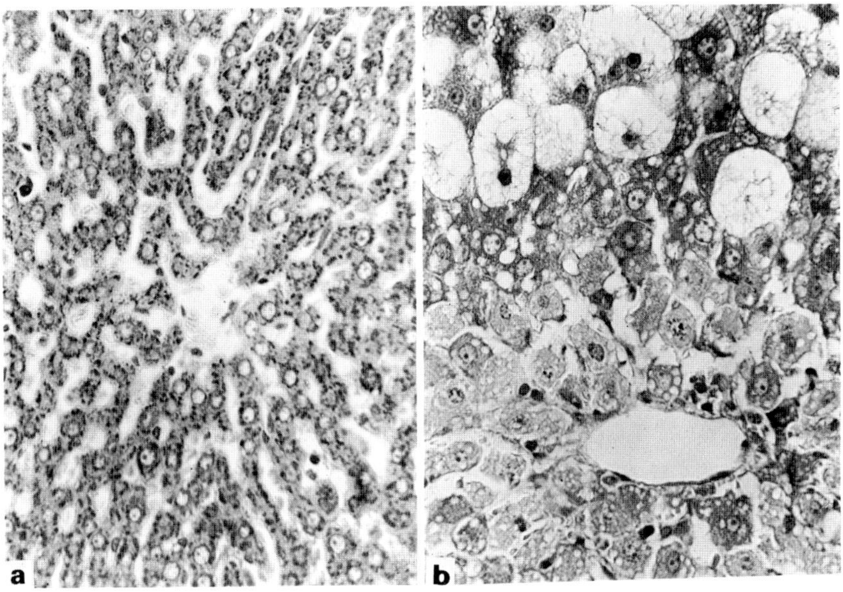

FIG. 7.14 Rat liver lobules stained by pyronin G which is specially adducted by RNA. ×335.

a. Hepatocytes of normal liver arrayed in trabeculae along sinusoids converging on central vein; basophilic granules of Berg in cytoplasm are intensely coloured.

b. Similarly situated hepatocytes from rat 24 h after injection of CCl_4 0.75 cl/100 g body weight; conspicuous loss of basophilic granules of Berg from cytoplasm of necrotic centrilobular cells and of midzonal hydropic cells. Dixon K. C. & McCullagh G. P. (1959) *Quart. J. exp. Physiol.*, **42**, 104.

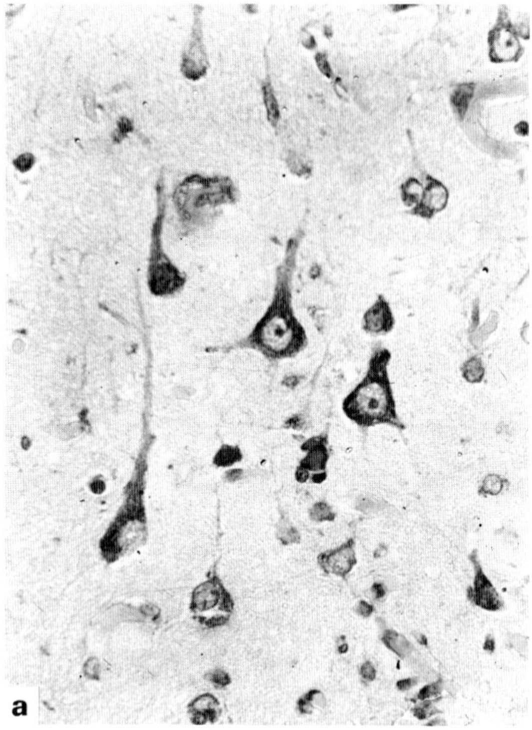

FIG. 7.15 *Right* and *left* frontal cortex from a patient who suddenly became comatose, with right hemiplegia, and died in 5 days after occlusion of left middle cerebral artery by thromboembolism. This also produced extensive zones of red infarction in left frontal and parietal cortex. Pyronin ×430.

a. Unaffected *right* frontal cortex; intensely coloured Nissl substance in cytoplasm of pyramidal cells.

synthesis of protein. Such basophilic zones, rich in RNA, typified by the granules of Berg (p. 46) in hepatic cells and the Nissl granules in neurones, are now known to be composed of arrayed cisternae of granular ER lying in parallel and covered on their outer surface by ribosomes. The anionic phsophate groups of RNA make these zones strongly basophilic and thus account for their intense colouration by cationic dyes like pyronin (Fig. 7.14a, p. 309), methylene blue and the metallic dye lake of haematoxylin. Disintegration or loss of these basophilic zones has long been regarded as a hallmark of cellular injury and death.

Chromatolysis in hepatic cells

Deficiency of protein in the diet of animals induces loss of these basophilic granules (seen by LM) and also disappearance of ribosomes from the granular ER of hepatic cells (p. 46). Detachment of ribosomes from granular ER in liver cells is an early consequence of ischaemia [2]. Moreover injection or feeding

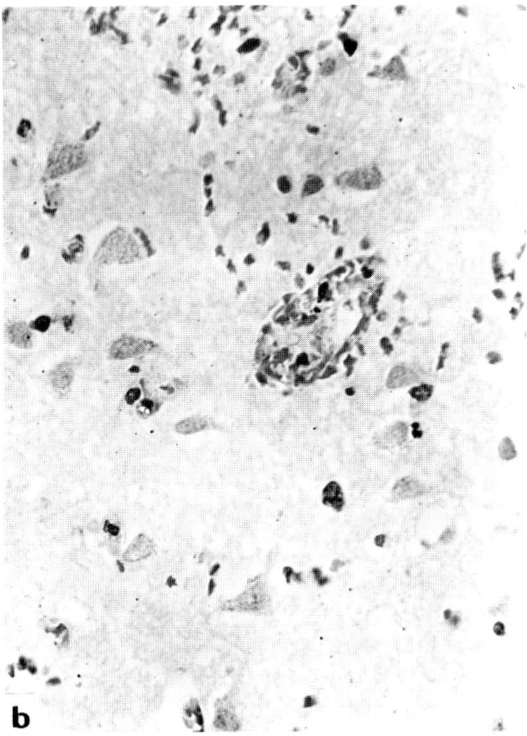

FIG. 7.15 cont.
b. Necrotic *left* frontal cortex; all Nissl substance lost from cytoplasm of shrivelled pyramidal cells (cell shadows). Dixon K. C. (1956) *J. Path. Bact.*, **71**, 37.

CCl_4 results in spectacular loss of basophilic granules stainable by pyronin from the centrilobular hepatic cells of rats (Fig. 7.14a, b); these cells also become necrotic. Observations by EM show that these changes are preceded by loss of ribosomes from the granular ER which then disintegrates [9].

Neuronal chromatolysis

Excessive activity causes temporary disintegration of Nissl substance; Nissl substance of motor neurones in the spinal cord of dogs disappears after excessive muscular exercise [49]. On recovery from fatigue this Nissl substance is restored. Similar loss of basophilic material stainable by gallocyanin-chrome alum, which specifically colours nucleic acids, occurs in the cytoplasm of cerebral neurones of human patients who die in acute delirium [50]. Section of axons causes temporary disintegration of Nissl granules in the neuronal cell bodies from which the severed axons arise (p. 111); this disintegration of Nissl granules (visible by LM) corresponds with disorganisation of cisternal arrays of granular ER and detachment of ribosomes visible by EM (p. 112).

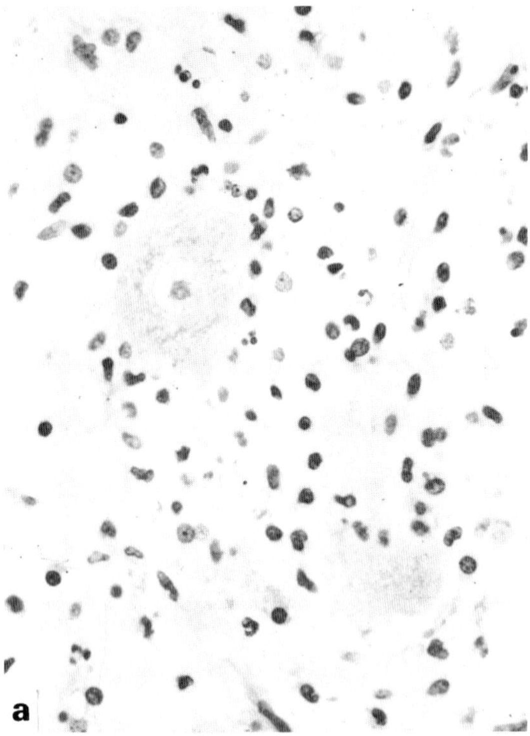

FIG. 7.16 Anterior horn cells from human spinal cord stained to show Nissl substance rich in RNA. Pyronin G ×335.

a. Motor neurones from child who died of paralytic spinomedullary poliomyelitis; nearly all Nissl substance has disappeared and neuronal cell bodies are surrounded by an exudate of phagocytic cells.

After short periods of ischaemia Nissl substance of neurones disappears temporarily. Thus after 15 min occlusion of the abdominal aorta of animals the Nissl substance of the spinal anterior horn cells slowly disappears in a few hours but is later completely reformed [33]; but after longer periods of ischaemia the Nissl substance is not reformed and the cells shrivel and die [34, 51].

Permanent disintegration of Nissl substance is characteristic of human cerebral neurones killed by ischaemia [36]. When RNA is lost from these necrotic neurones their cytoplasm is no longer coloured by pyronin which intensely stains RNA in the Nissl substance of normal neurones. Fig. 7.15a (p. 310) shows Nissl substance in normal pyramidal cells from the unaffected *right* frontal cortex of a man who died 5 days after occlusion of the *left* middle cerebral artery by thromboembolism; the Nissl substance is stained intensely by pyronin. Fig. 7.15b (p. 311) shows pyramidal cells similarly stained from the necrotic *left* frontal cortex of the same patient. The shrivelled necrotic neurones,

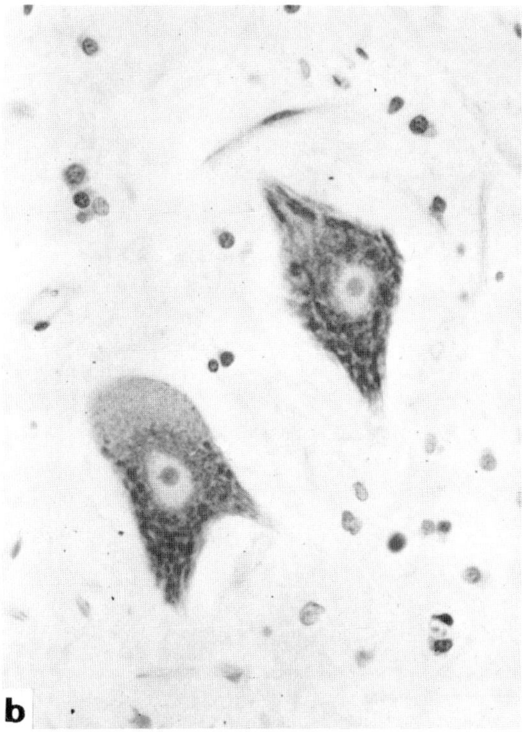

FIG. 7.16 cont.

b. Normal human motor neurones; neuronal cytoplasm contains prominent basophilic Nissl substance (a pale zone occupied by neuronal proteolipid is also visible in one of the cells). For comparison with Fig. 7.16a.

killed by ischaemia, have lost all Nissl substance stainable by pyronin from their cytoplasm.

Loss of Nissl substance and of cytoplasmic RNA is thus a characteristic feature of the phase of neuronal shrinkage of human cerebral neurones killed by ischaemia. Observations by EM on cerebral neurones of animals following injury by hypoxia [39] show that, during this phase of neuronal shrinkage, the cisternae of granular endoplasmic reticulum disintegrate and lose their attached ribosomes, which simultaneously become dispersed. These changes correlate with disappearance of Nissl substance visible by LM.

Similar disappearance of Nissl substance occurs in neurones injured by poliovirus. Fig. 7.16a shows cell bodies of motor neurones from spinal cord of a child who died from spinomedullary paralytic poliomyelitis. Most of the Nissl substance stainable by pyronin is lost from the neuronal cell bodies. For comparison normal spinal motor neurones stained by pyronin are shown in Fig. 7.16b. Even more complete loss of the Nissl substance from hypoglossal neurones in poliomyelitis is illustrated in Fig. 1.3a (p. 3). This disintegration of Nissl substance constantly occurs as a prelude to necrosis and shrinkage of neurones infected by poliovirus, although the nuclei of the motor neurones may at first appear intact (Figs 1.3a, 7.16a). Whether any of the chromatolytic infected neurones can ever recover is uncertain. Indeed phagocytic satellite cells are congregated around the spinal neurones seen in Fig. 7.16a; this may be a sign of chemotactic attraction of phagocytes to irreversibly injured neurones.

Mitochondrial swelling and disintegration

Mitochondria are highly sensitive to adverse conditions. In normal cells they are usually filamentous or sausage shaped. After cell injury they swell into spherical vesicles or agglutinate into clumps or are transformed into droplets of lipid before they finally break up into granules and disappear (chondriolysis).

Ischaemia is a potent cause of mitochondrial damage. Following occlusion of blood supply to liver the mitochondria swell (p. 294) and localised blebs may emerge from their surface after re-entry of flowing blood (Fig. 7.6) [22].

The mitochondria of myocardial fibres similarly swell as a result of ischaemia. This swelling is greatly magnified after reflow of blood into myocardium irreversibly injured by previous ischaemia. In this case dense bodies (Fig. 7.9) rich in calcium appear within the matrix of the swollen mitochondria [24, 52].

Membranes of mitochondria are sufficiently resistant to retain semipermeability even when the external cell membrane becomes fully permeable. This property, as we have seen, explains the microvacuolation described by Krogh [34] and by Brown & Brierley [38] in neurones irreversibly injured by ischaemia. Thus, when the cell membrane itself has become fully permeable, internal organelles including mitochondria may still swell by osmosis and then be converted into vacuolated cavities within shrunken necrotic cells (p. 290).

Mitochondria contain many of the enzymes concerned with cell respiration. By histochemical methods succinic dehydrogenase can be located in the myocardial mitochondria (sarcosomes) which are situated between the contractile fibrils. 6–24 h after coronary occlusion succinic dehydrogenase is lost from the mitochondria but the concentration of this enzyme temporarily increases in the A bands of the muscle fibrils [28]; later all traces of the enzyme disappear from the necrotic fibres.

Mitochondrial enzymes in brain also disappear after ischaemic injury. Gräff [53] showed that cytochrome oxidase disappears from the cytoplasm of neurones in infarcts. Similarly the mitochondrial enzymes NADH- and NADPH-tetrazolium reductases disappear from the cerebral cortex of rats following exposure to combined ischaemia and anoxia by the Levine technique (p. 67); initially the zones of enzyme activity became swollen after 0.5 h, and all enzyme activity disappeared after 24 h [54]. After such periods of anoxic ischaemia other mitochondrial enzymes in cerebral grey matter are also lost [55]; these enzymes include succinic, malic and glutamic dehydrogenases as well as ATPase and cytochrome oxidase.

Disintegration of other cytoplasmic components

Eventually dying cells become homogeneous and eosinophilic and lose their internal structure. If aqueous swelling and autolysis do not occur in the early phases of injury, then these amorphous cellular remnants may persist. But in the initial process of homogenisation cytoplasmic organelles are usually altered or lost; these include both specialised contractile proteins of skeletal and cardiac muscle as well as relatively resistant membranous components such as lysosomes.

Loss of contractile material from skeletal and cardiac muscle

When ATP disappears from *skeletal* muscle after death myosin combines with actin to produce the contraction and rigidity of *rigor mortis* (p. 81). Later rigor passes off owing to autolytic fragmentation of the myofibrils.

Injury due to ischaemia during life also destroys the fibrillar contractile material of skeletal muscle. When tourniquets are applied to the limbs of mice for 2 h the ischaemic leg muscles die and show the following sequence of changes after removal of the tourniquets [56]:

1. Saccules of ER and mitochondria swell and disintegrate.
2. Z discs between the sarcomeres disappear.
3. Contractile material disintegrates.

In typhoid fever zones of homogenisation appear in fibres of striated muscle. Here the fibres lose their striations and become glassy and eosinophilic. This change, which may only affect portions of the fibres, is called *Zenker's hyaline degeneration*.

As a result of ischaemia of *cardiac muscle* in animals, produced by arterial occlusion, 'contraction bands' (Fig. 7.7) become visible, in which the hypoxic fibres go into spasm. This phenomenon, like *rigor mortis* in skeletal muscle, may be due to loss of ATP. After more prolonged ischaemia this power of localised contractility is lost. Following ischaemic necrosis of human heart muscle in cardiac infarcts the striations may at first be plainly visible but later the necrotic fibres become homogeneous.

Deficiency of thiamine causes pronounced changes in the contractile material of myocardium in rats [57]. Foci of necrosis visible by LM appear among subendocardial fibres of left ventricle. By EM the mitochondria are seen to shrink and intense contraction bands develop in the myocardial fibres. Ultimately the myofibrillary structure is lost with formation of amorphous electron-dense masses. Such changes in myocardium produced by B_1-deficiency may account for heart failure and oedema in human beri-beri.

Lysosomes of injured cells

Rupture of lysosomes, with release of their enzymes, is probably only a late event in ischaemic damage. When liver cells are made ischaemic by ligating branches of the portal vein, circumscribed centrilobular foci of coagulative necrosis develop in 3 h [58]; these zones are eosinophilic and show loss of glycogen and of pyroninophilia, but *no change* is visible in the lysosomes. Limited dispersal of lysosomal acid phosphatase and esterase only commences 6 h after onset of ischaemia.

The lysosomes of cerebral neurones, detected by their high content of acid phosphatase, clump together and become swollen after ischaemia lasting for 1 h [59]. The enzyme is not released from the lysosomes into the cytoplasm after this period of ischaemia which causes irreversible injury to the neurones.

It is unlikely, therefore, that release of lysosomal enzymes initiates ischaemic necrosis or indeed contributes in any substantial degree to the irreversible injury produced by ischaemia.

However the granules of macrophages and of neutrophil polymorphs are lysosomes which play a highly important part in causing cellular damage and reactive inflammation in disease. This injury to lysosomes of macrophages by SiO_2 and of neutrophils by monosodium urate are basic determinants respectively in the pathogenesis of silicosis (p. 146) and of gout (p. 201). Also the release of lysosomal enzymes from neutrophils, which are attracted to the site of deposition of immune complexes (p. 209), is probably responsible for the synovial damage and erosion of articular cartilage in rheumatoid arthritis.

Degranulation and loss of lysosomes occurs very rapidly in neutrophils during the phagocytosis of bacteria; the lysosomes fuse with the phagosomes containing the bacteria, which then become exposed to the lysosomal hydrolases (p. 245). The bacterial walls are then digested *within* these fused phagolysosomes [60]. In this process the lysosomal enzymes are not released into the cytoplasm. The polymorphs are therefore unharmed and retain their motility.

On the other hand during degranulation of neutrophils by streptolysin O and streptolysin S the granules rupture directly into the cell sap and the released lysosomal enzymes then injure the cells with great rapidity (p. 227).

Rupture of lysosomes is, however, not a general prelude to the lethal activities of toxic substances. Indeed lysosomes appear to be among the most stable cellular components during the phases of lethal injury caused by some harmful compounds. Thus phagolysosomes labelled by fluorochrome, acridine orange or ferritin were produced in Chang human liver cells in culture, and were then observed following exposure to lethal concentrations of cyanide or iodacetate [61]. The cells were examined unfixed by phase contrast and by fluorescence microscopy and also, after fixation, by EM. Clumping of chromatin developed in 10 min, normal surface ruffling was lost in 20 min, vacuolation and swelling developed in 30–90 min, but rupture of lysosomes with dispersal of markers did not occur till *after* 4 h, during *post mortem* disintegration. It is clear, therefore, that lysosomal rypture with release of hydrolases cannot be a factor in promoting the early phases of lethal cell injury induced by these toxic substances.

Changes in neurofibrils: presenile dementia

Argyrophilic neurofibrils visible by LM in neurones are seen by EM to be composed of bundles of neurofilaments and microtubules. In the cerebral cortex of patients with Alzheimer's presenile dementia these neurofibrils become thickened and tortuous to form prominent neurofibrillary tangles; this change is seen by EM to involve aggregation of excessive neurofilaments [62]. Along with neurofibrillary change the cerebral cortex atrophies and neurones are lost. This presenile dementia usually commences in patients between 50 and 60 years of age with loss of memory and confusion progressing to complete mental deletion.

The cause of Alzheimer's presenile dementia is obscure. It is apparently not directly related to arterial occlusion and ischaemia as is 'arteriopathic dementia' (p. 345). Moreover, except for age of onset, there is no sharp distinction between Alzheimer's disease and the senile dementia of old age, in which similar cerebral changes are discernible [63]. Possibly in both these kinds of dementia deposition of excessive neurofibrils ultimately leads to diffuse neuronal necrosis and mental loss, but in Alzheimer's disease this change occurs precociously.

NUCLEAR DISINTEGRATION AND INJURY

Many of the adverse factors which destroy cytoplasmic structure simultaneously cause injury to the nucleus. Changes in the injured nucleus include:

1. Swelling; clumping and homogenisation of chromatin.
2. Pyknosis.
3. Karyorrhexis.
4. Karyolysis.
5. Karyokinetic injury.

Swelling; clumping and homogenisation of chromatin

Nuclear swelling

This is the first sign of injury in epidermal nuclei exposed to excessive heat (p. 115); later the chromatin marginates and clumps into crescentic masses attached to the nuclear membranes, or the nucleus is replaced by a swollen vacuole containing shrivelled chromatic remnants. Temporary swelling of neuronal nuclei follows section of axons (p. 111).

Clumping of chromatin

This is an early sequel to injury by ischaemia. Within 5 min of occlusion of branches of the coronary arteries in rabbits the nuclear chromatin of the cardiac muscle fibres clumps into masses attached to the nuclear membranes [23]; this change is at first reversible.

Homogenization of chromatin

Homogenization of chromatin in nuclei of thymocytes in culture along with loss of nuclear histones follow application of lethal doses of X-rays (p. 128). Neutrophil leucocytes suffer rapid and spectacular nuclear injury on exposure to streptolysin O; within a few minutes the nuclear lobes swell and fuse into a homogeneous spherical mass, while the cells round up and lose their motility (p. 227).

Swelling and homogenisation of nuclei in older leucocytes also rapidly follows

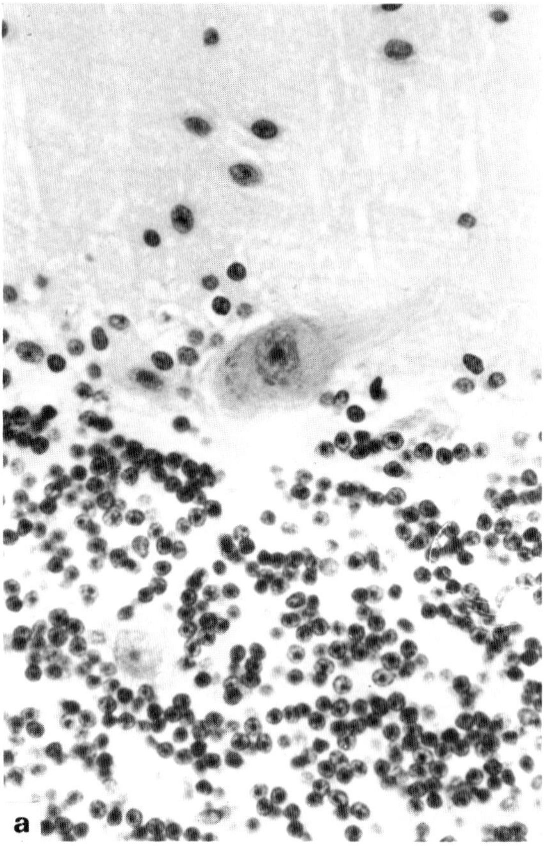

FIG. 7.17 Pyknosis of cerebellar granule cells. Cortex from left and right lateral lobes of cerebellum from a woman of 70 who died of heart failure due to coronary thrombosis; she also suffered from giddiness for 2 days before death, owing to thrombosis of *right* vertebral artery followed by infarction in right lateral lobe of cerebellum. × 510.

a. Unaffected granule cells and Purkinje cell from *left* lateral lobe of cerebellum; nuclear chromatin and nucleoli visible with clarity and definition.

their contact with LE factor present in serum of patients with SLE (p. 212). The swollen nuclear remnants are then ejected from the cells as naked LE bodies. These changes and the similar swelling and homogenisation of nuclei to form 'haematoxylin bodies' in the tissue of patients with SLE are the result of interaction of nuclear antigens with antinuclear antibodies; this interaction generates immune complexes with consequent activation of C in many tissues and is thus a dominant factor in the pathogenesis of SLE.

Pyknosis

In this process the nucleus shrivels and becomes homogeneous. Pyknotic nuclei appear dense (πυκνός, dense, thick) and are intensely stained by cationic dyes

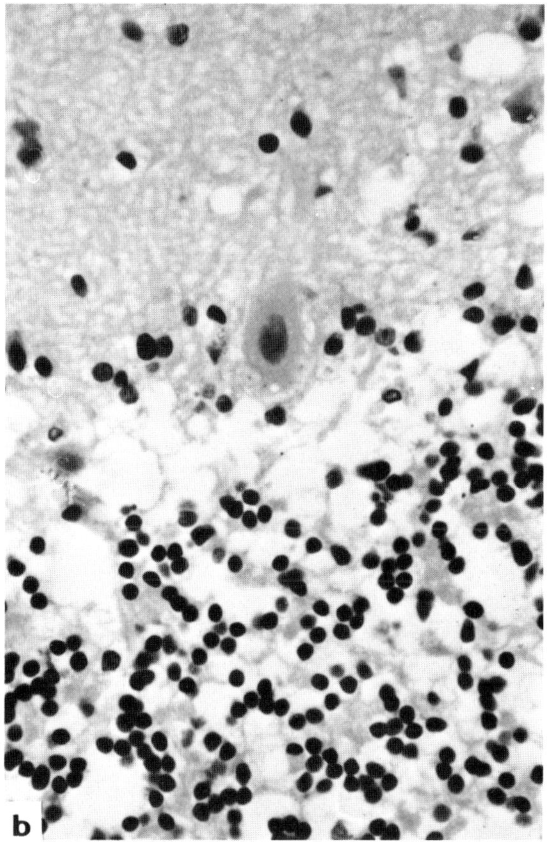

FIG. 7.17 cont.
b. Necrotic granule cells and Purkinje cell from right lateral lobe; nuclei contracted into darkly staining homogeneous remnants by synchronous pyknosis affecting every nucleus.

such as methylene blue and by basic dye lakes such as alum-haematoxylin (Fig. 7.17b). Pyknotic nuclei are strongly coloured by the Feulgen method for DNA (Fig. 7.18, p. 320). Intense colouration reflects a high concentration of stainable DNA within the contracted nuclei; there is no augmentation in the total quantity of nuclear DNA which remains unchanged or may actually be diminished [64].

Pyknosis, although a prominent event in cell death in disease, is continually occurring in health. The contracted 'ink spot' nuclei of the late normoblasts are the final pyknotic remnants resulting from progressive clumping and homogenisation of nuclear chromatin in the maturation of red cell precursors in the bone marrow. Although the nuclei are so strongly stained by basic dyes, the erythroblastic DNA is progressively lost during the normoblastic stage [65]. The pyknotic nuclei are either dissolved or expelled from the juvenile red cells, which commence their ephemerel extraosseous career as denucleated cytoplasmic saccules.

Pyknosis occurs frequently in cells as they die in the course of disease. It is a common event in ischaemic necrosis and may be particularly conspicuous after infarction of cerebellar cortex, where myriads of granule cell nuclei can simultaneously become pyknotic. Fig. 7.17a shows large numbers of normal granule cells from the unaffected *left* lateral lobe of the cerebellum of a patient with ischaemic heart failure and cardiac infarction, who died two days after the onset of giddiness and right facial palsy due to superadded occlusion of right vertebral artery by a thrombus. This caused infarction in *right* lateral lobe of cerebellum and consequent cerebellar malfunction. Fig. 7.17b shows numerous pyknotic granule cells from this necrotic zone in the *right* lateral lobe; all the nuclei are shrunken into darkly staining homogeneous remnants. Pyknosis can thus synchronously involve the entire population of necrotic granule cells as a singularly rapid and uniform consequence of irreversible nuclear injury.

Pyknosis is also a prominent lesion in granule cells of cerebellum of guinea pigs killed by large doses of radiation (p. 127).

Pyknosis is a common intermediate phase before the onset of karyolysis. For instance, during the caseous necrosis produced by tuberculosis, the nuclei of epithelioid cells (p. 239) may at first elongate and shrivel into pyknotic remnants

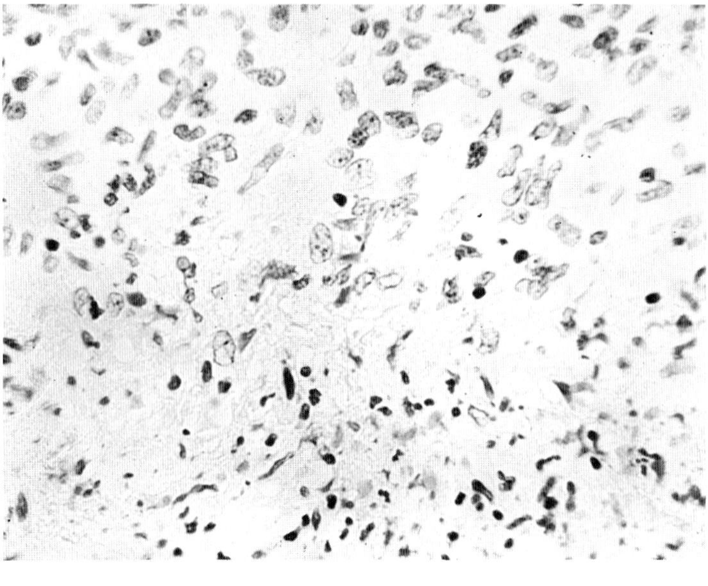

FIG. 7.18 Pyknosis in a tuberculous exudate. This exudate is composed of epithelioid cells and is situated around a caseous focus in the lung in fibrocaseous tuberculosis. Normal nuclei of active epithelioid cells are visible in upper part of the field. As these cells are killed, their nuclei contract into the intensely stained pyknotic remnants seen in the lower part of the figure. Feulgen method for DNA. ×440. Dixon K. C. (1958) *Amer. Rev. Tuberc.*, 77, 106.

rich in DNA before they ultimately disappear in the terminal karyolysis of caseation [66]. Fig. 7.18 shows epithelioid cells, from a caseous lesion in human pulmonary tuberculosis, stained by the Feulgen method for DNA. The nuclei in the lower half of the field show pyknotic shrinkage with intense colouration and concentration of DNA.

The condensation of pyknotic nuclei may involve coiling or collapse of partly uncoiled tenuous helices composed of DNA and protein into concentrated globular masses along with loss of structured water. The rapid action of heat in causing margination of chromatin and also pyknosis probably depends on such a process of condensation. Loss of nuclear water occurs in pyknosis which accompanies necrosis of cells caused by autotransplantation of liver tissue [64].

Karyorrhexis

In karyorrhexis (*κάρυον*, nut; *ῥῆξις*, break) the nucleus breaks up into granules of intensely staining debris. Like pyknosis karyorrhexis is usually an early event in necrosis.

Karyorrhexis typically occurs in the nuclei of necrotic neutrophils which have invaded infarcts or abscesses and are later killed themselves. Fig. 7.19 shows extensive karyorrhexis of nuclei of neutrophils in an infarct of the kidney where numerous neutrophils have invaded the interstitial tissue. Similar

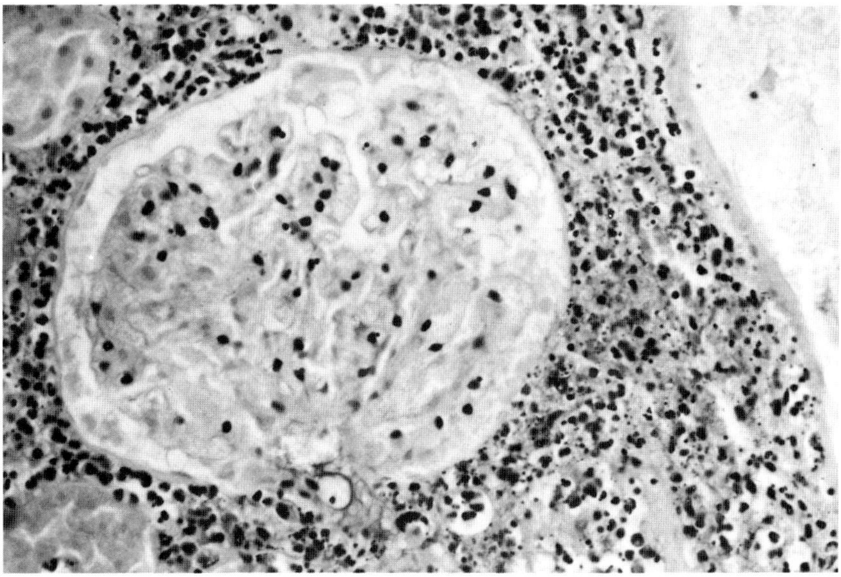

FIG. 7.19 Karyorrhexis of neutrophils in a renal infarct. The necrotic interstitial tissue between necrotic glomeruli and tubules is infiltrated by neutrophils which are also necrotic; some of the nuclei of these necrotic neutrophils are shrivelled by pyknosis and others are subdivided by karyorrhexis into numerous particles. The nuclei of the glomerular cells show both pyknosis and terminal karyolysis. × 330.

invasion of necrotic tissue by neutrophils occurs in cardiac infarcts. Indeed, fever frequently develops a few days after the onset of cardiac infarction as a result of release of pyrogens from neutrophils which invade the necrotic tissue and then themselves disintegrate.

Karyorrhexis may initially commence by aggregation of chromatin into coarse granules attached to the inner surface of the nuclear membrane; then the nucleus further disintegrates into a cluster of spherical granules which ultimately disappear. Fig. 7.20 shows this type of karyorrhexis in nuclei of the liver of a rat poisoned by CCl_4.

Otherwise karyorrhexis commences as a much more destructive process in which the nuclear chromatin is split into numerous minute particles. This kind of nuclear fragmentation is the usual fate of necrotic neutrophils and frequently occurs to an extreme degree when necrotic macrophages (epithelioid cells) disintegrate in the lesions of caseous tuberculosis. Fig. 7.21 shows this fragmentation in a caseous focus of the lung in human pulmonary tuberculosis: the nuclei are replaced by fine particles rich in DNA stainable by the Feulgen method. The nuclear remnants may persist for a considerable time before removal by autolysis.

The nature of karyorrhexis is obscure. One possibility is that the unravelled DNA of each chromosome of normal interphase nuclei becomes coiled by injury to form a separate spherical particle. This would account for the kind of

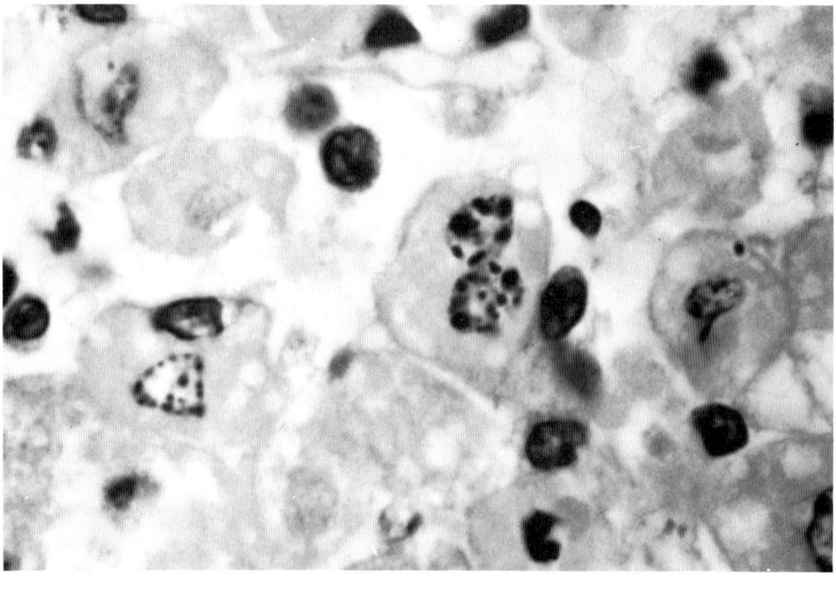

FIG. 7.20 Karyorrhexis in hepatocytes of a rat 1 day after injection of CCl_4 0.75 ml/100 g body weight. In the centre of the field is seen a binucleate hepatocyte; its two nuclei show synchronous karyorrhexis with fission into large particulate fragments. ×1300.

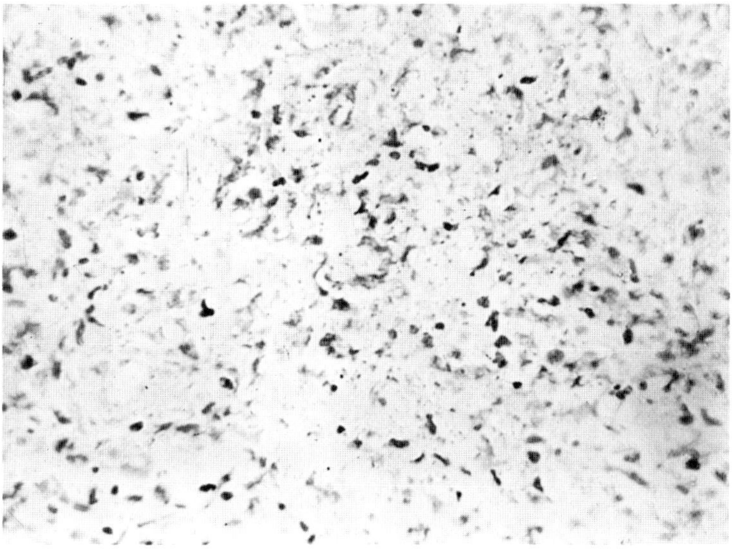

FIG. 7.21 Fibrocaseous tuberculosis of lung: extensive karyorrhexis adjacent to a caseous focus (from same lesion as Fig. 7.18). The nuclei of epithelioid cells have split into myriads of fine fragments rich in DNA. Feulgen. ×440. Dixon K. C. (1958) *Amer. Rev. Tuberc.*, **77**, 106.

karyorrhexis shown in Fig. 7.20, where nuclear remnants occur in clusters of spheroids no smaller than the Barr bodies of normal female nuclei. But in tuberculous exudates (Fig. 7.21) and after necrosis of polymorphs, where karyorrhexis may produce myriads of minute granules, each individual chromosome is probably subdivided into numerous fragments.

Karyolysis

In karyolysis (*κάρυον*, nut; *λύσις*, solution) the nucleus dissolves away; its capacity to be stained by basic dyes diminishes progressively and later the nucleus disappears altogether. Karyolysis can be either primary or secondary; thus karyolysis may be the initial change in nuclear disintegration, or it may be a sequel to pyknosis or karyorrhexis, when the intensely chromophilic products of these latter processes dissolve and vanish. Finally all stainable DNA disappears from the necrotic cells.

Disappearance of DNA in karyolysis may in part be due to hydrolysis by desoxyribonuclease, but may also depend on simple solution of DNA when no longer complexed with histone; such DNA may then diffuse out of the cells after lysis of their membranes. When mouse liver is incubated at 37° *in vitro*, no change in content of DNA occurs in the first 6 h. During the next 10 h the content of DNA falls by 20 per cent but still no loss of nuclei occurs. After further incubation, however, the number of visible nuclei and the content of

DNA both fall in parallel [67]. These observations indicate that DNA mainly disappears in karyolysis *after* lysis of nuclear membranes is completed.

Karyolysis in keratinisation

Karyolysis takes place continuously even in healthy cells. In the normal process

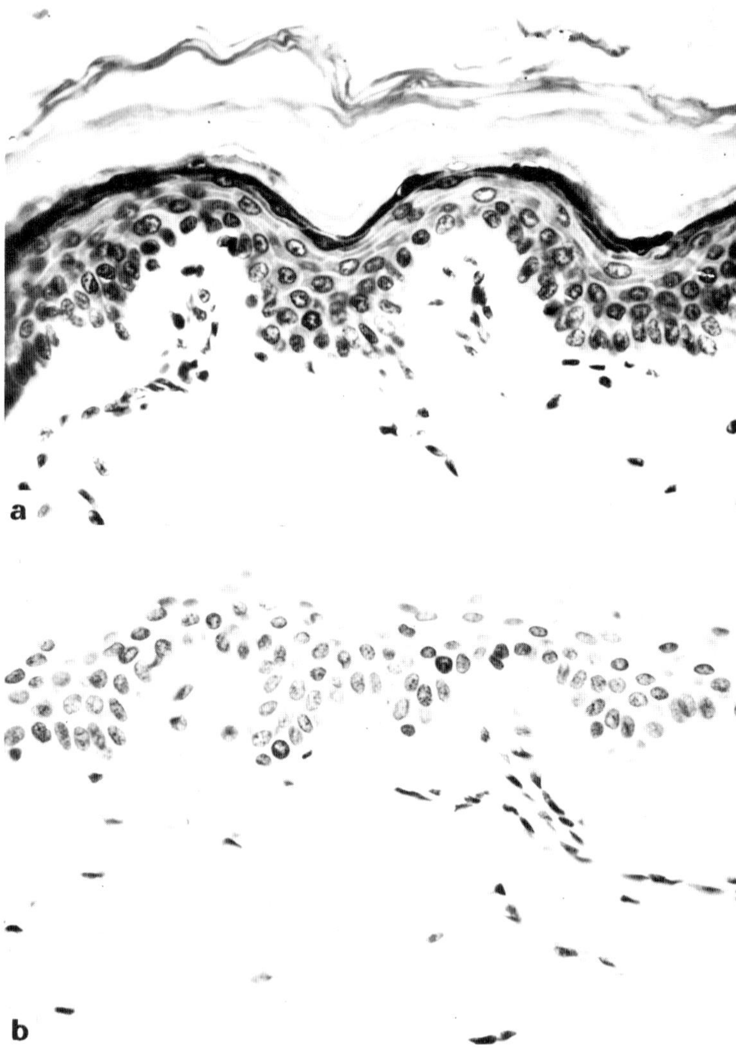

FIG. 7.22 Normal human epidermis. Loss of nuclei by karyolysis along with keratinization. × 390.

a. Loss of nuclei accompanied by formation of horny layer. H & E.

b. Adjacent section stained for DNA only; karyolysis and keratization involve loss of all DNA. Feulgen method for DNA. Dixon K. C. (1970) In *Biology of Skin,* p. 48, 50, ed. by R. H. Champion, T. Gillman, A. J. Rook & R. T. Sims. Blackwell, Oxford.

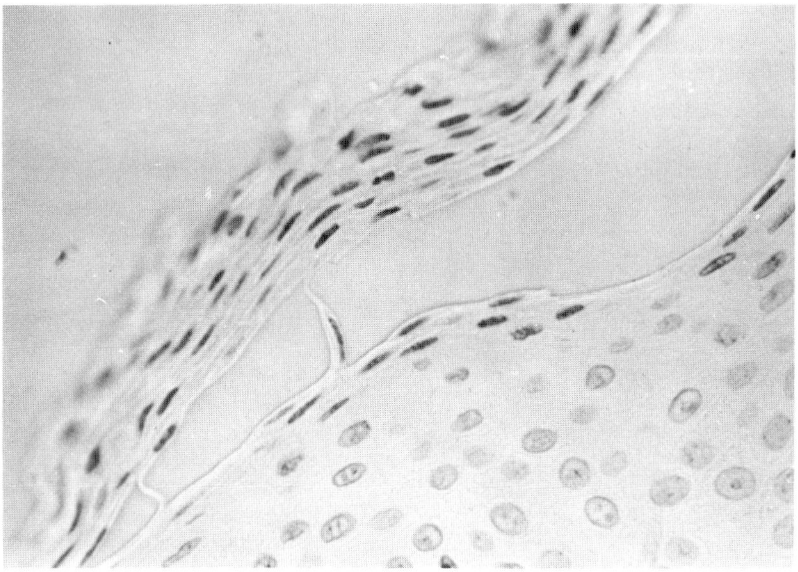

FIG. 7.23 Defects of karyolysis in psoriasis (see p. 326). Plaques of semi-cornified cells are formed in which the nuclei are not lost as in normal keratization; flattened nuclei rich in DNA are retained in imperfectly keratinized scales. Feulgen. ×510. Biopsy specimen courtesy of Dr C. H. Whittle.

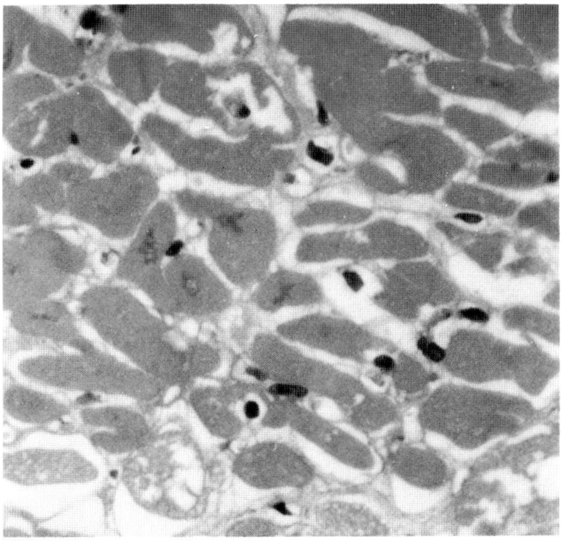

FIG. 7.24 Karyolysis in dying myocardial fibres from a zone of ischaemic necrosis in left ventricular muscle produced by coronary occlusion (see p. 328). Most of the myocardial nuclei have disappeared, but very faintly stained nuclear remnants are still discernible in some of the fibres. These contrast with dark pyknotic nuclei of the necrotic interstitial cells. ×510.

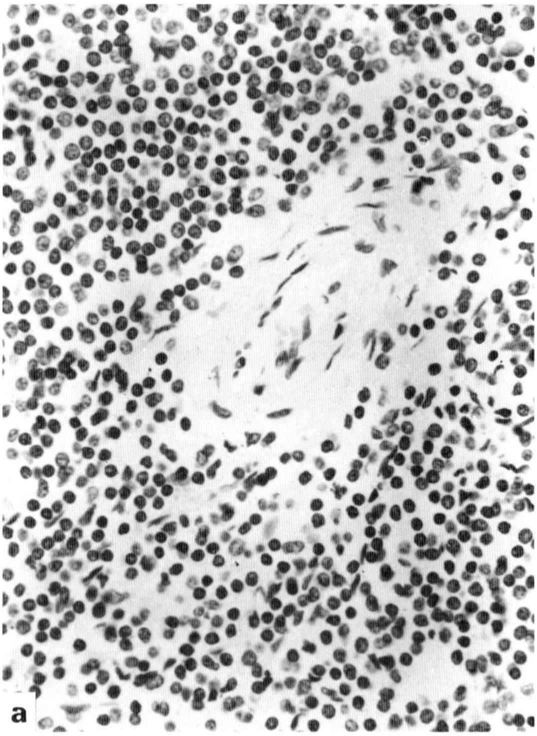

FIG. 7.25 Spleen containing a zone of ischaemic necrosis. Feulgen method for DNA. ×420.

a. Unaffected Malpighian corpuscle showing normal lymphocytic nuclei (with typical chromatin pattern) around a central vessel. For comparison with Fig. 7.25b on p. 327.

of keratinisation in human skin the cells of the stratum granulosum lose their nuclei by karyolysis at the same time as they are transformed into cornified scales of the horny layer. Fig. 7.22a shows this process of karyolysis in normal human skin stained by haematoxylin and eosin. This synchronous loss of nuclei from cells is accompanied by disapparance of all DNA stainable by the Feulgen method; Fig. 7.22b shows this disappearance of Feulgen-positive DNA from the nuclei of the tissue shown in Fig. 7.22a. This change in the keratinising epidermal cells may be due to progressive diminution in their supply of nutriments as they become further removed from the dermal capillaries.

Defect in epidermal karyolysis: psoriasis

In some disorders of the skin abnormal keratinisation can occur without karyolysis and the nuclei of epidermal cells are preserved in semi-cornified epidermal scales. This condition is called *parakeratosis*.

A common cause of extensive parakeratosis is the disease *psoriasis* which affects about 1 in 50 persons in Britain. In this disorder discoid red plaques

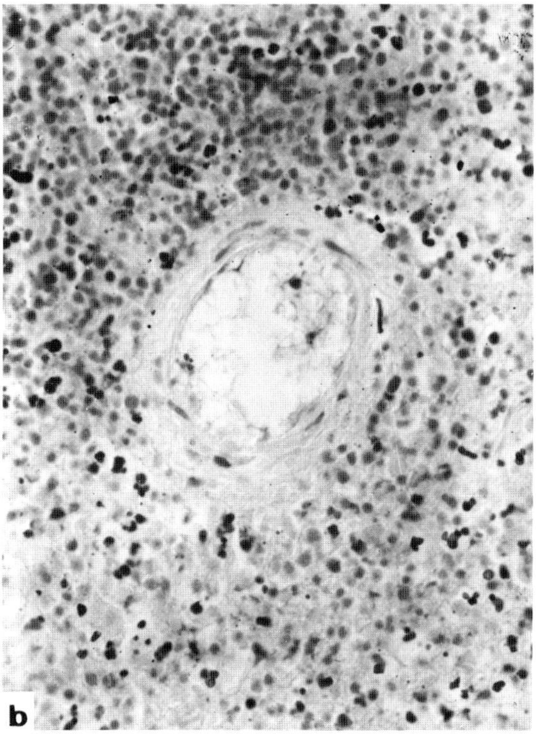

FIG. 7.25 cont.
b. Necrotic Malpighian corpuscle from infarct of same spleen; some of the lymphocytic nuclei are shrivelled by pyknosis, while others are losing DNA in terminal karyolysis.

covered by silvery scales appear in the skin. The epidermal cells proliferate and the number of cells in mitosis is increased, although the actual duration of the mitotic cycle is not shortened [68, 69]. This proliferation causes increase in formation of keratinocytes followed by excessive shedding of loosely adherent cornified scales. These scales readily become detached, leaving reddish patches no longer covered by horny layer, where the red colour of the dermis is visible through the transparent living Malpighian layer.

In psoriatic plaques the uppermost squamous cells are flattened as in the normal horny layer, but they separate from each other more readily than normal cornified cells, while their nuclei are retained as karyolysis is abolished. The stratum corneum in psoriatic lesions thus shows typical parakeratosis and consists of loose semi-cornified scales with persisting flattened nuclei rich in DNA stainable by the Feulgen method (Fig. 7.23, p. 325).

The loss of coherence of the horny layer in the lesions of psoriasis probably depends on disorder of the formative Malpighian layer. Indeed wide gaps containing microvilli are visible by EM between the Malpighian keratinocytes, while the formation of glycoprotein on the cell surfaces, as revealed by the periodic acid-methenamine technique, is also defective [70, 71]. These changes may also interfere with normal contact inhibition of growth (p. 465) and so promote intense proliferation.

Parakeratosis with abolition of epidermal karyolysis therefore appears to be a consequence of rapid proliferation along with separation and desiccation of the superficial cells. In this way diffusion or enzymatic fission of DNA may be arrested before karyolysis can be completed, so that compressed nuclear remnants persist in the cornified scales in the lesions of psoriasis (Fig. 7.23). These persistent nuclei appear to contain functional chromatin and they are surrounded by a zone of cytoplasmic tannophilic protein which is lost from normal keratinocytes [72]; this may indicate temporary retention of synthetic activity in these psoriatic scales.

Karyolysis in disease

Karyolysis is also the fate of nuclei in cellular death caused by disease. It is conspicuous in ischaemic necrosis of cardiac muscle fibres (Fig. 7.24, p. 325) and renal tubular cells (Fig. 7.29a). In these cells the nuclei progressively dissolve away (primary karyolysis) without any intermediate stage of pyknosis or karyorrhexis. But the nuclei of neutrophils which invade infarcts of heart or kidney (Fig. 7.19) usually undergo karyorrhexis before they ultimately disappear (secondary karyolysis).

In the necrotic cells of splenic infarcts pyknosis and karyolysis appear to occur together. Fig. 7.25a (p. 326) shows nuclei of normal splenic lymphocytes in a Malpighian corpuscle stained by the Feulgen method for DNA. Fig. 7.25b (p. 327) shows splenic lymphocytes from a necrotic Malpighian corpuscle in an infarct of the same spleen stained by the Feulgen method; in some of the lymphocytes the nuclei are shrivelled and DNA concentration is increased (pyknosis), while in others most of the DNA has disappeared (karyolysis).

In necrosis caused by *M. tuberculosis* karyolysis can occur directly without preliminary pyknosis or karyorrhexis. But frequently the latter processes intervene as a prelude to karyolysis. Fig. 7.26 shows the edge of a caseous focus in a lymph node (from the neck of a child who died of tuberculous meningitis), stained by the Feulgen method for DNA. Vesicular nuclei of epithelioid cells and giant cells are prominent and some of the former are shrivelled and stain more intensely owing to pyknosis, but the caseous debris in the lower left quadrant of the figure has lost all detectable DNA which has vanished in the terminal karyolysis of caseation.

Karyokinetic injury

Visible disorder of mitosis may arise directly from action of noxious agents on the mitotic chromosomes. Indeed during mitosis the cell is most sensitive to the lethal effects of electromagnetic radiation and of radiomimetic poisons (pp. 134 and 156). However, latent abnormality or injury often determines visible abnormality of karyotype, which only becomes unmasked when the individual

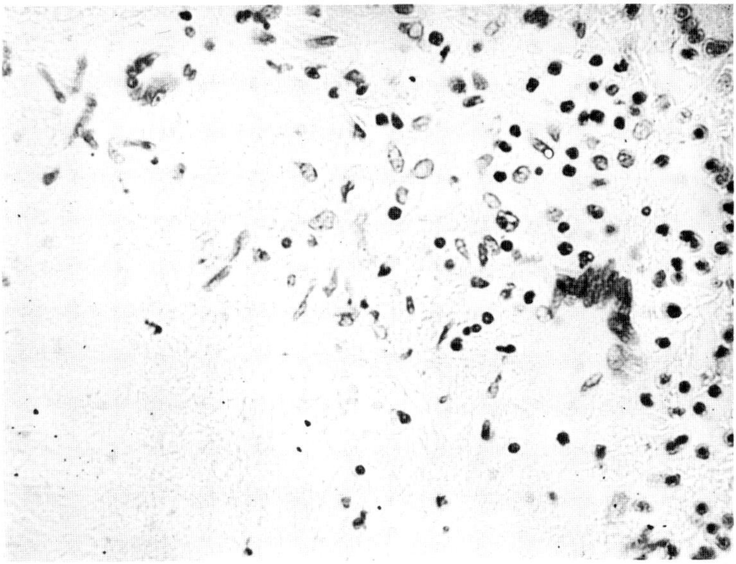

FIG. 7.26 Edge of a focus of caseous necrosis in an enlarged cervical lymph node from a child who died of tuberculous meningitis. Vesicular nuclei of epithelioid cells and giant cells are conspicuous and some of the former show pyknosis, but the caseous debris in the lower left quadrant of the field has lost all detectable DNA owing to intense terminal karyolysis. Feulgen. ×440.

chromosomes become visible during mitosis, although the actual injury may have been inflicted on the interphase nucleus.

Genomic abnormalities

Heteroploidy inherited by the zygote, as in Down's disease, affects all the cells of the body; this nuclear disorder, however, only becomes visible when the chromosomes are unmasked in mitosis (p. 34).

Clonal alterations of karyotype are usually present in malignant tumours (p. 38). Latent genomic changes may account for increased incidence of neoplasia (e.g. carcinoma of breast and thyroid) in persons exposed to radiation many years earlier. Possibly the development of neoplasia is potentiated only when a macromolecular alteration of DNA, caused by the original oncogenic agent, is unmasked by later onset of mitosis evoked by some fortuitous occurrence.

Similar instability of karyotype on a more extensive scale occurs in the rare inherited disability known as Bloom's syndrome (p. 470) in which there is a high incidence of four-armed quadriradials among the mitotic chromosomes of lymphocytes in culture from blood when stimulated by PHA. These quadriradials are formed by apposition of pairs of homologous chromosomes which probably results in exchange of chromatid segments at mitosis. This type of exchange may eventually produce chromosomal aberration with evolution of malignant neoplasia.

Aberrations in mitosis caused by radiation

These are considered in Chapter 4.

Karyokinetic poisons

The *radiomimetic poisons* such as aminopterin (p. 156) ape the effects of radiation; they cause clumping of chromosomes at metaphase and impede onset of anaphase. Colchicine is sometimes called a *spindle poison*; it is bound by mitotic spindle fibres and arrests mitosis at metaphase. Colchicine is a valuable tool in the study of human chromosomes; when it is added to cell cultures 1–2 h before fixation, many of the cells are trapped in metaphase and numerous mitotic chromosomes become available for chromosomal analysis.

Viral infection: effects on mitosis

Infection by viruses can cause conspicuous injury to dividing cells. Wildly *et al.* [73] found that herpes virus growing in culture of Hela cells causes arrest of mitosis at metaphase in a similar way to colchicine. But the mitoses arrested by

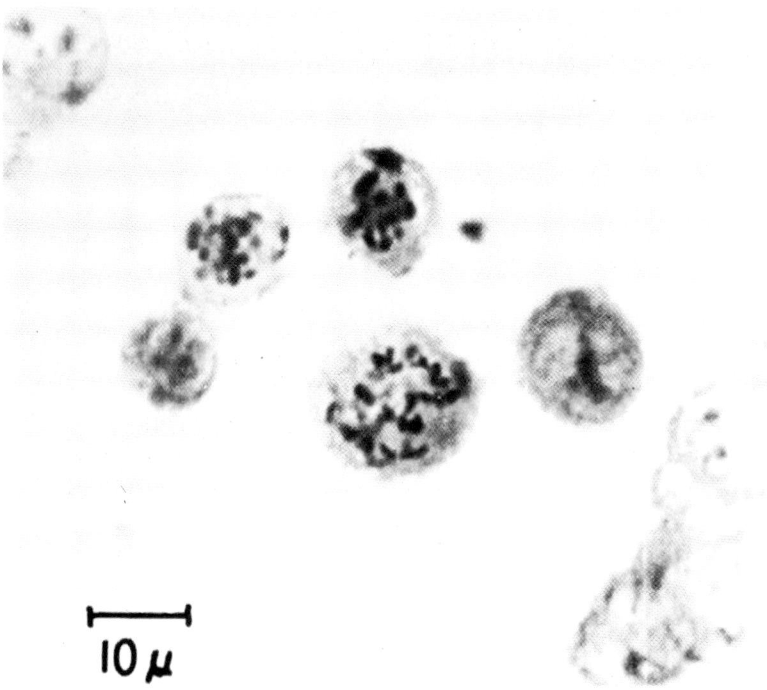

FIG. 7.27 Arrest of mitosis at metaphase in cells infected by herpes simplex virus. Hela cells infected in culture on cover slips: chromosomes become shorter and thicker and end up as spherical blobs, which may remain attached to the glass when the cells distintegrate. Gallocyanin-chromalum for nucleic acid. Courtesy of Professor P. Wildly, Dr. C. Smith, Dr A. A. Newton and Dr P. Dendy. Reproduced from *Virology* (1961) **15**, 486.

herpes infection, unlike those arrested by colchicine, do not persist; the chromosomes soon become shorter and thicker (Fig. 7.27) and finally contract into spherical blobs. Ultimately the cells disappear leaving chromosomal remnants still attached to the glass.

Viral infection can also cause chromosome breaks in dividing cells. Thus numerous chromosome breaks appear in lymphocytes cultured from the blood of patients with measles. Bizarre disintegration of chromatin in dividing cells occurs in cultured cells which form syncytia on infection with measles, NDV and herpes simplex [74]. This change, which is called pulverisation, involves fragmentation and unspiralling of chromatin. Observations using tritiated thymidine and autoradiography indicate that this pulverised material is genomic DNA in the synthetic (S) phase of mitosis, which is split up by viral infection into innumerable fragments [75].

Although some DNA tumour viruses do not at first cause visible change of karyotype in transformed mouse or hamster cell lines, abnormalities frequently develop on subculture. Thus SV_{40} causes gaps or breaks in chromosomes and the appearance of dicentrics when grown on dividing human skin fibroblasts; the fully transformed human fibroblasts show chromosomal abnormality at nearly all mitoses [76]. These observations suggested that the appearance of chromosomal abnormality, though not necessarily responsible for tumour progression, is very closely associated with the event of transformation to the neoplastic state.

REVERSIBLE INJURY AND DEATH

After these various kinds of injury to their cytoplasm or nucleus, the cells may recover or die; disintegration is thus reparable or irreparable.

Reparable disintegration

This may follow adverse conditions insufficient in duration or severity to cause lethal injury.

The nuclei of epidermal cells of skin become *temporarily* swollen following exposure for 1 min to water at 45–50°; but exposure to longer periods of heating (e.g. 1 h at 50°) or to higher temperatures (e.g. 1 min at 55°) causes permanent and irreversible nuclear injury followed by necrosis (p. 115).

Similarly, hepatic cells show temporary signs of injury, including loss of microvilli, formation of blebs and zones of weakness in cell membrane, disaggregation of polyribosomes into monosomes and cytoplasmic vacuolation, after occlusion of blood supply for 1 h or less; these cells recover completely if circulation is then restored (p. 79). But the hepatic cells are irreversibly injured and die after ischaemia lasting for 2 h, even though the circulation is restored [2]. Temporary loss of Berg granules and of ribosomes and RNA from hepatic cells also occurs in starvation (p. 46).

Neurones show temporary signs of injury following ischaemia or trauma, when damage is not sufficient to produce necrosis. Thus temporary swelling and loss of Nissl substance in cell bodies and dendrites may follow short periods of ischaemia which cause transient interruption of function (p. 312). The swelling of axons, which determines the formation of retinal cotton wool spots following ischaemia due to hypertensive attacks, also subsides completely when these lesions resolve (p. 305). The cell bodies of neurones swell and lose Nissl substance when their axons are cut, but later normal structure is recovered completely (p. 112). Even excessive muscular activity can cause temporary loss of Nissl substance from cell bodies of spinal anterior horn cells (p. 311).

Irreparable disintegration

Irreparable disintegration, accompanied by permanent cessation of activity and function, is synonymous with cell death or necrosis. A cell may be regarded as dying when disintegration has progressed beyond the point of possible return to the normal structure and equilibrium of life. Unfortunately we do not know where this point is; by inspecting a cell, after fixing it, we may not be able to discern whether *before fixation* it had or had not suffered irreparable damage.

Krogh [34] produced irreparable ischaemic injury in the anterior horn cells of the lumbar spinal cord of rabbits by compressing the abdominal aorta for 1 h (p. 301). The earliest changes visible by LM were just definable 1 h later; by then the Nissl substance was no longer sharp in outline, while small vacuoles appeared in the cytoplasm and the nucleus became shrunken. Later the Nissl substance disappeared completely and within 24 h the cells decomposed into faintly stainable shadows. Similar 'shadow cells' are visible following ischaemic necrosis of human cerebral cortex (Fig. 7.30a). Although such 'shadows' may still be rich in protein [40, 77], they are merely shrivelled remnants of the former cells (Fig. 7.30b).

Microvacuolation of irreversibly injured neurones in cerebral cortex can be detected even sooner by electron microscopy of cerebral tissue of animals killed immediately after exposure to hypoxia for 15–30 min [39]. This change is also followed by neuronal shrinkage with increase of electron-density in cytoplasm and formation of shadow cells with the same apparently inevitable march of cellular disintegration as is observable by LM.

It is clear therefore that, after a certain period of complete ischaemia, neurones suffer an irreversible lesion which leaves an irreparable though initially invisible imprint on them; this is followed by the most profound disintegration in the next 24 h. The nature of such latent though lethal injuries is obscure. It is possible that:

1. Proteins and lipids in membranes and other parts of the cell become so disarrayed as to be incapable of regaining their previous conformation when the supply of energy is restored; disintegration therefore continues. Thus irreversible change may occur in the proteins of membranes or fibrils when ATP is depleted by ischaemia (p. 93). In the absence of ATP active groups of fibrillar enzymic proteins like myosin, which can split ATP, may become exposed when not occupied and protected by their substrate. Such exposed groups may then interligate excessively with other proteins. Thus contractile effects similar to rigor mortis (p. 81) may cause multiple and irregular interligation which can never be disentangled even if ATP again becomes available. This may be a

common mechanism of irreversible change in cellular death whether affecting proteins in membranes or other parts of the cell.

2. Some unique sequence of nucleotides in nuclear DNA decomposes, thus eliminating the eventual transcription and translation of an essential cellular peptide which becomes expended; in this way one crucial macromolecular lesion may herald inevitable cellular death.

Although certain alterations in structure, including swelling of hepatocytes, astrocytes and neurones and clumping of chromatin in nuclei of myocardial fibres, become visible within 15 min of onset of ischaemia, these rapid changes are probably at first reversible. In fact the initial structural disarray which heralds the irreparable process of disintegration in dying cells has so far eluded definition.

FATE OF REMNANTS IN DEAD AND DYING CELLS

When cellular injury is irreparable what then is the final fate of the remnants? This is of three kinds:

1. Persistence.
2. Autolysis.
3. Heterolysis.

Persistence

Persistence of the remnants in a physically altered state but with little decomposition of protein or lipid is the commonest early sequel to necrosis.

Autolysis is probably prevented by two principal factors [77, 78]:

1. Lack of free 'unstructured' water available for hydrolysis of macromolecules.

2. Initial inaccessibility of catabolic enzymes to their substrates. Although DNA disappears early after necrosis along with loss of nuclei by karyolysis, protein is conspicuously retained in necrotic cells if they do not initially become swollen. This persistence of protein is characteristic of both coagulative necrosis and caseation [66].

Coagulative necrosis

As disintegration of lipoprotein membranes proceeds, the irreparably damaged cell becomes completely permeable: water cannot be absorbed by osmosis, but the micromolecular participants of living metabolism are lost from the cell by diffusion. The hydrolytic enzymes arc inactivated and the cell is transformed into a shrunken mass of denatured protein and lipid in which cell outline is remarkably preserved. This change in dying cells is called *coagulative necrosis* (p. 7). This type of cell death is a frequent consequence of irreparable damage caused by ischaemia.

Denaturation of protein involves unravelling of folded chains along with exposure of active groups and also their mutual aggregation. This change in coagulative necrosis was studied in pieces of rat liver transplanted into the peritoneal cavity of other (syngeneic) rats [79]. The transplanted liver cells then died owing to ischaemia. The optical density of transplanted liver tissue was measured at varying times after transplantation. Initially the optical density fell, probably because of mitochondrial swelling, but regained its original value in 4–5 h. Thereafter the optical density rose progressively. The tissue became *more opaque* along with denaturation and aggregation of protein.

This opacification of tissue during coagulative necrosis is specially prominent after infarction. The opaque dead cells do not transmit light but reflect it; this effect gives a whitish appearance to infarcts in kidney and spleen.

Unravelling of folded chains in protein molecules during denaturation along with exposure of cationic $-NH_3^+$ groups of lysine and arginine probably account for the eosinophilia of the dead tissue. Basophilia is not increased. Loss of basophilia is characteristic of the dead tissue owing to disappearance of RNA and of DNA, which accompanies chromatolysis in cytoplasm and karyolysis in the nuclei; in these changes loss of phosphate groups of nucleotides involves considerable diminution in power to bind basic dyes.

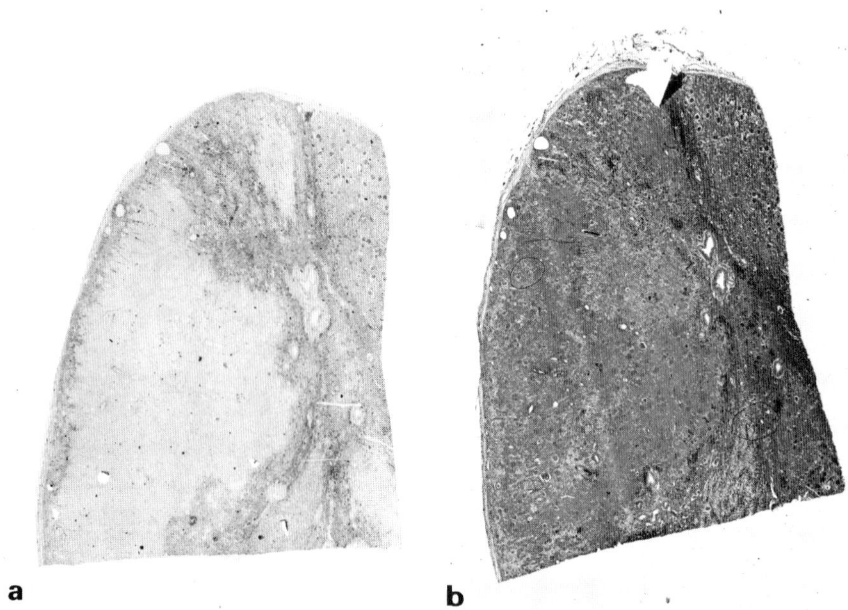

FIG. 7.28 Infarct of kidney.

a. Showing pallor due to loss of cytoplasmic and nuclear basophilia from necrotic zone. Pyronin. × 3.8.

b. Adjacent section stained for protein by coupled tetrazonium method. Retention of protein in necrotic zone. × 3.8. Dixon K. C. (1956) *J. Path. Bact.*, **71**, 37.

Another usual feature of coagulative necrosis is *shrinkage* of the dead cells. (Fig. 1.6 (p. 12) and Fig. 3.10 (p. 74) show this shrinkage of centrilobular hepatic cells killed by the general ischaemia of heart failure (p. 75). Similarly Purkinje cells of the cerebellum become shrivelled when killed by ischaemia (see Fig. 1.1a, p. 2, and 7.17b).

This shrinkage of necrotic cells may in part be due to mutual aggregation of unmasked charged groups which become exposed during denaturation of protein. But loss of water due to abolition of osmosis in the fully permeable dead cells and loss of bound water on disintegration of their membranes are probably more important factors in shrinkage of the dying cells.

Persistence of protein within the dead cells is a dominant feature of coagulative necrosis [77]. The dead cells retain this abundant cytoplasmic protein although RNA and DNA, which are stainable by basic dyes such as pyronin, disappear. Fig. 7.28a shows an infarct of the kidney stained by pyronin G: there is conspicuous loss of basophilic material from the necrotic zones. Fig. 7.28b shows the same renal infarct stained by the coupled tetrazonium method, which colours the phenolic groups of tyrosine within the tissue proteins: the necrotic tissue potently retains its content of protein, even though nucleic acids stainable by pyronin are lost.

The coupled tetrazonium method of Danielli is convenient for demonstrating cellular protein. By this technique tyrosine, tryptophane and histidine groups of cell proteins are first ligated with one of the two diazo groups of tetrazotised benzidine to form bright yellow compounds (I).

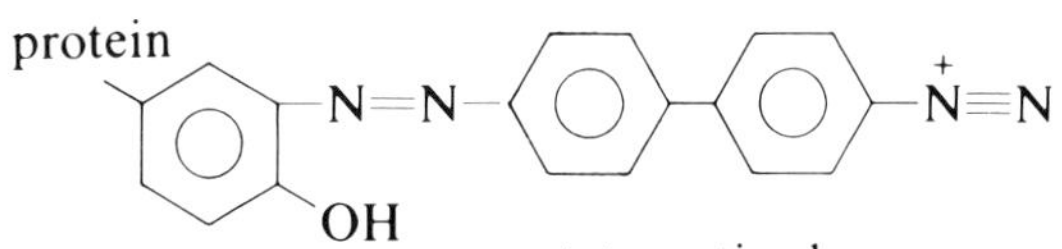

tyrosine group in protein — tetrazotized benzidine residue with one free diazo group

I

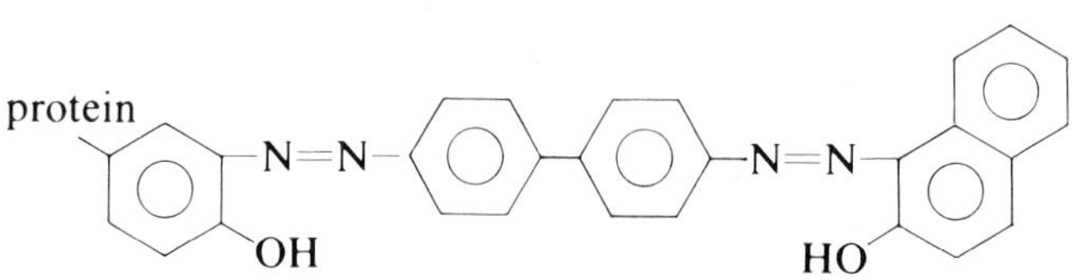

tyrosine group in protein — β-naphthol residue

II

These yellow compounds (I) still contain a free diazo group which, though firmly attached to the cell proteins, can then be coupled with β-naphthol to form an intense orange red dye (II). This dye is indissolubly ligated to the protein molecules in cells. This reaction involves a stoichoimetric covalent union of dye to protein; it is thus quite unlike ordinary staining in which variable quantities of ionised dyes are loosely held by charged regions (either anionic or cationic) in the cellular macromolecules.

In coagulative necrosis the outline of the dead cells is preserved and much of their protein stainable by the coupled tetrazonium method is retained, in spite of homogenisation and loss of internal structure. Fig. 7,29a shows (in a section stained by H and E) this homogenisation of necrotic renal tubular cells at the margin of the same infarct as shown in Fig. 7.28a and b. The renal tubular cells are homogenised and have lost their nuclei but the outline of the tubules is preserved. Fig. 7.29b shows similar necrotic renal tubules from the same renal infarct stained by the coupled tetrazonium method; the homogenised dead tubules are vividly coloured owing to abundance of protein retained in the necrotic tubules. This preservation of homogenised protein is typical of coagulative necrosis.

Protein may also be retained in the cell bodies of neurones of the cerebral cortex after ischaemic necrosis [77]. The necrotic pyramidal cells become angular and shrivelled, and they appear faint and shadowy in sections stained by H and E or basic dyes. This appearance is called Spielmeyer's ischaemic

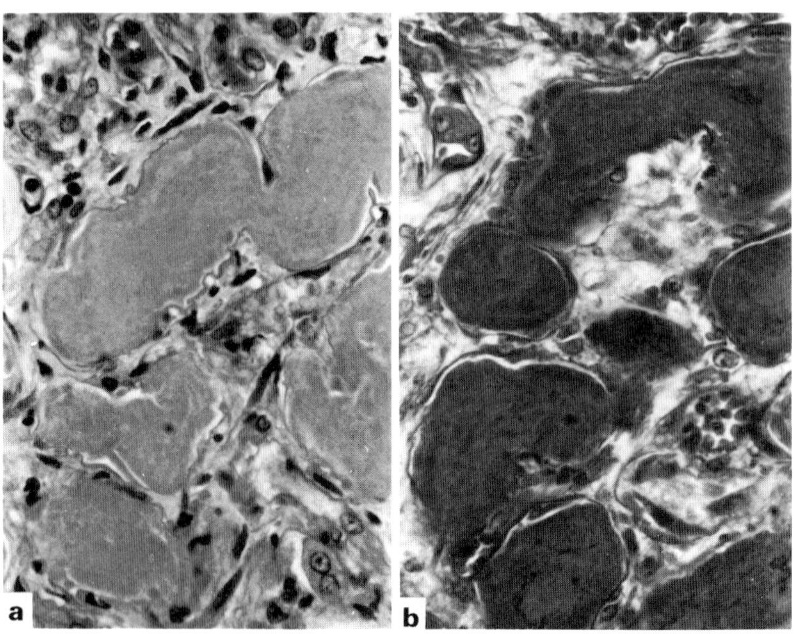

FIG. 7.29 Margin of renal infarct (shown in Fig. 7.28).

a. Complete loss of nuclei (karyolysis) in renal tubules; interstitial tissue unaffected. H & E. ×265.

b. Adjacent section. Conspicuous retention of protein in necrotic renal tubules. Coupled tetrazonium. ×265.

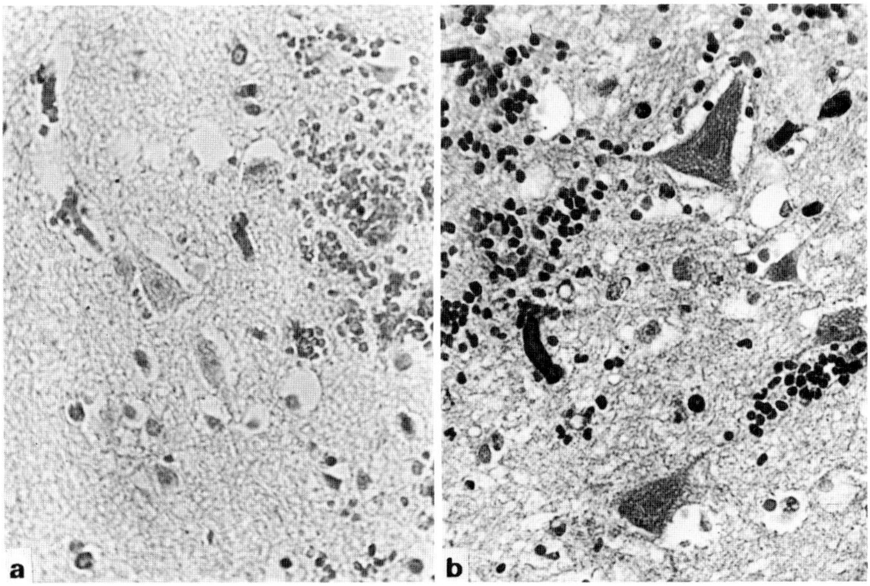

FIG. 7.30 Infarct of occipital cortex from a patient aged 84 who died in coma after a period of widespread ischaemia due to general anaesthesia and surgical shock, following repair of a femoral fracture. Several zones of red infarction were present in cerebral cortex.

a. Stained by pyronin G: conspicuous loss of basophilic Nissl substance from necrotic pyramidal neurones which appear as cell shadows. × 345.

b. Adjacent section stained by coupled tetrazonium method for protein; this reveals retention of abundant protein in the necrotic pyramidal cells. × 345. Dixon K. C. (1956) *J. Path. Bact.* **71**, 37.

change [36]. Fig. 7.30a shows these necrotic cell bodies stained by the basic dye pyronin G (which is specially adducted to RNA) in a zone of haemorrhagic infarction of human occipital cortex; the faintly coloured angular remnants of the pyramidal cells appear to have lost all cytoplasmic RNA. But, when stained by the coupled tetrazonium method, these phantom cells from the same zone of coagulative necrosis are strikingly revealed by their high content of protein, as shown in Fig. 7.30b.

Similar persistence of protein occurs in coagulative necrosis of centrilobular hepatic cells after injection of CCl_4 [80]; these cells die, their cytoplasmic RNA disappears (Fig. 7.31a), their nuclei show karyorrhexis (Fig. 7.20), but their cytoplasm remains rich in protein except in cells which become hydropic. Fig. 7.31a (p. 338) shows a liver lobule of a rat poisoned by CCl_4 stained by pyronin: the centrilobular cells are necrotic and have lost all cytoplasmic RNA stainable by pyronin. Fig. 7.31b shows the same hepatic lobule stained by the coupled tetrazonium method for protein: clearly there is no loss of protein from the centrilobular necrotic cells, although the midzonal hydropic cells retain hardly

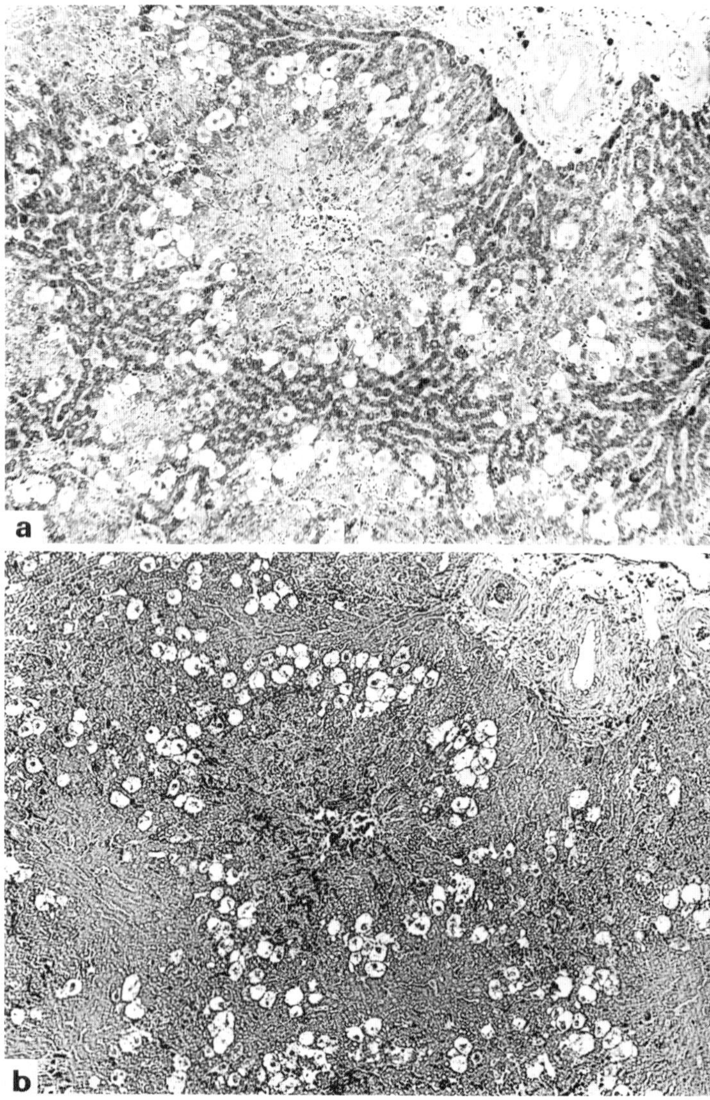

FIG. 7.31 Hepatic lobule of rat 1 day after injection of CCl_4 0.75 ml/100 g body weight. × 95.

a. Stained by pyronin: loss of basophilia due to RNA from necrotic centrilobular hepatocytes; midzonal cells are hydropic.

b. Adjacent section stained by coupled tetrazonium method for protein: conspicuous retention of protein in the necrotic centrilobular hepatocytes. Dixon K. C. & McCullagh G. P. (1957) *Quart. J. exp. Physiol.*, **42**, 104.

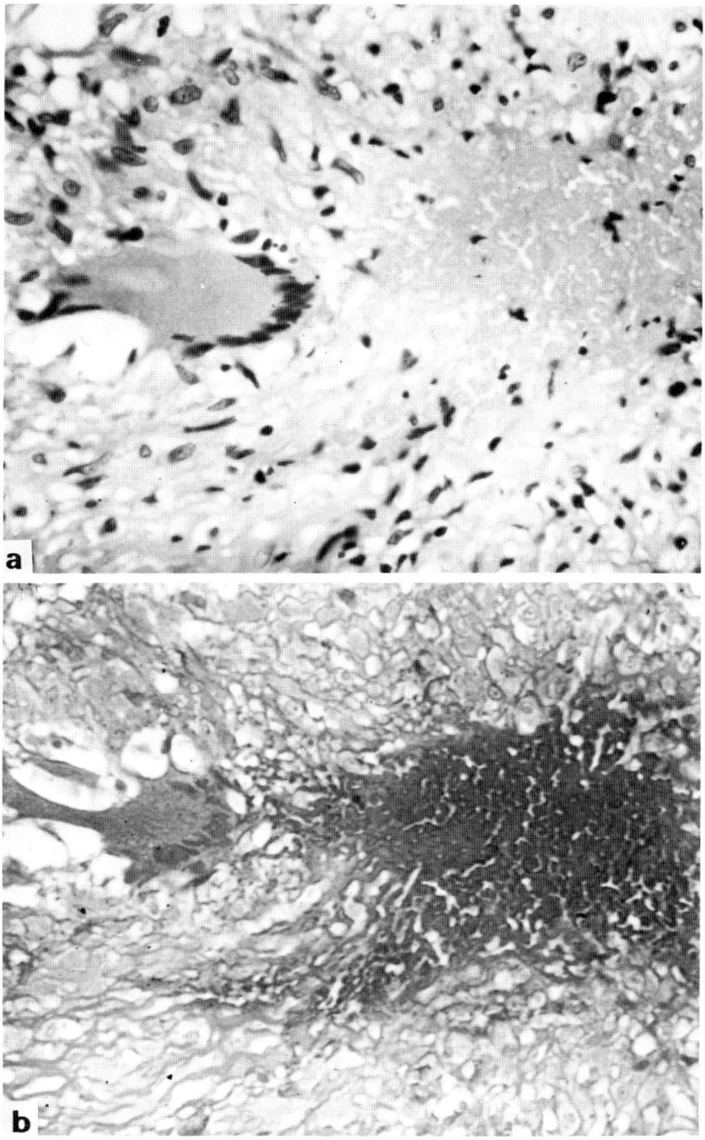

FIG. 7.32 Two adjacent sections from a tuberculous inguinal lymph node removed by biopsy from a child. The field illustrated shows the caseous centre of a tubercle surrounded by epithelioid cells and one large giant cell. × 410.

a. Loss of nuclei by karyolysis in central caseous zone. H & E.

b. Retention of protein in central caseous zone and in dying giant cell. Coupled tetrazonium method. From (1958) *Amer. Rev. Tuberc.* **77**, 106.

any protein. EM observations on dying hepatic cells injured by CCl_4 shows that the tubules of ER become aggregated to give electron opaque regions suggestive of membrane collapse [81].

The cellular homogenisation which is typical of coagulative necrosis as well as the cell shrinkage, which often occurs at the same time, may result from collapse of membranous organelles along with the compression and disintegration of their membranes, so as to form amorphous granular remnants in which cell contour is retained.

Caseous necrosis

Infection by tubercle bacilli can produce the most devastating and extensive lethal effects. Epithelioid cells of tuberculous exudates die and disintegrate along with tissue around them to form granular amorphous material of cheese-like consistency, in which both cellular structure and outline have vanished. This process is called caseation (p. 7).

Figs 7.32a and b (p. 339) illustrate two adjacent sections of a caseous focus in a tuberculous lymph node removed by biopsy from a child. In Fig. 7.32a (stained by H and E) there is disintegration of cell structure and outline and loss of nuclei from the eosinophil central zone of caseation, which is surrounded by epithelioid cells (p. 339) and a prominent giant cell. In spite of this complete disintegration and karyolysis the caseous central zone is rich in protein. This persistence of protein is strikingly conspicuous in Fig. 7.32b (stained by the coupled tetrazonium method), which shows intense colouration of the same caseous focus and also of the same dying giant cell. Persistence of protein is a cardinal feature of caseous necrosis [20, 66].

Exposure of cationic $-NH_3^+$ groups probably occurs in the denaturation of proteins involved in caseation. These electropositive loci selectively adsorb the anionic dye erythrosin (at pH 9·0) so that caseous material is intensely coloured by this dye. Fig. 7.33 shows a caseous focus and a large adjacent giant cell in a tuberculous lymph node prominently stained in this way by erythrosin.

Persistence of denatured protein and lipoprotein in dead cells and in the remnants formed by their destruction is thus a characteristic of both coagulative and of caseous necrosis. Similar persistence probably occurs in gummatous necrosis (p. 273). Such persistence emphasises the prevalence of macromolecular disarray as opposed to chemical fission as the principal event in the disintegration of dying cells.

Autolysis

Dissolution of cellular materials due to change in the cells themselves (*αὐτός*, self; *λύσις*, solution) may be a consequence of escape of these substances by diffusion or loss by enzymic fission, once the barriers of the living cell have disintegrated.

RNA and DNA usually disappear from necrotic cells despite persistence of protein. Ribosomes initially become detached from ER and are then dispersed in the cytoplasm. RNA is later lost from the dying cells. How far this loss is due

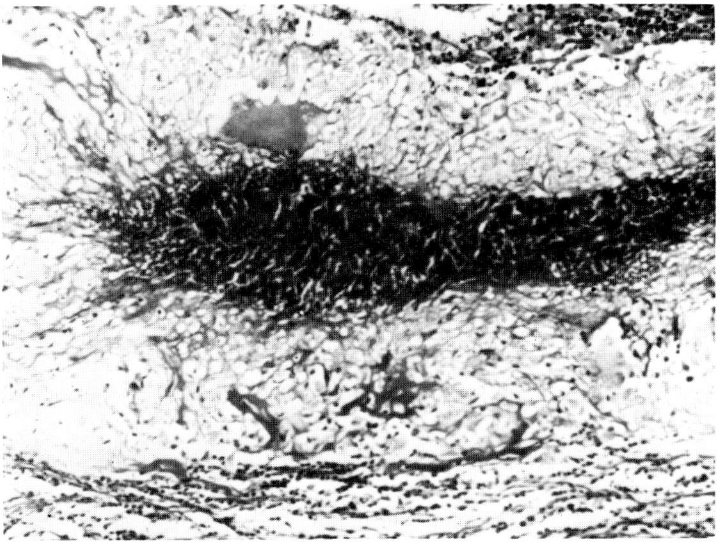

FIG. 7.33 Caseous focus in a tuberculous lymph node stained by erythrosin at pH 9.0; anionophilic protein in the caseous zone and in an adjacent necrotic giant cell is intensely coloured. × 165. From (1967) *Proc. roy. Soc. Med.* **60**, 271.

to diffusion of RNA out of the fully permeable cell remnants, or to enzymic fission by ribonuclease, is uncertain. Loss of DNA in karyolysis may also result from diffusion of DNA out of the fully permeable cell after release from attachment to histone, or may be a sequel to fission of DNA by desoxyribonuclease, once the nuclear membrane is destroyed. During autolysis of mouse liver *in vitro* loss of DNA due to fission by desoxyribonuclease only becomes appreciable after 6 h when nuclei commence to disappear [67].

Protein is more resistant to autolysis than nucleic acids. Autolysis of protein may depend on availability of free water absorbed into the dying cells before the proteolytic enzymes have become denatured. This process is minimal in rapidly killed cells, where semipermeability of the surface membrane is soon destroyed. When injury is not sufficiently severe to destroy this semipermeability, aqueous swelling may occur with entry of water into the injured cell (p. 289). Simultaneously the hydrolytic enzymes may become accessible to their substrates as intracellular compartments disintegrate. Hydrolysis of protein may then ensue along with visible loss of protein from the dying cells. Fig. 7.4 (p. 290) shows the swollen midzonal hepatocytes in rat liver injured by CCl_4 stained by the coupled tetrazonium method. The hydropic cells appear severely depleted of protein [80]. Similar loss of protein with rarefaction of cerebral cortex sometimes occurs as a sequel to ischaemic injury and swelling (p. 302). But the cells may be so rapidly killed that osmotic swelling cannot occur, and this fission of protein is impeded; later the hydrolytic enzymes become denatured and enzymic fission is precluded. Possibly proteins, unlike nucleic acids, cannot dissolve away from permeable dead tissue in the absence of initial enzymic hydrolysis.

Autolysis of protein is probably an important initiating event in demyelination both of transected nerves and in the lesions of demyelinating disease. This effect is considered with aggregation and disintegration of myelin lipids in chapter 8.

Phagocytic cells are specially endowed with capacity for autolysis and self demolition as well as for injuring other cells. This additional autolytic potential depends on the rich assortment of hydrolytic enzymes present in the granules or cytoplasmic vesicles (lysosomes) of phagocytes [82, 83]. When these granules are ruptured, release of hydrolases leads to irreversible cell injury and autolysis, while the liberated enzymes also damage other cells. Such autolytic effects along with injury to other tissues are prominent in the pathogenesis of silicosis (p. 146) and of gout (p. 202) and are probably also concerned in rheumatoid arthritis (p. 209). Moreover, the extremely rapid effect of streptolysin O in killing neutrophils is a direct sequel to rupture of cytoplasmic granules and is probably also determined by action of liberated hydrolases both on cytoplasmic and nuclear components of the cells (p. 227).

Autolysis may also occur in tuberculosis. Although caseous necrosis usually involves persistence of cheesy protein, sometimes this may become liquefied. This happens especially in pulmonary lesions with disastrous spread of infection; the liquefaction may result from activation of lysosomal cathepsin of

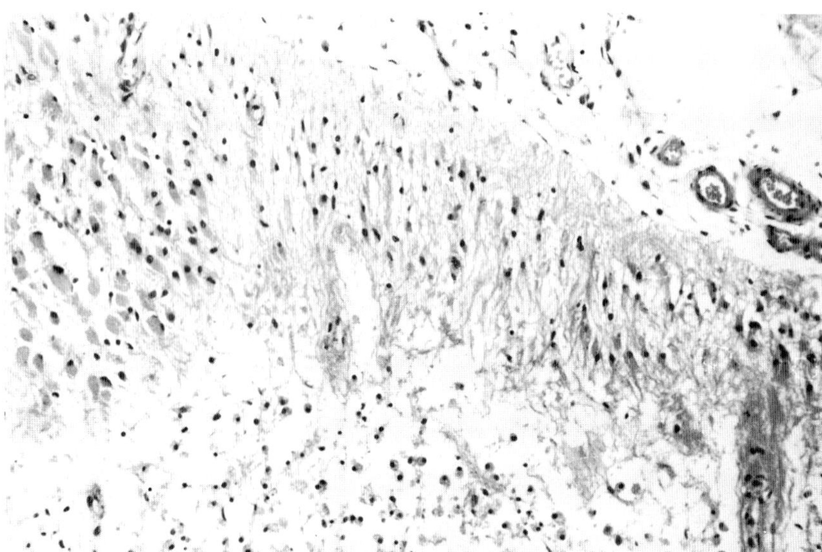

FIG. 7.34 Zone of ischaemic softening of cerebral grey matter near surface of occipital cortex. Cystic spaces containing cerebral macrophages are covered by a dense subpial array of proliferated astrocytic cells and fibres. H & E. × 130.

macrophages, which then autolyse themselves and also destroy the cells around them (p. 241).

Heterolysis

In this process injured or dead cells are consumed and destroyed by *other* cells of the body (*ἕτερος*, other; *λύσις*, solution).

Heterolysis of red cells occurs rapidly when they become coated with antibody containing exposed receptor sites for macrophages. Hepatic and splenic macrophages respectively engulf and destroy antibody-coated red cells after mismatched transfusions and in haemolytic disease of the newborn (p. 205).

Heterolysis is also a sequel to cell death. Thus, when motor neurones of spinal cord and medulla are killed by poliovirus, their surface is so altered that they attract phagocytes and become surrounded by neutrophils and macrophages in a few days (p. 255). Fig. 6.22b shows necrotic spinal anterior horn cells killed by poliovirus: the Nissl substance has disappeared and the shrivelled necrotic cells

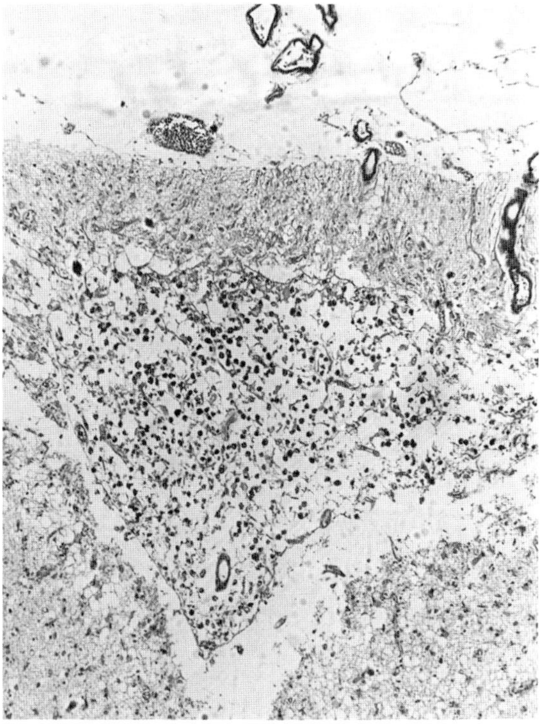

FIG. 7.35 Conical zone of softening in occipital cortex which is the end result of heterolysis of an infarct of grey matter, probably caused by occlusion of a cortical arteriole. The cavities in the softened cortex contain cerebral phagocytes filled with PAS-positive granules. PAS. × 71.

Dixon K. C. (1965). In *Neurohistochemistry*, p. 594, ed. by C. W. M. Adams.

are becoming enveloped by phagocytes which rapidly consume and destroy the cell remnants (neuronophagia, Fig. 6.22c, p. 255).

Heterolysis on a much more extensive scale occurs in cerebral tissue when patients survive the immediate effects of ischaemic or traumatic necrosis of groups of cerebral cells. In these lesions heterolysis of the dead neurones and glial cells is effected throughout the necrotic tissue by invading macrophages derived largely from microglia; in large zones of necrosis this process may last for weeks or months. As the dead cells are consumed the necrotic tissue liquefies into a soft spongy matrix composed of cystic spaces and necrotic remnants along with phagocytic cells. This process is called softening or malacia (μαλακός, soft); it is essentially a post-necrotic phenomenon.

When the process of softening occurs in lesions affecting cerebral *white matter* heterolysis of remnants of myelin is the principal event. This activity will be considered along with other aspects of demyelination in Chapter 8.

Softening of lesions in cerebral *grey matter* is a prominent sequel to ischaemic necrosis both in cerebral and cerebellar cortex. Cystic spaces produced by activity of phagocytes develop in the necrotic zones and enlarge progressively as microglial phagocytes consume the dead neurones and other necrotic cells. These zones of softening and cavitation are usually enveloped by a dense covering formed by proliferating astrocytic cells and fibres (Fig. 7.34). The cystic spaces contain phagocytes stuffed with granules of proteolipid which are

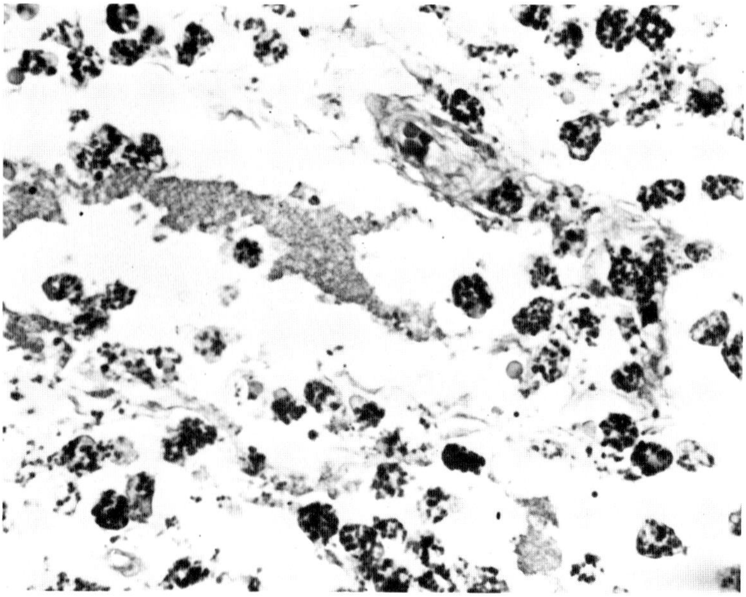

FIG. 7.36 Same tissue as in Fig. 7.35 showing cavities in softened cerebral cortex where phagocytes are consuming neuronal remnants. The phagocytes are filled by sudanophil granules. Sudan black. × 410.

probably indestructible remnants of the vanished neurones; these granules are coloured rose red by PAS [84].

Fig. 7.35 (p. 343) shows a conical zone of softening in occipital cortex stained by PAS. This lesion is the end result of localised ischaemic necrosis of a limited zone of cerebral cortex caused by the occlusion of a small cortical artery. Such ischaemic softening happens when patients survive long enough after vascular occlusion for cerebral phagocytes to destroy most of the necrotic cerebral cells. The central part of this softened cortex is then occupied by cystic spaces containing numerous microglial phagocytes which are darkly stained by PAS (Fig. 7.35) owing to intense colouration of the granules within them. Similar phagocytes in softened cerebral cortex are shown at higher magnification in Fig. 7.36 stained by Sudan black, which also colours the intraphagocytic granules intensely.

A small zone of softening, such as that shown in Fig. 7.35, can result from an isolated ischaemic lesion which of itself produces little or no clinical disability; if neuronal necrosis is more extensive or affects specialised areas of the cortex, then tragic loss of function may follow with paresis, urinary incompetence or coma, typical of apoplectic strokes. Widespread and extensive ischaemic necrosis of cerebral cortex can also produce disorder of memory and behaviour terminating in 'arteriopathic dementia'. If the patient lives long enough, in spite of hemiplegia, dementia or coma, then softening with heterolysis of the dead neurones by cerebral phagocytes similarly follows these more serious lesions. Finally granules of proteolipid (p. 405) within the phagocytes are the only remnants of the vanished neurones; these persist when all else is gone.

The thorns he spares when the rose is taken;
the rocks he leaves when he wastes the plain.
The wind that wanders, the weeds wind-shaken,
these remain.

Algernon Charles Swinburne.

REFERENCES

[1] SINGER S. J. & NICHOLSON G. L. (1972) The fluid mozaic model of the structure of cell membranes. *Science*, **175**, 720.
[2] BASSI M. & BERNELLI-ZAZZERA A. (1964) Ultrastructural cytoplasmic changes of liver cells after reversible and irreversible ischemia. *Exp. mol. Path.*, **3**, 332.
[3] CONWAY E. J. & MCCORMACK J. I. (1953) The total intracellular concentration of mammalian tissues compared with that of the extracellular fluid. *J. Physiol.*, **120**, 1.
[4] CONWAY E. J., GEOGHEGAN H. & MCCORMACK J. I. (1955) Autolytic changes at zero centigrade in ground mammalian tissues. *J. Physiol.*, **130**, 427.
[5] MUDGE G. (1951) Electrolyte and water metabolism of rabbit kidney slices: effect of metabolic inhibitors. *Amer. J. Physiol.*, **167**, 206.
[6] LEAF A. (1956) On the mechanism of fluid exchange of tissues *in vitro*. *Biochem. J.*, **62**, 241.
[7] ROBINSON J. R. (1960) Metabolism of intracellular water. *Physiol. Rev.*, **40**, 112.
[8] OBERLING C. (1959) The structure of cytoplasm. *Int. Rev. Cytol.*, **8**, 1.
[9] BASSI M. (1960) Electron microscopy of rat liver after carbon tetrachloride poisoning. *Exp. Cell Res.*, **20**, 313.

[10] GREEN H., BARROW P. & GOLDBERG B. (1959) Effect of antibody and complement on permeability control in ascites tumour cells and erythrocytes. *J. exp. Med.*, **110**, 699.

[11] LACHMANN P. J. (1975) In *Clinical Aspects of Immunology*, p. 329, ed. by P. G. H. Gell & R. R. A. Coombs. Blackwell, Oxford.

[12] BORSOS T., DOURMASHKIN R. R., & HUMPHREY J. H. (1964) Lesions in erythrocyte membranes caused by immune haemolysis. *Nature*, **202**, 251.

[13] LACHMANN P. J., MUNN E. A. & WEISSMANN G. (1970) Complement-mediated lysis of liposomes produced by reactive lysis procedure. *Immunol.*, **19**, 983.

[14] LACHMANN P. J., BOWYER D. E., NICOL P., DAWSON R. M. C. & MUNN E. A. (1973) Studies on the terminal stages of complement lysis. *Immunol.*, **24**, 135.

[15] KERR J. F. R. (1971) Shrinkage necrosis: a distinct mode of cell death. *J. Path.*, **105**, 13.

[16] KERR J. F. R., WYLLIE A. H. & CURRIE A. R. (1972) Apoptosis: a basic biological phenomenon with widespread implications in tissue kinetics. *Brit. J. Cancer*, **26**, 239.

[17] GILLMAN J. & GILLMAN T. (1949) Anoxia and the liver, with special reference to shock and chronic malnutrition. *Amer. J. dig. Dis.*, **16**, 348.

[18] BREWER D. B. & HEATH D. (1965) Electron microscopy of anoxic vacuolation in the liver cell and its comparison with sucrose vacuolation. *J. Path. Bact.*, **90**, 437.

[19] DIXON K. C. (1964) Rolled films of dying liver cells. *Brit. J. exp. Path.*, **45**, 481.

[20] DIXON K. C. (1967) Events in dying cells. *Proc. roy. Soc. Med.*, **60**, 271.

[21] TRUMP B. J., GOLDBLATT P. J. & STOWELL R. E. (1962) An electron microscopic study of early cytoplasmic alterations in hepatic parenchymal cells of mouse liver during necrosis *in vitro* (autolysis). *Lab. Invest.*, **11**, 986.

[22] CAJONE F., RAGNOTTI G., BERNELLI-ZAZZERA A. & BASSI M. (1971) State and function of liver polysomes during recovery from ischaemia. *Exp. molec. Path.*, **14**, 392.

[23] CAULFIELD J. & KLIONSKY B. (1959) Myocardial ischaemia and early infarction: an EM study. *Amer. J. Path.*, **35**, 489.

[24] KLONER R. A., GANOTE C. E., WHALEN D. A. & JENNINGS R. B. (1974) Effect of a transient period of ischemia on myocardial cells. 2. Fine structure during the first few minutes of reflow. *Amer. J. Path.*, **74**, 399.

[25] BOUCHARDY B. & MAJNO G. (1974) Histopathology of early myocardial infarcts. A new approach. *Amer. J. Path.*, **74**, 301.

[26] DERIAS N. W. & ADAMS C. W. M. (1979) The non-specific nature of the myocardial wavy fibre. *Histopath.*, **3**, 241.

[27] ADAMS C. W. M. (1967) in *Vascular Histochemistry*, p. 229, Lloyd-Luke, London.

[28] SCHNITKA T. K. & NACHLAS M. M. (1963) Histochemical alterations in ischaemic heart muscle and early myocardial infarction. *Amer. J. Path.*, **42**, 507.

[29] KENT S. P. (1966) Intracellular plasma protein: a manifestation of cell injury in myocardial infarction. *Nature*, **210**, 1279.

[30] VAN HARREVELD A. (1957) Changes in volume of cortical neuronal elements during asphyxiation. *Amer. J. Physiol.*, **191**, 233.

[31] VAN HARREVELD A. & SCHADÉ J. P. (1959) Chloride movements in cerebral cortex after circulatory arrest and during spreading depression. *J. cell comp. Physiol.*, **54**, 65.

[32] VAN HARREVELD A. (1961) Asphyxial changes in cerebellar cortex. *J. cell comp. Physiol.*, **57**, 101.

[33] TUREEN L. L. (1936) Effect of experimental temporary vascular occlusion on the spinal cord. 1. Correlation between structural and functional change. *Arch. Neurol. Psychiat . (Chic.)*, **35**, 789.

[34] KROGH E. (1945) Effect of acute anoxia on the large motor cells in the spinal cord. *Acta Jutlandica*, suppl. **17**.

[35] KROGH E. (1950) The effect of acute hypoxia on the motor cells of the spinal cord. Acta Physiol. scand., **20**, 263.

[36] Spielmeyer W. (1922) *Histopathologie des Nervensystems*. Springer, Berlin.
[37] Scholz W. & Hager H. (1959) Toxicity changes in the central nervous system: 2. Electronoptic studies on the earliest structural changes of the brain caused by hypoxidosis. *Tech. Rep. Contract AF 61*, USAF European Office.
[38] Brown A. W. & Brierley J. B. (1968) The nature, distribution and earliest stages of anoxic-ischaemic nerve cell damage in the rat brain as defined by the optical microscope. *Brit. J. exp. Path.*, **49**, 87.
[39] Brown A. W. (1977) Structural abnormalities in neurones. *J. clin. Path.* suppl. 30, **11**, 155.
[40] Dixon K. C. (1965) Ischaemia and the neurone. In *Neurohistochemistry*, p. 558, ed. by C. W. M. Adams. Elsevier, Amsterdam.
[41] Walker A. E., Diamond E. L. & Moseley J. (1975) The neuropathological findings in irreversible coma. A critique of the 'respirator brain'. *J. Neuropath.*, **34**, 295.
[42] Matakas F., Cervos-Navarro J. & Schneider H. (1973) Experimental brain death. 1. Morphology and fine structure of the brain. *J. Neurol. Neurosurg. Psychiat.*, **36**, 497.
[43] Spector R. G. (1961) Water content of the brain in anoxic ischaemic encephalopathy in adult rats. *Brit. J. exp. Path.*, **42**, 623.
[44] Alajouanine T., Hornet T. & Thurel R. (1936) L'aspect fenêtré de l'écorce cérébrale (contribution à l'étude des troubles circulatoires localisés à certaines couches cellulaires). *Rev. Neurol.*, **65**, 819.
[45] Dixon K. C. (1955) Cytochemistry of the cortical ground substance in apoplexy. *J. Path. Bact.*, **69**, 251.
[46] Ashton N. (1970) Pathophysiology of retinal cotton wool spots. *Brit. med. Bull.*, **26**, 143.
[47] Ashton N. (1959) Diabetic retinopathy, a new approach. *Lancet*, **2**, 625.
[48] Kerr J. F. R. *et al.* (1979) The nature of piecemeal necrosis in chronic active hepatitis. *Lancet*, **2**, 827.
[49] Mann G. (1895) Histological changes induced in sympathetic, motor and sensory nerve cells by functional activity. *J. Anat. Physiol.*, **29**, 100.
[50] Einarson L. & Krogh E. (1955) Variations in the basophilia of nerve cells associated with increased activity and functional stress. *J. Neurol. Neurosurg. Psychiat.*, **18**, 1.
[51] Marinesco G. (1896) Lésions de la moelle épinière consécutives à la ligature de l'aorte abdominale. *C. R. Soc. Biol. (Paris)*, **3**, 250.
[52] Slim A. C. & Jennings R. B. (1972) Myocardial calcium and magnesium in acute ischaemic injury. *Amer. J. Path.*, **67**, 417.
[53] Gräff S. (1912) Die naphtholblau-oxydasereaktion der gewebszellen nach untersuchungen am unfixierten präparat. *Frankfurt. Z. Path.*, **11**, 358.
[54] Becker J. D. (1961) The cytochemistry of anoxic-ischaemic encephalopathy in rats. 2. Alterations in the neuronal mitochondria identified by diphosphopyridine and triphosphopyridine nucleotide diaphorases. *Amer. J. Path.*, **38**, 587.
[55] Spector R. G. (1965) Enzyme chemistry of anoxic brain injury. In *Neurohistochemistry*, p. 547, ed. by C. W. M. Adams. Elsevier, Amsterdam.
[56] Moore D. H., Ruska H. & Copenhaver W. M. (1956) Electron microscopic and histochemical observations of muscle degeneration after tourniquet. *J. Biophys. Biochem. Cytol.*, **2**, 755.
[57] Davies M. J. & Jennings R. B. (1970) The ultrastructure of myocardium in the thiamine deficient rat. *J. Path.*, **102**, 87.
[58] Kerr J. F. R. (1965) A histochemical study of hypertrophy and ischaemic injury of rat liver with special reference to changes in lysosomes. *J. Path. Bact.*, **90**, 419.
[59] Becker J. D. & Baron K. D. (1961) The cytochemistry of anoxic-ischaemic encephalopathy. 1. Alterations in neuronal lysosomes identified by acid phosphatase activity. *Amer. J. Path.*, **38**, 161.

[60] HIRSCH J. G. (1962) Cinematographic observations on granule lysis in polymorphonuclear leucocytes with continuing locomotion of cells. *J. exp. Med.*, **116**, 827.
[61] HAWKINS H., ERICSON K., BIBERFIELD J. L. E. & TRUMP B. F. (1972) Lysosomes and phagosome stability in lethal cell injury. *Amer. J. Path.*, **68**, 255.
[62] TERRY R. D., GONATAS N. K. & WEISS M. (1964) Ultrastructural studies in Alzheimer's presenile dementia. *Amer. J. Path.*, **44**, 269.
[63] CORSELLIS J. A. N. (1976) Ageing and the dementias. In *Greenfield's Neuropathology*, 3rd Ed., p. 816, ed. by W. Blackwood & J. A. N. Corsellis. Arnold, London.
[64] LEUCHTENBERGER C. (1950) A cytochemical study of pyknotic nuclear degeneration. *Chromosoma*, **3**, 449.
[65] KORSON R. (1951) A microspectrophometric study of red cell nuclei during pyknosis. *J. exp. Med.*, **96**, 121.
[66] DIXON K. C. (1958) Protein and nucleic acid in caseous necrosis. *Amer. Rev.. Tuberc.*, **77**, 106.
[67] VAN LANCKER J. & HOLTZER R. L. (1962) The fate of nuclei, DNA and DNA-ase in the course of autolysis. *Lab. Invest.*, **12**, 102.
[68] BAUER F. W. & DE GROOD R. M. (1975) Impulse cytophotometry in psoriasis. *Brit. J. Derm.*, **93**, 225.
[69] HARDIE R. A. & HUNTER J. A. A. (1978) Dermatology: psoriasis. *Brit. J. Hosp. Med.*, **20**, 13.
[70] MERCER E. H. & MAIBACH H. I. (1968) Intercellular adhesion and surface coats of epidermal cells in psoriasis. *J. invest. Derm.*, **51**, 204.
[71] ORFANOS C. E., SCHAUENBERG-LEVER G., MAHRLE G. & LEVER W. F. (1973) Alterations of cell surface as a pathogenic factor in psoriasis. *Arch. Derm.*, **107**, 38.
[72] DIXON K. C., GRESHAM G. A. & WHITTLE C. H. (1962) Psoriasis: a disorder of necrosis. *Brit. J. Derm.*, **74**, 283.
[73] WILDY P., SMITH C., NEWTON A. A. & DENDY P. (1961) Quantitative cytological studies on Hela cells infected with herpes virus. *Virology*, **15**, 486.
[74] BLOOM A. D. (1972) Induced chromosome aberrations in man. *Advance. hum. Genet.*, **3**, 99.
[75] NICHOLS W. W. (1970) Virus induced chromosomal abnormalities. *Ann. Rev. Microbiol.*, **24**, 479.
[76] HARNDEN D. G. (1974) Viruses, chromosomes and tumors: the interaction between viruses and chromosomes. In *Chromosomes and Cancer*, p. 152, ed. by J. German. Wiley, New York.
[77] DIXON K. C. (1956) Persistence of protein in infarcts. *J. Path. Bact.*, **71**, 37.
[78] WELLS H. G. (1925) *Chemical Pathology*, 5th Ed., p. 83 and 443. Saunders, Philadelphia.
[79] MAJNO G., LA GATTUTA M. & THOMPSON T. E. (1960) Cellular death and necrosis: chemical, physical and morphological changes in rat liver. *Virchows Arch. path. Anat.*, **333**, 421.
[80] DIXON K. C. & MCCULLAGH G. P. (1957) Protein in dying liver cells. *Quart. J. exp. Physiol.*, **42**, 104.
[81] REYNOLDS E. S. & REE H. J. (1971) Liver parenchymal cell injury. VII Membrane denaturation following carbon tetrachloride. *Lab. Invest.*, **25**, 269.
[82] ALLISON A. C. (1978) Lysosomes in pathology. In *Recent Advances in Histopathology*, p. 69, ed. by P. P. Anthony & N. Woolf. Churchill Livingstone, Edinburgh.
[83] BAINTON D. F. (1973) Sequential degranulation of the two types of polymorphonuclear leucocyte granules during phagocytosis of micro-organisms. *J. cell. Biol.*, **58**, 249.
[84] DIXON K. C. (1953) Cytochemical changes in the necrotic grey matter of the brain. *J. Path. Bact.*, **66**, 251

CHAPTER 8

Intracellular Globulation and Aggregation

In this kind of derangement globules of liquid lipids, granular solids, or complex membranous micelles become visible in the affected cells.

These globules and aggregates are usually composed of substances which are sufficiently hydrophobic or insoluble to coalesce and form large multimolecular assemblies visible by LM or EM. These deposited materials include liquids such as fat and cholesterol esters as well as colloidal aggregates composed of proteolipids, glycolipids, polysaccharides and proteins.

Globulation or aggregation may be initiated within the cell by:

1. Interference with solubilisation or dispersion of hydrophobic or colloidal substances.

2. Accumulation of these substances in such excess that they cannot be held in solubilised or dispersed state. Interference with solubilisation may so retard utilisation and excretion that accumulation in excess becomes a consequence as well as a cause of deposition and may then determine further deposition (p. 357).

Interference with solubilisation or dispersion may be caused by lack of solubilising agents or by inherited structural defects in colloidal molecules, which are essential for their dispersion. Inherited defects in composition of the globin molecule lead to the formation of unstable haemoglobins which are hydrophobic and aggregate as visible inclusions within red cells (see Fig. 2.3, p. 25).

Accumulation in excess follows *either* acceleration of entry or formation, *or* retardation of utilisation and removal. Excessive ingress of fat in animals fed on fatty diets may thus produce spectacular fatty globulation in hepatic cells (see Fig. 8.4). Inert carbon particles or cytotoxic crystals like SiO_2 (in silicosis) may similarly be engulfed by macrophages and remain within them till their death. Massive synthesis and deposition of proteins and nucleic acids, as a result of viral replication and assembly, may determine the formation of conspicuous inclusion bodies either in cytoplasm or nucleus (see Figs. 6.25 and 6.29). Retardation of utilisation and excretion can be a disastrous consequence of inherited absence of lysosomal hydrolases, which are responsible for stages in the sequential catabolism of macromolecules such as glycolipids or polysaccharides; without catabolic enzymes these macromolecules may accumulate and bloat the cells into monstrous or bizarre forms (see Fig. 8.39).

In the ensuing chapter examples of intracellular globulation and aggregation and their harmful consequences will be discussed:

1. Fatty globulation and its mechanism.
2. Fatty globulation in disease.
3. Hepatic cirrhosis caused by intracellular globulation and aggregation.
4. Deposition of lipids in arterial walls: atherosclerosis.
5. Disintegration of meylin.
6. Aggregation and accumulation of complex lipids: Tay–Sachs disease.
7. Accumulation of polysaccharides in disease.
8. Excessive deposition of protein.

FATTY GLOBULATION

The appearance of visible droplets of fat (triglyceride) in the cytoplasm is one of the most prominent features of disordered cells. In health such droplets are usually sparse or absent in the normal cells of heart muscle, liver and kidney. However, even when no fat is discernible in a form capable of dissolving dyestuffs of the Sudan group, these cells may contain some invisible or concealed fat; this can be extracted from the tissues by mixtures of lipid solvents and estimated by chemical methods.

The lipocytes of areolar tissue, on the other hand, are filled by droplets of liquid fat which have the capacity to dissolve the Sudan dyes. This visible fat displays the properties of a liquid which forms a separate phase from the rest of the cytoplasm.

Cells which in health contain little or no visible fat may in disease contain spherical droplets of liquid fat in abundance; this fat, like that of the lipocytes, is in a form capable of being coloured by the Sudan dyes and may conveniently be termed globular fat. This appearance of globular fat is referred to as fatty change or fatty globulation.

State of cellular fat

Fats and oils are not soluble in water but in the cell, as in plasma, they may be solubilised so as to be invisible by LM. Triglycerides (TG), being hydrophobic, are prevented from solution in water by enormous interfacial forces. Invisible fat can only be dissolved by a process called solubilisation. Solubilisation was defined by McBain [1] as the spontaneous passage of molecules of a substance insoluble in water into a dilute aqueous solution of a solubiliser to form a thermodynamically stable solution. A solubiliser can only act in this way if it can form micelles (or clusters) of aggregated molecules, which then dissolve within them the water-insoluble oil. In this way an oil can be held in stable solution in water.

Micellar fat

Substances which in aqueous solution are capable of aggregating to form clusters or micelles contain both polar and non-polar groups. These molecules are termed amphipathic to indicate their duality of affinity; they contain both a hydrophilic (polar) portion which tends to dissolve in water and a lipophilic (non-polar) portion which tends to dissolve in oil and to be excluded from contact with water [2]. Such amphipathic substances are concentrated at surfaces and interfaces where they exert profound effects on surface behaviour. For this reason they are also called surfactants to denote their intense surface activity, upon which also depends their capacity to form micelles.

An amphipathic substance with a polar group and a non-polar hydrocarbon chain of the type shown in Fig. 8.1 exists only as single molecules in very dilute aqueous solution. Such compounds are attracted to surfaces, and when their concentration rises the tendency to aggregation becomes irresistible, so that micelles or clusters are formed. In these micelles the hydrophilic polar part is in contact with water, but the hydrophobic non-polar part is occluded internally within the micelles (Fig. 8.1).

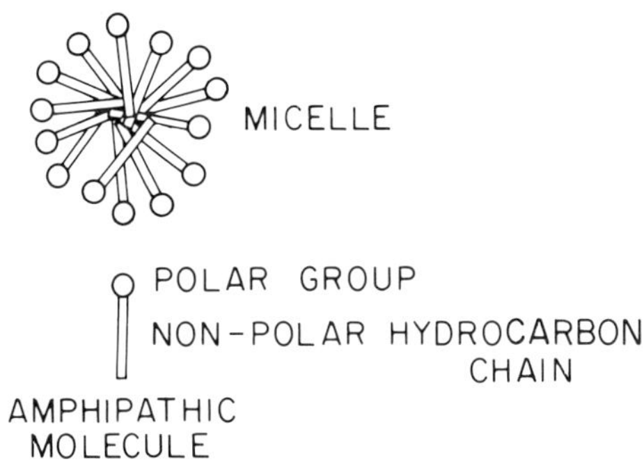

FIG. 8.1 Single amphipathic molecule (below), and micelle (above) composed of a cluster of aggregated amphipathic molecules. From (1973) *Histochem. J.* **5**, 363.

Hydrophobic substances can dissolve in the inner parts of these micellar clusters. In this way fats and oils can be solubilised by amphipathic soaps to form stable solutions in which no liquid droplets are visible by LM. It is likely that fats in the body can similarly be solubilised within micelles composed of amphipathic phospholipids and protein and can thus be held in optically invisible form both in cells and in plasma. This solubilised or *micellar fat* includes very low density lipoprotein (VLDL) of plasma and similar micelles of liver cells which, although invisible by LM, can enlarge enough to be discernible by EM. Such micelles (diameter 30–80 nm) are found within the Golgi and ER vesicles of rat liver [3] and have been separated and shown to contain tryglyceride, phospholipid, cholesterol and protein and to have a chemical composition resembling that of VLDL from plasma of the same rats [4].

Moreover these hepatic particles form lines of identity with VLDL on immunodiffusion in agar against antibody to VLDL; these particles may therefore be the direct precursors of VLDL. Micellar fat in cells may, like VLDL, consist of a central core of hydrophobic neutral lipids surrounded by a surface film of protein and polar lipids [5] or it may be composed of laminar and vesicular micelles of these amphipathic substances in which hydrophobic triglyceride molecoles are separately solubilised (Fig. 8.2).

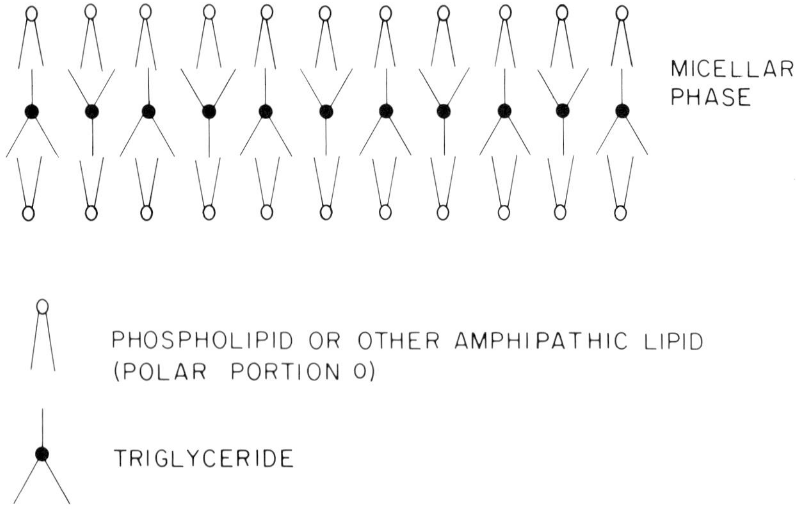

FIG. 8.2 Possible disposition of triglyceride (TG) molecules in micellar or hidden fat. When large enough to be seen by EM such micelles may extend to form multimolecular assemblies or to cover aqueous vesicles. For simplicity portions of peptide chains which may contribute to solubilization of TG are not shown.

Globular fat

When visible globules of fat are present in cells they exist either as single spheres surrounded by cytoplasmic pellicles, as in areolar tissue, or as separate globules forming the oil phase of an emulsion in which the surrounding cytoplasm constitutes the aqueous phase. Whether the globules are large or small depends on the capacity of the amphipathic surfactants in the cell to act as emulsifiers and form closely packed molecules arrayed as a condensed film at right angles to the oil/water interface (Fig. 8.3). In this way a stable emulsion can be formed.

Emulsification and solubilisation are entirely distinct processes. An amphipathic surfactant such as a soap can emulsify an oil, but the surfactant, provided it can form micelles, can also solubilise the oil. However, the property of forming an effective unimolecular film, on which emulsification depends (Fig. 8.3), may not be possessed by cellular surfactants, which nevertheless can solubilise and occlude hydrophobic molecules when these are present in limited

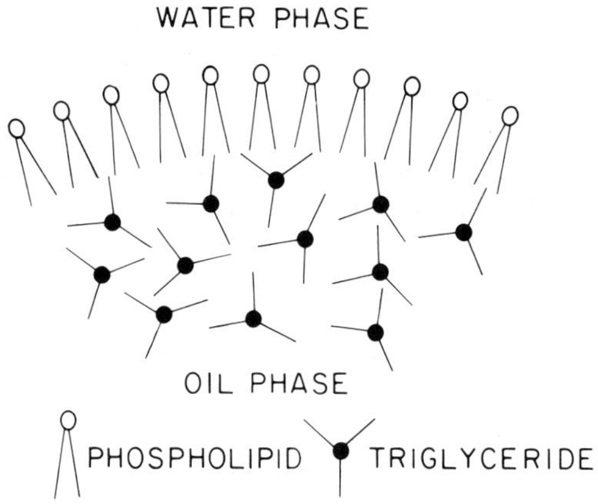

FIG. 8.3 Possible disposition of triglyceride molecules in globular or visible fat.

amount. Thus an amphipathic substance may be efficient as a solubiliser but inadequate as an emulsifier; in this case relatively large globules of fat appear once an oil phase is formed.

When the quantity of hydrophobic fat in cells exceeds the limited amount which can be solubilised in micelles or lipoprotein complexes, a third (oil) phase suddenly appears where before there was only an aqueous phase and a micellar

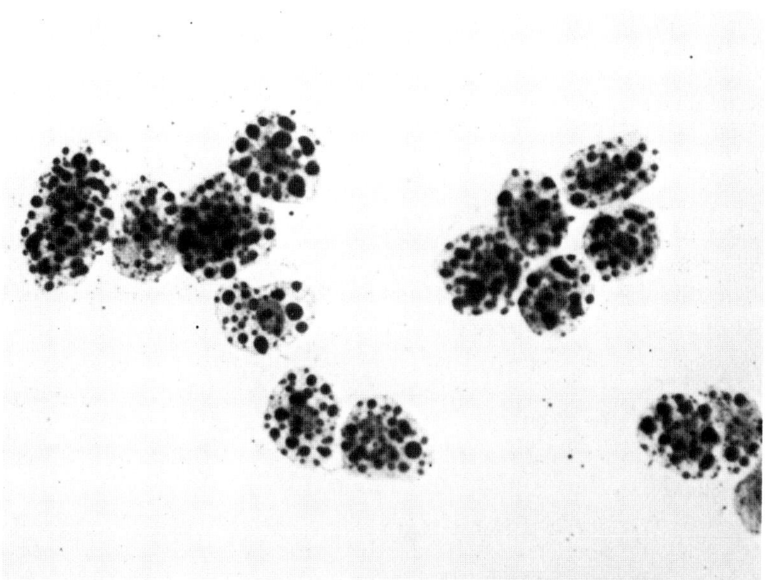

FIG. 8.4 Hepatocytes in a rolled film of liver from a rat fed on margarine and water for 3 days: each cell contains numerous globules of sudanophil lipid. Fixation formol-saline, stained Sudan III–IV & H. × 400.

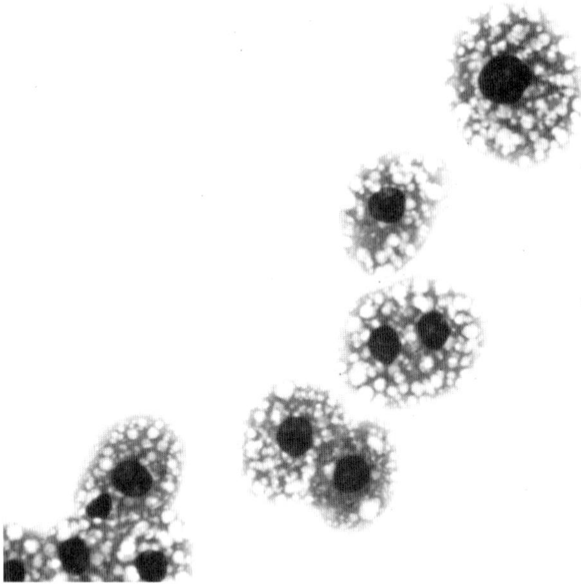

FIG. 8.5 Hepatocytes in a rolled film of same tissue shown in Fig. 8.4: each cell is filled by spherical vacuoles from which globular lipid has been dissolved by fixation in ethanol. H & E. × 400. Dixon K. C. & King A. J. (1970) *Histochem. J.*, **4**, 111.

phase. This oil phase is composed of visible droplets. Such emulsions are formed rapidly in the liver cells of rats fed with margarine as their sole food for 1–3 days. This abrupt and spectacular formation of an oil phase is shown by LM in Fig. 8.4 and 8.5 and by EM in Fig. 8.6a. Since the cellular amphipathic solubilisers are not necessarily good emulsifiers, the establishment of this oil phase may be followed by coalescence of microdroplets to form relatively large globules with minimum interfacial surface. The droplets of fat probably enlarge by coalescence until each can be completely enclosed by a unimolecular film of phospholipid and other amphipaths which can hold the hydrophobic TG out of contact with water.

Determinants of fatty globulation

The ratio of fat to phospholipid may thus play a critical part in determining whether globules of fat occur in a cell or not. Excess of fat beyond the amount which can be solubilised in lipoprotein micelles causes globular fat to appear. Similarly lack of phospholipid or of the proteins which participate in the formation of micelles promotes the same transition from micellar to globular fat. As soon as globular fat makes its appearance there exists a potential equilibrium between it and micellar fat (Fig. 8.7).

In some normal cells this equilibrium is not reached, since all the triglycerides

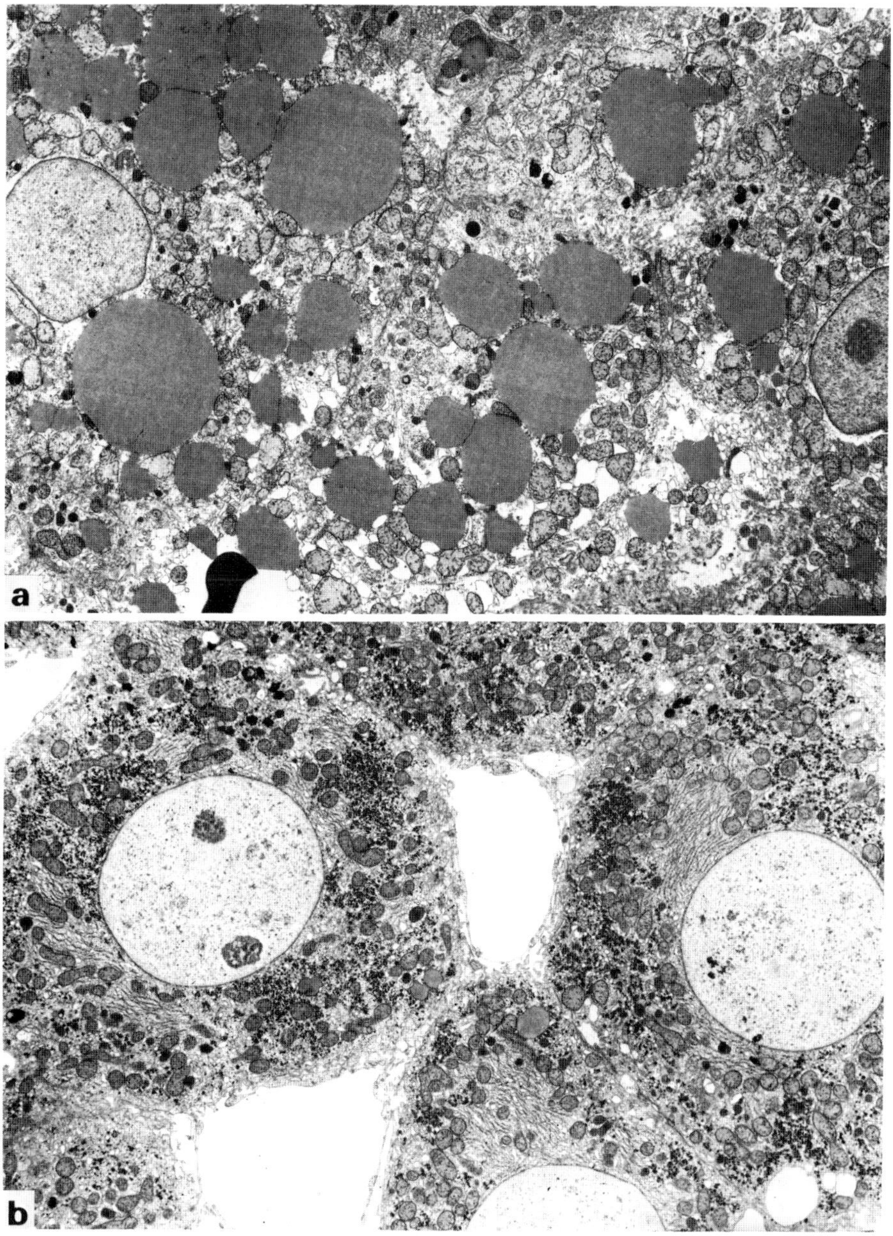

FIG. 8.6a Hepatocytes from liver of rat fed on margarine for 3 days. Fixed OsO_4. EM × 3000. The cytoplasm of each of two adjoining hepatocytes contains prominent spheroidal droplets of globular lipid 0.5–5 μm in diameter. Part of a blackened red cell is seen in a sinusoid at the lower margin of field. (b) Hepatocytes from liver of rat fed on stock diet. Fixed OsO_4. EM × 3100. Courtesy of Dr B. M. Herbertson & Mrs Jean Wardle).

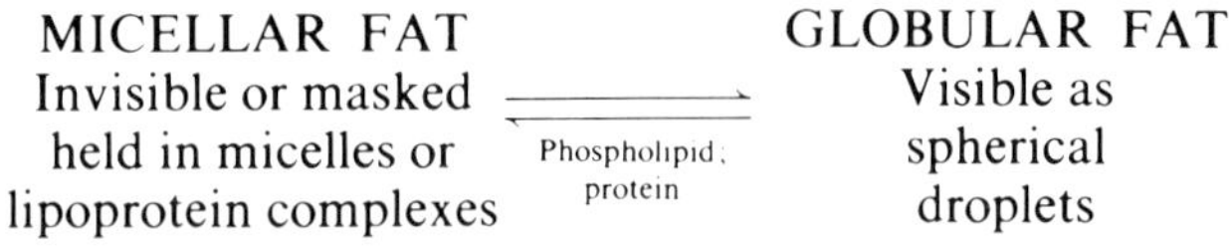

FIG. 8.7 Equilibrium between micellar and globular fat.

are solubilised. This is probably the situation in healthy cells of heart muscle and kidney and in the majority of liver cells. In lipocytes of adipose tissue, on the other hand, an equilibrium between micellar and globular fat is usually in operation [6, 7]; in these cells fat is located in two cellular compartments, a small compartment containing micellar fat associated with other cytoplasmic constituents, and a large compartment of visible globular fat which ultimately expands into a single large globule surrounded by a tenuous film of cytoplasm.

Visible globular fat is temporarily at least outside the zone of active transport and metabolism. Micellar fat, on the other hand, is readily available for transport out of the cell and also for participating in enzymic reactions within the cell. Experiments with lipocytes in adipose tissue support this concept of the dynamic reactivity of micellar fat. Thus centrifugal fractionation of lipocytes previously exposed to [I-^{14}C] palmitate, supplied as a complex with serum albumin, shows that the solubilised cytoplasmic fat rapidly incorporates the

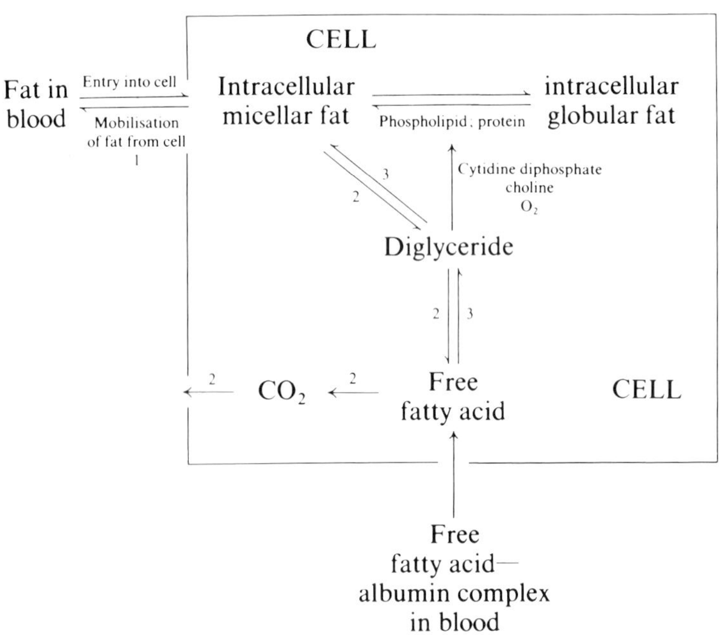

FIG. 8.8 Intracellular relation between micellar and globular fat. Micellar fat is probably the form which is (1) transported from the cell, (2) hydrolysed and oxidised, and (3) formed *de novo* from free fatty acid and carbohydrate.

radioative palmitate, while the lighter globular fat in the supernatant assimilates it only slowly. Moreover the solubilised micellar fat of the cytoplasm has a much more rapid turnover than the fat present in the supernatant liquid globules.

This dynamic position of micellar fat in cellular economy is illustrated in Fig. 8.8. Micellar fat is probably the form in which fat is:

1. Transported out of the cell (route 1).
2. Hydrolysed to free fatty acid (FFA) and then oxidised (route 2).
3. Formed *de novo* in the cell from FFA (route 3).

The concept of an equilibrium between micellar and globular fat, as well as the realisation that micellar fat is the form used in mobilisation and metabolism, helps to envisage the mechanisms of fatty globulation in disease [8]. Visible droplets of fat are probably formed when a certain ratio of fat to phospholipid and protein is surpassed or if the action of these solubilisers is impeded. It is thus clear that fatty globulation can arise in two principal ways:

1. By interference with solubilisation of fat, either from diminution in available phospholipid and protein, or annulment of their solubilising power.
2. By quantitative excess of fat above the amount that can be solubilised in micelles or lipoprotein complexes.

Interference with solubilisation of fat

As solubilised or micellar fat is the form which is metabolised within the cell and excreted from it, interference with solubilisation will clearly cause a rapid accumulation of fat, so long as fat is being formed within the cell; this fat will then aggregate into lipid globules as it cannot be solubilised. Thus, if the cell continues to synthesise TG *de novo* from FFA or carbohydrate, then defect in solubilisation will ultimately cause very substantial deposition. Indeed fatty change produced by cell injury is generally most prominent in those cells where damage is not so severe as to annul synthetic mechanisms [9].

Interference with solubilisation results from lack of solubilisers or from inhibition of their solubilising power.

Lack of solubilisers

The ability of an amphipathic substance to form micelles is lost when its concentration falls below a critical micellar concentration. At this level clusters cannot form and thus solubilisation within them is abolished. Thus when solubilising substances are in very low concentration fat aggregates into liquid globules. Phospholipids and proteins are probably the most important cellular solubilisers for fat.

Deficiency of phospholipid may result from lack of phospholipids themselves in the diet or from lack of choline or inositol which provide integral parts of phospholipid molecules. Lack of choline in the diet of mice and rats causes intense fatty globulation in liver and heart muscle [10, 11]. Moreover a diet high in fat causes a slight increase of triglycerides (TG) in liver of rats; the same diet, if lacking in choline, evokes an enormous increase in TG [12]. Probably the synthesis of phospholipid from choline is responsible for solubilisation of TG in micelles, which contain *both* phospholipid and protein and are similar in composition to VLDL. Thus the presence of phospholipid enables TG to be utilised in metabolism and transport. Proteins may replace choline in the diet because methionine in the proteins can provide labile methyl groups necessary for the synthesis of choline. Lack of protein may thus contribute to lack of phospholipid and so cause defect in solubilisation.

Since protein as well as phospholipid is probably an essential constituent of micelles (or lipoproteins) which solubilise fat, *lack of protein* may itself impede solubilisation. Lack of protein may thus cause fatty globulation quite apart from its action in retarding synthesis of phospholipids. Thus, when rats are fed a diet deficient in protein, globules of fat rapidly appear in the periportal hepatic cells, even when the diet is supplemented by choline [13]. Moreover, fatty globulation due to lack of protein commences in the periportal cells of the hepatic lobules in contrast to fatty globulation due to lack of choline, which is initially centrilobular in position. Visible fatty globulation also occurs in the livers of malnourished children in tropical countries (p. 368). Lack of protein in the diet may thus interfere with the hepatic synthesis of 'acceptor' protein, which is necessary for formation and excretion of fat in plasma lipoptoteins elaborated by the liver [14]; this protein is probably an essential participant in the solubilisation of TG to form micellar fat which is then excreted from the liver as VLDL (pre-β-lipoprotein).

Hypoxia may also diminish the supply of solubilisers. Thus the synthesis of phospholipid measured by incorporation of ^{32}P into tissue lipids of liver slices is inhibited by anoxia and also by cyanide which eliminates respiration [15]. Hypoxia probably interferes with synthesis of cytidine diphosphate choline which is the essential donator of activated choline needed for the synthesis of phospholipid. Hypoxia may also retard the synthesis of protein, another participant in the solubilisation of fat.

Lack of solubilisers may thus be an important factor in fatty globulation.

Inhibition of solubilising power

Impairment of the ability of phospholipid to form micelles may be responsible for conversion of micellar to globular fat [8, 16]. Micelles of an amphipathic substance can in fact only form when its concentration reaches a certain level—the critical micellar concentration. Any factor which raises the critical micellar concentration of an amphipath diminishes its solubilising power by restricting the capacity to form micelles.

Carbon tetrachloride (CCl_4) administered to rats causes lipoperoxidation of the lipids in the microsomal fraction of rat liver [17] this change may occur in the phospholipids of the ER. Recknagel [18] suggested that this lipoperoxidation interrupts the formation and excretion of lipoprotein by the ER cisternal system. However, decrease in hydrocarbon chain length of an amphipathic substance by even one CH_2 group doubles the critical micellar concentration and so halves the efficacy of the amphipath as a solubiliser. In this way cleavage or

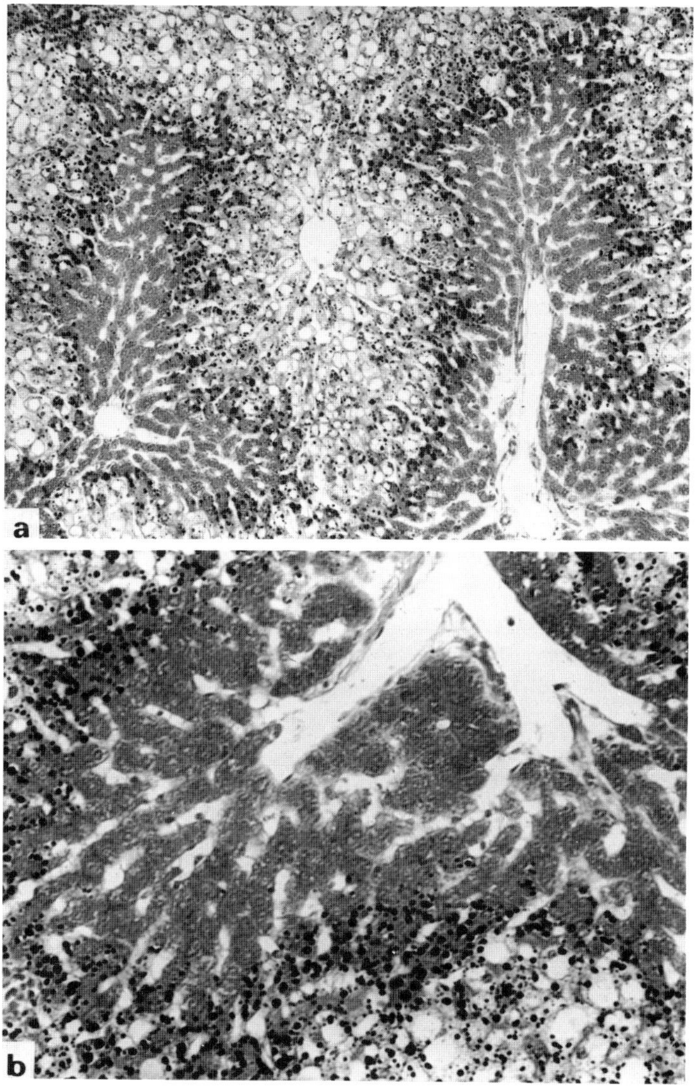

FIG. 8.9 Wax-embedded section from rat fed approximately 2.5 g of CCl_4 over 2 days. Fixative contained OsO_4 which has blackened the globules of liquid lipid; counterstained with pyronin.

a. × 100. Numerous droplets of blackened lipid are prominent in the outer midzonal cells. Some lipid droplets are also visible in the hydropic centrilobular cells.

b. × 190. Periportal part of hepatic lobule showing sharp transition from unaffected periportal cells to midzonal cells with conspicuous globules of lipid; this may indicate how a small defect in solubilization can determine substantial fatty globulation. Dixon K. C. (1958) *Quart. J. exp. Physiol.*, **43**, 139.

conformational change of phospholipids caused by lipoperoxidation may prevent the formation of micelles and so impede the formation and excretion of micellar fat [8]; some of the fat which cannot be solubilised would then aggregate into a third phase composed of visible liquid globules. Since globular fat cannot be excreted, a quantitative increase in fat then ensues, provided fat continues to be formed in the cells.

As protein and phospholipid probably act as co-solubilisers of fat within lipoprotein micelles, inhibition of solubilising power of phospholipid by CCl_4 may simultaneously exclude protein as well as fat from the micelles. This disruption of micellar structure may account for the combined aggregation of anionophilic protein along with fat globules (see Fig. 8.48), which may occur in centrilobular hepatocytes of rats poisoned by CCl_4 [19].

The effect of CCl_4 in causing fatty globulation in the liver is usually confined to the midzonal and centrilobular hepatic cells; this change seldom occurs in the periportal cells (Fig. 8.9a). This difference may reflect the relatively high content of microsomal oxygenases in the centrilobular cells and the resultant oxidation within them of CCl_4 to a toxic intermediary (p. 164). The sharp transition from midzonal cells containing conspicuous fatty globules to periportal cells with no visible fat (Fig. 8.9b) may indicate how a small defect in solubilising power may determine substantial fatty globulation.

When animals are fed on diets rich in fat, the addition of *cholesterol* increases TG in the liver cells and also stimulates the formation of visible droplets of lipid [12, 20]. This effect may depend on the known action of cholesterol in antagonising the power of phospholipid to form fine emulsions of oil in water. But this effect of cholesterol on an emulsified fat, when an *oil phase* is *already* present, is very different from the stabilising action of cholesterol on micellar fat which is solubilised by phospholipid and cholesterol in VLDL. There is accordingly a paradox that cholesterol may take part in solubilisation of fat in phospholipid or lipoprotein micelles, but the presence of cholesterol, superadded to gross excess of fat or other hydrophobic lipid, promotes further lipid globulation and may increase the size of emulsion globules. This difference probably depends on two distinct potentialities of amphipathic substances; first to act as solubilisers, and second to act as emulsifiers [8, 21]. In the former activity cholesterol and phospholipid are apparently synergic but in the latter they are antagonistic. This antagonistic action of cholesterol may thus become apparent when either fat or cholesterol esters are present in such excess as to necessitate the presence of an oil phase; then the advent of extra cholesterol may antagonise the formation of a fine emulsion of microglobules of oil in water. A coarse emulsion may thus result which cannot readily pass into solubilised form. This antagonistic action of cholesterol may contribute to fatty globulation in both diabetes (p. 369) and atherosclerosis (p. 388).

Initial excess of fat

As soon as fat accumulates in excess of the amount that can be solubilised in micelles, visible globules are formed as an extra oil phase. Such quantitative increase in fat arises in two principal ways: by acceleration of entry or formation, and by retardation of removal.

Acceleration of entry or formation of fat

Excessive entry of preformed fat may determine substantial fatty globulation in neutrophils and macrophages when they ingest dead cells containing fat or free fat droplets in necrotic tissues. Neutrophils which invade cardiac infarcts may become filled with fat globules after ingesting fat droplets previously formed in hypoxic myocardial fibres.

Excessive entry of fat also accounts for intense fatty change most prominent in the periportal zones of liver lobules in rats fed on diets with very high content of fat [12, 20, 22]. This fatty change (visible by LM) is accompanied by quantitative increase of fat and the appearance of small osmiophilic particles (100–250 nm in diameter seen by EM) in the periportal hepatic cells. This observation suggested that chylomicrons are directly absorbed from the blood by liver cells to form globules of fat, and that this mechanism is responsible for the disappearance of the normal lipaemia which usually occurs after food. Minute particles of latex can similarly be taken up by the liver cells.

Globules of liquid fat in enormous numbers appear in the liver cells of rats fed on margarine as their sole food [23]. This fatty globulation is more intense in the periportal that the centrilobular cells and can be observed both in sections and films of hepatic tissue1–3 days after commencement of feeding margarine. Very substantial quantitative increase in triglycerides occurs along with this conspicuous visible fatty globulation [24]. Fig. 8.10 shows a film of liver from a

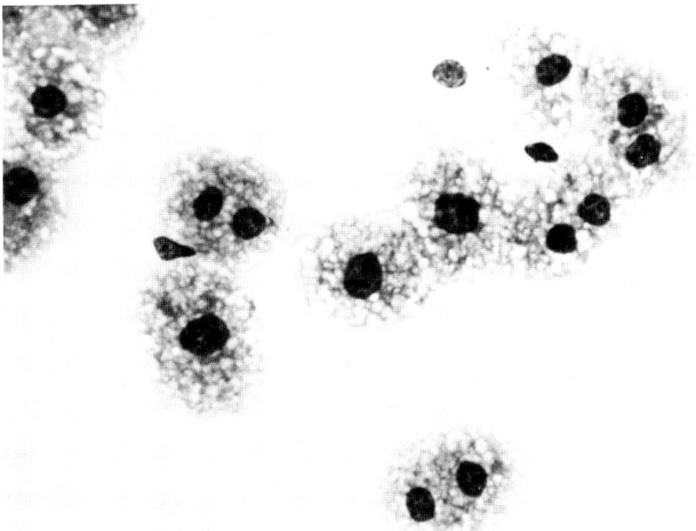

FIG. 8.10 Hepatocytes in a rolled film of liver from a rat fed on margarine and water for 16 h. Fixation ethanol. H & E. × 510.

rat fed for 16 h on margarine. Thus when fat enters the cell in an amount in excess of that which can be solubilised and removed, an oil phase containing liquid fat may rapidly occupy a large part of the cytoplasm.

Excessive formation of fat within the cell may also be a potent factor in causing quantitative increase followed by fatty globulation [25]. Such excessive synthesis probably mainly occurs as a result of *hypoxia* or *lack of choline*.

Hypoxia stimulates the formation of fat from free fatty acid (FFA) in liver and heart muscle. The cells of both these tissues remove FFA from blood and utilise it as a major metabolic substrate. The FFA in liver may also be derived from chylomicrons of the blood which can be hydrolysed at the surface of hepatic cells to liberate FFA; the latter is then absorbed. Inside hepatic cells and cardiac muscle fibres. FFA has three major fates:

1. Oxidation to CO_2 (route 1).
2. Conversion to phospholipid (route 2).
3. Conversion to fat (route 3).

It is clear from Fig. 8.11 that hypoxia obstructs route 1. Moreover, since oxygen is necessary for synthesis of cytidine diphosphate choline (CDC), hypoxia also obstructs route 2. With metabolism along routes 1 and 2 thus impeded, hypoxia effectively diverts the metabolism along route 3, so that the formation of fat is substantially accelerated in hypoxic cells with resultant fatty globulation within them.

Lack of choline, by inhibiting the synthesis of CDC, may also divert the

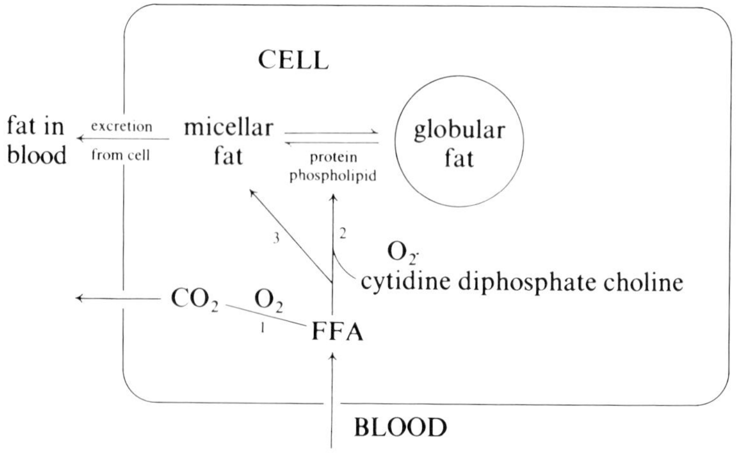

FIG. 8.11 Major intracellular fates of free fatty acid (FFA) in liver cells and cardiac muscle fibres:

1. Oxidation to CO_2 (route 1).
2. Conversion to phospholipid (route 2).
3. Conversion to micellar fat (route 3).

metabolism of FFA away from route 2 along route 3. Indeed the addition of CDC to homogenates of rat liver impedes synthesis of fat as measured by the incorporation of ^{14}C-labelled glycerol into liver TG. Thus lack of choline may contribute to fatty globulation by accelerating the formation of fat as well as by interfering with its solubilisation.

Retardation of removal of fat

Provided fat is being *formed* within the cell, then retardation of utilisation causes quantitative increase and so promotes the appearance of globular fat. Interference with solubilisation is probably one of the most important causes of retardation of utilisation, irrespective of whether fat is being excreted, unchanged in lipoprotein micelles, or is being removed by metabolism. The secondary surplus of fat produced by such retardation of removal results in further visible globulation in addition to any immediate effect produced by direct coalescence of solubilised fat.

In liver cells minute particles of solubilised lipid (possibly lipoprotein complexes) are visible by EM within the tubules of ER, where TG is probably synthesised [26]; these micellar particles appear to emigrate from the hepatic cells by passing along the tubules to the exterior. But if solubilisation is impeded then TG would become aggregated into droplets too large to be excreted.

Aggregation or collapse of tubules of ER in hepatocytes, which rapidly follows administration of CCl_4 by stomach tube to rats (p. 163), may directly interrupt excretion of lipoprotein micelles along tubules and so promote globulation of fat. However lipoperoxidation of phospholipids may quite independently interfere with solubilisation of TG and thus determine globulation. Moreover it is possible that the actual route of excretion of lipoprotein from the liver is by the microtubular system [27] rather than along the tubules of ER.

Retardation of excretion or metabolism of fat, no matter how generated, can only augment the total amount of fat in the cell, if fat is actually being formed or absorbed. When cell damage is so severe as to interrupt formation of fat from FFA or carbohydrates, retardation of removal cannot produce a surplus of fat and thus cause globulation. This explains why dead and dying cells in zones of ischaemic or toxic necrosis often contain less visible fat than is present in adjacent injured but surviving cells [9]. In the latter cells formation of TG from FFA continues or is even augmented (see Fig. 8.14a and b).

FATTY GLOBULATION IN DISEASE

The cells of the body in disease are frequently exposed to conditions which cause intracellular globulation of fat. Indeed disease may interfere with solubilisation and excretion of fat and also accelerate the formation and entry of fat, so as to cause extensive coacervation of hydrophobic triglycerides.

Diseases and disorders particularly conducive to fatty globulation include (a) cellular hypoxia, (b) malnutrition, (c) diabetes, (d) excessive consumption of fat or lipogenic substances and (e) infection and toxaemia.

Cellular hypoxia

Hypoxia, which is a common cause of fatty globulation usually results from generalised ischaemia in heart failure, local ischaemia due to arterial occlusion, or severe anaemia.

Liver

In congestive cardiac failure the flow of blood along the hepatic sinusoids is retarded, and when it reaches the centrilobular cells it is depleted of oxygen; the centrilobular cells may then receive so little oxygen that they shrivel and die, while the partially hypoxic midzonal cells show conspicuous fatty globulation. Two factors probably contribute to this fatty change. First, the hypoxia may cause intracellular lack of phospholipid and protein owing to interference with synthesis and thus interfere with solubilisation of fat. Secondly, hypoxia inhibits

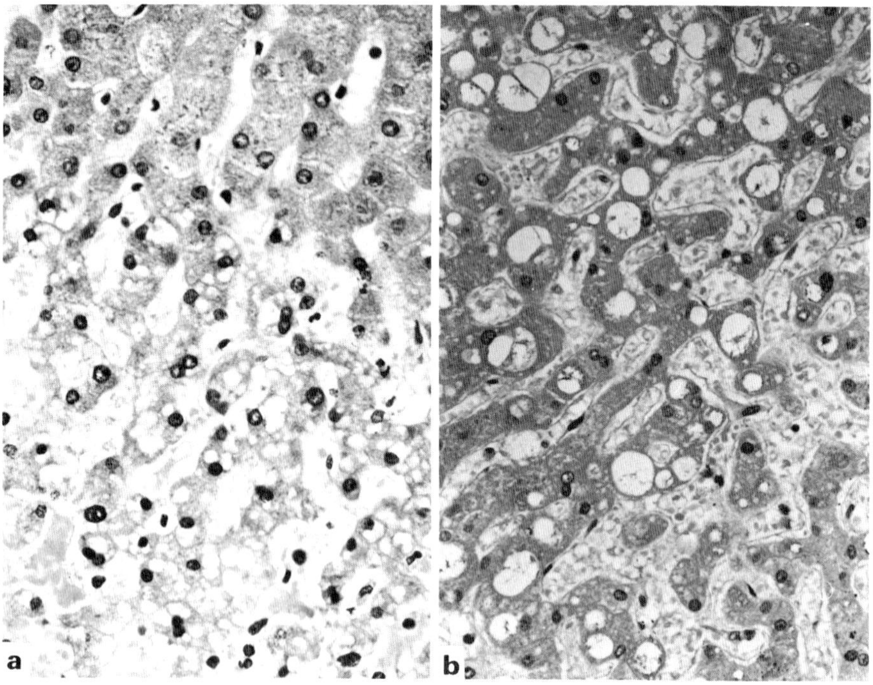

FIG. 8.12 Fatty globulation in midzonal hepatic cells induced by hypoxia due to cardiac failure. H & E. × 265.

a. Upper part of field shows unaffected periportal hepatocytes at the periphery of hepatic lobule; lower part of the field shows more hypoxic midzonal hepatocytes with conspicuous fatty change. From a woman of 76 who died of heart failure due to ischaemic cardiac disease.

b. Hypoxic midzonal hepatocytes containing large vacuoles due to fat; these cells are separated by intensely dilated (congested) sinusoids. Heart failure has caused slowing of circulation with hypoxia and congestion. From a woman of 52 who died of acute heart failure due to haemopericardium following pericardial metastases from bronchial carcinoma.

the oxidation of FFA and also retards its conversion to phospholipid; the metabolism of FFA is therefore diverted along route 3 in Fig. 8.11 to form an excess of neutral fat. Moreover in these midzonal cells, which may show intense fatty globulation, the hypoxia is not severe enough to kill the cells and so interrupt conversion of FFA to fat, as happens in the most profoundly anoxic centrilobular cells which contain less fat. The typical 'nutmeg' liver of congestive heart failure thus shows a tripartite pattern: the most hypoxic centrilobular cells are necrotic and shrivelled (see Fig. 3.10b, p. 74), the partly hypoxic midzonal cells are fatty (Fig. 8.12a), while the well-oxygenated peripheral cells are unaffected (Fig. 8.12a). This dependence of fatty globulation in the midzonal hepatocytes on *limited* hypoxia is further illustrated in Fig. 8.12b; this shows conspicuous fatty change in midzonal hepatocytes along with gross dilation and congestion of the adjacent sinusoids which reflect the extreme retardation of microcirculation produced by terminal cardiac failure.

Cardiac muscle

Hypoxia is also a common cause of fatty globulation in cardiac muscle fibres. As in liver sinusoids there is progressive depletion of oxygen from the blood as it passes along the capillaries which supply the cardiac fibres. Thus the fibres near the arteriolar ends of the capillaries are best supplied with oxygen, while the fibres placed near the termination of capillaries in venules receive more hypoxic blood. When the flow of blood is retarded as a result of chronic progressive coronary occlusion (p. 75) or when the oxygen content of the blood is greatly diminished as in pernicious anaemia, patchy regions of fatty globulation develop in the most hypoxic fibres. These zones of fatty fibres have a creamy appearance which can be seen through the transparent endocardium as pale flecks contrasting conspicuously with the red brown colour of the unaffected cardiac muscle; this appearance is called 'thrush breast'. Fig. 8.13 shows this speckled distribution of fatty change in papillary muscles of the right ventricle of a woman of 81 with very severe pernicious anaemia who died of acute cardiac failure. In such hypoxic heart muscle systolic contraction of the heart diminishes tissue oxygenation still further, since during each systole the capillaries become temporarily closed. This occlusive effect is greatest nearest to the ventricular cavities where intracardiac pressure during systole is highest [28]. For this reason visible fatty globulation is more pronounced in the inner than the outer portions of ventricular muscle; in these visibly fatty parts there is quantitative increase of extractable fat [29].

Fatty globulation in ischaemic heart muscle of human patients suffering from coronary occlusion is sometimes very prominent at the margins of regions where more severe hypoxia has caused necrosis. Between the necrotic and unaffected fibres there is a zone of partial hypoxia where the fibres show intense fatty change. This progressive transition from necrotic to fatty and then to normal fibres is typically evident where an infarct approaches the endocardium [9]. In this situation sufficient oxygen can diffuse from the intraventricular blood to maintain the fibres nearest to the endocardial surface; between the latter

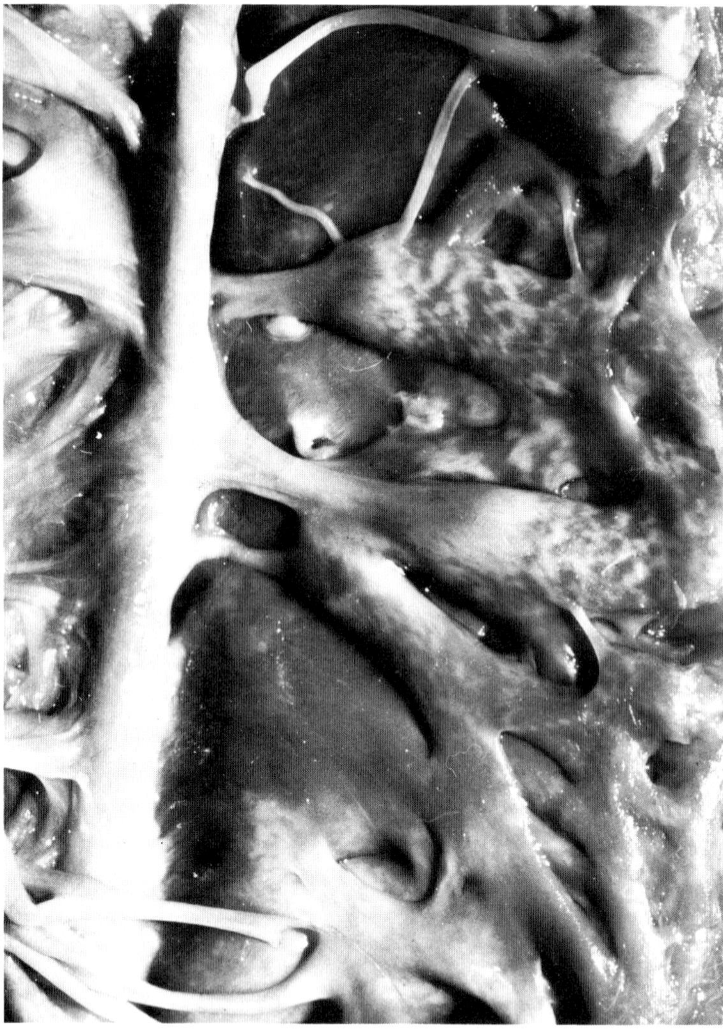

FIG. 8.13 Patchy zones of fatty globulation in papillary muscles of right ventricle. From a woman of 81 with severe pernicious anaemia (rbc 1.2×10^{12}/l, Hb 4.0 g/dl) who died of acute heart failure. The most hypoxic zones of myocardium have a creamy appearance visible through the transparent endocardium as pale flecks ('thrush breast'), contrasting with the red brown colour of unaffected heart muscle. Courtesy of Professor G. A. Gresham.

heatlhy fibres and the necrotic fibres in the infarct there is an intervening zone of partially hypoxic fibres which show conspicuous fatty globulation (Fig. 8.14).

Such fatty change may however be succeeded by more serious injury; this can develop suddenly when coronary occlusion becomes more complete. Then the fatty fibres become necrotic, softened and friable. This change in cardiac muscle

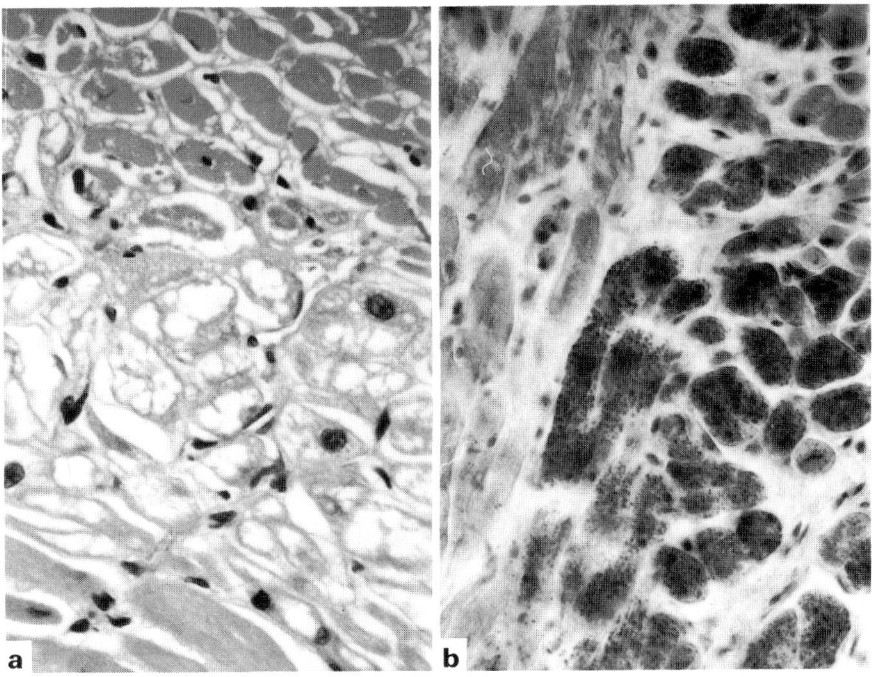

FIG. 8.14 Fatty globulation in zones of limited hypoxia between myocardial infarcts and adjacent endocardium. Sufficient oxygen can diffuse from ventricular cavity to maintain the myocardial fibres nearest to the endocardium. Between these unaffected fibres and the necrotic fibres of the infarct there is an intervening zone of partially hypoxic fibres which may show intense fatty globulation.

a. Transition from normal fibres nearest to endocardium (at lower border) through fatty fibres (midfield) to homogeneous necrotic fibres of an infarct (upper border). H & E. × 400.

b. Transition from subendocardial fatty fibres to necrotic fibres of an infarct (at left of field). Sudan III–IV & H. ×265.

was vividly described by William Stokes in 1854: 'the substance of the ventricle was softened, most easily broken by the finger, and of a pale yellowish colour . . . the scalpel was greased in cutting the muscular substance'. If the patient survives for a few days these necrotic fatty fibres become surrounded by polymorphs which themselves are filled with globules of fat as they consume the dead cardiac muscle.

Fatty globulation in cardiac muscle is a rapid sequel to ischaemia. Thus globulation with quantitative increase in fat is prominent in hypoxic myocardial fibres of dogs after ligation of the anterior descending branch of the left coronary artery [30]. Following such arterial occlusion in dogs droplets of fat appear within the dying myocardial fibres within 2–4 h; later the fat disappears and is then confined to fibres at the periphery of the infarct in a 'narrow reversibly damaged zone' [31].

Fatty globulation is thus a frequent sequel to hypoxia in both cardiac and hepatic cells. In these cells where FFA is such an important metabolic substrate, globulation may principally depend on diversion of the metabolism of FFA by hypoxia. This diversion can only occur (Fig. 8.11) provided the cells remain alive, so that esterification of FFA by glycerophosphate can still take place. It is thus clear that the most intensely fatty cells occur in intermediate zones of partial hypoxia situated between necrotic and unaffected cells.

Fatty globulation caused by malnutrition

Acute starvation

As soon as starvation causes fall in blood sugar, secretion of catecholamines, TSH and ACTH result in activation of the hormone sensitive lipases of the lipocytes. This effect is mediated by the adenylcyclase system and is followed by hydrolysis of fat in the lipocytes with rise in FFA of blood.

The liberated FFA is attached to serum albumen in the blood and is transported to the liver where it is resynthesised to TG [32]. Starvation thus causes increase in quantity of fat in liver and visible fatty globulation in hepatic cells.

By feeding mice with linseed oil labelled with deuterium Barret, Best & Ridout [33] succeeded in fattening mice with depot fat labelled by deuterium. The animals were then starved or injected with anterior pituitary extract; this caused rapid discharge of depot fat followed by accumulation of hepatic fat labelled with deuterium. These experiments showed, in a novel manner, that fat deposited in the liver during starvation contains fatty acids derived from depot fat.

Much of the fat which appears in liver cells in starvation is probably formed by synthesis from FFA but some of this fat may enter the liver cells as fat itself, since fasting can cause lipaemia as well as increase of FFA in blood [34].

Chronic malnutrition

Grossly enlarged fatty livers are common among malnourished children of tropical countries who suffer kwashiorkor (p. 46). This disease is primarily caused by deficient intake of protein. The accumulation of hepatic fat is accompanied by conspicuous globulation of sudanophil lipid in the liver cells [35] and the fat content of the liver may reach 50 per cent of wet weight [36].

Probably deficiency in dietary protein deprives the liver cells of an essential solubiliser required for the solubilisation of TG. Without this solubilising protein (or peptide), micellar fat (VLDL) cannot be formed and the hepatic cells can no longer excrete TG. Intense fatty globulation with gross accumulation of TG then follows. When these malnourished children are given food containing adequate protein, then fat is solubilised and excreted by the liver followed by a rise in TG and of lipoprotein in the serum [35, 37].

Fatty globulation in diabetes

Uncontrolled diabetes is a potent cause of accumulation of fat in the liver. Diabetes also increases the incidence of atherosclerosis in which lipids are deposited in arterial walls.

Lack of insulin is an important determinant in causing fatty globulation in the liver in diabetes both in animals and in man. Thus, following pancreatectomy, the liver of animals may become extremely fatty. Best [38] found 25 per cent of fat in the liver of a pancreatectomised dog. Similarly when the β-cells of pancreatic islets are killed by injection of alloxan into rats, conspicuous fatty globulation may occur in liver [16].

Lack of insulin is also responsible for fatty globulation in the liver of human patients suffering from the juvenile-onset type of diabetes (p. 437). In this severe form of diabetes β-cells are usually absent from the pancreas and no insulin is secreted (p. 432).

Lack of insulin probably causes fatty globulation in the liver by increasing concentration of FFA in blood. This effect has two basic determinants:

1. Without insulin glycerophosphate is not formed by glycolysis of glucose in lipocytes, so that FFA cannot be esterified to form depot fat, and FFA therefore accumulates in the blood.
2. Without insulin adrenalin acts unchecked in stimulating lipolysis, and TG is thus excessively hydrolysed to FFA.

In the absence of insulin therefore the lipocytes cannot store fat. The juvenile-form of diabetes is thus a severe wasting disease which causes increase in concentration of FFA in blood [39] followed by excessive entry of FFA into the liver. In the hepatic cells, however, glycerokinase, which is absent in lipocytes, catalyses the synthesis of TG from FFA and glycerol. Accumulation of TG may then follow.

In the milder type of diabetes which occurs in middle aged corpulent patients insulin is not deficient (p. 433). In these patients the over-enlarged fat depots probably discharge excess of FFA into the blood and this may also be esterified in the liver with resultant formation of globular fat.

Another determinant of fatty globulation in the cells of diabetic patients may be excess of cholesterol. Hypercholesterolaemia is usual in all forms of diabetes. Since cholesterol (p. 360) antagonises the emulsifying action of phospholipid, the fine emulsion necessary to initiate solubilisation may not form. Thus solubilisation may be inhibited and this effect may increase globulation of fat in the liver of diabetics. This antagonistic action of cholesterol on the emulsifying action of phospholipid may also accelerate the deposition of hydrophobic lipids in arterial walls and thus account for the high incidence of atherosclerosis in diabetes (p. 388).

Finally lipaemia which is common in uncontrolled diabetes [40] may further accelerate hepatic fatty globulation, as chylomicrons may be directly absorbed into liver cells.

Excessive consumption of fat and carbohydrate: corpulence

When people eat too much then fat deposits enlarge.

Overeating coupled with lack of exercise results in a small net daily surplus of intake of fat and fat-forming substances over their utilisation. The net balance y fine one, but if it is continuously positive over the years men and arge into unsightly ovoid objects encased in masses of subcutaneous at is stored in the cells of adipose tissue.

people become obese more rapidly than others. In obese human adults essive volume of the fat depots is determined by (1) abnormally high er of lipocytes, and (2) increase in their size.

Hirsch *et al.* [41] estimated the total number of lipocytes and also their size in non-obese and in obese human adults. In the non-obese the average number is of the order of 27×10^9 lipocytes containing an average of 0.61 μg lipid/cell, while in the obese the order is 77×10^9 lipocytes with 0.91 μg lipid/cell. Observations on children indicate that increase in the *number* of lipocytes is determined by excessive feeding during the *first* year of postnatal life. On the other hand increase in the weight of lipid/cell and therefore in the size of the lipocyte can arise from overfeeding at any phase in life. The sensitive period during which the number of lipocytes can be increased occurs both in children and young animals. During this phase overfeeding of children can cause considerable obesity; this is rarely seen in completely breast-fed children [42]. In adult life the number of lipocytes is constant and changes in their size alone account for variation in adiposity.

Clearly, if the number of lipocytes is increased by excessive feeding in infancy, the tendency to corpulence is a permanent threat. Extreme corpulence probably results from an abnormally high number of lipocytes initially generated by hyperplasia in childhood, coupled with persistent overeating even to a small extent throughout a long period of adult life. Reduction of weight in such obese adults is followed by diminution in average size of the cells, but the hypercellularity persists. Thus corpulence is determined by a combination of (a) multiplication of lipocytes during infancy, succeeded by (b) periods of lipocytic enlargement in later life, when the overnumerous lipocytes enlarge into bloated vesicles of fat. But if the number of lipocytes is stabilised during the formative period at a relatively low number, the possibility of corpulence is greatly diminished, even though fat and carbohydrate are later consumed in amounts which would cause adiposity in adults with larger numbers of adipocytes.

In corpulent patients the weight of excessive adipose tissue can exert extremely harmful effects. Hypertrophy of adipose tissue, like hypertrophy of myocardium and of striated muscle, increases the weight of the body to be lifted and moved but, unlike hypertrophy of the latter tissues, increase of adipose tissue in no way assists the added contractile action of myocardium and striated muscle which such increase of body weight compels. Thus ischaemic heart failure may be aggravated by coincident corpulence which increases the work of an already defective myocardium and thereby depletes still further its supply of oxygen.

Another complication of prolonged adiposity is intense hepatic fatty change [43]; eventually this may lead to hepatic cirrhosis (p. 374).

Infection and toxaemia

Intracellular fatty globulation frequently occurs in the liver of patients who die as a result of acute bacterial infection. Prolonged fever with resultant anorexia and malnutrition is probably the principal determinant of this kind of fatty change.

In gas gangrene globules of lipid are visible in the necrotic muscle fibres and their content of fat is increased [44]. This globulation with accumulation doubtless depends on action of the α-toxin of *Clostridium welchii* (p. 225), which decomposes phospholipid and thus interferes with solubilisation and at the same time liberates hydrophobic liquid diglyceride.

Intense fatty change may be visible in the myocardial fibres of patients dying of diphtheria; the cells contain emulsions of fine droplets of fat. This fatty globulation may depend on the action of the exotoxin of *Corynebacterium diphtheriae* in preventing the synthesis of protein and so depriving the cells of essential solubilisers responsible for forming lipoprotein micelles. The fatty change in the myofibres may be responsible for defect of function which finally results in acute heart failure or cardiac arrest.

Centrilobular necrosis and fatty change are visible in hepatic lobules of human patients who die following ingestion of CCl_4 given for treatment of hookworm infection [45]. In animals CCl_4 causes intense fatty change in liver lobules, most marked in the midzonal cells (p. 360). Another organic poison which can cause intense hepatic fatty change in man is ethanol. This is oxidised in the body to products which can provide energy to cells by exergonic catabolism. Ethanol is therefore both a food and a poison. Whether its harmful effects are due to direct toxicity or to indirect action in diminishing utilisation of other nutriments is considered in the next section.

Fatty globulation and injury caused by ethanol

Acute effects

Early events induced in man and animals by ingestion of ethanol include conspicuous fatty globulation in hepatic cells as well as stupor or coma which may be produced by gross excess.

In rats visible fatty globulation and increase in content of TG in liver rapidly follow ingestion of ethanol [46, 47]. Within 8–16 h of a single dose of 6 g ethanol/kg given to rats conspicuous fatty globulation becomes visible in hepatic cells along with enlargement of mitochondria [48]. This acute fatty change is at first mainly in the periportal zones of liver lobules and disappears after 36 h. In human liver pronounced fatty globulation develops within 3–10 days of ingestion of large doses of ethanol; this change is also accompanied by enlargement of mitochondria followed later by their degeneration [49].

This rapid development of hepatic fatty globulation after ingestion of ethanol probably depends on:

1. Oxidation of ethanol itself via acetaldehyde and acetic acid to acetyl CoA, which is then synthesised to higher fatty acids (FFA) and thence to fat (TG). This oxidation of ethanol to acetaldehyde is catalysed by alcohol dehydrogenase in the cytoplasm of hepatocytes and requires simultaneous reduction of NAD^+ to NADH.

$$\underset{\text{ethanol}}{CH_3CH_2OH} \xrightarrow[\text{alcohol dehydrogenase}]{NAD^+ \;\; NADH + H^+} \underset{\text{acetaldehyde}}{CH_3CHO}$$

2. The above reaction depletes the cellular reserves of NAD^+ necessary for oxidation of FFA which therefore accumulates and is converted to TG. Moreover the increase in production of NADH accelerates reduction of dihydroxyacetone phosphate to glycerol-1-phosphate which then becomes available to combine with FFA, derived from oxidation of ethanol, and produce more TG by providing the glycerol as well as the fatty acid portions of the molecule.

$$\underset{\text{dihydroxyacetone phosphate}}{P\text{–}OCH_2\text{–}\underset{\underset{O}{\|}}{C}\text{–}CH_2OH} \xrightarrow[\text{glycerol 1-phosphate dehydrogenase}]{NADH + H^+ \;\; NAD^+} \underset{\text{glycerol-1-phosphate}}{P\text{–}OCH_2\text{–}\underset{\underset{OH}{|}}{CH}\text{–}CH_2OH}$$

3. High concentration of ethanol within cells may interfere with solubilisation of TG by phospholipid and so promote globulation of fat.

4. Injury to mitochondria may interfere with oxidation of FFA and so promote further synthesis of TG (Fig. 8.11).

Prolonged effects of ethanol

Excessive consumption of ethanol continued over long periods can lead to severe injury both to myocardial fibres and to hepatic cells.

In human *myocardium* damage usually only becomes revealed after excessive consumption of ethanol for many years [50]. Cardiomyopathy may then result in dyspnoea, dysrhythmia and tachycardia terminating in lethal heart failure. Globules of triglyceride are visible by LM between the myofibrils in the cardiac muscle cells; EM shows increase in number of lysosomes and also formation of dense intramitochondrial inclusions.

In the *liver* in man prolonged effects of excessive consumption of ethanol include:

1. *Persistent fatty globulation.* The liver and its cells become enlarged by intracellular globules of fat. The fat is usually present as a single large globule in each cell, but in some cells the cytoplasm may appear foamy due to smaller droplets [51]; fatty cysts are produced by rupture of swollen cell membranes and coalescence of globules. This fatty globulation is a readily reversible process and fat disappears when intake of ethanol ceases.

2. *Alcoholic hepatitis.* This usually only develops after excessive consumption of ethanol for at least 10 years. The affected patients develop fever, nausea, vomiting and abdominal pain followed in some patients by lethal hepatic failure [52]. The liver is enlarged and infiltrated with neutrophils and lymphocytes.

This enlargement is caused by cellular swelling due to globules of fat and also increase of cell protein. Many of the centrilobular cells contain hyaline masses of eosinophilic protein called Mallory bodies or alcoholic hyaline (p. 417). The mitochondria become swollen into giant forms and their cristae disappear; this effect may interrupt oxidation of FFA and so lead to accumulation of FFA with diversion of metabolism to form TG.

3. *Alcoholic cirrhosis*. This dreaded complication of chronic alcoholism in man only arises after high consumption of ethanol persisting for 10 years or more [53]. At first a fine microlobular portal cirrhosis develops in which hepatic tissue becomes subdivided by fibrous partitions into small regular nodules (Fig. 8,15a). Later some nodules enlarge further by differential regeneration. Cirrhosis eventually produces disastrous obstruction of hepatic circulation with ascites, haemorrhage from dilated oesophageal veins or hepatic failure terminating in coma. In some patients hepatocellular carcinoma develops from regenerating nodules, though this neoplasm in fact occurs most commonly in parts of the world where no ethanol is consumed.

Nature of lesions produced by ethanol

Ethanol given in large doses to man or animals thus rapidly induces conspicuous fatty globulation in the liver probably by increasing the synthesis of TG and also possibly by interfering with solubilisation and excretion of TG.

Prolonged excessive intake of ethanol in man also produces hepatic enlargement with intense fatty globulation in liver cells which may eventually be followed by alcoholic hepatitis and cirrhosis. There is no doubt that these lesions are sequels of prolonged consumption of ethanol. But how far ethanol *per se* is directly responsible for these lesions is uncertain. If a man drinks half a bottle of gin a day, he may not wish to eat much food, and his intake of protein and other potential solubilisers of fat may thus be insufficient to prevent prolonged fatty globulation terminating in cirrhosis.

This question of induced deficiency of lipotropic factors was emphasised by Best *et al.* [54]; they showed that ethanol, given to rats over long periods, conditioned a deficiency of lipotropic factors which results in gross hepatic fatty deposition followed by cirrhosis. However, these effects of ingestion of ethanol were entirely prevented by adequate supplies of dietary choline.

Experiments on baboons, however, indicate that prolonged consumption of ethanol alone can produce hepatic fatty globulation, hepatitis and eventually cirrhosis, even in animals which are consuming an entirely adequate diet [55]. Mallory bodies similar to those found in livers of human alcoholics were also found in the livers of these animals. In fact the whole spectrum of alcoholic injury appears to be caused by ethanol in the absence of nutritional deficiency.

On the other hand, in rats fed with large amounts of ethanol for 5–6 months, no fatty globulation, nor hepatitis, nor cirrhosis develops provided adequate amounts of protein and lipotropic factors are consumed [48]. Rats fed large amounts of ethanol in their water are disinclined to eat sufficient food, *unless* their fluid intake can be raised [48]. This object was attained by feeding sucrose together with ethanol in water; this mixture has great appeal to rats and results in adequate consumption of fluid and food along with large amounts of ethanol. On this diet hepatic fatty globulation was prevented, although Mallory hyaline bodies eventually were formed.

These results re-emphasise that fatty globulation and consequent cirrhosis in man following prolonged consumption of excess of ethanol may in part depend on defective intake of protein and other lipotropic agents. In any case efforts to remove hepatic fat and prevent further irreversible injury by cirrhosis should always ensure adequate supply of lipotropic nutriments as well as elimination of alcoholic intake.

This view that alcoholic cirrhosis and other hepatic lesions caused by prolonged alcoholism are in part determined by lack of nutriments is reinforced by observations on patients treated for gross obesity by jejuno-ileal by-pass [43]. Although the livers of many of these obese patients show fatty change before operation, the surgical introduction of jejunal by-pass is often followed by other hepatic lesions strikingly similar to those occurring in alcoholic liver disease; these lesions include centrilobular necrosis, infiltration with neutrophils, development of Mallory bodies, and cirrhosis. This similarity suggests a possible common pathway in liver disease caused by ethanol and that caused by jejunal by-pass.

HEPATIC CIRRHOSIS CAUSED BY INTRACELLULAR GLOBULATION AND AGGREGATION

Fatty globulation, if prolonged, may be followed by harmful subdivision of the liver into nodules separated by fibrous trabeculae which obstruct portal circulation; this fibrosis is called cirrhosis.

In man this hepatic cirrhosis is commonly a sequel to prolonged storage of fat in the liver cells as a result of alcoholism, diabetes, obesity, nutritional defect or pernicious anaemia. In rats similar hepatic cirrhosis is produced by chronic fatty globulation caused by diets deficient in choline [56, 57].

An important factor in the pathogenesis of cirrhosis is swelling of fat-filled hepatocytes followed by bursting of the bloated cells [58, 59]. Fibrosis then follows. This involves active fibrogenesis with increase in collagen, estimated by content of hydroxyproline [60]. This process is accompanied by regeneration of small nodules of hepatic cells separated by fibrous trabeculae producing micronodular cirrhosis (Fig. 8,15a). Such micronodular change is usual in alcoholic cirrhosis, in which hyaline masses of eosinophilic protein (Mallory bodies) as well as globules of fat are frequently visible in the enlarged hepatocytes (p. 373 and Fig. 8.46).

As well as fibrogenesis, collapse of pre-existing peri-sinusoidal connective tissue contributes to the fibrous septa which separate the regenerated nodules of cirrhotic liver (Fig. 8.15b). When rupture of bloated cells is extensive whole lobules may disappear with condensation of their connective tissue into fibrous bands [59] along with regeneration of remaining hepatic cells into large irregular pseudolobules. The latter are then separated by trabeculae of connective tissue

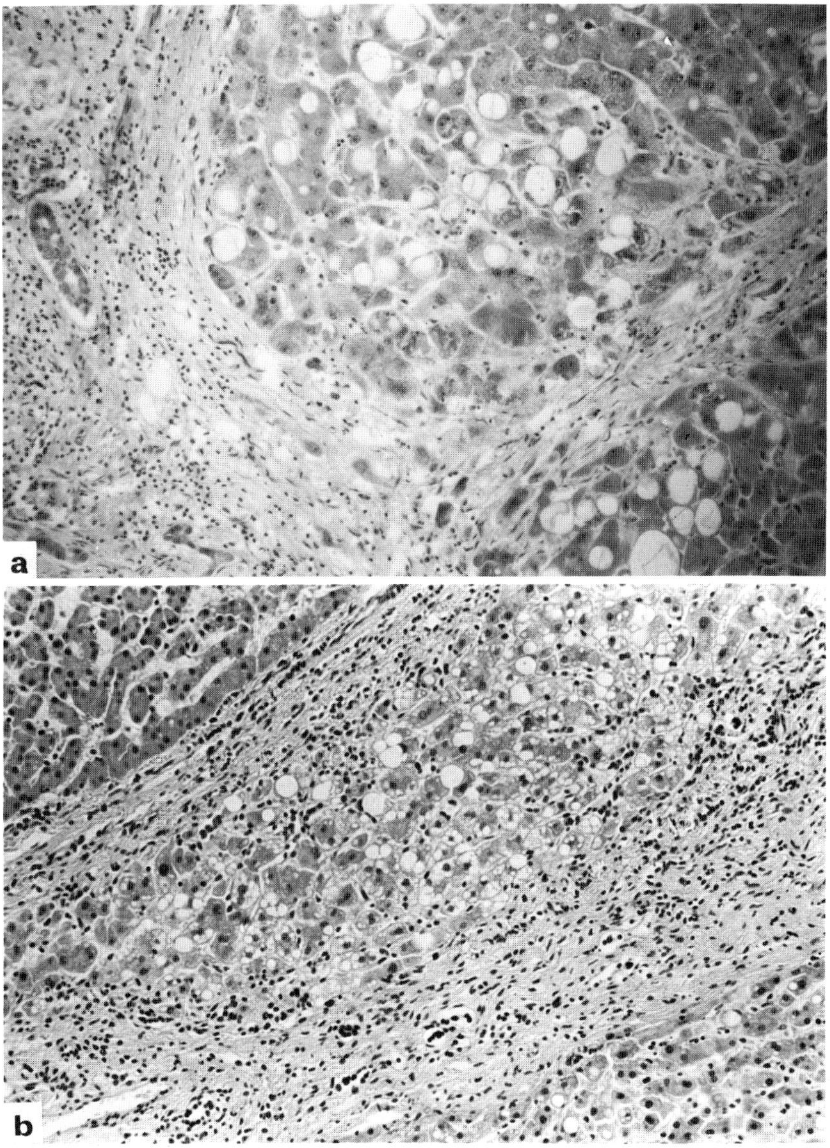

FIG. 8.15 Hepatic cirrhosis associated with fatty change.

a. Micronodular cirrhosis of type usually found after prolonged excessive intake of ethanol. Parts of two small ovoid nodules of hepatocytes are present (at right of field); they are separated by a fibrous septum. Many of the hepatocytes are bloated by fat and Mallory bodies can be seen in some of them (lower centre). × 130.

b. Collapse of hepatic lobule after rupture and loss of fatty hepatocytes. Fibrous septa, formed from collapsed perisinusoidal connective tissue with added fibrogenesis, enclose the remnant of a fatty hepatic lobule. The hepatic cells bloated with fat are being eroded at interface with surrounding fibrous tissue; this erosion depends on bursting of the swollen hepatocytes. The intense lymphocytic infiltration of the fibrous tissue is characteristic of adjacent piecemeal necrosis. × 130.

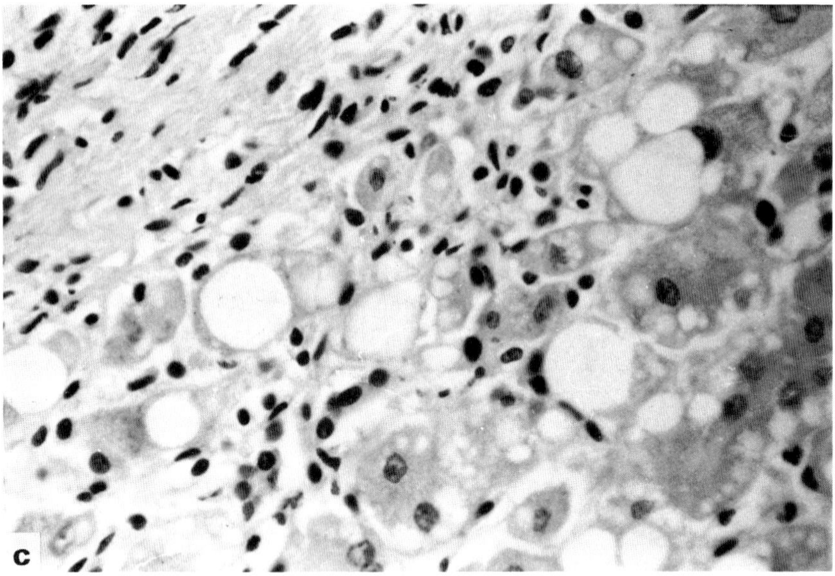

FIG. 8.15 cont.
c. Group of fatty hepatocytes at an interface with fibrous tissue from same field as (b). Some of the swollen hepatocytes have burst and have coalesced to form fatty cysts enclosed by fused cellular remnants. Lymphocytic infiltration is prominent. × 510.

containing fatty cysts enclosed by coalescent remnants of burst hepatic cells (Fig. 8,15c).

At the interfaces between these fibrous trabeculae and the surviving liver cells some of the hepatocytes individually shrivel, degenerate and disappear. This process is accompanied by infiltration of the fibrous trabeculae with lymphocytes (Fig. 8.15b, c) and may depend on the necrotising action of T-lymphocytes sensitised by cell-mediated hypersensitivity to antigenic materials in the cells. This effect, in addition to bursting of fat-filled cells, may contribute to the destruction of hepatocytes which precedes cirrhosis.

Cirrhosis may also follow prolonged deposition of substances other than fat in hepatic cells. Thus cirrhosis is a usual sequel to accumulation of metalloprotein complexes in liver of patients with haemochromatosis, hepatolenticular degeneration and Indian childhood cirrhosis, in which iron or copper complexes are aggregated in the cells (p. 415); whether rupture of cells by insoluble deposits or some allergic mechanism is responsible for loss of hepatocytes and subsequent fibrosis is uncertain.

Besides following intracellular deposition of fat or metalloprotein in hepatic cells, cirrhosis may be a serious consequence of persistent infection by hepatitis B virus (p. 269). This produces proliferation of fibrous trabeculae infiltrated with lymphocytes along with gradual elimination of adjacent hepatic cells. The disappearance of these cells which become enveloped by lymphocytes is called piece meal necrosis and may follow injury by contact with sensitized lymphocytes [61, 119]; the resultant cirrhosis is characterised by large and irregular nodules of hepatocytic regeneration separated by thick fibrous septa. This cirrhosis is much coarser than the finely nodular lesions which follow chronic alcoholism and fatty change.

Results of cirrhosis

The regenerated nodules of cirrhotic liver may at first contribute to hepatic function, but later, portal circulation, becomes irretrievably retarded by obliteration of the microvascular connections in the condensed septa which replace collapsed hepatic lobules. This vascular obstruction causes *portal hypertension* with the harmful sequels of ascites and oesophageal haemorrhage. Portal hypertension can also induce portacaval anastomosis which deprives the liver of much of its normal blood supply. This may produce hepatic failure with encephalopathy and terminal coma (p. 449).

DEPOSITION OF LIPIDS IN ARTERIAL TISSUE

Nature of atherosclerosis

In this common arterial disorder raised patches of proliferated tissue develop in the intima of arteries along with deposition of visible lipid globules and crystals within the thickened zones. This process is called atherosclerosis (*ἀθάρα*, porridge; *σκληρός*, hard), a word which indicates that the thickened plaques are hard and are composed internally of gruel-like material. These plaques have sharply defined edges and are seen as raised creamy patches on the inner surface of the arterial wall.

In human atherosclerosis the most conspicuous deposition of lipid occurs in the deepest parts of the intima adjacent to the internal elastic lamina (Fig. 8.16, p. 378). However, deposition may be more widespread and extend into the more superficial intima (Fig. 8.17) or even into the media. Immediately internal to these zones of lipid deposition intense proliferation of smooth muscle cells and fibrous tissue develops; the resulting 'fibrous caps' cause remarkable unilateral thickening of the arterial wall which eventually produces eccentric narrowing of the lumen (Fig. 8.17) with consequent ischaemic injury. Atherosclerosis tends to be most prominent in the aorta, coronary and cerebral arteries. Ischaemic injury due to occlusion of the coronary and cerebral arteries by atherosclerosis is the commonest cause of sudden death in man.

These mounds of proliferated intima enclosing within them zones of lipid deposition are called *fibro-lipid plaques*; they are the essential lesions of atherosclerosis. Atherosclerosis thus involves both proliferation of the intimal tissue and deposition of lipids in the thickened zones [62]. We shall briefly consider both these features.

Tissue proliferation

These swollen zones of intima are formed by intense proliferation of connective

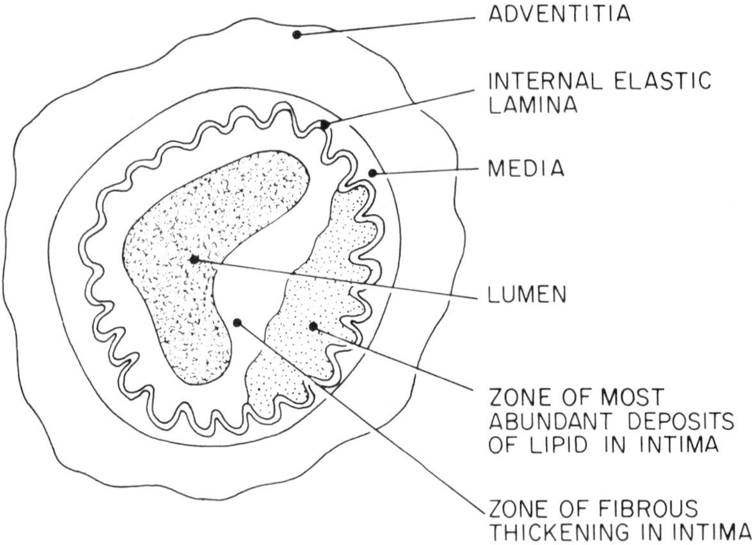

FIG. 8.16 Atherosclerosis in an artery. Eccentric proliferation of intimal tissue is coupled with deposition of both intracellular and extracellular lipids. These deposits are often most abundant in the external part of the intima.

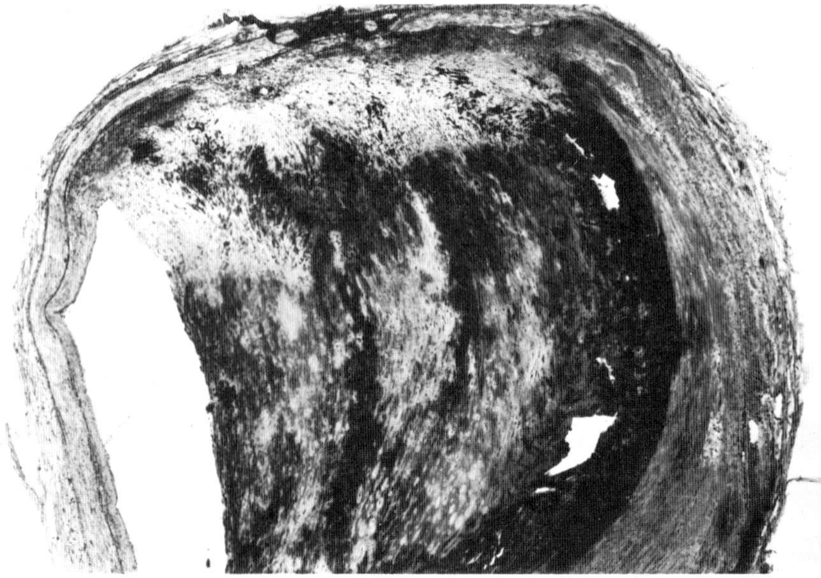

FIG. 8.17 Extensive atherosclerosis in a coronary artery from a diabetic man of 73 who died from left ventricular failure caused by severe IHD terminating in cardiac infarction. Frozen section. Sudan III–IV & H. $\times 35$.

tissue composed of cells and intercellular material. The cells are elongated, stellate or spherical and usually contain droplets of hydrophobic lipid. The elongated cells are possibly derived from smooth muscle, since in some of them myofibrils are visible by EM [63]. Bundles of collagen are present between the cells. This collagen, when extracted, has the electrophoretic properties of type I collagen, present in tendon, bone and skin, and different from type III collagen present along with smooth muscle in arterial media.

Since many of the cells in the plaques lack myofibrils and also form type I instead of type III collagen, they differ markedly from normal smooth muscle; it seems likely therefore that they either have become transformed or are derived from fibrocytes rather than smooth muscle cells [64].

Monoclonal origin of atherosclerotic plaques

The cells which form these mounds of useless tissue in atherosclerotic plaques show intense cellular proliferation of an aberrant type and thus appear to be transformed both in structure and behaviour in the manner of neoplastic cells.

Such an origin by neoplastic transformation caused by mutation of a single cell is suggested from results obtained by electrophoretic analysis of isozymes of enzyme glucose-6-phosphate dehydrogenase (G-6-PD) extracted from the lesions [65–67]. G-6-PD is a polymorphic X-linked gene product (p. 471). Female cells potentially contain two forms of G-6-PD derived from two separate X-allelic loci situated in the two X-chromosomes. In accordance with the suppressed-X (Lyon) hypothesis one of the variants is suppressed in each *post-embryonic* female cell and its progeny. But, owing to random suppression in embryonic cells, every normally developed female tissue contain both variants in approximately equal amounts. Among the large number of variant isozymes of G-6-PD known to exist are the common B variant and the more rapidly electromigrating A variant, which is present in a substantial proportion of negroes. About 40 per cent of negro women are heterozygons for these two forms and their normal tissues contain *both* isozymes A and B, each coded from one of their two X-chromosomes. Normal aortic tissue from 98 per cent of these women contains (as expected) both isozymes A and B, but only A or B *alone* is found in 75 per cent of atherosclerotic plaques present in the aortic intima of these same women.

Thus the majority of intimal plaques are apparently derived from one post-embryonic cell, and, therefore, from a single clone of cells. Such monoclonal origin (Chapter 9) suggests that neoplastic transformation is responsible for the proliferation of an aberrant population of cells which have the singularly harmful tendency of causing arterial occlusion.

Deposition of visible lipids in atherosclerotic lesions

Lipids visible in *atherosclerotic plaques* are both intracellular and extracellular. The intracellular deposits are composed of liquid cholesterol esters (CE) and triglycerides (TG). The extracellular deposits similarly contain liquid globules of CE and TG, but in addition include solid crystals of cholesterol (C) and CE and also amorphous masses of phospholipid (Adams, 1967).

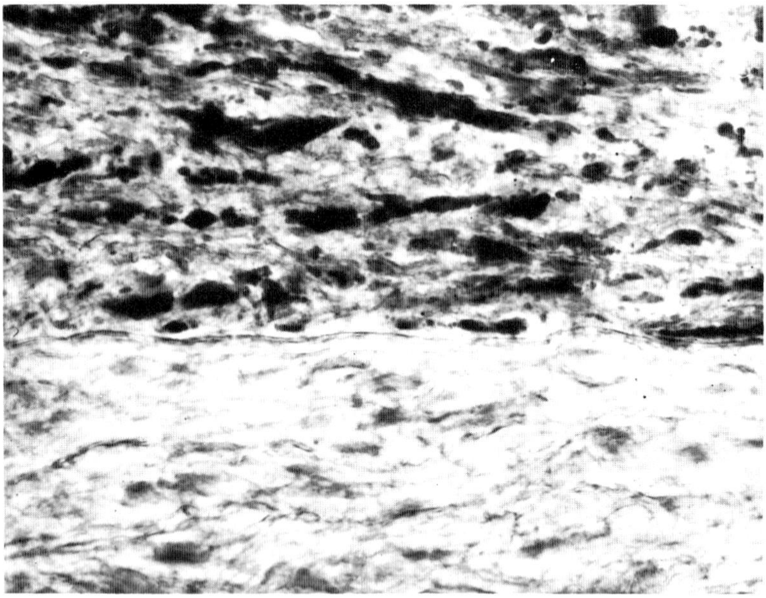

FIG. 8.18 Atherosclerosis (subclavian artery). Deposition of sudanophil lipid in elongated intimal cells immediately inside internal elastic lamina. Frozen section. Sudan III–IV & H. × 400. From Dixon, K. C. (1961) *Amer. J. Path.*, **39**, 65.

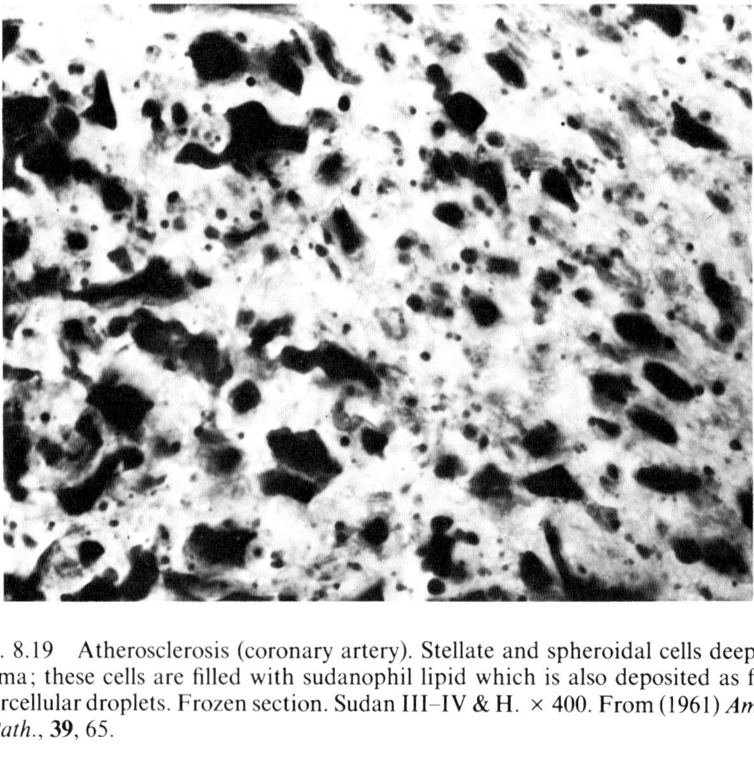

FIG. 8.19 Atherosclerosis (coronary artery). Stellate and spheroidal cells deep in intima; these cells are filled with sudanophil lipid which is also deposited as fine intercellular droplets. Frozen section. Sudan III–IV & H. × 400. From (1961) *Amer. J. Path.*, **39**, 65.

The intracellular globules of lipid are visible within elongated, stellate or spheroidal cells (Fig. 8.18 and 8.19) mainly derived from smooth muscle or other local cells. The absence of catalase from these cells makes it unlikely that many of them are derived from reticuloendothelial phagocytes [69]. Intracellular globules of lipid are specially prominent in elongated intimal cells immediately inside the internal elastic lamina [70]; these lipid-laden cells may sharply demarcate the outer limits of the fibrolipid plaque (Fig. 8.18 and 8.20). Elongated cells (possibly smooth muscle) containing lipid may also be present in the superficial parts of the fibrolipid plaque (Fig. 8.21). Stellate and spheroidal lipocytes and also extracellular lipid are commonly situated in degenerate connective tissue in the outer intima.

Liquid droplets of globular lipid (CE and TG) in frozen sections are strongly stained by the red Sudan dyes (Fig. 8.18, 8.19 and 8.20), but the lipid droplets are removed by the process of embedding in wax, so that sections of wax-embedded tissues merely contain clear cells (Fig. 8.22, p. 383) or intercellular lacunae from which globular lipid has been extracted.

The solid crystals of cholesterol and CE cannot be coloured by Sudan dyes and, although present in frozen sections, can only indistinctly be discerned (Fig. 8.23a); but these crystals are anisotropic [68] and become visible as brilliantly illuminated needles and flakes when the same sections are viewed between polaroid glasses (Fig. 8.23b, c). Crystals of cholesterol and CE are of course absent from sections of wax-embedded tissues but spaces from which these acicular crystals have been extracted are seen as needle-shaped clefts which are prominent in the deeper parts of atherosclerotic plaques (Fig. 8.24, p. 386).

Lipid-filled cells also occur in more superficial *fatty streaks* present in normal intima of unthickened arteries of children and young adults. These fatty streaks are also present in the intima of older patients where fibrolipid plaques occur as well. Indeed Virchow [71] emphasised that fatty cells in arterial walls occur in whitish streaks or spots (*weissliche Flecke*) as well as in the depths of atheromatous foci (*Heerde*); these *Heerde* are now called plaques. In the fatty streaks zones of thickened collagen enclose within them elongated lipid-laden cells which are situated in fusiform clefts [72]. The relation of fatty streaks to atherosclerotic plaques is uncertain.

Determinants of atherosclerosis

The mechanism of cellular proliferation and of coincident deposition of lipids in these fibrolipid plaques is unknown. Indeed it is uncertain whether proliferation of cells or deposition of lipids is the initial event in this complex process. Presumably the deposition of hydrophobic lipids, as in other instances of this phenomenon, depends on either (a) interference with solubilisation or (b) accumulation of hydrophobic substances in too great excess to be solubilised. Moreover several factors are known to influence the incidence of atherosclerosis and these give some clues to its mechanism. These factors will briefly be considered.

Site, age and sex

As already indicated three of the commonest sites for human atherosclerosis are

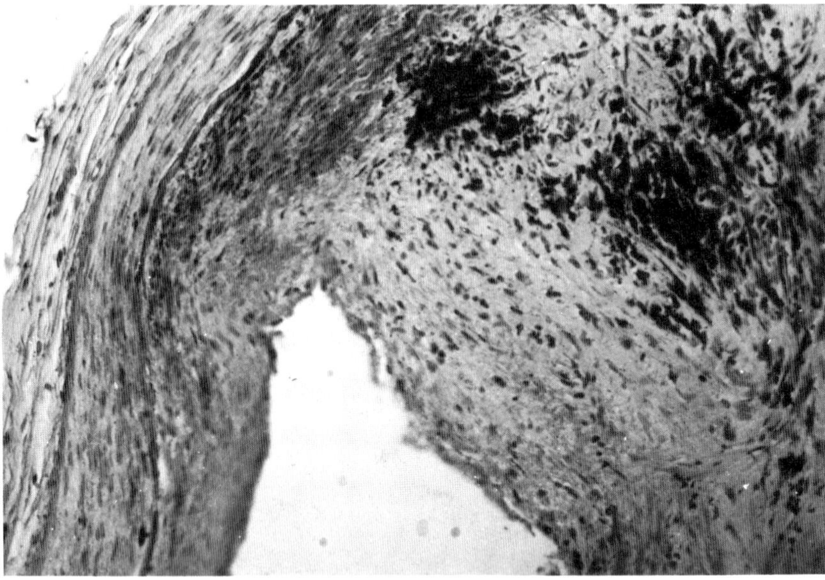

FIG. 8.20 Atherosclerosis (coronary artery). Upper part of same section as shown in Fig. 8.17. Location of sudanophil lipid deep in intima and also immediately inside internal elastic lamina. Sudan III–IV & H. × 130.

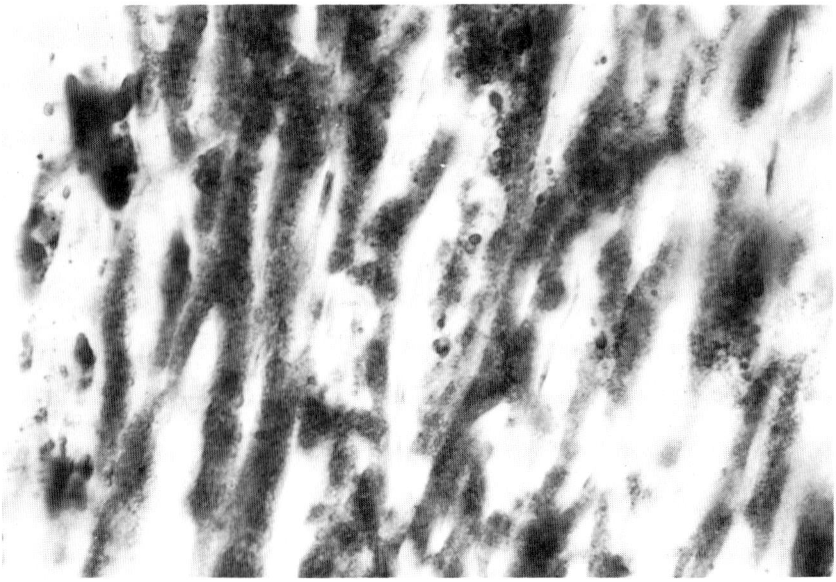

FIG. 8.21 Atherosclerosis (coronary artery). Same section as shown in Fig. 8.17. Fine lipid droplets present in elongated cells (possibly smooth muscle) which are situated in fibrolipid cap of thickened intima. Sudan III–IV & H. × 510.

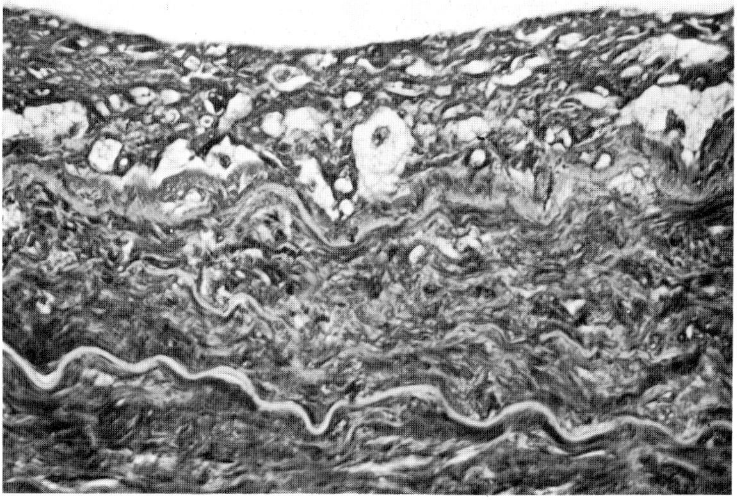

FIG. 8.22 Arterial intima thickened by atherosclerosis from same vessel as shown in Fig. 8.18, but from tissue embedded in wax. This extracts the lipids from cells previously filled by lipid globules and converts the cells into empty vacuolated cavities. OTA method for protein. × 400. From (1961) *Amer. J. Path.*, **39**, 65.

the aorta and the coronary and cerebral arteries. The site of lesions probably correlates with those parts of the arterial wall where flow is sluggish and shear is low, and presumably where lipids discharged from the tissue are only slowly removed by the blood [73]. Atherosclerosis increases with age and becomes appreciable much earlier in men than in women, in whom severe atherosclerosis is rare before the menopause.

Intimal hypoxia

The deepest layer of the intima, immediately within the internal elastic lamina, is probably the most hypoxic part of the arterial wall and is commonly the site of the most abundant deposition of lipids in atherosclerotic plaques. In this hypoxic zone cells containing sudanophil lipid (Fig. 8.18) are prominent as well as intercellular crystals of birefringent lipid (Fig. 8.23b). Hypoxia in the outer intima and also the adjacent media may become even more severe in atherosclerotic plaques where the effective distance through which oxygen must diffuse is *increased* by cellular proliferation and fibrosis or by mural thrombosis [70].

Intimal hypoxia may initiate globulation of cholesterol esters (CE) and TG by interfering with synthesis of solubilising protein. Although intimal cells in atherosclerosis can synthesise phospholipid [68], the type of phospholipid synthesised (sphingomyelin) may not be an effective solubiliser.

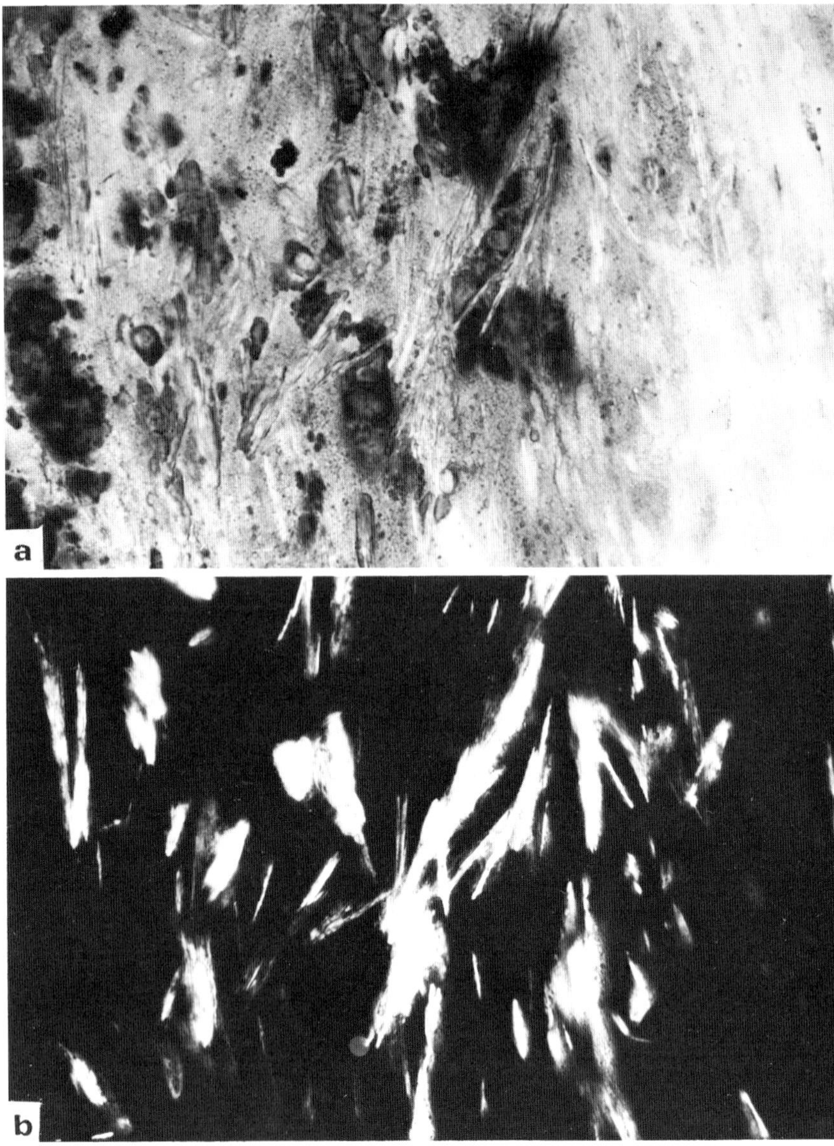

FIG. 8.23 Birefringent solid deposits of cholesterol and CE deep in thickened intima of an atherosclerotic plaque (same section as shown in Fig. 8.17). × 330.

a. Viewed by direct transmitted light: sudanophil liquid lipids are darkly coloured, while some uncoloured solid deposits of lipid are also visible as indistinct crystalline forms.

b. Same field as (a), viewed between polaroid glasses: birefringent deposits of cholesterol and CE become brilliantly illuminated as anisotropic acicular crystals.

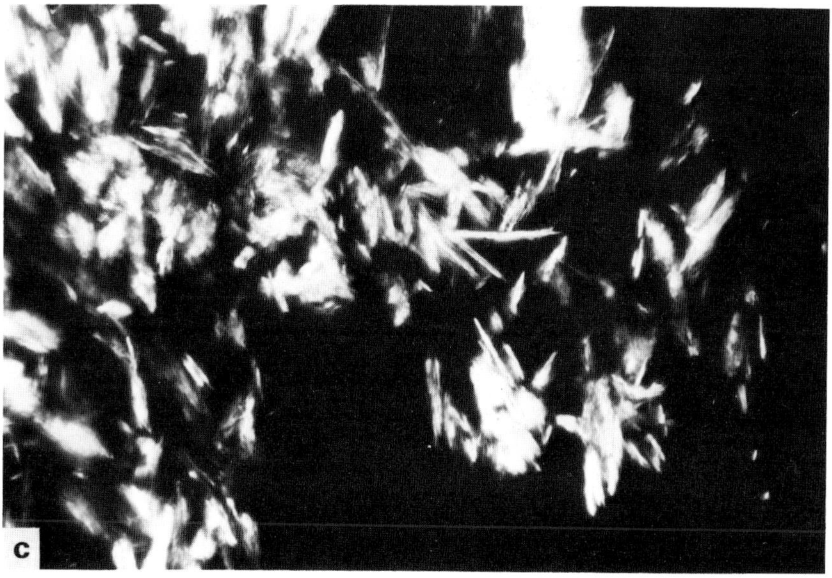

FIG. 8.23 cont.
c. Near field to (b), also viewed between polaroid glasses: more abundant birefringent crystalline flakes as well as needles are prominent.

But hypoxia probably exerts a bigger effect in forming visible deposits of hydrophobic lipids by promoting their synthesis in excess. Hypoxia, by inhibiting oxidative catabolism of acetyl-CoA (Fig. 8.25) may thus cause accumulation of acetyl-CoA and its precursor FFA within the intimal cells and so provide excess of the ingredients necessary for forming cholesterol and its esters. In this way hypoxia may deflect metabolism along an alternative path so that, instead of being oxidised to CO_2, FFA is converted into cholesterol and cholesterol esters (Fig. 8.25, p. 387).

C and CE may thus be formed in too great excess to be solubilised completely in micelles. This may result in formation of visible globules of CE and also micellar particles of LDL containing CE, C and protein. LDL is found in raised concentration in the gelatinous covering of atherosclerotic plaques [74]. Finally the cells containing these deposits may be ruptured and CE and C then accumulate as extracellular globules and crystals within the most hypoxic parts of the plaques (Fig. 8.23b, c). These products may then stimulate fibrosis and so induce further intimal thickening and hypoxia; this may perpetuate a progressive cycle of thickening and lipid deposition [68].

When the concentration of FFA in plasma is raised the formation of C and CE in hypoxic intimal cells is likely to be accelerated even more (Fig. 8.25). In this way the extent of atherosclerotic lesions may be aggravated in diabetes by excess of FFA in the plasma.

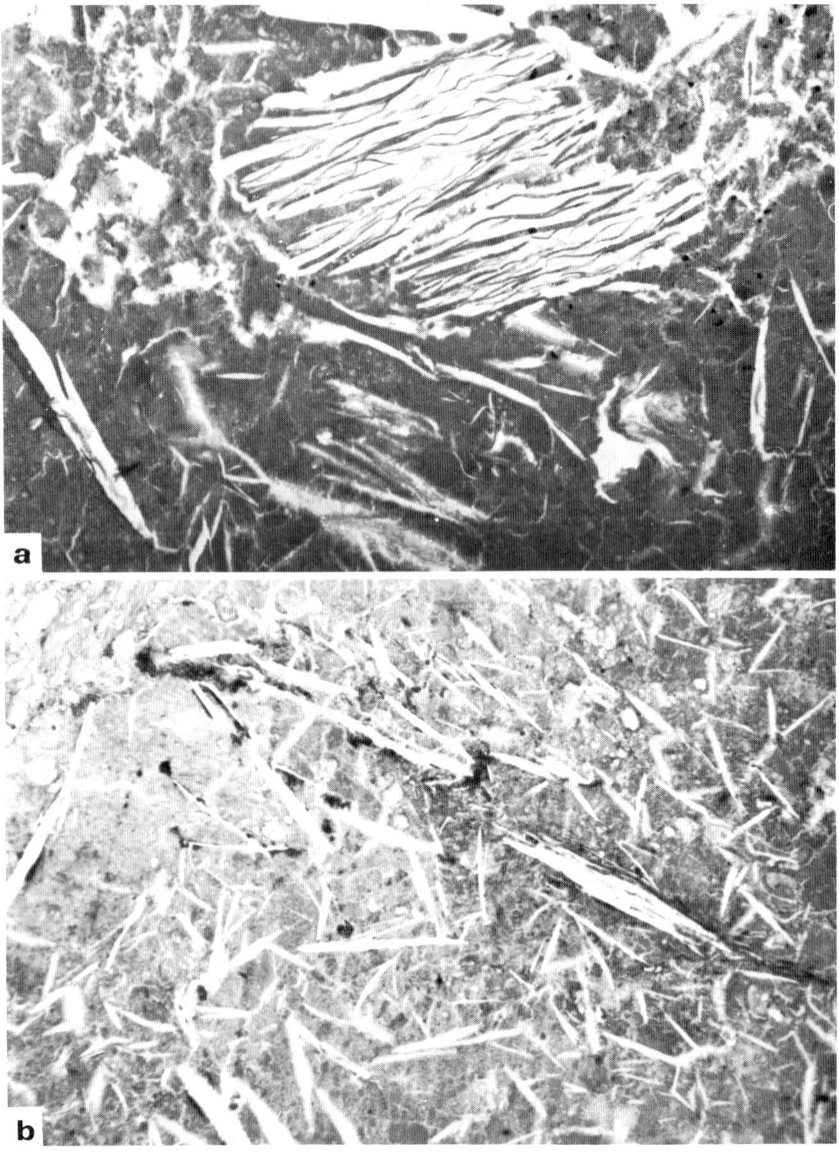

FIG. 8.24 Crystal spaces visible in atherosclerotic plaque from a coronary artery embedded in wax. Acicular spaces previously occupied by crystals of cholesterol and CE form laminar clefts deep in the intima.
a. H & E. × 330.
b. Tannoferric method for protein. × 330.

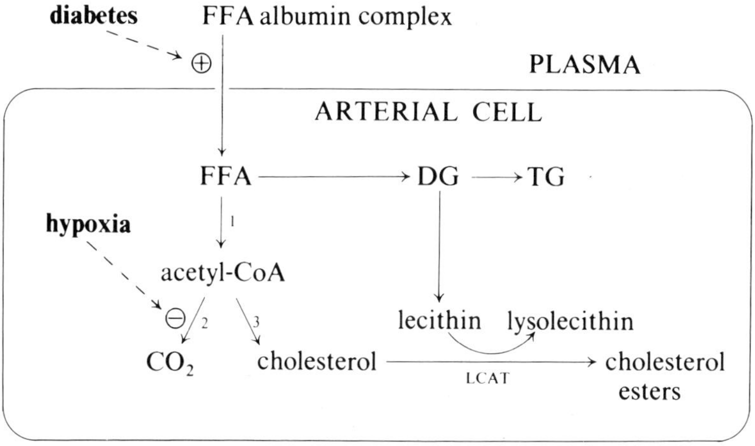

FIG. 8.25 Effect of hypoxia and of diabetes in stimulating the formation of cholesterol and cholesterol esters in arterial cells. By retarding oxidation of acetyl-CoA to CO_2 (route 2) hypoxia deflects metabolism along alternative path (route 3) and increases formation of cholesterol. In diabetes concentration of FFA is increased so that metabolism along routes 1 and 3 is accelerated; this also increases formation of cholesterol.

FFA	free fatty acid
DG	diglyceride
TG	triglyceride
LCAT	lecithin-cholesterol acyltransferase

Mural thrombosis and intimal thickening

Thickening of the arterial intima by organisation of mural thrombi probably also contributes to human atherosclerosis. Von Rokitansky in 1852 [75] suggested that deposition of fibrin from the blood on the arterial wall initiates atheromatous thickening. Duguid [76] considered that this process consists of continuous deposition of fine films of fibrin followed by local inflammation and organisation so that zones of granulation tissue form at the sites where fibrin was originally deposited. Duguid presented considerable evidence to show that zones of mural organisation are in direct continuity with typical atherosclerotic plaques. In this process deposition of lipids may occur in hypoxic cells within the granulation tissue itself or in outer intimal cells which become more hypoxic as their distance from the arterial lumen is increased by the overlying organising thrombus. Indeed, thrombosis followed by organisation may be an important factor in the development of hypoxia of intimal cells with resultant globulation of hydrophobic lipids.

Intimal thickening is also promoted by a mitogenic agent liberated from platelets which adhere to damaged arterial endothelium. These adherent platelets release a heat stable protein of low molecular weight which makes cells pass from G_0 phase to G_1 phase [77]. This mitogenic agent stimulates proliferation of smooth muscle cells in culture. *In vivo* endothelial injury in arteries of monkeys is followed by release of this mitogenic agent. Medial smooth muscle cells then pass through fenestrae in the internal elastic lamina and are stimulated to proliferate within the intima. Thickening of the intima in this way may also contribute to hypoxia in the outermost intimal cells. Adherence of platelets to zones of endothelial injury may thus lead to the lesions of atherosclerosis. Clumping of platelets may further be amplified by local liberation of aggregating agents such as ADP (p. 192) and thromboxane A_2, a prostaglandin which can be generated by platelets [77a].

Possible role of hypersensitivity

Extensive atherosclerosis develops in allografts of rabbit aorta [78]. Similarly coronary arteries in a human transplanted heart showed intense and uniform intimal deposition of lipids along with severe occlusive coronary disease within 20 months of cardiac transplantation [79]. Gresham suggested that atherosclerosis in such transplanted arteries is induced by allergic formation of immune complexes with subsequent aggregation of platelets. The development of atheroma in transplants may indicate that hypersensitivity to other foreign antigens is also concerned in atherogenesis.

Excess of cholesterol in plasma and tissues

The incidence of coronary heart disease (CHD) is raised in persons with excess of cholesterol or of TG in the plasma [80]. Excess of these lipids may therefore be concerned in causing atherosclerosis which is the prime determinant of CHD.

Hypercholesterolaemia is usual in diabetes and in hypothyroidism. Patients with these diseases often suffer from severe and precocious atherosclerosis. Indeed diabetes abolishes the usual sex difference in the incidence of atherosclerosis. Thus diabetic men have 2–3 times more CHD, and diabetic women have 5–6 times more CHD than corresponding non-diabetics. However this increase in concentration of C and CE in plasma in diabetes may be a secondary consequence of increase in FFA with excessive entry of FFA into cells (p. 387). This may be followed by stimulation of intracellular synthesis and deposition of C and CE with later release of these lipids into the plasma (Fig. 8.25).

When rabbits are fed on diets containing added cholesterol, cellular plaques containing C and CE are formed in arterial walls [68, 81]. These plaques consist of masses of spheroidal cells bloated by droplets of lipid, which occur immediately beneath the intimal endothelium [82]. These intimal lesions are at first almost entirely cellular and lack the intense fibrosis so typical of human atherosclerosis. Fibrosclerotic lesions more comparable to human athersclerosis can be produced in rabbits by feeding beef fat rich in saturated TG [83].

The plaques in arterial walls of rabbits fed with cholesterol are formed at sites where the flow of blood is rapid and where the shear is great, in contrast to the plaques of human atherosclerosis which occur where the flow is slowest (p. 383). Increase in the entry of lipid or lipoprotein from the blood rather than retardation of removal from the arterial wall is thus likely to be responsible for these lesions in arteries of rabbits fed excess of cholesterol.

But the location of plaques in human atherosclerosis at arterial sites, where blood moves slowly and shear is low, suggests that diminished removal and excessive synthesis in the plaques are the dominant determinants of deposition of C and CE in the human lesions. The presence of excess of cholesterol in plasma and tissue fluids may, however, increase deposition of lipids and impede their removal, since cholesterol can antagonise the action of phospholipids in forming fine emulsions of hydrophobic lipids and thus may prevent solubilisation (p. 360). This effect is likely to be greatest where removal of solubilised lipid and flow of blood are slowest.

Another possibility is that increase of low density lipoprotein (composed of micelles rich in C and CE) in the plasma is followed by excessive entry of these micelles into arterial cells and that atheromatous deposition of C and CE then ensues [84]. This hypothesis, however, does not account for the paramount location of human atherosclerosis at arterial sites where flow of blood is slowest (see above).

Probably the most injurious effect of hydrophobic deposits of C and CE in atherosclerotic lesions is their capacity to excite reactive fibrosis; this further thickens the arterial intima and thus increases hypoxia along with further deposition of hydrophobic lipids, so that atherosclerosis becomes a self perpetuating process [68]. This process may be exacerbated by deficiency of plasma *high* density lipoprotein which apparently promotes the normal removal of C from arterial walls [84a].

Hypertension

This also increases the risk of CHD. This risk is greater at all levels of blood pressure for smokers than non-smokers. The effect of hypertension is sometimes cited as evidence that atherosclerosis is determined by excessive entry of lipoproteins containing C, CE and TG into arterial walls from the blood. But hypertension results in intimal and medial fibrosis and elastosis as well as medial muscular hypertrophy. Such thickening doubtless increases hypoxia of the arterial wall [70] and may thus equally account for increase in deposition of hydrophobic lipids followed by further atherosclerosis. Moreover cardiac hypertrophy caused by hypertension also increases the risk of ischaemic damage to the myocardium.

Smoking

The risk for smokers of dying from CHD is about twice that for non-smokers. This risk is tragically increased in men between 35–44; among a group of British doctors of this age group the mortality from CHD among smokers was five times that of non-smokers.

This cardiotoxic action of smoking may be due to two ingredients of tobacco smoke, CO and nicotine. The resultant injury probably depends on:

1. Effect of CO in causing intimal hypoxia and thus increasing the severity of atherosclerosis; Astrup *et al.* [85] found that CO increased the content of

cholesterol in aortic tissue of rabbits fed with cholesterol above that of control animals not exposed to CO.

2. Direct effect of CO in producing cardiac hypoxia by combining with myoglobin, Hb and cytochrome (p. 152).

3. Action of nicotine in stimulating secretion of catecholamines and thus needlessly increasing cardiac activity and myocardial hypoxia.

Mechanism of human atherosclerosis: summary

The two principal phenomena of atherosclerosis, namely cellular proliferation and deposition of hydrophobic lipids, are almost certainly interlinked. When one of these processes becomes established, it indirectly initiates the other, so that progressive intimal enlargement ultimately leads to arterial occlusion.

These two sequential processes may interact as follows:

1. Cellular proliferation, caused by transformation with monoclonal growth or by organisation of mural thrombi, increases intimal thickness and thus causes hypoxia in deeper layers of intima.

2. Intimal hypoxia then produces intracellular accumulation of hydrophobic C, CE and TG (Fig. 8.25) followed by intracellular and extracellular deposition of these hydrophobic lipids; this effect is paramount in the most hypoxic zones where the presence of extracellular deposits then excites further cellular proliferation and fibrosis.

Thus process 1 excites process 2 which in turn re-excites process 1 *seriatim*. Atherosclerosis thus becomes self perpetuating.

But one main point of ignorance remains: the origin of the hydrophobic lipids deposited in human atherosclerotic lesions is uncertain. *Does* the lipid enter along with increase in filtration from the plasma of VLDL (carrying TG) and of LDL (carrying C and CE), *or* is the lipid formed by aberrant metabolism of intimal cells, which is primarily initiated by hypoxia?

Possibly both these processes contribute: thus the composition of extracellular lipids within the plaques indicates origin from plasma lipids [74], but the zonal preponderance of intracellular lipids deposited in the outer intima suggests that hypoxia is also a determinant of deposition [70].

DISINTEGRATION OF MYELIN: GLOBULATION OF MYELIN LIPIDS

Myelinated fibres of neurones are encased in sheaths composed of the compressed cell membranes of Schwann cells and oligodendrocytes wound around the internodal segments of the axons. The lipids of myelin consist of sphingomyelin, cerebroside, lecithin and free cholesterol; these amphipathic molecules are orientated at right angles to the surface in bimolecular arrays to form laminar micelles bounded by adherent films of protein. Myelin thus consists of adjacent cell membranes compressed en masse to form stacks of parallel laminar micelles. Changes in disintegrating myelin accordingly provide a large scale model of events in the disintegration of single cell membranes.

Lipids in demyelination: Marchi reaction

When myelin disintegrates the hydrophilic amphipathic lipids of the myelin sheath are replaced by hydrophobic globular lipids and crystals. A valuable method of distinguishing these products of degeneration from the original normal myelin is the Marchi reaction in which the tissues are treated with a mixture of osmium tetroxide (OsO_4) and $KC10_3$ in aqueous solution.

OsO_4 alone in aqueous solution dissolves both in lipids of normal myelin as well as in the products of its disintegration such as cholesterol esters (CE). This dissolved colourless OsO_4 is reduced by the ethylenic bonds in these lipids to form black lower oxides of osmium one of which is OsO_2. This black osmium

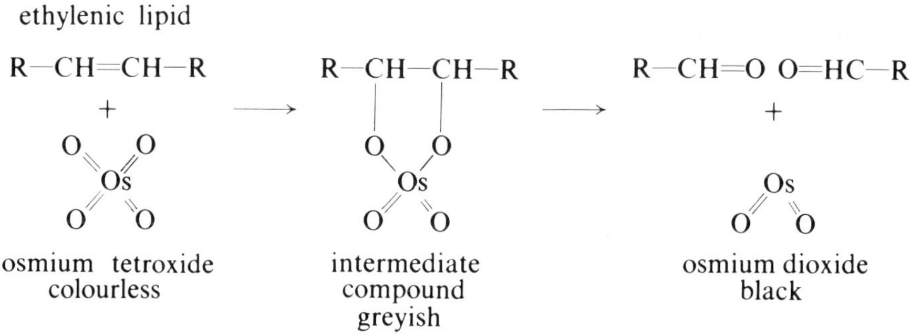

dioxide is still held in solution in the oxidised lipids which therefore appear black. Moreover the blackened oxidised lipids are insoluble in lipid solvents. Thus myelin and the products of its degeneration, such as CE, are both blackened by OsO_4 and are retained in sections of wax embedded tissues.

But when myelin is treated with an aqueous solution containing $KC10_3$ *as well as* OsO_4, the $KC10_3$ also dissolves in the hydrophilic myelin and effectively *prevents* the reduction of OsO_4 to black OsO_2. On the other hand $KC10_3$ cannot dissolve in hydrophobic lipids such as CE. Therefore a mixture of $KC10_3$ and OsO_4 still blackens droplets of CE in degenerating myelin, although this mixed reagent cannot blacken normal myelin. This is the basis of the Marchi reaction [86]; it differentiates hydrophilic lipids which remain uncoloured from hydrophobic lipids including fats and CE which are coloured black. Thus normal myelin which does not blacken (Marchi negative) is conveniently distinguished from degenerating myelin which blackens (Marchi positive).

Sudan IV also distinguishes between the lipids of normal and disintegrating myelin, since it only faintly stains hydrophilic micellar lipids of normal myelin but colours intensely the hydrophobic globular lipids formed in demyelination. Sudan black, however, intensely colours both normal and disintegrating meylin.

Injury to myelin

This complex laminar assembly of compressed cell membranes which encases each myelinated axon is readily injured by poisons or disease, and it also cannot survive destruction of the axon which it encloses. This injury often results in complete disintegration of the myelin sheath, a process which is called demyelination.

The commonest causes of demyelination are:

1. Localised or direct injury to myelin itself by harmful substances (such as Pb^{++} or diphtheria toxin) or in the course of demyelinating diseases such as multiple sclerosis. This is called *primary degeneration* and often involves damage to the myelin of individual Schwann cells to produce segmental degeneration of myelin restricted to the zone between two nodes of Ranvier; such change occurs in lead poisoning (p. 149) and in diphtheritic neuropathy (p. 224). In multiple sclerosis isolated plaques of degeneration of myelin may also occur in localised zones of lysis marked by absorption of antibody and complement (p. 206).

2. Extensive indirect injury as a result of division or compression of the axon proximal to the site of degeneration (p. 108) or by death of neuronal cell body from which the axon arises. This is called *secondary degeneration*, as the initial lesion of axon or cell body may be far removed from much of the subsequent degeneration of the myelin sheath distal to the point of initial injury. This kind of demyelination in white matter of brain or spinal cord may occur in myelinated fibres following injury to grey matter in which their cell bodies are situated. Such damage suggests that substances formed in the cell body (and which pass down the axon) are necessary for the survival of oligodendrocytes and Schwann cells and their membranous laminae.

Process of demyelination

Demyelination is conveniently considered in two sequential phases (Fig. 8.26). In the first the injured myelin disintegrates. In the second the remnants are ingested by phagocytes and further altered by intraphagocytic metabolism.

First phase of demyelination

Retraction of myelin from nodes of Ranvier and enlargement of the Schmidt–Lautermann incisurae follow within a few minutes of crushing a myelinated nerve (p. 110). These effects may be determined by alteration in the conformation of arrayed lipids in the massed membranes of the myelin sheath and they appear to spread from the site of trauma.

Following section of the sciatic nerve in rats autolysis of protein in the distal segments of the myelin sheaths is the first detectable chemical event in the demyelination of Wallerian degeneration. This change involves activation of proteases in the myelin sheath and loss of basic protein stainable by trypan blue at pH 5.0 [87, 88]. Loss of this basic protein from the myelin sheaths of the severed axons is detectable one day after section and increases progressively for several days (Fig. 8.27). The loss of protein in the disintegrating myelin sheaths is pronounced before any chemical changes are detectable in the lipid components.

Similarly in multiple sclerosis enhancement of proteolytic activity and loss of basic protein (Fig. 8.28) are early events in the formation of plaques of

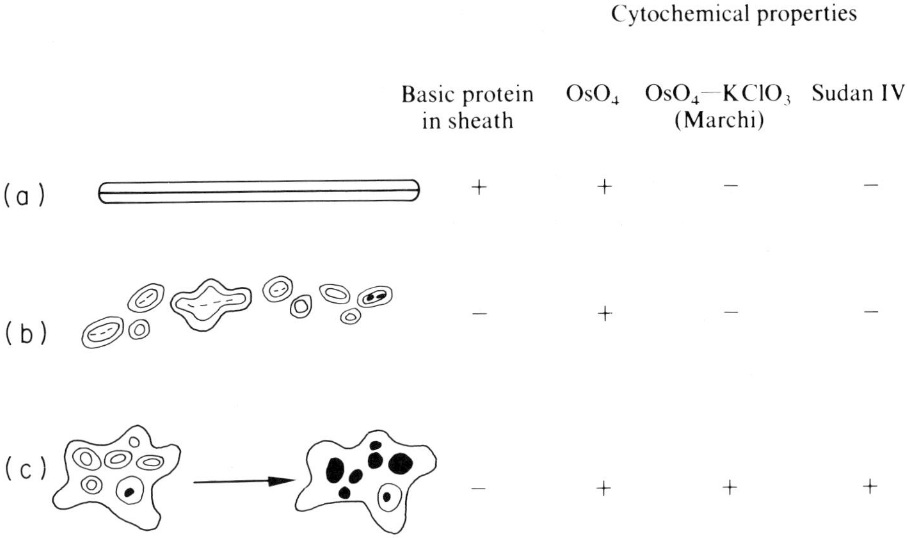

FIG. 8.26 Histochemistry of demyelination. a. Intact myelinated fibres, b. first phase, c. second phase. Disintegration of myelinated fibre involves preliminary fragmentation of myelin along with loss of its basic protein (first phase), followed by phagocytosis of myelin fragments and intraphagocytic conversion of hydrophilic myelin lipids to hydrophobic cholesterol esters (second phase). These changes occur following axonal section (Wallerian degeneration), after ischaemic necrosis, and during demyelination in the plaques of multiple sclerosis. Finally the macrophages disintegrate (not showin in figure) leaving extracellular lipid droplets, granules and crystals.

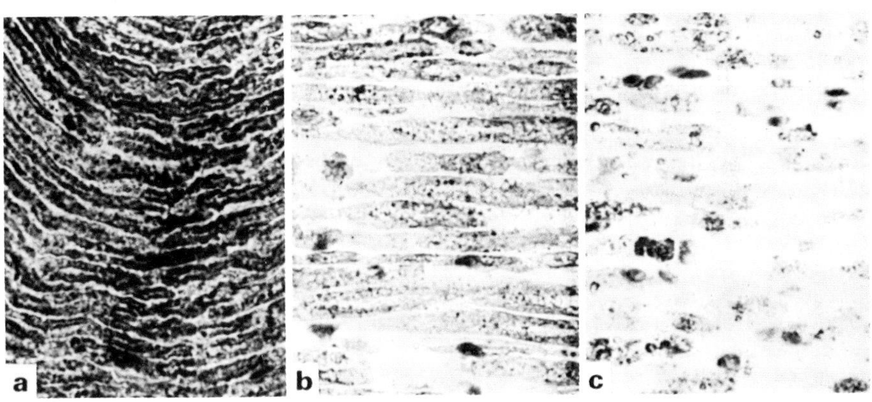

FIG. 8.27 First phase of demyelination. Loss of basic protein of myelin in sciatic nerves of rats following axonal section: trypan blue at pH 5.0. × 240.

a. Normal distribution of basic protein in myelin sheaths of intact nerve.

b. Loss of protein one day after section.

c. Loss of protein six days after section.

Courtesy of Dr J. F. Hallpike, Professor C. W. M. Adams & Dr O. B. Bayliss. Reproduced from *Histochem. J.* (1970); **2**, 323.

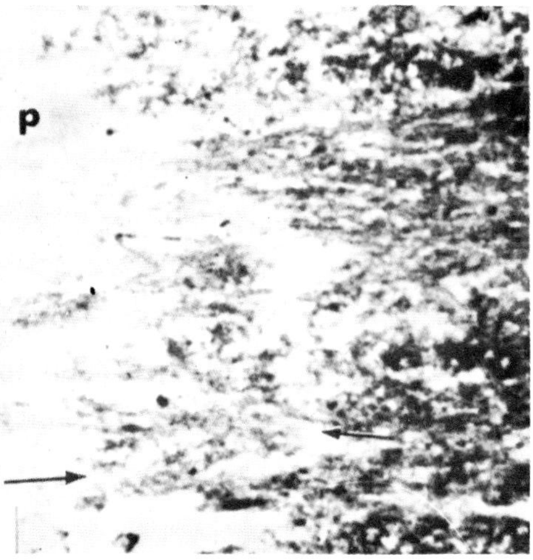

FIG. 8.28 Loss of basic protein from myelin in a plaque (p) produced by multiple sclerosis. Staining diminished at edge of plaque (between arrows). Trypan blue at pH 5.0. × 45. Courtesy of Dr J. F. Hallpike, Professor C. W. M. Adams & Dr O. B. Bayliss. Reproduced from *Histochem. J.* (1970), **2**, 323.

degeneration in myelinated tracts in cerebral white matter [88] and occur before chemical changes in the lipids are detectable.

Progressive changes in the physical state of myelin occur very rapidly after traumatic injury to nerves. Almost immediate retraction of myelin [89] (p. 110), distal to the site of a crush injury, later extends down the nerves. This retraction also follows section of nerves; the myelin sheath (below the plane of section) then becomes swollen, assumes a wavy outline, and breaks up into ellipsoids and spheres [90]. Fig. 8.29 shows these successive changes of Wallerian degeneration in sciatic nerves of mice 1–7 days after transection of the nerves.

Similar swelling and fragmentation of myelinated fibres is visible in cerebral white matter subjacent to zones of ischaemic necrosis in cerebral cortex. Thus, after infarction of the cortex with destruction of perikarya and dendrites of pyramidal cells, demyelination extends into the underlying white matter as the fibres emanating from the dead cell bodies undergo Wallerian degeneration. Fig. 8.30 shows fragments of degenerating myelinated fibres in white matter subjacent to a cortical infarct stained by Sudan black, with normal fibres for comparison; the degenerating myelin sheaths are swollen and fragmented into vesiculated tubules and spheroids, while phagocytes which initiate the second phase of demyelination (see below) have already ingested some of the fragments. Traumatic injury to cerebral tracts also causes swelling and fragmentation of myelinated fibres in cerebral white matter distal to the plane of injury.

How ischaemic necrosis of cell body or trauma to the fibre initiates these changes in myelinated fibres is obscure. Presumably death of the axon is followed by disintegration of the surrounding myelin sheath. But in multiple

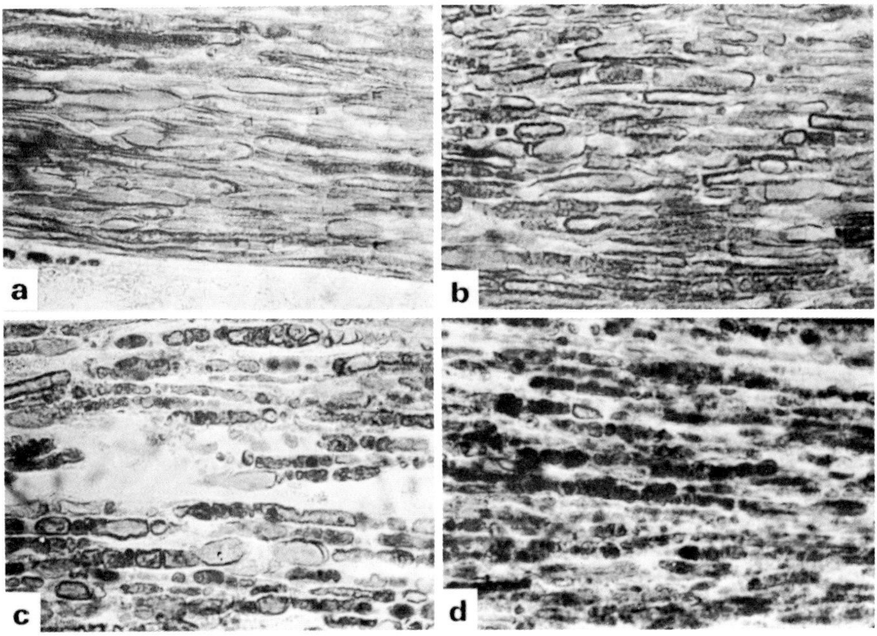

FIG. 8.29 First phase of demyelination. Early changes of Wallerian degeneration in distal portions of severed sciatic nerves of mice. Fixation and staining by buffered OsO_4. Time after transection: a. 1 day; b. 2 days; c. 4 days; d. 7 days.

The myelin sheath swells, contracts, and successively breaks down into ellipsoids, ovoids and spheres although the lipids remain chemically unaltered. Courtesy of Professor M. Wolman. Reproduced from *Pathology of the Nervous System* (1968) vol. 1, p. 764, ed. by J. Minckler. McGraw Hill, New York.

sclerosis injury to the myelin probably precedes axonal damage and this may happen following trauma also.

However the spectacular changes in physical state of disintegrating myelin are almost certainly related to autolysis of protein. Adams [88] suggested that loss of protein so changes the basic skeleton of each myelin lamella, that vertically arrayed lipid molecules lose their attachments and then reaggregate to produce the ellipsoidal globules into which myelin is at first transformed. Another possibility is that hydrolysis of protein during autolysis raises osmolality inside lacunae between the myelin laminae which then reassume cellular osmotic activity and so become swollen. Further fission along the period lines of myelin with fusion of these spaces may thus result in formation of large cavities covered by myelin lamellae which constitute the 'ellipsoids' and 'ovoids' of the disintegratiing myelin sheath.

While these profound changes in the physical state of myelin occur during the first phase of demyelination, no alteration in the chemical properties of the disintegrating lipids is detectable. Moreover the myelin in these fragmenting

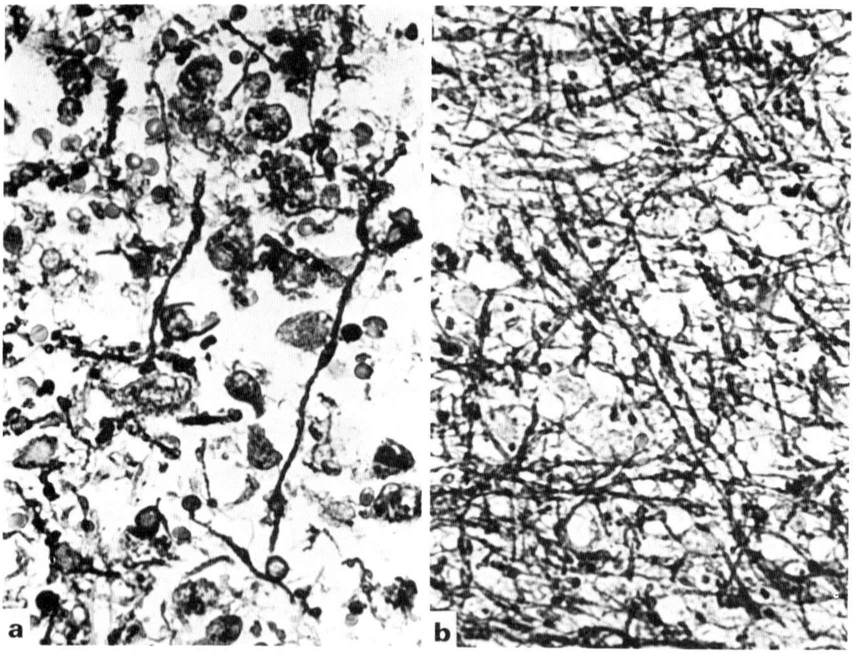

FIG. 8.30 Degeneration of cerebral white matter in a diabetic woman of 61 following ischaemic necrosis of overlying occipital cortex due to embolism about three months earlier. This patient had ischaemic heart disease which resulted in formation of thrombi adherent to necrotic endocardium in left ventricle. Detachment of one of these thrombi probably caused the cerebral embolism with infarction of occipital cortex; after necrosis of cell bodies in cortex their myelinated fibres in subjacent white matter degenerated. Wax section, Sudan black. × 385.

a. Myelinated fibres are fragmented and vesiculated; many of them have already been destroyed by invading macrophages, which initiate second phase of demyelination.

b. Unaffected myelinated fibres for comparison with above. Dixon K. C. & Gresham G. A. G. (1974) *Acta neuropath.* **28**, 55.

ellipsoidal remnants at first remains Marchi negative and retains the other cytochemical properties of normal myelin.

In the first phase of demyelination, which usually last about 7 days, basic protein of the myelin sheath is thus decomposed by autolysis. At the same time the lipids show spectacular physical changes by swelling and disintegrating into ellipsoidal fragments; the chemical composition of the myelin lipids is unaltered.

Second phase of demyelination

In this phase macrophages invade the disintegrating myelin and transform the meylin lipids from hydrophilic laminar micelles into hydrophobic globules (Fig. 8.26c). An early stage in the second phase of demyelination is seen in Fig. 8.30a, which shows disintegration of myelin in cerebral white matter; the myelin sheaths coloured by Sudan black are already broken into tubular and spheroidal fragments, between which are macrophages containing disintegrating fragments of myelin. At first the fragments of myelin within the macrophages are finely granular but are unaltered in cytochemical nature; then this myelin is transformed into globules of hydrophobic lipid which are Marchi positive and are coloured by Sudan IV (sudanopositive stage of Spielmeyer). Histochemical methods used by Petrescu show that these liquid globular lipids within the macrophages are composed of cholesterol esters [91, 92]. In Wallerian degeneration following section of nerves this conversion of hydrophilic to hydrophobic lipid occurs 7–21 days after axonal section, but this process may take much longer in degeneration of cerebral white matter after ischaemic necrosis.

The decomposition of myelin fragments within the phagocytes involves reaction between lecithin and free cholesterol to form cholesterol esters (CE); this is mediated by the enzyme lecithin cholesterol acyl transferase (LCAT).

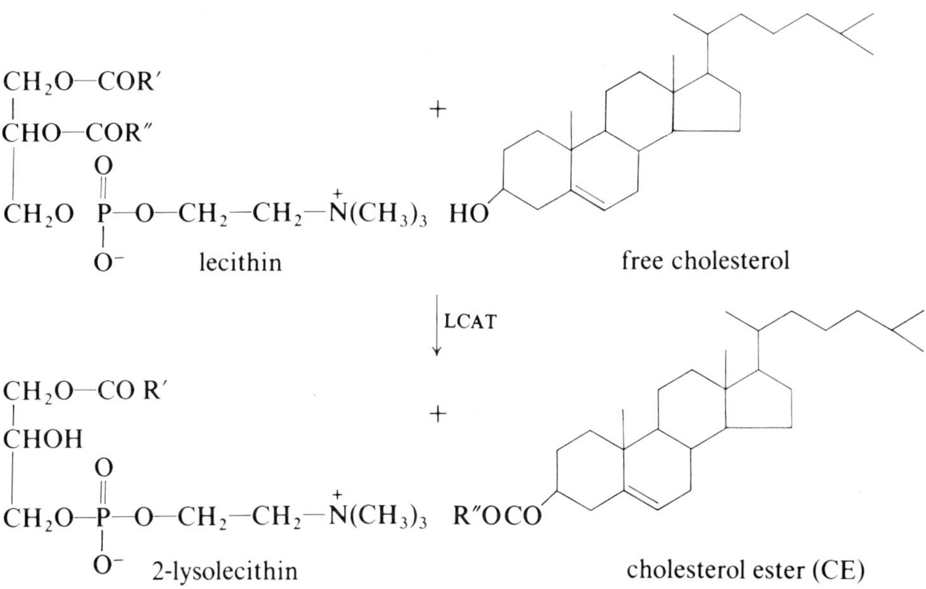

The substrates of this reaction (lecithin and free cholesterol) are amphipathic constituents of myelin micelles and are accessible to *both* OsO_4 ans $KClO_3$ and are therefore Marchi negative. The products of the reaction (CE) are, on the other hand, hydrophobic and dissolve OsO_4 but *not* $KClO_3$, and are therefore Marchi positive.

This same change of hydrophilic laminated myelin lipids into CE occurs wherever myelin degenerates in peripheral nerves or in cerebral white matter, whether as a result of ischaemic damage, trauma or demyelinating disease such as multiple sclerosis. Fig. 8.31 shows massed lipomacrophages within a focus of demyelination in cerebral white matter from a patient who died of acute necrotising leucoencephalitis possibly due to viral infection. The tissue was

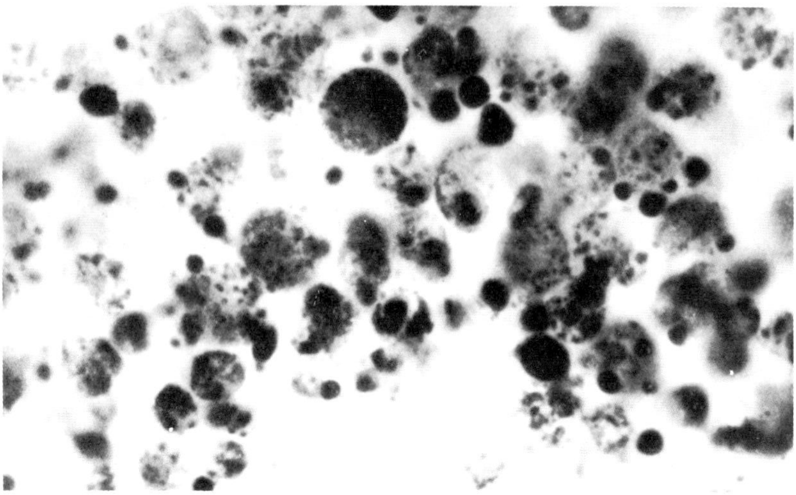

FIG. 8.31 Second phase of demyelination. Conversion of myelin fragments to hydrophobic CE within cerebral lipomacrophages. These cells are massed in a focus of demyelination of cerebral white matter from a patient with acute leucoencephalitis (possibly due to viral infection).

The macrophages contain granules of hydrophobic CE blackened by OsO_2 and paler granules of disintegrating myelin. OTAN method of Adams. Courtesy of Dr A. Petrescu. Reproduced from *Wien. Z. Nervenheilk.* (1969), Suppl II, 38.

stained by the OTAN method of Adams. This employs OsO_4 to reveal hydrophobic lipids which become blackened by OsO_2 (Marchi positive), and OsO_4 and α-naphthylamine which give a brown colour to the hydrophilic lipids of myelin when the power to reduce OsO_4 to OsO_2 is inhibited by $KClO_3$ (Marchi negative). The hydrophobic CE within the lipomacrophages is seen as blackened granules and globules; the hydrophilic lipids of unaltered myelin appear as paler granules, while the background is uncoloured owing to complete destruction of myelin [92].

Transformation of hydrophilic myelin lipids into hydrophobic CE within the lipomacrophages is thus the predominant event in the second phase of demyelination [91].

Finally the macrophages disintegrate and discharge their enclosed lipids into the tissue spaces, where remnants of myelin persist as Marchi positive globules and needle-like crystals both composed of CE.

The process of demyelination thus consists of two principal sequential events:

1. Autolysis of protein with loss of stability in myelin micelles followed by swelling and fragmentation of the myelin sheath.
2. Phagocytosis of myelin fragments by lipomacrophages with subsequent intraphagocytic conversion of hydrophilic phospholipids and free cholesterol

into hydrophobic cholesterol esters; later these hydrophobic remnants may be released from dying macrophages.

AGGREGATION AND ACCUMULATION OF COMPLEX LIPIDS

Fragments from the complex lipids of cell membranes may also become aggregated when the laminar micelles of the cell surface and organelles are disorganised, or when these lipids accumulate in excess because of inherited lack of specific enzymes required for their metabolic removal.

The following examples of visible deposition of complex lipids will be considered:

1. Perennial accumulation of lipofuscin in neurones.
2. Deposition of a similar pigmented lipid in cerebral macrophages which erode necrotic grey matter.
3. Swelling of neuronal cell bodies owing to accumulation of ganglioside GM_2 due to inherited enzymic defect in amaurotic family idiocy.

Neuronal lipofuscin

Neurones have no replacements and their metabolic activity is lifelong. Even without overt injury or functional impairment time alone can exert an effect on neurones by causing progressive deposition within them of clusters of yellowish brown granules of lipofuscin or 'wear and tear' pigment. The deposition of this proteolipid is universal in mankind and may be related to the uniquely extensive surface membranes of neurones which become disarrayed and aggregated throughout the perennial course of neuronal life.

Such disorganisation of membranes may account for formation of this brownish hydrophobic lipid which accumulates as a spectacular constituent in human neurones as age advances. Indeed Ramon y Cajal suggested that this pigmented lipid is responsible for the usual pale brownish colour of human grey matter. Similar though less prominent pigmented lipids are also deposited in myocardial and hepatic cells.

Prominent masses of neuronal lipofuscin are present, as clusters of granules, in pyramidal cells of cerebral cortex, in spinal anterior horn cells and in neurones of the hypoglossal nuclei from middle age onwards. In the neuronal cell bodies of the inferior olivary nucleus, however, this deposition commences in younger persons and, by early middle age, these cells contain abundant and uniform clusters of coarsely granular particles of lipofuscin. The granules of lipofuscin in neurones of human brain and spinal cord are readily visible in sections of wax-embedded tissue in which they are intensely coloured by staining with PAS [93].

These granules in human neurones are lipophilic and dissolve fat soluble dyes. Although not readily extracted by lipid solvents, the lipid portion of these granules can partly be removed by exhaustive extraction with lipid solvents.

Neuronal lipofuscin contains protein as well as lipid and is therefore termed a proteolipid, i.e. a substance which behaves physically as a lipid but in which protein is present. Owing to polymerisation or bonding to protein, the lipid of neuronal lipofuscin is retained in wax-embedded sections where its presence is revealed by colouration with Sudan black (Fig. 8.32) and with mixed Sudan III and IV. The granules are also coloured by the coupled tetrazonium method for protein (Fig. 8.33) and by paraldehyde-fuchsin after oxidation with $KMnO_4$ (Fig. 8.34); they are faintly coloured by pyronin but give an intense rose red colour with PAS (Fig. 8.35).

This reaction with PAS probably indicates the presence of vicinal hydroxyl groups. These may be formed by prolonged lipoperoxidation of ethylenic groups in membrane lipids, followed by detachment of oxidised lipid fragments as hydrophobic aggregates.

Some granules of lipofuscin are associated with lysosomal enzymes such as acid phosphatase and β-galactosidase which suggests that the granules may be engulfed by lysosomes [94]. By EM large granules of neuronal lipofuscin exhibit a complex structure of vesicles (probably lipid vacuoles) bordering on granular or fibrillar electron-dense material; both components are enclosed by a membrane [95].

A material very similar to human neuronal lipofuscin appears in neurones of rats and monkeys fed on diets deficient in vitamin E, probably as a result of autoxidation in the absence of this vitamin (p. 50). Einarson [96] suggested that

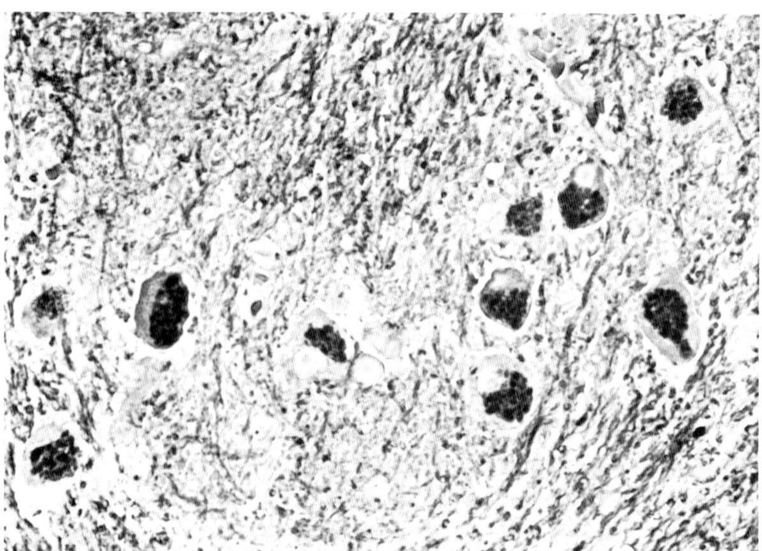

FIG. 8.32 Clusters of large granules of lipofuscin in cell bodies of neurones of inferior olivary nucleus from a man of 62. Lipofuscin intensely blackened, remainder of cytoplasm faint grey, nuclei unstained. Sudan black. × 420. From (1970) *Histochem. J.*, **2**, 151.

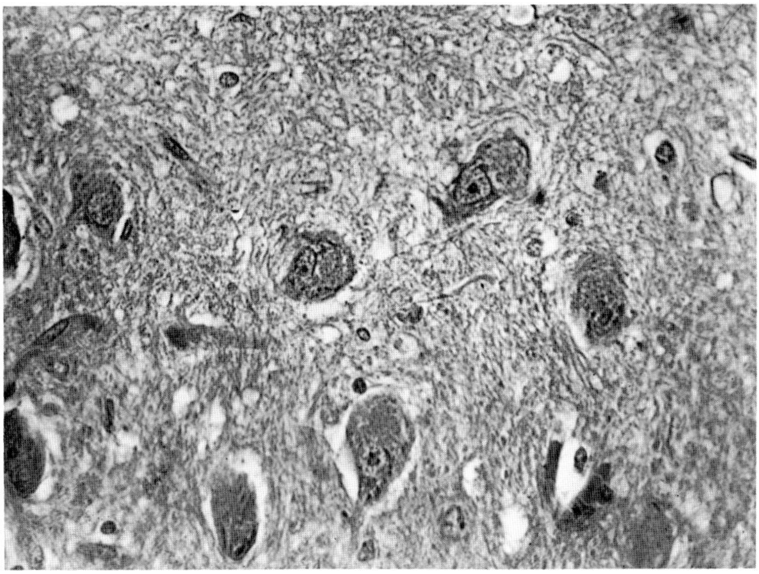

FIG. 8.33 Cell bodies of olivary neurones from a man of 49. Coupled tetrazonium method for protein. × 420.

Nissl substance around nuclear membranes and at extreme periphery of cells is intensely coloured. Clusters of lipofuscin granules, which are also coloured, occupy much of the cytoplasm of the cell bodies. Nucleoli are deeply stained. From (1970) *Histochem. J.*, **2**, 151.

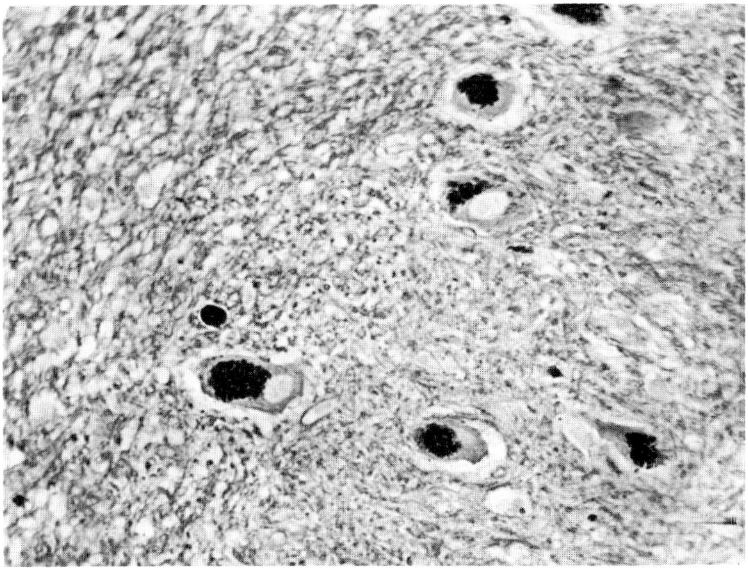

FIG. 8.34 Cell bodies of olivary neurones from a man of 49. Paraldehyde fuchsin after pre-treatment with $KMnO_4$. × 420.

Cell bodies contain clusters of lipofuscin granules which stain purple, cytoplasm violet, nuclei almost uncoloured. A small intercellular amyloid body is also coloured purple. From (1954) *Quart. J. exp. Physiol.*, **39**, 129.

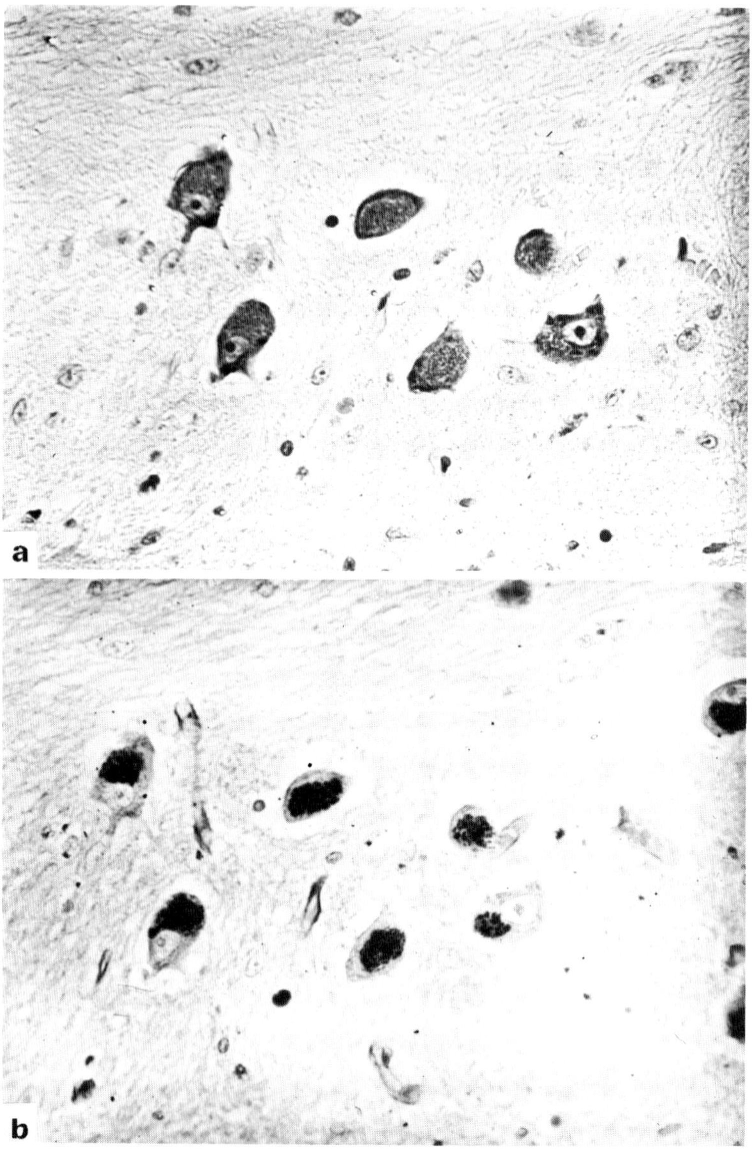

FIG. 8.35 Olivary neurones from a man of 49 successively stained by pyronin G and PAS. × 420.

a. Nissl substance displaced to periphery of cells by large clusters of granular lipofuscin. Nissl substance very dark, lipofuscin much paler. Pyronin G.

b. Same cells as in (a) after decolorisation and treatment by PAS which selectively colours the granules of lipofuscin a deep rose red. From (1954) *Quart. J. exp. Physiol.*, **39**, 129.

similar autoxidation over longer periods of time accounts for deposition of lipofuscin in human neurones as age advances. Autoxidation of ethylenic groups in arrayed lipids of cell membranes may thus cause partial disintegration with aggregation of discarded fragments as hydrophobic granules which accumulate throughout the entire span of neuronal life. This process may be specially prominent in neurones because of their exceptionally extensive surface membranes [9].

Proteolipid in cerebral macrophages

Conspicuous pale brown granules of proteolipid are formed in phagocytes which consume dead neurones of cerebral grey matter after necrosis caused by ischaemia or trauma (p. 344). If a patient survives infarction of a zone of cerebral cortex, then phagocytic cells erode the dead grey matter to form cystic cavities where the remnants of the dead neurones and their processes are finally destroyed by heterolysis (see Fig. 7.35).

The granules of proteolipid formed in these phagocytes have properties very similar to those of neuronal lipofuscin [97, 98]. The granules are pale brown in colour and are retained in wax-embedded sections. They are intensely coloured by Sudan black (Fig. 8.36), by paraldehyde-fuschin after oxidation with $KMnO_4$

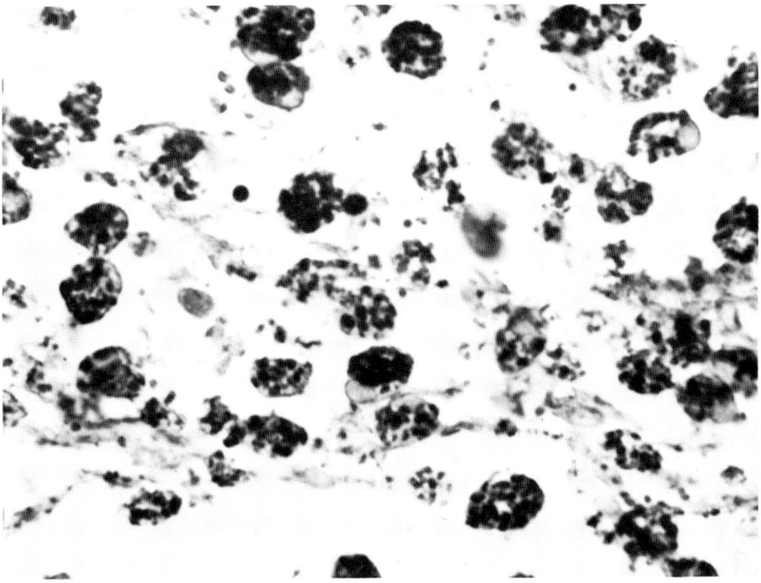

FIG. 8.36 Cerebral macrophages in zone of cystic softening of right occipital cortex from a woman of 63. This lesion was initiated by partial occlusion of right posterior cerebral artery by a thrombus some months before death from coronary thrombosis. The cells contain prominent granules of sudanophil proteolipid which are probably the final remnants of the vanished neurones. Sudan black. × 650. From (1967) *Proc. roy. Soc. Med.*, **60**, 271.

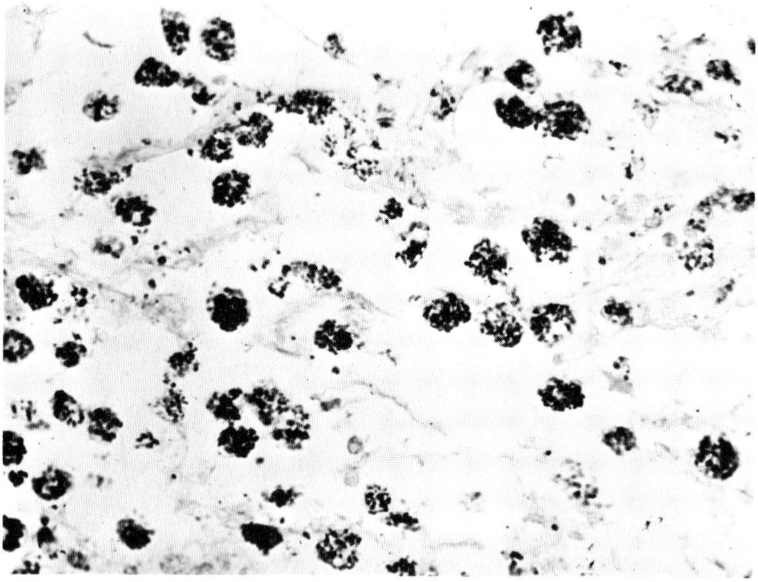

FIG. 8.37 Necrotic occipital cortex from the same ischaemic lesion as shown in Fig. 8.36. Cerebral macrophages filled with granules stained deep purple by paraldehyde-fuchsin after pre-treatment with $KMnO_4$. × 420.

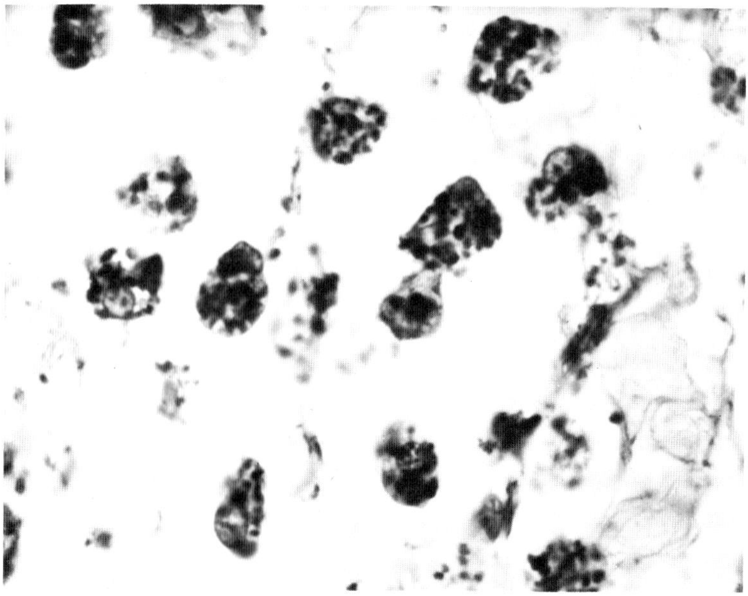

FIG. 8.38 Necrotic occipital cortex from same lesion as shown in Fig. 8.36. Cerebral macrophages filled by granules stained rose red by PAS. × 1020.

(Fig. 8.37) and by PAS (Fig. 8.38); they are also coloured by the coupled tetrazonium method for protein. Although usually brownish in colour they do not contain ferric iron.

These brownish granules of proteolipid formed in macrophages which consume necrotic *grey matter* are not present in the lipomacrophages of necrotic *white matter* in which products of destruction of myelin predominate; the latter are cholesterol esters not proteolipids and are largely removed from the tissue by the process of embedding in wax.

The proteolipid present in macrophages which consume necrotic grey matter is thus clearly very similar to neuronal lipofuscin in its cytochemical properties. This similarity may indicate a like mechanism of formation. Just as lipofuscin appears to be formed inside neurones by partial disintegration and discard of fragments from the immense expanse of neuronal surfaces during the course of life, so also, when neurones are killed by ischaemia, their uniquely extensive membranes may become disarrayed and release hydrophobic proteolipid fragments [99]. When neurones are destroyed *en masse* more substantial quantities of neuronal membranes are likely to disintegrate than during the more gradual process of ageing. Much of this disintegration may progress within the macrophages. Ultimately a hydrophobic remnant derived from the enormously extensive axo-dendritic surfaces of the dead neurones may persist as PAS-positive granules within the macrophages in the softened grey matter.

Amaurotic family idiocy (Tay-Sachs disease)

Gangliosides, which are the dominant glycolipids of cerebral grey matter, are normally degraded by sequential fission inside lysosomes by a series of specific hydrolases. Inherited deficiencies of these ganglioside-splitting enzymes are responsible for a number of ganglioside storage diseases [100]. One of these is Tay-Sachs diseases (G_{M2} gangliosidosis type 1), in which the sphingolipid G_{M2} ganglioside accumulates in cerebral neurones.

This disorder, caused by a rare recessive gene occurring principally among Ashkenazi Jews, starts with the onset of motor weakness at 3–6 months of age, followed by blindness, spasticity, convulsions and decerebrate rigidity leading to death in early childhood. The cerebral neurones swell into grotesque forms bloated by abundant glycolipid (Fig. 8.39). This change occurs in the cell bodies and also the apical dendrites of pyramidal cells which develop bizarre swellings filled with lipid. The ganglion cells of the retina are also filled by the deposits, which give a creamy appearance to the retina; but as the optic fibres degenerate the central fovea becomes more translucent than usual, so that the intensified red reflex of the choroid causes the foveal area to appear as a 'cherry red' spot on a creamy retinal background. Under EM the cytoplasm of the cerebral neurones is seen to be filled with laminated spheroids; these membranous cytoplasmic bodies (MCBs) are about 1 μm in diameter and have a laminar periodicity of 5–6 nm [101]. Acid phosphatase is enclosed within these MCBs and they are therefore regarded as enlarged lysosomes. By LM these bodies appear as vesicles (Fig. 8.40) with PAS-positive rims [102]. MCBs isolated from cerebral tissue by centrifugation of homogenates contain large quantities of

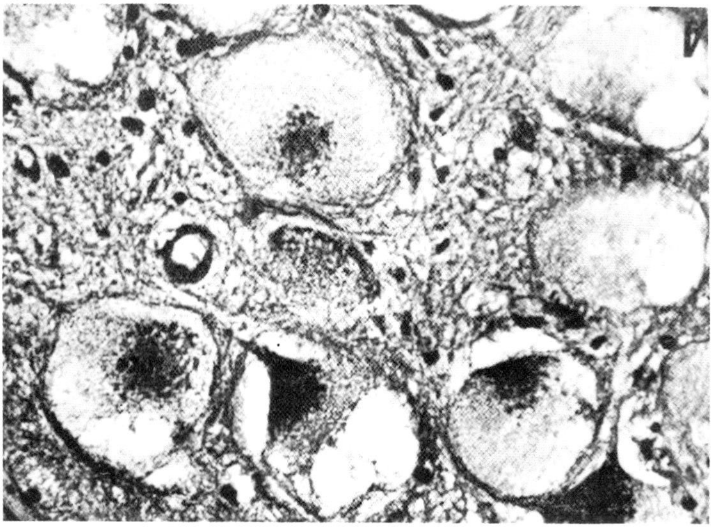

FIG. 8.39 Swollen ganglion cells from medulla oblongata of a patient with Tay-Sachs disease (infantile form of amaurotic family idiocy). The neuronal cell bodies are swollen by deposits of ganglioside G_{M2}. H & E. × 800. Courtesy of Professor M. Wolman. Reproduced from Proceedings of the Vth international Congress of Neuropathology. *Excerpta med.* (*Amst.*) (1965) **100**, 116.

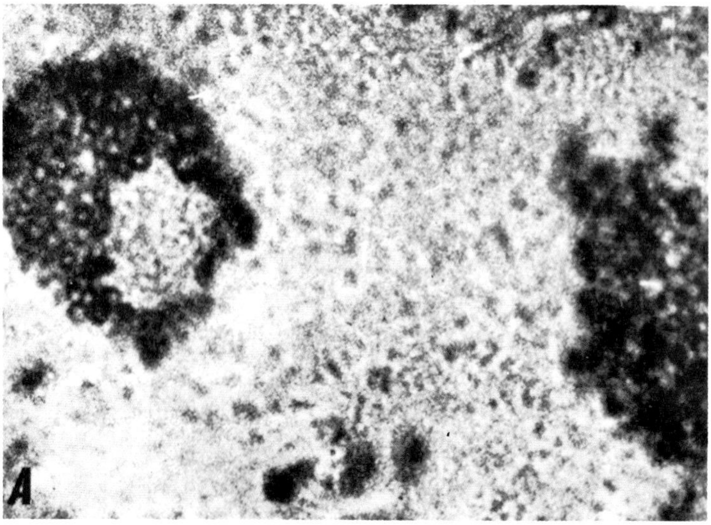

FIG. 8.40 Ganglion cells from cerebral cortex of a patient with Tay-Sachs disease. Semi-thin epon-embedded tissue fixed with OsO_4. Stained PAS. × 1350. Neuronal cytoplasm filled by vesicles with PAS-positive rims. Courtesy of Professor M. Wolman. Reproduced from Proceedings of the Vth international Congress of Neuropathology. *Exerpta med.* (*Amst.*) (1965) **100**, 116.

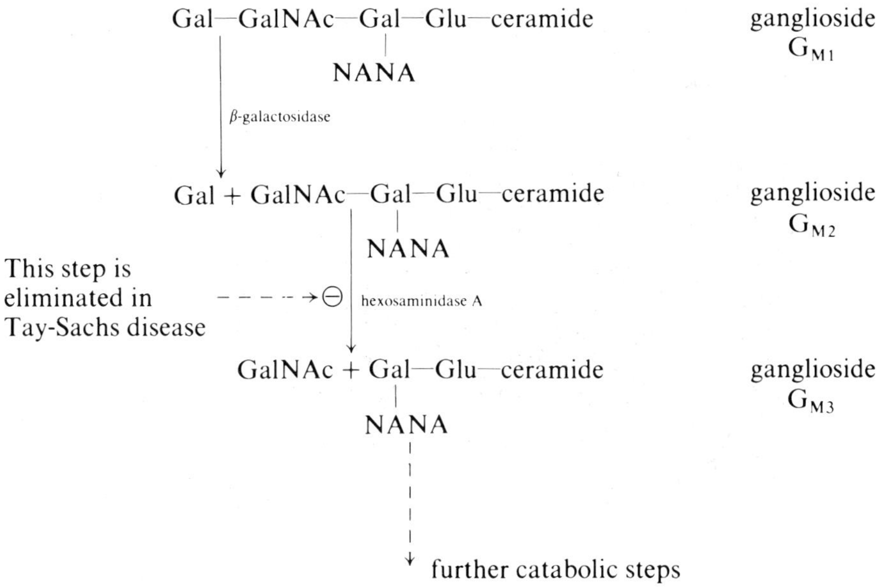

FIG. 8.41 Enzymic defect in Tay-Sachs disease. Brain gangliosides G_{M1} and G_{M2} are normally degraded by sequential loss of sugar residues. Absence of hexosaminidase A in Tay-Sachs disease arrests release of GalNAc from G_{M2}; this causes accumulation of G_{M2}.

Gal	galactose residue
GalNAc	N-acetylgalactosamine
NANA	N-acetylneuraminic acid
Glu	glucose residue

ganglioside G_{M2}, the concentration of which is raised 100- to 300-fold in cerebral tissue from these patients.

The excess of G_{M2} is almost certainly determined by the absence of enzyme hexosaminidase A which occurs in normal brain and other tissues. This enzyme is responsible for splitting off N-acetylgalactosamine from this ganglioside component of brain. This fission is an obligatory step in the sequential degradation of cerebral gangliosides (Fig. 8.41). The lysosomal fraction of normal brain and other tissues contains two hexosaminidases A and B which can split off this terminal N-acetyl-galactosamine from G_{M2}. These two enzymes can be separated by starch-gel electrophoresis as component A is more negatively charged than component B. Component A is entirely absent from tissues in Tay-Sachs disease, although component B and other lysosomal enzymes are increased probably as a result of lysosomal stimulation by excess of G_{M2}. Component A appears to be mainly responsible for normal catabolism of G_{M2}.

This absence of hexosaminidase A causes deposition of G_{M2} in gross excess so as to inflate the lysosomes, and the neurones which contain them, into balloon-like monstrosities; the change is followed by degeneration of axons and disintegration of their myelin sheaths resulting ultimately in paresis, coma and death. During the course of the disease neuronal necrosis is followed by gliosis which ultimately produces considerable cerebral enlargement.

ACCUMULATION OF POLYSACCHARIDES

Glycosaminoglycan storage diseases: gargoylism

Glycosaminoglycans (GAGs) are normally formed in cells by disintegration of proteoglycans of connective tissue (formerly called mucopolysaccharides). Proteoglycans are macromolecules consisting of a central protein core to which are attached numerous GAG chains. Normally these GAG fragments are degraded by sequential action of lysosomal enzymes. But if one of these enzymes is absent, the whole sequential process is interrupted and polymeric GAG fragments accumulate in the lysosomes. In these GAG storage diseases the lysosomal catabolism of two GAG polymers *dermatan sulphate* and *heparan sulphate*, singly or together, is interrupted by absence of one of the lysosomal enzymes necessary for the sequential fission of these sulphated GAGs. These polymers then accumulate in cells including those of connective tissue where their presence during early development induces severe facial and skeletal deformity. In these disabilities *glycolipids* also accumulate in cerebral neurones and thus in addition cause mental retardation.

These disorders are inherited and are typified by Hunter's syndrome (X-linked recessive) and Hurler's syndrome (autosomal recessive). In both these conditions malfunction of connective tissue cells is accompanied by gross abnormality in development with facial, bony and cardiovascular malformations usually coincident with mental defect. The enlarged head with coarse features, protruding tongue, flattened nose bridge and widely spaced eyes led to the term gargoylism which is applied to both diseases. In Hurler's syndrome, in which accumulation of GAG produces the most severe defects, clouding of the cornea is an additional sign of deposition of GAG. Hepatocytes and connective tissue cells are commonly swollen and vacuolated by enlarged lysosomes containing deposits of GAGs. These substances consist of sulphated uronic acid-hexosamine polymers which are detached from their proteoglycan cores with or without a few residual amino acids. These polymers include dermatan sulphate, which contains units of sulphated iduronic acid conjoined with sulphated N-acetylgalactosamine residues with high net negative charges (Fig. 8.42), and also heparan sulphate, another similar sulphated GAG [103]. These strongly anionic polyglycans are visible within connective tissue cells and also in blood lymphocytes, as 'metachromatic' granules, which are stained red by the kationic dye toluidine blue. These anionic GAGs are excreted in the urine of patients and can be detected by forming precipitates with cationic reagents such as cetyl pyridinium bromide.

Fibroblasts of normal skin when grown *in vitro* contain very few metachromatic granules. But similarly cultured fibroblasts from patients with Hunter's or Hurler's syndrome accumulate abundant cytoplasmic metachromatic granules

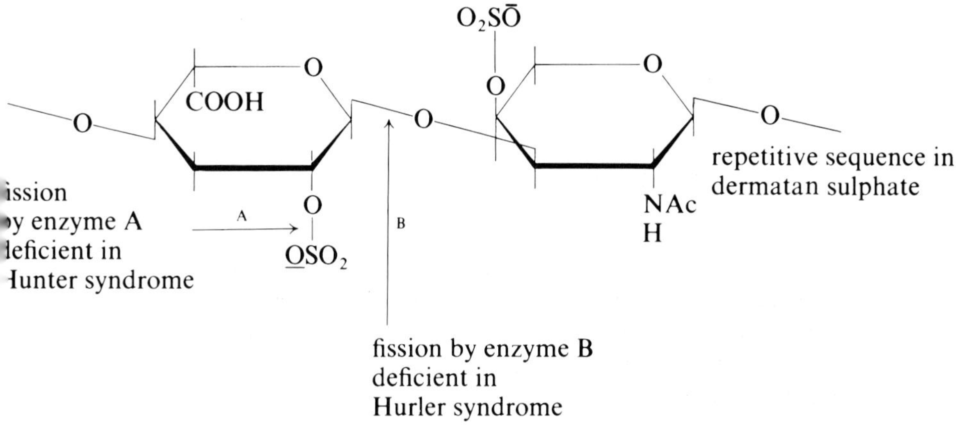

FIG. 8.42 Enzymic defects in Hunter's syndrome and in Hurler's syndrome. In these disorders sulphated GAGs, such as dermatan sulphate, cannot be degraded and so accumulate within lysosomes as metachromatic granules. Dermatan sulphate contains in its chain of sugar units a repetitive sequence of sulphated iduronic acid joined to sulphated N-acetylgalactosamine. Successive action of enzyme A (a sulphatase) and enzyme B (an iduronidase) is responsible for catabolism of GAG chains containing this sequence. If either of these enzymes is absent dermatan sulphate accumulates. Enzyme A is absent in Hunter's syndrome, while enzyme B is absent in Hurler's syndrome.

containing dermatan sulphate and heparan sulphate which are coloured pink by toluidine blue [104]. The normal fission of dermatan sulphate depends on the successive action of a sulphatase (enzyme A in Fig. 8.42) and an iduronidase (enzyme B in Fig. 8.42). In the absence of *either* of these enzymes accumulation of dermatan sulphate and heparan sulphate occurs [103]. One of these enzymes A is deficient in Hunter's syndrome; this splits off sulphate groups (Fig. 8.42). The other enzyme B is deficient in Hurler's syndrome; this hydrolyses the iduronic acid-galactosamine linkage (Fig. 8.42).

The fibroblasts of normal connective tissue secrete both these enzymes into the surrounding fluid. The enzymes are then reabsorbed into the fibroblasts by selective pinocytosis, and the fluid containing them is then concentrated within phagolysosomes, which *only then* can degrade the GAGs completely. In the absence of *either* enzyme necessary for this step by step degradation of the polyglycan chains, GAG remnants, such as dermatan sulphate, accumulate in the cells. Indeed admixture of normal skin fibroblasts with a culture of fibroblasts from one of these patients provides sufficient amounts of both enzymes to prevent this accumulation of GAGs, which is also suppressed in mixed cultures of cells from a 'Hunter' patient added to those from a 'Hurler' patient [105]. Absence of one of these two enzymes in the cells of patients with either Hunter's or Hurler's disease is also responsible for excretion of these GAGs in the urine, which enables diagnosis in young children before morphological defects become apparent.

The accumulation of GAG in cultured human skin fibroblasts is conveniently followed by measuring the rate of incorporation of radioactive $^{35}SO_4$ into GAG extracted from the cells [105, 106]. This rate is relatively low in normal fibroblasts but is enormously greater in fibroblasts grown from the skin of patients with either Hunter's or Hurler's syndrome. By using cultures of fetal fibroblasts from amniotic fluid this excessive rate of incorporation can be detected in antenatal life if the fetus is affected by either of these diseases; thus prenatal diagnosis of these disabilities is possible.

The presence of these GAG residues, which accumulate in the swollen lysosomes of fibroblasts and osteoblasts, apparently produces severe malformation in developing connective tissue and bone of young children and thus accounts for the disfiguring deformities of gargoylism. Accumulation of GAGs in hepatic and splenic cells is associated with enlargement of liver and spleen with abdominal distension and umbilical hernia in affected children.

In gargoylism (both Hunter and Hurler types) gangliosides also accumulate within neurones as well as GAG in connective tissue and hepatic cells. Granules containing these complex glycolipids are thus prominent in the neuronal cell bodies of both brain and spinal cord (Fig. 8.43a) and they form characteristic swellings shaped like rugby footballs in the apical dendrites of cerebellar Purkinje cells (Fig. 8.43b). These granules are coloured intensely by Sudan black and PAS; by EM they appear as distended lysosomes bounded by a single membrane with internal transverse lamellae which give these organelles a striped appearance ('Zebra bodies') [107]. The accumulation of these granules rich in ganglioside within the neurones is probably caused by concomitant lack of β-galactosidase (Fig. 8.41) which is generally deficient in cells of patients with gargoylism. The mental retardation of children with gargoylism is probably determined, as in Tay-Sachs syndrome, by distension of neurones with copious lipid deposits. No adequate explanation has been advanced as to why this inherited absence of enzymes which split GAG can result in lack of β-galactosidase in neurones followed by accumulation of gangliosides.

Glycogen storage diseases

In these disorders glycogen is deposited in cells owing to inherited deficiency of various intracellular enzymes which are either directly or indirectly responsible for its degradation. Such glycogen accumulates in visible deposits *either* free in the cytoplasm, as in glycogenosis type 1 (von Gierke's disease), *or* sequestered within lysosomal vesicles as in glycogenosis type 2 (Pompe's disease). Glycogenosis types 1 and 2 will briefly be considered as examples of these disabilities, which are in general caused by abnormal autosomal recessive genes.

Glycogenosis type 1

This inherited disorder of infancy is characterised by enlargement of liver and kidney due to excessive deposits of glycogen. Affected children fail to grow and suffer from severe hypoglycaemia (as low as 0.6 mmol glucose/litre of blood), hyperlipidaemia and ketosis.

The intracellular deposition of glycogen is due to congenital absence of

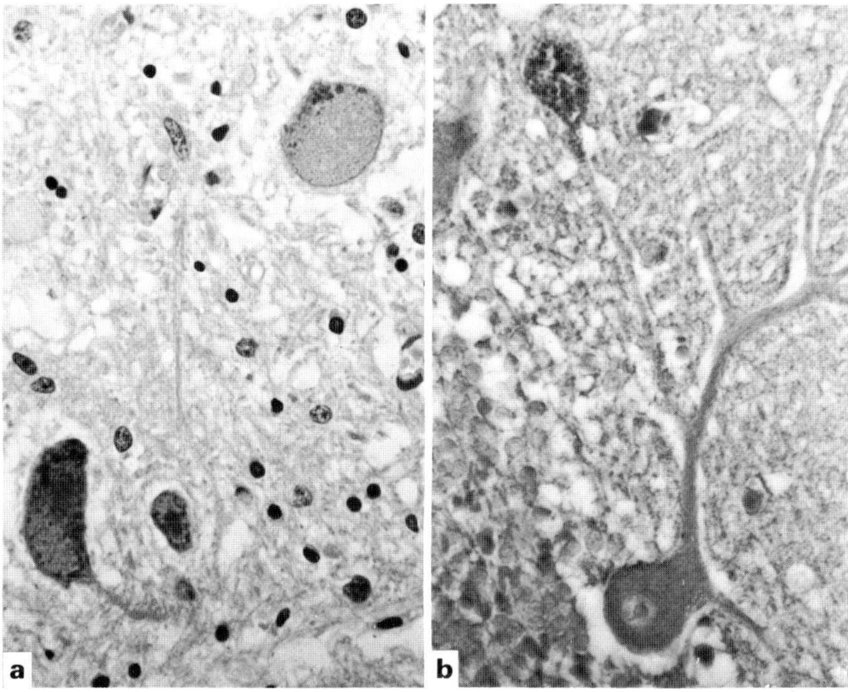

FIG. 8.43 Spinal cord and cerebellum from a boy of 9 with Hurler's syndrome (gargoylism with severe mental defect and corneal opacification).

a. Cell bodies from spinal neurones distended by deposits of glycolipid. Wax-embedded tissue. H & E. × 415.

b. Purkinje cell from cerebellum. Large ellipsoid swelling filled with blackened granules of glycolipid is visible on branch of an apical dendrite. Wax-embedded tissue. Sudan black. × 415.

enzyme glucose-6-phosphatase. This also results in abolition of normal mechanism of release of glucose from hepatic cells into the blood. In the absence of this enzyme glucose-6-phosphate accumulates and this accelerates synthesis of glycogen within the cells as well as arresting the release of glucose (Fig. 8.44). The hepatic cells are swollen by accumulation of glycogen, and they may also contain fine droplets of fat. The hypoglycaemia may result in convulsions and mental retardation.

Glycogenosis type 2

This inherited disability results in cardiomegaly with severe cyanosis and dyspnoea along with profound muscular weakness which develop within the first few months of life. Glycogen is found in gross excess within cardiac and skeletal muscle fibres, in liver cells and in medullary neurones. EM shows that this glycogen is not free within cell cytoplasm but is enclosed in large irregular

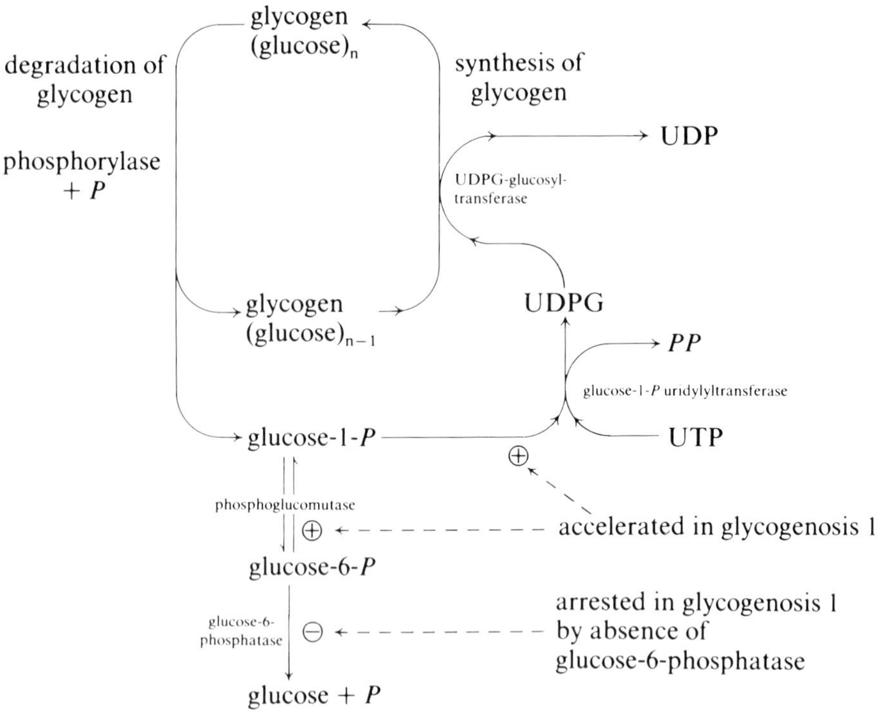

FIG. 8.44 Glycogenosis type 1. Absence of glucose-6-phosphatase in hepatic cells causes excessive synthesis and accumulation of glycogen by increasing concentration of glucose-6-*P* and indirectly of glucose-1-*P*. Liberation of glucose is grossly retarded.

UTP	uridine triphosphate
UDP	uridine diphosphate
UDPG	uridine diphosphate-glucose
P	phosphate
PP	pyrophosphate

vacuoles bounded by unit membranes identical to those which normally cover lysosomes. The hepatic cells contain grossly enlarged misshapen lysosomes filled with microgranules of glycogen. In skeletal muscle fibres these enlarged lysosomes stuffed with glycogen displace the contractile fibrils which remain visible only at the edge of the fibres. Cardiac muscle is similarly deformed. Eventual compression or displacement of myofibrils by these swollen lysosomes probably accounts for the profound muscular and cardiac malfunctions which are responsible for death in early childhood.

The basic abnormality in Pompe's disease is absence of acid maltase, which is a normal lysosomal hydrolase. This enzyme hydrolyses the α-1-4 maltose linkage (Fig. 8.45). Unlike phosphorylase, which degrades glycogen and is free in the cytoplasm, acid maltase is confined to lysosomes and only degrades glycogen which has been taken up by these phagocytic organelles. This enzyme is absent from the lysosomes of all cells in Pompe's disease.

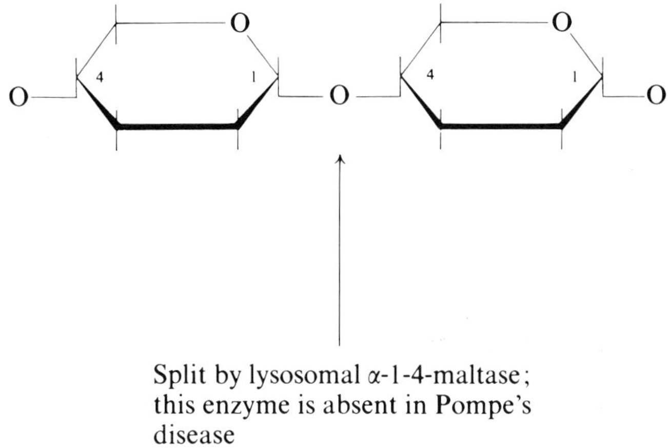

FIG. 8.45 Glycogenosis type 2. Absence of lysosomal α-l-4-maltase prevents normal fission of principal link between glucose residues of glycogen. Glycogen then accumulates in lysosomes which expand into large irregular saccules; this causes swelling of cells, including hepatocytes and fibres of cardiac and skeletal muscle.

Glycogen is composed of chains containing 12–18 glucose residues joined by 1-4 linkages which branch by attachment to other 1-4 chains through occasional 1-6 interconnections. Interference with fission of the principal 1-4 junction results in gross accumulation of glycogen within the lysosomes. The cells become swollen by enlarged and irregular lysosomal sacs which ultimately result in disastrous malfunction of both cardiac and skeletal muscle fibres.

Deposition of glycogen in diabetes

Excessive deposition of glycogen is conspicuous in some cells of diabetic patients. Although lack of insulin impedes entry of glucose into skeletal muscle, it does not interfere with penetration of glucose into liver nor pancreatic islets. In diabetic hyperglycaemia glucose may enter these organs and form glycogen, which is deposited in the pancreatic insular cells and also as characteristic 'vacuoles' within the nuceli of hepatocytes. These vacuoles represent spaces from which glycogen has been dissolved during the fixation and preparation of sections.

DEPOSITION OF PROTEIN

Disorders of cells can produce visible deposits in which protein is the principal constituent. Such deposition may be due to aggregation of original cellular protein or may result from excessive entry or formation of abnormal protein.

Inherited defects in assembly or stability

Inborn errors may interfere with synthesis of a particular component of a protein so that the product formed is unstable and aggregates as a hydrophobic visible deposit. Such inclusions of aggregated protein may be actively harmful to the cells which contain them.

In β-thalassaemia (p. 24) deficiency of β-chains of globin results in accumulation of free α-chains which become denatured and aggregate as large hydrophobic inclusions within erythroblasts; the inclusions damage the cell membranes and shorten the life of both the erythroblasts and of any red cells which develop from them. Acid hydrolases probably derived from lysosomes can be detected in the inclusions; this suggests that lysosomes may fuse with or envelop these aggregates of denatured protein [108]. In α-thalassaemia (p. 24) deficiency of α-chains of globin results in accumulation of free β-chains or free γ-chains which can combine with haem to form respectively $Hb\beta_4$ or $Hb\gamma_4$. These pigments are also unstable and readily denature to produce inclusions. $Hb\beta_4$, also called HbH, is denatured rapidly *in vitro* in the presence of brilliant cresyl blue which strongly colours the precipitated pigment granules (see Fig. 2.3, p. 25).

Inherited instability of the red cell enzyme glucose-6-phosphate dehydrogenase (p. 28) indirectly results in denaturation of haemoglobin to methaemoglobin, which precipitates to form irregular aggregates attached to the inner surface of the red cell membranes. These inclusions are called Heinz bodies and they are also coloured by brilliant cresyl blue. All such inclusions of protein within erythrocytes shorten their life span and promote haemolytic anaemia.

Action of metals: metalloprotein complexes

Metals can aggregate and chelate with proteins so as to deposit insoluble metalloprotein complexes visible within cells; complex-forming metals include iron, copper and lead.

Iron

Iron is stored within cells in soluble macromolecules of ferritin visible by EM and also in brown granules of insoluble haemosiderin visible both by LM and EM.

Ferritin is a macromolecular complex of protein and hydrated ferric oxide with an electron-dense core rich in iron surrounded by a shell of protein. Each particle is approximately 10 nm in diameter and its electron-dense core contains hydrated ferric oxide in the polymeric form $(O{=}Fe{-}OH)_x$. The amount of $O{=}Fe{-}OH$ varies: fully loaded molecule of ferritin contains 26 per cent Fe, that is, up to 4000 atoms of iron per molecule associated with about 24 units of protein each with MW of 18 500D [109]. These macromolecules of ferritin are dispersed in the cytoplasm as a colloidal solution either free or in vesicles called siderosomes.

When the concentrations of ferritin rises excessively the particles coalesce to form brown aggregates of haemosiderin visible by LM. Haemosiderin of this type consists of granules approximately 100 nm in diameter which are seen by EM to be composed of compact masses of ferritin molecules. Haemosiderin may also consist of compact masses of ferritin cores which have been stripped of their protein shells. Both types of haemosiderin are seen by LM as brown granules and both contain complexes of hydrated ferric oxide $(O{=}Fe{-}OH)_x$ which reacts with $K_4Fe(CN)_6$ to form ferric ferrocyanide (Prussian blue). Both types of ferritin may occur free in cytoplasm or in siderosomes. In cells where granular haemosiderin is visible by LM particles of free ferritin are also usually visible by EM in the cytoplasmic matrix.

Haemosiderin is formed in macrophages when they ingest red cells and then disintegrate the liberated haemoglobin. This process is greatly accelerated in various forms of haemolytic anaemia and also following repeated transfusion of blood. In haemolytic anaemia abundant granules of haemosiderin generally occur in reticuloendothelial cells of bone marrow, spleen and liver, while after repeated blood transfusion haemosiderin is also deposited in cells of organs such as liver and pancreas.

Generalised deposition of haemosiderin (haemosiderosis), which affects the parenchymal cells of organs such as liver, heart and pancreas, is called *haemochromatosis*. Familial studies indicate that the so-called *idiopathic* form of haemochromatosis is an inherited disability. In this disease granules of haemosiderin are deposited in the hepatocytes of liver and also in the cells of heart muscle and pancreas. Hepatic deposition culminates in severe cirrhosis, while myocardial and pancreatic siderosis lead respectively to heart failure and diabetes. Deposition of haemosiderin in the skin is usually accompanied by excessive formation of melanin to give a bronzed appearance; hence the term 'bronzed diabetes' is applied to the disease. The excessive storage of iron is reflected by elevation of serum iron and increase in hepatic iron concentration. Whereas the total body content of iron is normally about 5 g, in idiopathic haemochromatosis the liver alone may contain 30–40 g. The actual cause of this excessive storage of iron is obscure; it is apparently a slow process, as the disease first appears in men between 40–60 years of age. Women are very rarely affected, probably because prolonged accumulation of iron is lessened by menstrual loss of blood.

Acquired haemochromatosis can follow repeated blood transfusions (see above) and also occurs among Bantu men in Africa. These men ingest large amounts of iron by using iron cooking utensils and their intake is further increased by drinking alcoholic liquor stored in iron containers. The resultant haemochromatosis affects both liver and pancreas and is followed respectively by cirrhosis and diabetes. Women are notably exempt from this form of haemochromatosis.

Copper

Accumulation of excessive copper within cells is probably the principal direct cause of *hepatolenticular degeneration* (Kinnier Wilson's disease). In this inherited disorder transmitted by an autosomal recessive gene a copper protein complex is deposited in liver cells and also probably in the neurones of the corpus striatum in the brain. In the liver this eventually produces cirrhosis, and in the brain, degeneration of the striatal neurones follows with tremor, rigidity and some degree of dementia. The corpus striatum is shrunken, and the disappearance of neurones from the lentiform nucleus is accompanied by gliosis and sometimes cavitation; the atrophic grey matter may also become brick coloured probably as a result of deposition of copper protein complexes. The content of copper in the putamen is grossly increased. Copper also accumulates in golden brown granules deposited in a circular zone of the corneal limbus within Descemet's membrane [109a]. These granules produce a brown annular deposit visible in the deepest part of the outer cornea, called the Kayser–Fleischer ring.

The basic determinant of Wilson's disease is probably a congenital deficiency of caeruloplasmin, the α_2-globulin-copper complex of normal plasma. This globulin carries the copper of the plasma as a blue metalloprotein complex. Without caeruloplasmin there is a rise of free copper in the plasma along with excessive entry of Cu^{++} into cells and tissues. Increase of copper content of liver tissue together with fall in the level of caeruloplasmin in serum are useful diagnostic criteria of Wilson's disease.

Hepatic deposition of a copper-protein complex also occurs in *Indian childhood cirrhosis*. This extensive intralobular pericellular fibrosis coupled with hepatic enlargement is not uncommon among Indian children aged 1–3 years. Affected children often become jaundiced as the disease progresses, and usually die within a few months of onset of illness. The hepatic cells contain hyaline inclusions identical with Mallory bodies (p. 417) and they also contain dark brown granules stainable by orcein [110]. These granules are probably enlarged lysosomes containing a copper-protein complex [111]. The total copper content is greatly increased from the normal range 15–60 μg/g dry weight to levels around 1400 μg/g in livers of these children [112]. This disease occurs mainly among children in middle class homes, and is thus unlikely to be determined by dietary deficiency. Moreover Indian children outside India are not affected, so that an inherited defect can hardly be concerned. Whether the intake of copper depends on absorption of this metal from cooking utensils, or food, or from some other environmental source is uncertain. But, as in Wilson's disease, the deposition of a copper protein complex in liver cells appears to be a dominant factor in causing hepatic cirrhosis in this highly lethal malady of childhood.

Lead

Pb^{++} form complexes with protein which are deposited as intranuclear inclusion bodies in tubular cells in the kidneys of human patients and animals poisoned by lead; indeed the formation of these complexes, in which lead is sequestered in an indiffusible form, serves as a valuable protective mechanism from the harmful action of ionic lead (p. 148).

Prominent basophilic particles are visible in red cells stained by Leishman's method in blood films from human patients or animals after intake of lead. These particles are confined to reticulocytes which still retain ribosomes and they are only seen when the red cells are slowly dried in air. Observations by EM show that these basophilic particles are composed of aggregated ribosomes [113]. This aggregation is probably determined by previous reaction between ribonucleoprotein and Pb^{++} to form a metalloprotein complex. This basophilic stippling is an important diagnostic feature of lead poisoning.

Fe^{+++}, Cu^{++} and Pb^{++} can thus all form visible metalloprotein complexes within cells. These complexes sequestrate such potentially toxic ions as indiffusible and relatively harmless aggregates. But prolonged deposition of iron and copper complexes in hepatic cells leads to cirrhosis, and similar deposition in the corpus striatum causes degeneration of cerebral neurones.

Action of organic poisons

These substances, unlike metals, do not form macromolecular complexes with proteins, but they may aggregate proteins in cells by damaging lipoprotein micelles or membranes in which proteins are component parts.

Mallory bodies (alcoholic hyaline)

Hyaline eosinophilic deposits rich in protein are present in the cytoplasm of hepatic cells in human alcoholic patients suffering from cirrhosis [114]. These bodies which appear as a coarse hyaline meshwork or as smaller spherical deposits are called Mallory's alcoholic hyaline (Fig. 8.46, p. 418). These bodies are also formed in the hepatocytes of patients with alcoholic hepatitis which precedes cirrhosis (p. 373). Similar hyaline inclusions develop in hepatic cells of rats fed excessive amounts of ethanol; even when fatty change and subsequent cirrhosis in rats fed with ethanol are prevented by feeding abundant lipotropic factors, these hyaline bodies are still formed if sufficient ethanol is consumed [48].

Observations by EM on hepatocytes in human patients with alcoholic liver disease show that alcoholic hyaline is a fibrillar deposit without a limiting membrane [115–117]. Mallory bodies contain arginine-rich basic protein and may be formed in association with ribosomes or RER and thus be deposited at their site of synthesis [116] by the toxic action of ethanol.

The mechanism of formation of Mallory bodies is obscure. Very similar hyaline bodies are formed in the liver cells of patients with Wilson's disease and with Indian childhood cirrhosis, while apparently identical deposits occur in the liver of obese patients after treatment by jejuno-ileal by-pass (p. 374). Mallory bodies cannot therefore be regarded as diagnostic of poisoning by ethanol. However aggregation of protein previously arrayed in cellular micelles may be determined by a variety of harmful agents including ethanol.

Protein inclusions produced by CCl_4

Following injection of CCl_4 into rats hyaline inclusion bodies rich in protein appear in the cytoplasm of the centrilobular hepatic cells (Fig. 8.47). This change is probably a prelude to necrosis and involves aggregation of protein along with denaturation to an acidophilic material stainable by the anionic dyes eosin and erythrosin [19]. Later these eosinophilic bodies expand and occupy much of the cytoplasm of the injured centrilobular cells. Fat may then be deposited along with the protein to form globules of lipid surrounded by

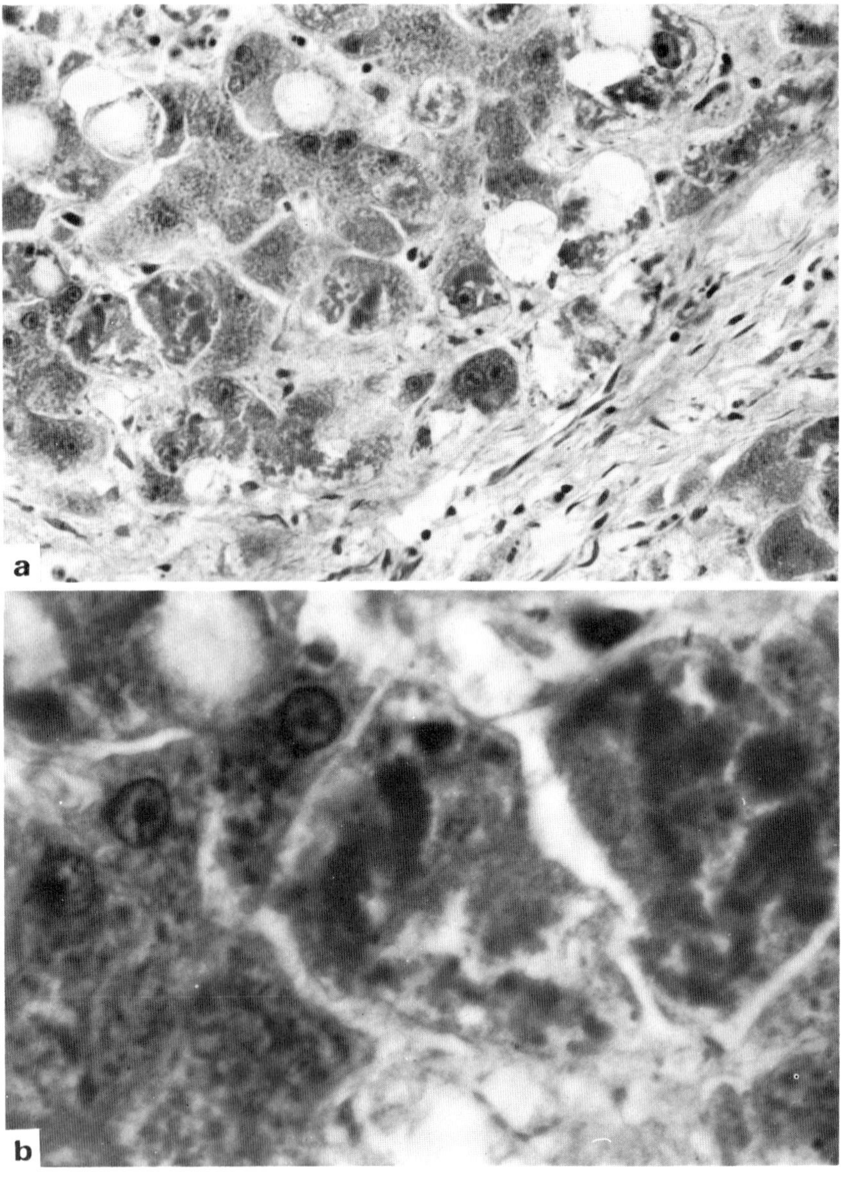

FIG. 8.46 Mallory's hyaline bodies in alcoholic micronodular cirrhosis. From liver of a patient with hepatic cirrhosis and portal obstruction which caused ascites and terminal oesophageal venous haemorrhage. (From same liver as shown in Fig. 8.15a.)

a. Some of the hepatic cells are bloated by globules of fat. Hyaline bodies are seen as a granular cytoplasmic meshwork in hepatocytes at lower left of field. $\times$ 330.

b. Part of same field. Prominent hyaline eosinophilic bodies visible in two enlarged hepatocytes. $\times$ 1300.

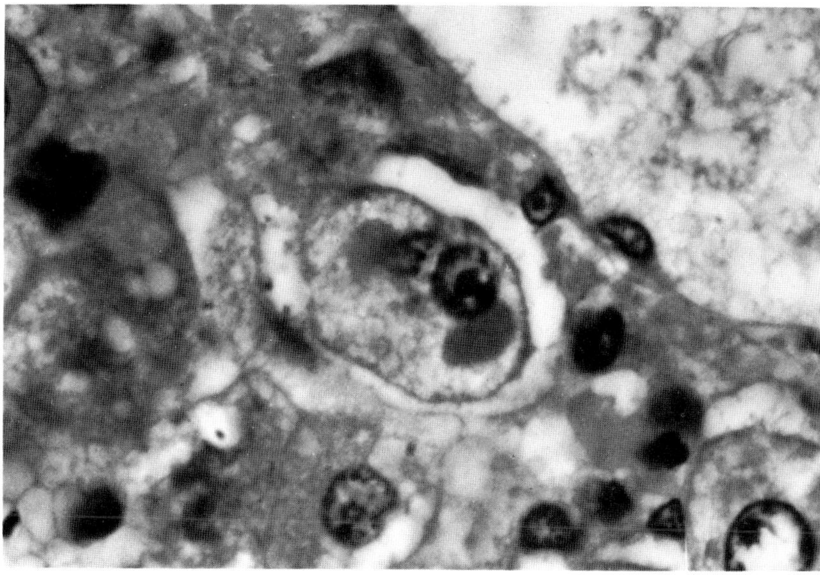

FIG. 8.47 Aggregation of anionophilic protein in cytoplasm of centrilobular hepatic cells of rat 24 h after injection of CCl_4 (0.75 ml/100 g body weight). A cell near the central vein of a liver lobule contains two large eosinophilic inclusions of denatured protein. H & E. × 1300.

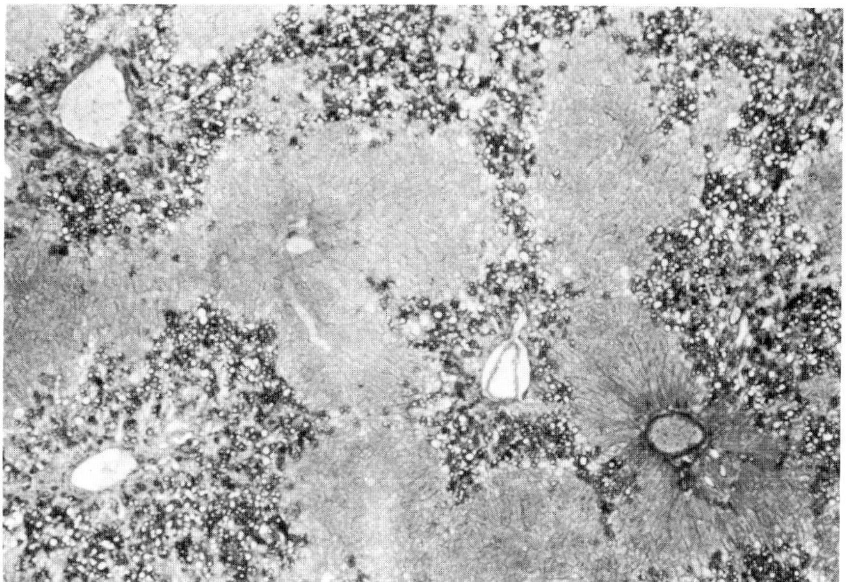

FIG. 8.48 Abundant deposits of anionophilic protein along with fat in cytoplasm of centrilobular hepatic cells of rat 44 h after injection of CCl_4 (0.75 ml/100 g body weight). Spaces from which globules of lipid have been extracted are seen to be enclosed by thickened shells of protein. Oxidized tannin-oxazine (OTO) method for protein. × 70. Dixon K. C. (1962) *Quart. J. exp. Physiol.*, **47**, 7.

thickened rims of anionophilic protein (Fig. 8.48). This change may be initiated by lipoperoxidation of phospholipid by activated CCl_4 (p. 164) which disarrays lipoprotein micelles and so interferes with normal excretion of fat as micellar VLDL. This would account for accumulation of both protein and fat.

Observations by EM on hepatic cells of rats poisoned by CCl_4 show that the cisternae of ER coalesce rapidly into condensed aggregates [118]. The hyaline inclusions seen by LM may be formed by further condensation and denaturation of the protein derived from the disintegrated membranes of ER.

Excessive entry of protein

After intraperitoneal injection of egg white into animals the egg ovomucoid, a glycoprotein, is excreted through the renal glomeruli and is later reabsorbed by the renal tubules. During the process of reabsorption the tubular cells contain conspicuous granules of glycoprotein which stain intensely with PAS.

Similarly in human renal disease which causes proteinuria, hyaline eosinophilic droplets of protein may be seen in the cells of the convoluted tubules owing to absorption of protein which has entered the glomerular filtrate.

Phagocytic cells can ingest remnants rich in protein. Macrophages which erode necrotic cerebral grey matter contain prominent granules of proteolipid (p. 403). Phagocytes can enclose the entire nuclei of lysed or vanished cells; ingested homogenous masses rich in protein and DNA are visible in neutrophils and monocytes of blood treated with serum containing the LE factor of SLE (p. 212).

Another mode of entry of cell remnants containing protein is phagocytosis of membrane-bound cell fragments originally formed by *apoptosis* (p. 292). Thus, following various forms of cell injury including ischaemia and damage by cell-mediated immunity (as after infection by hepatitis-B virus), injured hepatic cells cast off condensed membrane-bound fragments by budding [119]. These fragments and their contained organelles are then ingested both by other hepatic cells and by macrophages. Eventually the fragments become homogenised into eosinophil cytoplasmic inclusions rich in protein which are called Councilman bodies.

Excessive formation of protein

Immunoglobulins

Large amounts of immunoglobulins with binding sites for specific antigen are synthesised within plasma cells on re-exposure to the same antigen (p. 203). When immunoglobulins with these binding sites are being formed in the plasma cells they can be detected by preliminary treatment with excess of the same antigen followed by pin-pointing of the adsorbed antigen with fluorescent antibody (sandwich technique). Sometimes the fabrication of antibody within plasma cells is so great that hyaline masses of immunoglobulin (Russell bodies) are deposited in the cytoplasm. These masses are strongly coloured by PAS [119a].

Amyloid

This glassy gelatinous protein is deposited between cells in liver, kidney and spleen usually following chronic infection, rheumatoid arthritis or other disease associated with prolonged immunoglobulinaemia. It is believed that precursors of amyloid are formed from immunoglobulins within phagocytes [120, 121] and are then excreted into the intercellular spaces, where they condense as translucent aggregates almost entirely composed of protein. Amyloid accumulates around hepatic sinusoids, and in the basement membranes of renal tubules and glomerular capillaries. Prominent glassy deposits of amyloid sometimes infiltrate the Malpighian corpuscles of the spleen ('sago spleen'). The darkness of these glassy zones depends on power to transmit light in contrast to other tissues which reflect it.

Amyloid is intensely stained by Congo red to give birefringent complexes which are brilliantly illuminated by polarised light. By EM amyloid is seen to be composed of laterally aggregated fibrils with a diameter of 7.5 nm and a longitudinal periodicity of 10 nm. The fibrils show X-ray diffraction patterns that indicate 'a cross-β pleated sheath conformation' of their peptide chains; this structure may account for the tinctorial and optical properties of amyloid when stained by Congo red [121].

The most harmful effects of amyloid are determined by its action on the kidneys. Deposition of amyloid at first injures the glomeruli so that albumin can filter into the tubules. This is followed by the nephrotic syndrome with albuminuria and oedema, which may terminate in chronic renal failure and uraemia as the glomeruli become converted into amyloid masses.

Viral protein

Inclusion bodies rich in protein (see Fig. 6.26, p. 259) are formed in many cells by viral infection. These aggregates, which are produced either in cytoplasm or in the nucleus, are usually present in the zones of assembly where viral structure is elaborated (p. 264). The proteins contained in these deposits include the so called 'early' viral proteins, which are enzymes concerned with viral synthesis, as well as the structural proteins of the infective particles themselves. Sometimes cytoplasmic inclusions may occupy a large part of the cell which then becomes filled with enzymic and structural proteins necessary for the assembly of the invader. Such massive inclusions with the appearance of ground glass (p. 270) occur among groups of hepatic cells in biopsy specimens from healthy carriers of hepatitis B virus; these inclusions are also coloured by orcein and are probably rich in viral proteins. The same cells contain abundant hepatitis B surface antigen detectable by immunofluorescence [122, 123].

REFERENCES

[1] McBain J. W. (1942) Solubilisation and other factors in detergent action. In *Advances in Colloid Science*, Vol. 1, p. 99, ed. by E. O. Kramer. Interscience, New York.

[2] Hartley G. S. (1936) *Aqueous Solutions of Paraffin-Chain Salts: A Study in Micelle Formation*, p. 44. Hermann, Paris.

[3] Hamilton R. L. & Lequire V. S. (1967) Electron microscopy of very low density lipoprotein (VLDL) secretion and early fatty liver. *Fed. Proc.*, **26**, 575.

[4] Mahley R. W., Hamilton R. L. & Lequire V. S. (1969) Characterisation of lipoprotein particles isolated from the Golgi apparatus of rat liver. *J. Lipid Res.*, **10**, 433.

[5] Schumaker V. N. & Adams G. H. (1969) Circulating lipoproteins. *Am. Rev. Biochem.*, **38**, 113.

[6] Kerpel S., Shafrir E. & Shapiro B. (1961) Mechanism of fatty assimilation in adipose tissue. *Biochim. biophys. Acta* (*Amst.*) **46**, 495.

[7] Stein Y. & Stein O. (1961) Metabolic activity of rat epididymal fat pad labelled selectively by an *in vivo* incubation technique. *Biochem. biophys. Acta*, **54**, 555.

[8] Dixon K. C. (1973) Solubilisation and cellular fatty change. *Histochem. J.*, **5**, 363.

[9] Dixon K. C. (1970) Hydrophobic lipids in injured cells. *Histochem. J.*, **2**, 157.

[10] Wilgram G. F., Hartroft W. S. & Best C. H. (1954) Dietary choline and the maintenance of the cardiovascular system in rats. *Brit. med. J.*, **2**, 1.

[11] Best C. H. (1956) The Croonian lecture. The lipotropic agents in the protection of the liver, kidney, heart and other organs of experimental animals. *Proc. roy. Soc. B.*, **145**, 151.

[12] Ashworth C. T., Sanders E. & Arnold N. (1961) Hepatic lipids. Fine structural changes in liver cells after high-fat diet, high cholesterol and choline-deficient diets in rats. *Arch. Path.*, **72**, 625.

[13] Best C. H., Hartroft W. S., Lucas C. C. & Ridout J. H. (1955) Effects of dietary protein, lipotropic factors and re-alimentation on total hepatic lipids and their distribution. *Brit. med. J.*, **1**, 1439.

[14] Roheim P. S., Miller L. & Eder H. E. (1965) The formation of plasma lipoproteins from apoprotein in plasma. *J. biol. Chem.*, **240**, 2994.

[15] Chaikoff I. L. (1942) The application of labelling agents to the study of phospholipid metabolism. *Physiol. Rev.*, **22**, 291.

[16] Dixon K. C. (1958) Fatty deposition: a disorder of the cell. *Quart. J. exp. Physiol.*, **43**, 139.

[17] Recknagel R. O. & Ghoshal A. K. (1966) Lipoperoxidation as a vector of carbon tetrachloride hepatotoxicity. *Lab. Invest.*, **15**, 132.

[18] Recknagel R. O. (1967) Carbon tetrachloride hepatotoxicity. *Pharmacol. Rev.*, **19**, 145.

[19] Dixon K. C. (1962) Deposition of protein in damaged liver cells. *Quart. J. exp. Physiol.*, **47**, 7.

[20] Ashworth C. T., Wrightman F. & Buttram V. (1961) Hepatic lipids. Comparative study of effect of high fat, choline-deficient and high cholesterol diets upon serum and hepatic lipids. *Arch. Path.*, **72**, 620.

[21] Smith R. L. (1960) The micelle form. Original lectures. *3rd International Congress of Surface Activity, Cologne*, p. 242, Universitätsdruckerei, Mainz.

[22] Ashworth C. T., Stembridge B. A. & Sanders E. (1960) Lipid absorption, transport and hepatic assimilation studied with electron microscopy. *Amer. J. Physiol.*, **198**, 1326.

[23] Dixon K. C. & King A. J. (1972) Fatty globulation in the liver of fat-fed rats studied by rolled films. *Histochem. J.*, **4**, 111.

[24] Bowyer D. E. & Dixon K. C. Unpublished observations.

[25] PEREZ-TAMAYO R. (1961) *Mechanisms of Disease: An Introduction to Pathology*, p. 22. Saunders, Philadelphia.
[26] STEIN O. & STEIN Y. (1965) Fine structure of the ethanol-induced fatty liver in the rat. *Israel J. med. Sci.*, **1**, 378.
[27] ORCI L., LE MARCHAND Y., SINGH A., ASSIMACOPOULOS-JEANNET F., ROUILLER C. & JEANRENAUD B. (1973) Role of microtubules in lipoprotein secretion by the liver. *Nature*, **244**, 30.
[28] PAYLING WRIGHT G. (1958) *An Introduction to Pathology*. Longmans, London.
[29] DIBLE J. H. (1934) Is fatty degeneration of the heart muscle a phanerosis? *J. Path. Bact.*, **39**, 197.
[30] HACK M. H. & FERRANS V. J. (1960) Nitrogen-free plasmalogen observed in infarcted myocardium of the dog. *Circulation*, **8**, 738.
[31] SCHNITKA T. K. & NACHLAS M. M. (1963) Histochemical alterations in ischaemic heart muscle and early myocardial infarction. *Amer. J. Path.*, **42**, 507.
[32] STEINBERG D. (1967) The dynamics of free fatty acid mobilisation and utilisation. *Prog. biochem. Pharmacol.*, **3**, 139.
[33] BARRET H. M., BEST C. H. & RIDOUT J. H. (1938) A study of the source of liver fat using deuterium as an indicator. *J. Physiol.*, **93**, 367.
[34] FREDRICKSON D. S. & GORDON R. S. (1958) Transport of fatty acids. *Physiol. Rev.*, **38**, 585.
[35] FLORES H., PAK N., MACCIONI A. & MONCEBERG F. (1970) Lipid transport in kwashiorkor. *Brit. J. Nutr.*, **24**, 1005.
[36] GARROW J. S., FLETCHER K. & HALLIDAY D. (1965) Body composition in severe infantile malnutrition. *J. clin. Invest.*, **44**, 417.
[37] SCHWARTZ R. & DEAN J. F. A. (1957) The serum lipids in kwashiorkor. 1. Neutral fat, phospholipids and cholesterol. *J. trop. Pediat.*, **3**, 23.
[38] BEST C. H. (1946) Factors affecting fat transport in the animal body. *Amer. J. dig. Dis.*, **13**, 155.
[39] BIERMAN E. L., DOLE V. P. & ROBERTS T. N. (1957) An abnormality of nonesterified fatty acid metabolism in diabetes mellitus. *Diabetes*, **6**, 475.
[40] RICKETTS H. T. (1959) Endocrinology (diabetes). *Ann. Rev. Med.*, **10**, 145.
[41] HIRSCH J., KNITTLE J. L. & SALANS L. B. (1966) Cell lipid content and cell number in obese and non-obese human adipose tissue. *J. clin. Invest.*, **45**, 1023.
[42] BROOK G. G. D. (1973) Fat children. *Brit. J. Hosp. Med.*, **10**, 30.
[43] GALAMBOS J. T. (1976) Jejuno-ileal bypass and nutritional liver injury. *Arch. Path. Lab. Med.*, **100**, 229.
[44] MACFARLANE R. G. & MACLENNAN J. D. (1945) The toxaemia of gas gangrene. *Lancet*, **2**, 328.
[45] CAMERON G. R. & KARUNARATNE W. A. E. (1936) Carbon tetrachloride cirrhosis in relation to liver regeneration. *J. Path. Bact.*, **42**, 1.
[46] ASHWORTH C. T., JOHNSON C. F. & WRIGHTSMAN F. J. (1965) Biochemical and morphologic correlations of hepatic protein synthesis in acute ethanol intoxication in rats. *Amer. J. Path.*, **46**, 757.
[47] DI LUZIO N. R. (1966) A mechanism of acute ethanol-induced fatty liver and the modification of liver injury by antioxidants. In *Biochemical Pathology*, p. 50, ed. by E. Farber & P. N. Magee. Williams & Wilkins, Baltimore.
[48] PORTA E. A., KOCH O. R. & HARTROFT W. S. (1970) Recent advances in molecular pathology: a review of the effects of alcohol on the liver. *Exp. molec. Path.*, **12**, 104.
[49] RUBIN E. & LIEBER C. S. (1967) Early fine structural changes in the human liver induced by alcohol. *Gastroenterology*, **52**, 1.
[50] BRIGDEN W. (1977) Alcoholic cardiomyopathy. *Brit. J. Hosp. Med.*, **18**, 122.
[51] MACSWEEN R. N. M. (1978) Alcoholic liver disease. In *Recent Advances in Histopathology 10*, p. 193, ed. by P. P. Anthony & N. Woolf. Churchill Livingstone, Edinburgh.
[52] HEATON K. W. (1977) Alcoholic liver disease. *Brit. J. Hosp. Med.*, **18**, 118.

[53] RUBIN E. & LIEBER C. S. (1975) Relation of alcoholic liver injury to cirrhosis. *Clinics in Gastroenterology*, **4**, 247.

[54] BEST C. H., HARTROFT W. S., LUCAS C. C. & RIDOUT J. H. (1949) Damage produced by feeding alcohol or sugar and its prevention by choline. *Brit. med. J.*, **2**, 1001.

[55] RUBIN E. & LIEBER C. S. (1974) Fatty liver, alcoholic hepatitis and cirrhosis. *New Engl. J. Med.*, **290**, 128.

[56] HARTROFT W. S. (1950) Accumulation of fat in liver cells and in lipodiastemata preceding experimental fatty liver and cirrhosis. *Anat. Rec.*, **106**, 61.

[57] ROGERS A. E. & NEWBERNE P. M. (1973) Animal model of human disease: alcoholic or nutritional fatty liver and cirrhosis in lipotrope-deficient male rats. *Amer. J. Path.*, **73**, 817.

[58] HARTROFT W. S. (1953) Diagnostic significance of fatty cysts in cirrhosis. *Arch. Path.*, **55**, 63.

[59] HARTROFT W. S. (1954) The sequence of pathologic events in the development of experimental fatty liver and cirrhosis. *Ann. N. Y. Acad. Sci.*, **57**, 633.

[60] POPPER H. & UDENFREUND S. (1970) Hepatic fibrosis: correlation of biochemical and morphological investigations. *Amer. J. Med.*, **49**, 707.

[61] BIANCHI L. *et al.* (1977) Acute and chronic hepatitis revisited. *Lancet*, **2**, 914.

[62] ADAMS C. W. M. (1964) Arterosclerosis in man, other mammals and birds. *Biol. Rev.*, **39**, 372.

[63] GEER J. C., MCGILL H. C. & Strong J. P. (1961) The fine structure of human atherosclerotic lesions. *Amer. J. Path.*, **38**, 263.

[64] MCCULLOUGH K. A. & BALLIAN G. (1975) Collagen characterisation and cell transformation in human atherosclerosis. *Nature*, **258**, 73.

[65] BENDITT E. P. & BENDITT J. M. (1973) Evidence for a monoclonal origin of human atherosclerotic plaques. *Proc. nat. Acad. Sci* (*Wash.*), **70**, 1753.

[66] BENDITT E. P. (1977) Implications of monoclonal character of human atherosclerotic plaques. *Amer. J. Path.*, **86**, 693.

[67] PEARSON T. A., KRAMER E. C., SOLEZ K. & HEPTINSTALL R. H. (1977) The human atherosclerotic plaque. *Amer. J. Path.*, **86**, 657.

[68] ADAMS C. W. M. (1967) *Vascular Histochemistry*. Lloyd-Luke, London.

[69] ADAMS C. W. M., BAYLISS O. B. & TURNER D. R. (1975) Phagocytes, lipid removal and regression of atheroma, *J. Path. Bact.*, **116**, 225.

[70] DIXON K. C. (1961) Deposition of globular lipid in arterial cells in relation to anoxia. *Amer. J. Path.*, **39**, 65.

[71] VIRCHOW R. (1859) *Die Cellularpathologie in ihrer Begründung auf Physiologische und Pathologische Gewebelehre*, 2nd Ed., pp. 309 and 327. Hirschwald, Berlin.

[72] GRESHAM G. A. & HOWARD A. N. (1961) The histogenesis of the atherosclerotic 'fatty streak'. *J. Atheroscler. Res.*, **1**, 413.

[73] CARO C. G., FITZGERALD J. M. & SCHROTER R. C. (1971) Atheroma and arterial wall shear. Observation, correlation and proposed shear dependent mass transfer mechanism for atherogenesis. *Proc. roy. Soc. B.*, **177**, 109.

[74] SMITH E. B. (1977) Molecular interactions in human atherosclerotic plaques. *Amer. J. Path.*, **86**, 665.

[75] VON ROKITANSKY C. (1852) *A Manual of Pathological Anatomy*, Vol. 4, p. 272 (translated by G. E. Day). The Sydenham Society, London.

[76] DUGUID J. B. (1946) Thrombosis as a factor in the pathogenesis of coronary atherosclerosis. *J. Path. Bact.*, **58**, 207.

[77] ROSS R., GLOMSET J. & HARKER L. (1977) Response to injury in atherogenesis. *Amer. J. Path.*, **86**, 675.

[77a] MITCHELL J. R. A. (1981) Prostaglandins in vascular disease: a seminal approach. *Brit. med. J.*, **1**, 590.

[78] GRESHAM G. A. (1980) *Reversing Atherosclerosis*. Thomas, Illinois.

[79] THOMSON J. G. (1969) Production of severe atheroma in transplanted human heart. *Lancet*, **2**, 1088.
[80] ROYAL COLLEGE OF PHYSICIANS (1976) Report on prevention of coronary heart disease. *J. roy. coll. Phycns Lond.*, **10**, 213.
[81] ANITSCHKOW N. (1913) Über die veranderungen der kaninchenaorta bei experimenteller cholesterinsteatose. *Beitr. path. Anat.*, **56**, 379.
[82] COOK R. P. & MCCULLAGH G. P. (1939) A comparative study of cholesterol metabolism and its relation to fatty infiltration, with particular reference to experimental cholesterol atheroma. *Quart. J. exp. Physiol.*, **29**, 283.
[83] GRESHAM G. A. & HOWARD A. N. (1962) Atherosclerosis produced by semisynthetic diet with no added cholesterol. *Arch. Path.*, **74**, 1.
[84] GOLDSTEIN J. L. & BROWN M. S. (1977) Atherosclerosis: the low density lipoprotein receptor hypothesis. *Metabolism*, **26**, 1257.
[84a] MILLER G. J. & MILLER N. E. (1975) Plasma-high-density-lipoprotein concentration and the development of ischaemic heart disease. *Lancet*, **1**, 16.
[85] ASTRUP P., KJELDSEN K. & WANSTRUP J. (1967) Enhancing influence of carbon monoxide on the development of atheromatosis in cholesterol-fed rabbits, *J. Atheroscler. Res.*, **7**, 343.
[86] ADAMS C. W. M. (1958) Histochemical mechanisms of the Marchi reaction for degenerating myelin. *J. Neurochem.*, **2**, 178.
[87] HALLPIKE J. F., ADAMS C. W. M. & BAYLISS O. B. (1970) Histochemistry of myelin. XI. Loss of basic protein in early myelin breakdown and multiple sclerosis plaques. *Histochem. J.*, **2**, 323.
[88] ADAMS C. W. M. (1972) *Research on Multiple Sclerosis*. Thomas, Springfield, Illinois.
[89] WILLIAMS P. L. & HALL S. (1971) Prolonged *in vivo* observations of normal peripheral nerve fibres and their acute reactions to crush and deliberate trauma. *J. Anat. (Lond.)*, **108**, 394.
[90] WOLMAN M. (1968) Myelin structure, ultrastructure and degeneration. In *Pathology of the Nervous System*, p. 758, ed. by J. Minckler. McGraw Hill, New York.
[91] PETRESCU A. (1966) Contributions histochimiques à l'étude des lipides dans les lésions demyélinisantes. *Ann. Histochim.*, **11**, 237.
[92] PETRESCU A. (1969) Histochemistry of lipids in multiple sclerosis. *Wien. Z. Nevernheilk*, Suppl. II, 38.
[93] DIXON K. C. & HERBERTSON B. M. (1950) Clusters of granules in human neurones. *J. Path. Bact.*, **62**, 335.
[94] Hirsch H. E. (1970) Enzyme levels of individual neurones in relation to lipofuscin content. *J. Histochem. Cytochem.*, **18**, 268.
[95] WOLMAN M. (1975) Biological peroxidation of lipids and membranes. *Israel J. med. Sci.*, suppl., **11**, 147.
[96] EINARSON L. (1962) Cellular structure of the central nervous system of vitamin E-deficient monkeys. In *Aging Round the World*, Vol. 3, p. 131, ed. by N. W. Shock. Columbia University Press, New York.
[97] DIXON K. C. (1965) Ischaemia and the neurone. In *Neurohistochemistry*, p. 558, ed. by C. W. M. Adams. Elsevier, Amsterdam.
[98] DIXON K. C. & GRESHAM G. A. (1974) Remnants of necrotic grey matter. *Acta neuropath. (Berl.)*, **28**, 55.
[99] DIXON K. C. (1967) Events in dying cells. *Proc. roy. Soc. Med.*, **60**, 271.
[100] O'BRIEN J. S. (1972) Ganglioside storage diseases. *Advanc. hum. Genet.* **3**, 39.
[101] TERRY R. D. & WEISS M. (1963) Studies in Tay-Sachs disease. II. Ultrastructure of the cerebrum. *J. Neuropath.*, **22**, 18.
[102] WOLMAN M. (1965) Histochemistry of the lipidoses. Proceedings of the Vth international Congress on Neuropathology. *Excerpta Medica International Congress Series*, **100**, 116.
[103] NEUFELD E. F. (1974) The biochemical basis for mucopolysaccharidoses and

mucolipidoses. In *Progress in Medical Genetics*, Vol. 10, p. 81, ed. by A. G. Steinker & A. G. Bearn. Grune & Stratton, New York.

[104] DANES B. S. & BEARN A. G. (1965) Hurler's syndrome: demonstration of an inherited disorder of connective tissue in cell culture. *Science*, **149**, 987.

[105] NEUFELD E. F. & FRATANTONI J. C. (1970) Inborn errors of mucopolysaccharide metabolism. *Science*, **169**, 141.

[106] FRATANTONI J. C., HALL C. W. & NEUFELD E. F. (1968) Hurler and Hunter syndromes: mutual correction of the defect in cultured fibroblasts. *Science*, **162**, 570.

[107] ALEU F. P., TERRY R. D. & ZELLWEGER H. (1965) Electron microscopy of two cerebral biopsies in gargoylism. *J. Neuropath.*, **24**, 304.

[108] ALLISON A. C. (1978) Lysosomes in pathology. In *Recent advances in Histopathology, 10*, p. 69. Churchill Livingstone, Edinburgh.

[109] RICHTER G. W. (1978) The iron-loaded cell—the cytopathology of iron storage. *Amer. J. Path.*, **91**, 363.

[109a] PEARSE A. G. E. (1972) *Histochemistry: theoretical and applied*, 3rd ed. Vol. 2, p. 1147. Churchill Livingstone, Edinburgh.

[110] PORTMANN B., TANNER M. S., MOWAT A. P. & WILLIAMS R. (1978) Orcein-positive liver deposits in Indian childhood cirrhosis. *Lancet*, **1**, 1338.

[111] POPPER H., GOLDFISCHER S., STERNLIEB I., NAYAK N. C. & MADHAVAN T. V. (1979) Cytoplasmic copper and its toxic effects: studies in Indian childhood cirrhosis. *Lancet*, **1**, 1205.

[112] TANNER M. S., MOWAT A. P., PORTMANN B. & WILLIAMS R. (1979) Increased hepatic copper concentration in Indian childhood cirrhosis. *Lancet*, **1**, 1203.

[113] JENSEN W. N., MORENO G. D. & BESSIS M. C. (1965) An electron microscopic description of basophilic stippling in red cells. *Blood*, **25**, 933.

[114] MALLORY F. B. (1911) Cirrhosis of the liver: five different types of lesions from which it may arise. *Bull. Johns Hopk. Hosp.*, **22**, 69.

[115] YOKOO H., MINICK O. T., BATT F. & KURT G. (1972) Morphologic variants of alcoholic hyalin. *Amer. J. Path.*, **69**, 25.

[116] HORVATH E., KOVACS K. & ROSS R. C. (1973) Subcellular features of alcoholic liver lesion: alcoholic hyaline. *J. Path.*, **110**, 245.

[117] KAHN L. B. (1973) Ultrastructure of human alcoholic hyaline: a brief review. In *Liver*, p. 152, ed. by S. J. Saunders & J. Terblanche. Pitman Medical, London.

[118] REYNOLDS E. S. & REE H. J. (1971) Liver parenchymal cell injury. VII Membrane denaturation following carbon tetrachloride. *Lab. Invest.*, **25**, 269.

[119] KERR J. F. R. *et al.* (1979) The nature of piecemeal necrosis in chronic active hepatitis. *Lancet*, **2**, 827.

[119a] PEARSE A. G. E. (1949) The nature of Russell bodies and Kurloff bodies: observations on the cytochemistry of plasma cells and reticulum cells. *J. clin. Path.*, **2**, 81.

[120] COHEN A. S. (1965) The constitution and genesis of amyloid. *Int. Rev. exp. Path.*, **4**, 159.

[121] GLENNER G. G. & PAGE D. L. (1976) Amyloid, amyloidosis and amyloidogenesis. *Int. Rev. exp. Path.*, **15**, 1.

[122] HADZIYANNIS S., GERBER M. A., VISSOULIS C. & POPPER H. (1973) Cytoplasmic hepatitis B antigen in 'ground-glass' hepatocytes of carriers. *Arch. Path.*, **96**, 327.

[123] PORTMANN B., GALBRAITH R. M., EDDLESTON A. L. W. F., ZUCKERMAN A. J. & WILLIAMS R. (1976) Detection of HBsAg in fixed liver tissue: use of a modified immunofluorescent technique and comparison with histochemical methods. *Gut*, **17**, 1.

CHAPTER 9

Derangements of Metabolism, Behaviour and Growth

Visible changes in structure of cells, such as disintegration of fabric or aggregation of contents are, as emphasised in the preceding chapters, some of the most prominent features of disease. But pathogenic cellular defects may be responsible for disease by altering metabolism or behaviour without producing overt structural alteration or injury in the affected cells. Such disorders, however, almost certainly reflect changes in structure or conformation at a molecular level and they may also indirectly induce visible effects, such as fatty change or atherosclerosis occurring as a consequence of diabetes.

Cellular defects associated with such microscopically invisible lesions will now be illustrated by a short account of some derangements of metabolism, behaviour and growth.

METABOLIC DEFECTS OF CELLS

Many defects of metabolism cause accumulation of soluble substances in tissue fluids. Indeed elevation in the concentration in blood or urine of solutes, which are insufficiently absorbed or excessively liberated by cells, is a most conspicuous indicator of metabolic disease. But it is well to remember that such accumulation usually reflects more fundamental derangements in the cells themselves than in the surrounding fluids.

Thus the hyperglycaemia of diabetes reflects failure of cells to absorb or utilise glucose. The hyperbilirubinaemia of hepatocellular jaundice indicates damage to liver cells which fail to absorb bilirubin from the blood or fail to conjugate and excrete it into the bile ducts. Hepatitis viruses thus cause jaundice. Similarly acceleration or deflection of cellular metabolism can promote excessive formation of substances which are then released from disordered cells into the blood or urine. In this way excessive lipolysis of TG in the lipocytes in diabetes releases large quantities of FFA into the blood, while retardation of oxygenation of phenylalanine to tyrosine in phenylketonuria causes accumulation of phenylalanine with deflection of its metabolism to form phenylpyruvic acid which is then excreted in the urine.

Metabolic defects of the cell include:

1. Retardation of absorption by the cell.
2. Acceleration, retardation or diversion of chemical processes within the cell.
3. Retardation of excretion of substances by the cell.

Retardation of absorption by the cell

Intestinal cells fail to absorb Ca^{++} when not supplied by activated products of Vitamin D. This effect, which results in rickets, depends on lack of Ca-binding carrier in the jejunal cells (p. 49).

Similarly the enterocytes of the terminal ileum cannot absorb cobalamin (vitamin B_{12}) in the absence of intrinsic factor secreted by the gastric parietal cells; this defect causes pernicious anaemia (p. 57).

Absorption of amino acids by intestinal enterocytes and by renal tubular cells depends on inherited carrier substances each of which transports a group of amino acids across the absorbent epithelial cells. One of these groups of co-migrant amino acids includes cystine and the basic diaminoacids lysine, arginine and ornithine. The similar behaviour of these four amino acids may depend on the presence within each of them of two positively charged amino groups separated by a chain of 4–6 atoms.

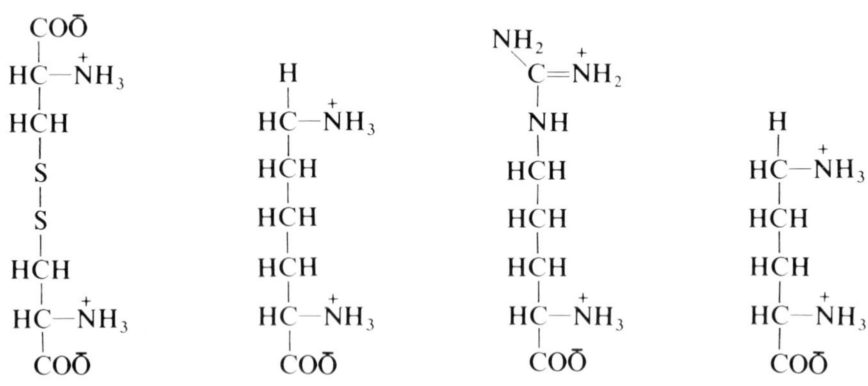

cystine lysine arginine ornithine

These four amino acids are probably each transported across epithelial cells by the same carrier protein. In the hereditary disease *cystinuria* all four are not absorbed by the renal tubules and are therefore excreted in the urine [1]. Of these, cystine alone is relatively insoluble and is precipitated in the urine and may also be deposited to form renal stones in the urinary tract.

Although such inherited defect in absorption of amino acids affects the intestinal mucosa as well as renal tubules, this does not usually cause deficiency disease; this protection from deficiency is probably due to the capacity of jejunal epithelium to absorb *unhydrolysed* peptides containing all the necessary amino acids, even though some of the individual aminoacids in the free state cannot be absorbed [2].

Retardation of absorption of glucose into striated and cardiac muscle and also into lipocytes is a prominent effect of lack of insulin. This defect of penetration of glucose into cells is a major determinant of hyperglycaemia in diabetes (p. 434).

Acceleration, retardation and diversion of metabolism within the cell

These changes in rates of metabolic reactions may depend on alteration either in quantity or activity of enzymes or in concentration of their substrates. Enzyme quantity may be increased by induction of enzyme synthesis, Enzymic activity may be diminished by hereditary defects in structure (p. 20). Enzymic activity may also be increased or diminished by feed-back mechanisms exerted by products of metabolism which alter the structure or conformation of the enzyme proteins.

The resulting acceleration or retardation in rates of metabolic reaction may exert harmful effects by:

1. Causing accumulation of metabolites which are toxic in excess.
2. Suppressing reactions, which are themselves necessary for cellular activity or survival, or which form as their products the substrates for further essential reactions.

Increase in concentration of a metabolite, which may be toxic in excess, arises when its formation is accelerated or its disposal is retarded so that rate of formation outpaces rate of removal. Moreover such accumulation may divert metabolism along an alternative path by accumulation of a by-product such as phenylypyruvic acid in phenylketonuria (p. 26).

Harmful acceleration of metabolism

Substantial acceleration of normal metabolism occurs in patients with Graves' disease. This acceleration is caused by excessive induction of enzyme synthesis. In these patients the serum contains *human specific thyroid-stimulating immunoglobulin* which becomes bound by an antigen on the thyroid cells and then stimulates them to excrete increased amounts of thyroxine (T_4) and triodotyrosine (T_3) into the plasma. T_4 and T_3 then act on the nuclei of cells in many organs including the liver and induce increase in synthesis (transcription) of mRNA, rRNA and tRNA. These RNAs move into the cytoplasm where they induce synthesis (by translation) of many enzymic proteins such as respiratory enzymes and RNA-polymerases. This results in gross increase in cellular oxidation and generation of heat, which ultimately leads to severe wasting.

In various forms of porphyria the rate of synthesis of ALA-synthase is increased and the quantity of this enzyme in hepatic or erythropoietic cells is augmented so that excessive quantities of ALA and of porphobilinogen (PBG) accumulate (p. 167). PBG may then condense to harmful porphyrins which cause injurious sensitisation of the skin to light and also cerebral and neural disorders (p. 196). This induction of ALA-synthase may be greatly increased by barbiturates.

Induction of enzyme synthesis may also be responsible for conversion of various foreign substances to oncogenic agents not normally produced by metabolism in the body. Thus benz(a)pyrene and other aromatic hydrocarbons can induce synthesis of microsomal oxygenases which then oxygenate these or other hydrocarbons to actively oncogenic epoxides. Induction of this kind of metabolic reaction may be of paramount importance in the initiation of neoplasia (p. 174).

Activation of enzymes *already present* in the cell may be responsible for acceleration of metabolism in disease. Thus the hormone-sensitive lipase of lipocytes is normally present in an inactive form which can be activated by phosphorylation mediated by cAMP; cAMP is itself formed from ATP by adenylcyclase (p. 150) when exposed to the uninhibited action of catecholamines (Fig. 9.1). This action of catecholamines is opposed and suppressed by insulin [3, 4]. In diabetes, therefore, when insulin is deficient, the formation of cAMP is stimulated and hormone-sensitive lipase is converted into its active phosphorylated form, which causes the fission of TG with release of FFA into the plasma (Fig. 9.1).

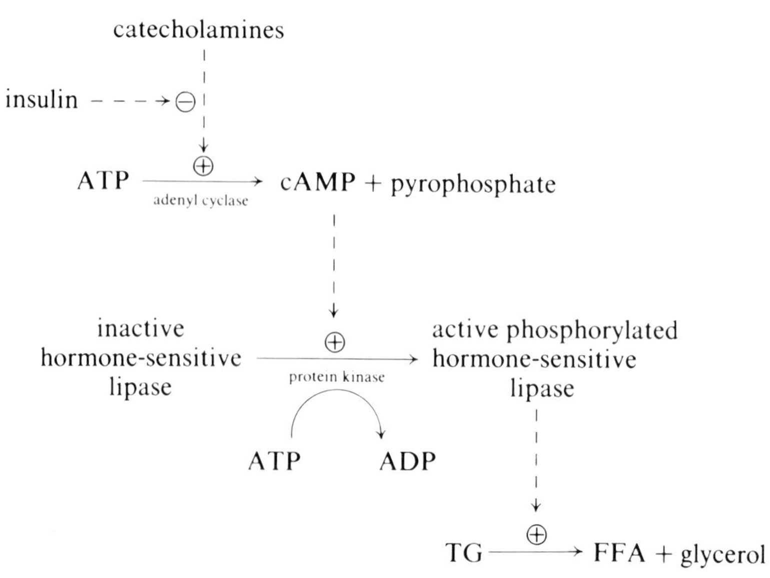

FIG. 9.1 Action of catecholamines in accelerating lipolysis by increase in activity of lipase. This effect is suppressed by insulin but becomes dominant when supply of insulin is deficient in diabetes. In starvation also increase in secretion of catecholamines increases lipolysis. Thus in both starvation and diabetes level of FFA in plasma rises.

Increase in concentration of *substrates* of metabolic enzymic reactions can also accelerate formation of potentially harmful products. Thus the accumulation of uric acid (HU) in gout is associated with increase in rate of conversion of ^{15}N-glycine to ^{15}N-HU. This probably results from increase in concentration of precursors of HU, such as hypoxanthine or xanthine, when alternative paths for their utilisation are eliminated (see Fig. 6.2, p. 199); increase in concentration of precursors then causes acceleration in formation of the harmful product. Similarly, rise in concentration of FFA in plasma (after excessive lipolysis in adipose tissue) augments the concentration of FFA in liver cells; this is followed by excessive synthesis in the liver of TG and of ketone bodies, each of which is a product of metabolism of FFA. This sequence of events occurs during starvation and in diabetes (p. 368).

Harmful retardation of metabolism

Retardation or suppression of metabolic reactions can also be highly injurious.

Hypoxia, by suppressing exergonic cellular oxidation of glucose and other metabolites, deprives the cells of their principal source of energy and is the basic determinant of ischaemic injury. Although hypoxia may cause diversion of oxidative carbohydrate catabolism to anaerobic glycolysis, the products formed are not actively toxic. But this alternative path usually cannot supply sufficient energy to prevent cellular injury (p. 85).

Deficiency of thiamine retards the oxidative decarboxylation of pyruvate to acetyl-CoA and so also interrupts the principal pathway in the oxidative catabolism of glucose (p. 51).

$$\text{glucose} \longrightarrow \text{pyruvate} \xrightarrow[\ominus]{\text{lack of thiamine}} \text{acetyl—CoA} + CO_2$$

This inhibition results in accumulation of pyruvate in cells and in blood; the excess of pyruvate is not itself actively harmful, but suppression of the oxidative fission of pyruvate deprives both cardiac and cerebral cells of an important source of energy and further damages them by interrupting supply of acetyl-CoA.

Suppression or retardation of metabolism may also result in accumulation of substances which are actively harmful. Inherited lack of phenylalanine 4-monooxygenase suppresses oxidation of phenylalanine to tyrosine and causes accumulation of phenylalanine which interferes with normal myelination in the developing brain (see Fig. 2.4, p. 27). Similarly, suppression of catabolism of G_{M2} in Tay-Sachs disease (owing to inherited absence of hexosaminidase A) results in accumulation of this ganglioside in cell bodies of cerebral neurones; this is followed ultimately by degeneration of axons in brain and retina with resultant idiocy and blindness (p. 405 and Fig. 8.41). Retardation of disposal of a normal metabolite also accounts for the lesions of hereditary protoporphyria (p. 197).

Harmful diversion of metabolism

Products formed by diversion of metabolism may also be harmful. Such diversion along an alternative path generally follows retardation with accumulation of a metabolite. When hypoxia retards oxidation of FFA, diversion of its metabolism to form TG or cholesterol may be important factors in fatty globulation (p. 362) and atherogenesis (p. 385). Similarly, interruption in the normal path of conversion of porphobilinogen to haem may cause accumulation of porphyrinogens, which then are oxidised to harmful porphyrins as in porphyria variegata (p. 196).

Retardation of excretion by the cell

Starvation may diminish the formation of albumin by hepatic cells so that they excrete less albumen and this results in hypoalbuminaemia and oedema (p. 46). Less severe lack of protein in chronic malnutrition interrupts the formation and excretion of VLDL from liver cells and also promotes gross fatty globulation within them (p. 368). Retardation of metabolism within cells can therefore result in diminished excretion of metabolic products.

Defects of metabolism thus include derangements in absorption, sequential interconversion, and excretion of cellular nutriments and their products. These kinds of derangement are specially common and prominent in diabetes mellitus.

Diabetes mellitus and its injurious effects

Diabetes mellitus is a disease in which metabolic disorder of cells produces both hyperglycaemia and glycosuria. This derangement affects about 4 per cent of mankind. Many diabetic patients suffer little disability but some of them develop gross hyperglycaemia and polyuria with severe wasting. Without treatment such patients may deteriorate rapidly with severe dehydration and lethal hyperosmolar coma. In other patients more chronic arterial disease becomes established which leads to cardiac or cerebral ischaemia, renal disease or retinopathy with blindness.

Diabetes mellitus occurs in two principal types; these are called type-1 (juvenile-onset type) and type-2 (maturity-onset type). However, some patients have signs intermediately between those of the two types.

Type-1 diabetes (juvenile-onset)

This generally commences in children or young adults. It is characterised by severe wasting of the body, owing to rapid depletion of fat stores with discharge of TG from lipocytes, and by *absence* or *very low concentration* of insulin in the blood [5, 6]. Treatment with insulin is life-saving for these patients who (without insulin) may suddenly pass into hyperosmolar coma. These patients also suffer from ketoacidosis with fall of plasma pH and over-breathing. Injection of insulin rapidly lowers the level of blood sugar and enables return to a normal active life. These patients have an increased incidence of arterial and renal disease later in life; these later complications can probably be averted by controlled treatment with insulin.

In patients with type-1 diabetes, who die soon after the onset of the disease, the number of β-cells in the pancreatic islets is usually less than 10 per cent of normal, while in patients who survive longer, β-cells disappear completely [7]. Inflammatory exudate containing lymphocytes and plasma cells is often visible in the islet tissue; this may indicate allergic destruction of β-cells in this type of diabetes.

Type-2 diabetes (maturity-onset)

This is usually a disease of middle age. These patients are obese and their fat stores may be saturated. They usually eat much carbohydrate and fat, sometimes to gross excess. The blood plasma of these patients contains substantial amounts of insulin [8]. Moreover, treatment with insulin has little effect on the level of blood sugar; there is thus apparently no shortage of insulin. Although severe ketoacidosis does not usually develop in these patients, their blood sugar may be high and they may pass into hyperosmolar coma especially following infection or surgical operations.

Pathogenesis of diabetes mellitus

Diabetes mellitus may have several causes and this multiple origin obscures the initial events in pathogenesis. Possible determinants include:

1. *Genetic factors*. These clearly influence the incidence of type-2 diabetes; about half the children of two parents with this type of disease develop mild diabetes by the age of 60. Inheritance of type-1 disease is less clear; it may depend on a recessive gene which is only expressed when other factors such as infection or hyperphagia overtax the pancreatic β-cells.

2. *Injury to insular β-cells*. Loss of β-cells in pancreatic islets is the paramount defect in type-1 diabetes. In normal persons injection of glucose is followed by prompt release of insulin. This response is sluggish in patients with type-1 diabetes and also in their apparently normal monozygotic twins [9]. This sluggish response may indicate an inherited defect in production or secretion of insulin by the β-cells, which is later followed by necrosis. An autoallergic mechanism may be concerned in the destruction of β-cells, and this may account for infiltration of the islets by lymphocytes [7]. The basic cause for loss of β-cells in most patients with severe diabetes is unknown. However, destruction of β-cells by fibrosis in haemochromatosis (p. 415) and by invasive carcinoma can also result in diabetes by abolishing the cellular source of insulin.

3. *Microangiopathy*, including thickening of capillary and venular basement membranes, is a common occurrence in diabetes and may precede or determine metabolic defects. Microangiopathy in skeletal muscle (assessed by EM) is also detectable in 50 per cent of non-diabetic persons whose parents are both diabetic [10]. This suggests that microangiopathy antedates the development of diabetes and is more likely to be a cause than an effect of injury to the β-cells; microangiopathy has been observed in the islet tissue of diabetics. A contrary view is that microangiopathy is a sequel to hyperglycaemia and results from excessive synthesis of glycoprotein in vascular basement membranes steeped in saccharine fluid.

4. *Corpulence.* Excessive enlargement of lipocytes may be the determining factor in diabetes of maturity-onset in corpulent patients. In these adipose diabetics lipolysis is accelerated. This stimulation in catabolism of TG may result from increase in accessibility of lipolytic enzymes following gross distension of cytoplasmic film of lipocytes by enlarged globules of TG; this may cause adsorption of enzyme proteins on the enlarged oil/water interface followed by increase in liberation of FFA (p. 369).

Metabolic derangements in diabetes

There are two principal metabolic lesions:

1. Retardation of uptake and metabolism of glucose by cardiac and striated muscle and also by lipocytes; this results in hyperglycaemia.
2. Acceleration of lipolysis of TG to FFA in lipocytes along with increase in uptake and metabolism of FFA in many tissues; this is followed by excessive formation of ketone bodies and cholesterol.

1. *Retardation of entry and metabolism of glucose.* In type-1 diabetes this is the paramount metabolic lesion and is a direct consequence of lack of insulin (Fig. 9.2). Insulin is necessary for the transport of glucose into both cardiac and striated muscle and also into lipocytes (p. 96). Entry and metabolism of glucose are so much suppressed in type-1 diabetes that the usual rise of blood pyruvate which follows injection of glucose in normal persons is abolished [11] and the removal of glucose from arterial blood by peripheral tissues is retarded [11a].

In type-2 diabetes, even though insulin is present in the blood and the usual rise in blood pyruvate after injection of glucose still occurs, the entry of glucose into cells is severely retarded. This restriction of entry of glucose in type-2 diabetes is probably a consequence of the inhibiting action exerted by FFA and ketone bodies which are present in the blood owing to excessive lipolysis. This inhibitory effect of fatty acids on the metabolism of glucose was discovered by observations on metabolism of perfused rat hearts [12]. In this tissue addition of palmitate or β-hydroxybutyrate to the perfusing fluid *in the presence of insulin* diminishes uptake of glucose and also its conversion to hexose phosphates.

This effect of FFA and ketone bodies in preventing uptake and metabolism of glucose is the principal cause of hyperglycaemia in type-2 diabetes in which there is no deficiency of insulin; the same mechanism may also augment hyperglycaemia in type-1 diabetes. The suppression of uptake of glucose may result from blocking by FFA and ketone bodies of the receptors in cell membranes which are concerned with transport of glucose. The phosphorylation of glucose and its conversion to fructose-diphosphate may also be inhibited by FFA. This interruption of the metabolism of glucose may be due to feed-back inhibition of phosphofructokinase by citrate, which is formed as a product of oxidation of FFA and ketone bodies [13].

2. *Acceleration of lipolysis and liberation of FFA from lipocytes.* In diabetes there is gross increase in the concentration of FFA in plasma owing to liberation

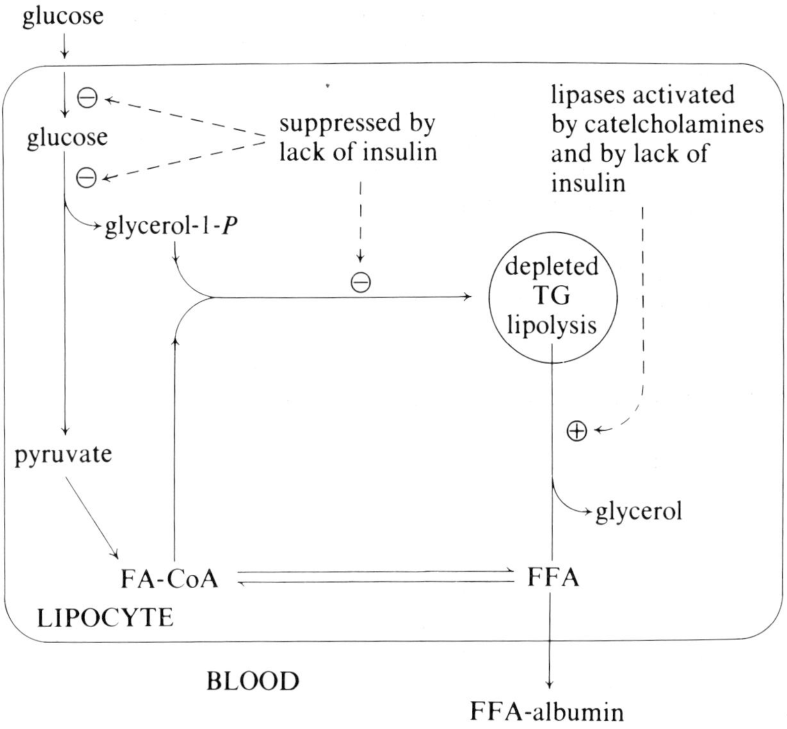

FIG. 9.2 Metabolic derangements in lipocytes caused by lack of insulin in type-1 diabetes. Retardation of entry and metabolism of glucose suppresses formation of glycerol-1-*P* and so prevents synthesis of TG from glycerol-1-*P* and FA-CoA. Removal of restrictive effect of insulin on activation of hormone-sensitive lipase by catecholamines results in stimulation of lipolysis.

of FFA from lipocytes [14]; this increase is greatest in patients with ketosis. Injection of insulin causes a dramatic fall in concentration of both FFA and glucose in the blood of these patients and this precedes the elimination of ketosis by many hours.

In type-1 diabetes this release of FFA from lipocytes into blood depends on two factors: (a) lipolysis is accelerated owing to activation of hormone-sensitive lipases by catecholamines *in the absence of insulin* (p. 430 and Fig. 9.1); and (b) the conversion of FFA to TG within lipocytes becomes retarded when glycerol-1-phosphate ceases to be formed on account of suppression of metabolism of glucose in absence of insulin (Fig. 9.2). Both these factors summate to cause depletion of fat depots and discharge of FFA into the blood and make type-1 diabetes a severely wasting disease.

In type-2 diabetes excessive FFA can be released into the blood from the enlarged lipocytes of obese patients. When lipocytes are grossly distended with globular fat, amphipathic proteins, including lipase, may be adsorbed on the extended oil/water interfaces so as to reduce interfacial tension to a minimum.

Lipase in such a situation may become highly accessible to ester linkages of TG with resultant lipolysis and release of FFA into the blood. This FFA then may exert an inhibiting effect on uptake and metabolism of glucose by lipocytes and other cells so that hyperglycaemia becomes established even in the presence of insulin.

The metabolic lesions in diabetes thus produce two principal effects:

1. Hyperglycaemia.
2. Rise in concentration of FFA in blood.

Both of these effects are potentially injurious: their consequences will now be considered.

Harmful consequences of hyperglycaemia: hyperosmolar coma

In untreated diabetics the blood sugar may rise to very high levels such as 1000 mg/dl blood (55 mmol/l) or more. These patients are usually confused, drowsy or frankly comatose; they commonly suffer from air hunger and also become dehydrated as a result of polyuria. In many of these patients the plasma contains substantial amounts of ketone bodies and its pH is lowered. For this reason the condition was called *keto-acidotic coma*.

But in many drowsy or comatose diabetics with intense hyperglycaemia there is little or no ketonaemia and the plasma pH is not lowered. Moreover, in all patients with severe hyperglycaemia, *both with and without keto-acidosis*, the degree of stupor parallels the hyperosmolality of the plasma and not the severity of the acidaemia; the depression of consciousness is thus apparently caused by hyperosmolality and not by keto-acidosis [15, 16]. For this reason stupor or coma in diabetic patients with severe hyperglycaemia is now usually called *hyperosmolar coma*; it is probably directly related to dehydration and shrinkage of cerebral cells owing to intense hyperosmolality of the extracellular fluid principally caused by high concentration of glucose.

This view is supported by observations on animals following intravenous infusion of other solutes such as urea, mannitol, NaCl and sucrose. When the osmolality of the plasma is thus raised from the normal level of about 290 mosmol/l to above 400 mosmol/l, stupor or coma develops, irrespective of solute used. Death usually follows when this level reaches 435–450 mosmol/l [17].

Besides glucose, ketone bodies doubtless contribute to hyperosmolality of the plasma in diabetes both directly and by their effect in inhibiting uptake of glucose by cells and so increasing hyperglycaemia (p. 434).

The concentration of *acetone* in plasma of comatose diabetic patients sometimes rises as high as 10 mmol/l. However, treatment with insulin in most cases rapidly restores consciousness and lowers the level of blood sugar *before* the concentration of acetone falls appreciably; moreover, the concentration of acetone in the plasma is low in many comatose diabetic patients [18].

Clearly therefore diabetic coma is not directly related to concentration of acetone in the plasma but is primarily determined by exposure of cerebral tissue to hyperosmolar extracellular fluid.

Although treatment with insulin uniformly lowers the level of blood sugar and usually restores consciousness in patients with diabetic coma, in some patients coma may persist or deepen and they may die in a few days with hyperpyrexia. The brain in these cases is swollen and shows extensive neuronal necrosis; the neuronal cell bodies in deeper layers of cerebral cortex and globus pallidus are converted into 'unstainable shadows' (p. 332) and capillaries are dilated and their endothelium is damaged [19]. These changes are probably caused by superadded cerebral ischaemia which develops during the preceding period of hyperglycaemia and is primarily determined by terminal *hypotension* and heart failure; this then results in extensive neuronal swelling and necrosis (p. 302).

Prolonged hyperglycaemia has other injurious but usually less immediate effects. Thus, when blood glucose rises above 11 mmol/l, glucose appears in the sweat and also in inflammatory exudates; these fluids then become ideal media for bacterial and fungal growth. Under these conditions infection by *Staphylococcus pyogenes* can produce severe boils and *Candida albicans* may colonise skin of axilla, groin or vulva causing intense pruritus. Hyperglycaemia may also determine the onset of cataract in elderly diabetics; this may depend on opacification of the lens fibres by deposition of polysaccharides synthesised by lens epithelial cells after prolonged immersion in sugary fluid.

How far hyperglycaemia contributes to diabetic angiopathy is undetermined (p. 440).

Harmful consequences of rise in concentration of FFA in blood

Excess of FFA in the blood exerts, as we have seen, a suppressive action on entry and metabolism of glucose in many tissues. But excessive entry of FFA into diabetic liver cells has specially harmful consequences which will now be considered.

In liver cells increase in entry of FFA is followed by increase in production of fatty acyl-CoA(FA–CoA); this results in accumulation of both TG and acetyl-CoA (Fig. 9.3).

This excessive formation of TG in liver in diabetes depends on the presence of glycerol kinase in hepatic cells; this enzyme catalyses the formation of glycerol-1-phosphate (glycerol-1-*P*) from glycerol and ATP. Glycerol-1-*P* can thus be formed in hepatic cells in diabetes, although its formation in other cells, such as lipocytes, is suppressed by inhibition of glycolysis in absence of insulin (Fig. 9.2). Thus intense fatty globulation can occur in the liver in diabetes (Fig. 9.3) and may eventually lead to cirrhosis. Hepatic cirrhosis is discussed on p. 374 and its harmful cerebral effects on p. 451.

Besides TG the other main product of FFA, which enters liver in diabetes, is acetyl-CoA (Fig. 9.3). This has three principal fates:

1. Oxidation to CO_2.
2. Conversion to ketone bodies which are released into the blood and produce ketonaemia and acidosis.
3. Synthesis to cholesterol which in the long term is a most injurious product.

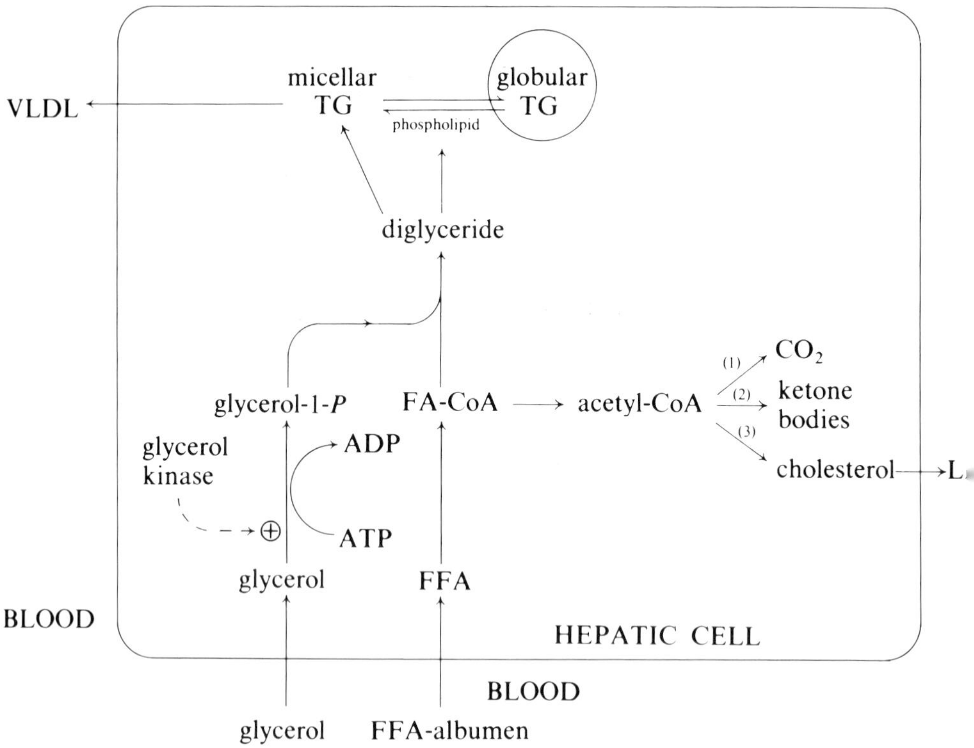

FIG. 9.3 Consequences of excessive entry of FFA into hepatic cells in diabetes. Harmful effects include fatty globulation, formation of ketone bodies and excessive formation of cholesterol.

Cholesterol is then excreted from the liver both as free cholesterol and cholesterol esters mainly carried in LDL fraction of plasma. This excessive amount of total cholesterol formed by the liver accounts for the typical hypercholesterolaemia of diabetes.

Cholesterol is probably also formed excessively from FFA in other cells such as those of the arterial intima in diabetes (see Fig. 8.25). This intra-arterial synthesis of cholesterol as well as uptake of cholesterol from LDL probably both contribute to the high incidence of atherosclerosis in diabetes.

Thus excess of FFA in the plasma in diabetes acts as a potential determinant of both hepatic cirrhosis and of atherosclerosis.

Diabetic vascular disease

The most harmful concomitant of polonged diabetes is vascular disease. This arises in two principal forms, atherosclerosis and microangiopathy (Fig. 9.4). Atherosclerosis was discussed in Chapter 8; microangiopathy will now be considered.

Diabetic microangiopathy affects both capillaries and venules (p. 433). The principal lesion is thickening of basement membrane (BM) with accumulation

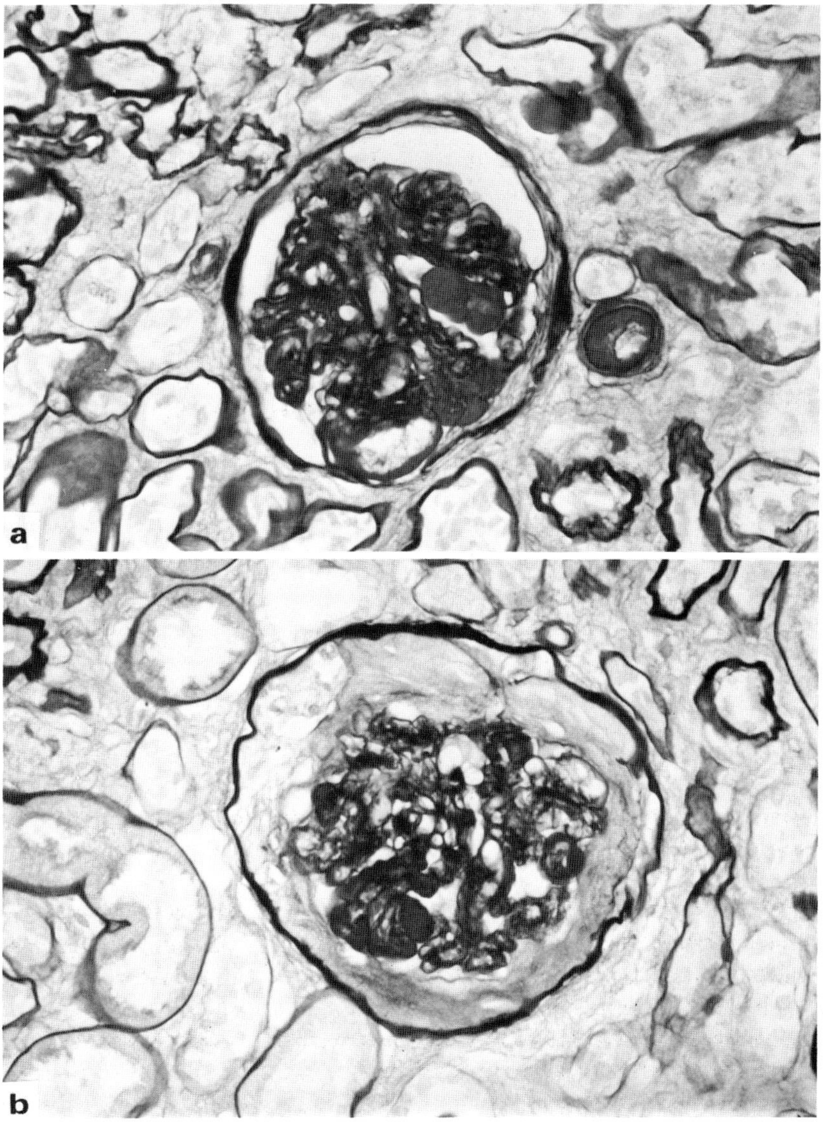

FIG. 9.4 Diabetic glomerulosclerosis. Kidney from a man of 35 who had diabetes mellitus for 12 years. He later suffered from chronic heart failure due to ischaemic myocardial fibrosis associated with severe coronary atherosclerosis and also from hypertension. Terminally he developed oedema and retinopathy with rise in blood urea. He died in coma. PAS. × 330.

a. Diffuse thickening of basement membrane of glomerular capillaries and round hyaline nodules of PAS-positive material near glomerular periphery; a micro-aneurysm is visible at lower pole of glomerulus.

b. More severe nodular change in glomerular tuft, also sclerosis of Bowman's capsule.

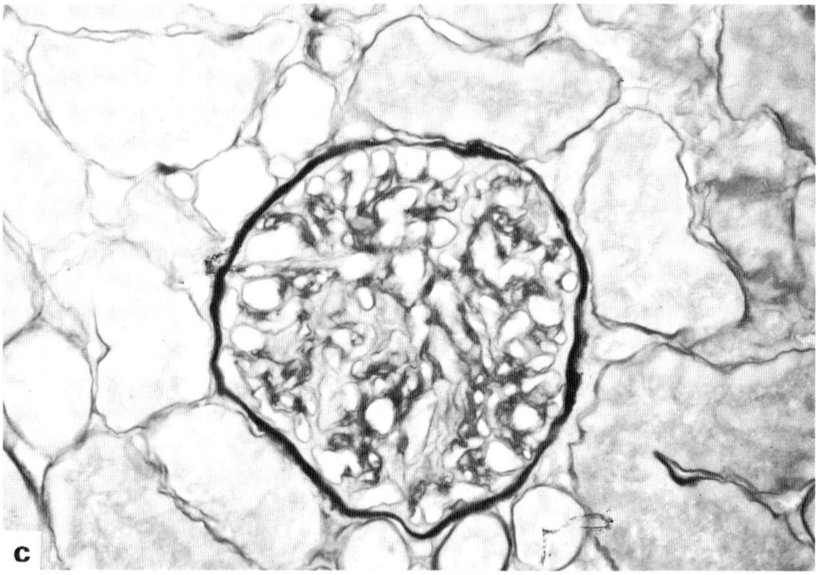

FIG. 9.4 cont.
c. Glomerulus from a normal kidney. PAS. × 330.

of hyaline glycoprotein stainable by PAS (Fig. 9.4). Observations by EM on capillaries in human quadriceps femoris muscle removed by biopsy showed thickening in nearly all diabetic patients examined [10, 20]; this thickening of BM in muscle capillaries may however be much less frequent in younger diabetics [21]. But conspicuous renal and retinal microangiopathy, visible by LM, is common after prolonged diabetes at all ages.

Renal microangiopathy (*diabetic glomerulosclerosis*) is the principal cause of renal disease in diabetes. This sclerosis involves diffuse thickening of the capillary BM in the glomeruli along with nodular thickening extending into the mesangial spaces; these nodules are called Kimmelstiel–Wilson lesions. Both the nodules and the diffuse thickening of the BM contain PAS-positive glycoprotein (Fig. 9.4). Some of the glomerular capillaries enlarge into microaneurysms, while later the whole glomerulus becomes sclerosed (Fig. 9.4). These lesions are responsible for albuminuria and oedema, followed by chronic renal failure and hypertension which may terminate in uraemic coma or cerebral haemorrhage. Proteinuria is the clinical hallmark of this 'diabetic nephropathy' and the prognosis is worst when the excretion of protein is greatest; there is also an increased risk of atherosclerosis in these patients. It is uncertain how far good control of sugar level in the blood affects the prognosis of patients with these renal lesions, or indeed whether the thickening of capillary BM by glycoprotein is in any way related to hyperglycaemia.

Retinal microangiopathy is also a common occurrence in diabetes. This causes thickening of BM and the formation of microaneurysms in retinal venules. Retinal oedema, due to leakage of plasma through diseased capillaries and venules, is apparently largely responsible for loss of visual acuity and blindness. Development of new blood vessels (retinitis proliferans) may further impair vision.

Microangiopathy is thus a highly injurious concomitant of diabetes; whether it is a determinant or a consequence of the metabolic lesions is still obscure.

DEFECTS OF CELLULAR BEHAVIOUR AND FUNCTION

In this kind of derangement behaviour and function of cells are altered without concomitant visible changes in structure. Such disorder probably depends, however, on cellular lesions at a macromolecular level.

Some aberrations of this nature will be considered in cells of the central nervous system, where profound malfunction can occur without overt changes in microscopic appearance.

Coma caused by hypoxia

Both consciousness and cerebral electrical activity are rapidly abolished by hypoxia (p. 86). These effects occur within about 10 seconds of arrest of supply of O_2 to the brain; irreversible injury follows more slowly.

This elimination of consciousness is probably a consequence of neuronal hypoxia, which inhibits oxidative phosphorylation and thus grossly retards the formation of exergonic agents such as ATP. Fission of ATP provides energy for active transport of ions necesssary for maintaining ionic gradients upon which electrical activity depends. Without ATP, continuation of nerve impulses within the brain (p. 86), which are an essential part of consciousness, is precluded. Lack of ATP later causes irreversible structural injury which permanently eliminates nervous activity.

Besides interfering with oxidative phosphorylation and synthesis of ATP, hypoxia may also suppress oxygenation necessary for forming neurotransmitters (p. 456); this effect may contribute to the coma caused by hypoxia [22]. But the irreversible injury to neurones by anoxia, which is followed by permanent coma, probably depends on structural damage to neuronal membranes caused by elimination in supply of ATP (p. 93).

Inhibition of respiration caused by coma

Coma due to causes other than hypoxia is also accompanied by depression of respiration.

In patients with severe diabetes the oxygen consumption of the brain varies inversely with the depth of diabetic coma and is diminished by 40 per cent in deeply comatose patients [23]. This might imply that diabetic coma is itself caused by a fall in consumption of O_2, but the initial coma is almost certainly a direct result of hyperosmalality due to hyperglycaemia (p. 436).

Indeed, decrease in uptake of O_2 by the brain occurs in all conditions of coma or semi-coma regardless of cause, whether due to hypoxia, trauma, hyperglycaemia, narcotics or renal or hepatic disease [24]. The O_2 uptake of normal human brain is approximately 3.3 ml/100 g brain/min. In coma, irrespective of cause, this is diminished to values between 1.5–2.3 ml/100 g brain/min. The constancy of this effect suggests that coma itself may determine diminution in uptake of oxygen, and that this is linked with interruption of neuronal electrical activity and function.

Electrical changes on the surface of neurones depend on waves of surface depolarisation involving entry of Na^+ followed by exit of K^+ [25, 26]. This efflux of K^+ to the exterior during activity may have profound metabolic consequences since K^+ exert a remarkable effect in stimulating both respiration and aerobic glycolysis of cerebral grey matter *in vitro* [27]. Thus waves of increased glycolytic metabolism initiated by expelled K^+ may be closely related to the passage of impulses [28]. External K^+ liberated from excited neurones may induce much of the normal respiration and aerobic glycolysis of brain *in vivo*. External K^+ are actively transported back into neurones after passage of impulses, while Na^+ which have entered the cells are at the same time expelled; thus resting ionic gradients are restored [28a]. This active transport of ions stimulates respiration and may act as a pacemaker for respiration and glycolysis. Indeed, when the uptake of K^+ by slices of cerebral cortex *in vitro* is inhibited by the cardiac glycoside ouabain, the rate of oxygen uptake is simultaneously diminished [29, 30].

The energy for this active transport of K^+ into the neurone and Na^+ out of it is provided by fission of ATP by membrane-bound ATPase. Fission of ATP diminishes its concentration and so retards its normal action in limiting glycolysis and respiration by allosteric inhibition of the enzyme phosphofructokinase [6]. Hence active transport of K^+ into the cell increases glycolysis and respiration by lowering concentration of ATP.

The addition of K^+ *in vitro* to slices of cerebral cortex simulates these effects by accelerating both aerobic glycolysis and respiration. Fig. 9.5 shows that this

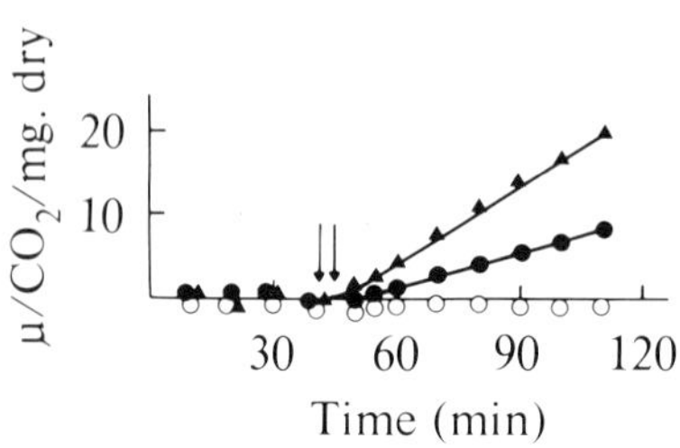

FIG. 9.5 Rapid action of K^+ in stimulating aerobic glycolysis of slices of rabbit cerebral cortex in glucose-bicarbonate-Ringer. Each series of points first shows a very low rate of aerobic glycolysis up to the period between the arrows; at this point NaCl and KCl were added to give final additional concentration of Na^+ and K^+ in mmol/litre as follows:

O—O—O	Na^+ 40	K^+ O
●—●—●	Na^+ 10	K^+ 30
▲—▲—▲	Na^+ 0	K^+ 40

Dixon K. C. (1949) *J. Physiol.* **110**, 87.

effect of K^+ on aerobic glycolysis rapidly follows addition of K^+ and proceeds continuously when external concentration of K^+ is raised. Similar increase in glycolysis and respiration stimulated by external K^+ *in vivo* may generate sufficient energy to replenish the cellular level of ATP, as it is consumed in restoring the normal resting ionic gradients after activity.

Neuronal electrical activity, followed by restoration of ionic gradients coupled with utilisation of ATP, accordingly accelerates aerobic glycolysis and respiration owing to temporary fall of intracellular concentration of ATP. But when electrical activity is supressed as in various forms of coma, this utilisation of ATP and consequent acceleration of glycolysis and respiration is eliminated. Coma, no matter how caused, thus diminishes the rate of cerebral uptake of O_2.

In contrast to diminution of uptake of oxygen which is an automatic consequence of neuronal *inactivity*, excessive nervous *activity*, during episodes of anxiety or grave fear, correspondingly increases uptake of O_2 by human brain from 3.3 to 5.0 ml O_2/mg brain/min [31]. During these episodes of excitement augmentation of nervous activity may promote ionic movement so as to raise extraneuronal K^+ and thus increase active transport of ions coupled with consequent increase in glycolysis and uptake of O_2.

The rate of cerebral respiration thus reflects changes in neuronal activity in disease or stress which are not necessarily accompanied by visible alteration in cellular structure.

Cerebral malfunction due to trauma

Two of the most prominent sequels of cerebral trauma are coma and amnesia.

Coma

Consciousness is apparently determined by neuronal activity in the reticular formation of the midbrain which continually alerts activity in the cerebral cortex. After transection of the brain-stem at mid-collicular level, even without damage to the cortex or its blood supply, animals behave as if asleep [32]. The process of consciousness is abolished when messages from the reticular formation fail to reach the cortex. Memory and intelligence almost certainly reside entirely in the cerebral cortex, but the conscious state is a function of the mesencephalic reticular formation which constantly alerts the cortex (p. 114).

In human brain traumatic transection of long fibres in cerebral white matter may follow injuries which cause shearing of the cerebral substance (p. 113); these injuries can produce *permanent* stupor or coma when they dissever connection between reticular formation and the cortex. Similar permanent loss of consciousness, hypersomnia and coma may follow interruption of mesencephalic connections owing to lesions caused by local haemorrhage or neoplasm.

Cerebral concussion can also produce coma by *temporary* suppression of neuronal activity in the reticular formation. Concussion in animals depresses electrical activity both in reticular formation and in cerebral cortex but the depression in the reticular formation is far greater and more prolonged than in the cortex. Often there is no macroscopic evidence of cerebral damage, although in some neurones, especially in the reticular formation, the Nissl substance shows central chromatolysis (p. 114). Loss of consciousness due to concussion is only temporary provided axonal connection between reticular formation and cortex remains intact.

Cerebral concussion and memory

As well as causing coma concussion can interrupt the cataloguing of events into memory. The temporary coma produced by concussion outlasts the period of violence and is generally succeeded by amnesia of the immediately preceding events.

This *retrograde amnesia* indicates that neuronal processes concerned with recent happenings are less indelibly impressed in memory than long past experiences. Any reasonable view of the molecular basis of concussion and of memory should account for this impermanence of recent memory traces.

Possibly repetitive patterns of electrical activity at neuronal surfaces are determined by mutually aligned and complementary mosaics of lipid and protein molecules which provide the physical basis and continuity of consciousness, memory and thought. Incoming impulses may temporarily mould these lipid patterns. Then if such a temporarily formed lipid pattern can find a complementary peptide pattern among the hereditary peptides of the cell, this peptide pattern becomes aligned in the membrane. In this way the peptide may be temporarily removed and debarred from exerting a *repressor effect* which may previously have suppressed its own synthesis [33]. The synthesis of this specific peptide pattern by genomic transcription followed by translation is thereby evoked. Thereafter the peptide pattern is instrumental in recreating the complementary lipid pattern in the cell membrane and also the original pattern of electrical activity. By this type of resonance with potential peptide patterns, coded by the neuronal genome, external impressions may evoke memory and thought which are limited by the capacity of the genome to initiate the fabrication of various peptide patterns.

Following this view the transient coma of concussion may be due to temporary disalignment of lipid membrane patterns. Only when the lipid patterns become specifically remoulded by their complementary peptides can consciousness return. The retrograde amnesia after concussion may depend similarly on interruption of mutual alignment of a *newly* moulded lipid pattern with the minute amounts of complementary peptide originally present, *before* fabrication of the new specific peptide pattern has become evoked. In this way a recent memory trace may be erased before a permanent record becomes established. Intoxication by ethanol can similarly erase recent memory traces before permanent records are imprinted.

Defects of neurotransmission

Disorders of neuronal behaviour can arise from deficiency in supply and reception of neurotransmitters which are normally released by the terminals of presynaptic fibres and are bound by receptors of post-synaptic neurones or other excitable cells.

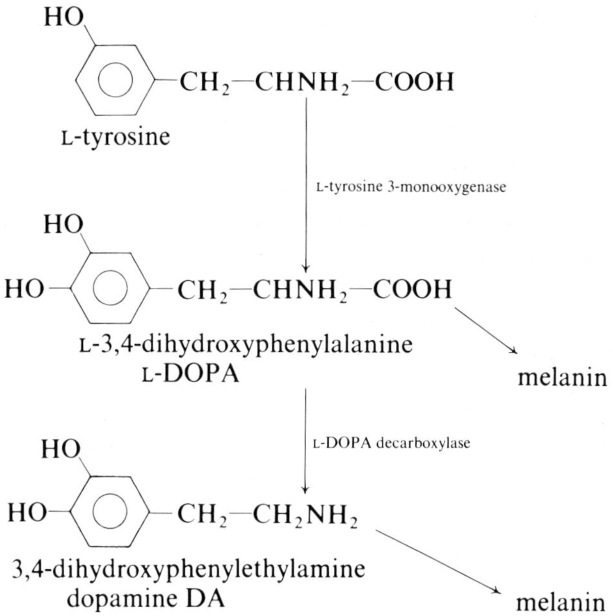

FIG. 9.6 Formation of dopamine and melanin in neurones of substantia nigra (SN) and locus caeruleus (LC). When these neurones die, dopamine is no longer formed and the dopaminergic receptors in the corpus striatum cease to be activated by the nigrostriatal fibres; this results in Parkinson's disease.

Defect in secretion of dopamine (DA)

A relatively common example of such defect is Parkinson's disease (paralysis agitans). In this malady paralysis, rigidity and tremor are produced by malfunction of neurones in the corpus striatum following destruction of dopamine-forming neurones in the substantia nigra (SN) and locus caeruleus (LC), which normally activate the specific dopaminergic receptors in the striatal cells.

In health the intact neurones of the SN and LC synthesise dopamine (3,4-dihydroxyphenylethylamine, DA) from tyrosine as shown in Fig. 9.6. L-3,4-dihydroxyphenylalanine (DOPA) is formed as an intermediary in this biosynthesis of DA. Any excess of DOPA or DA in neurones of SN and LC is transformed into dark granules of melanin which gives these cells their characteristic dark colour. DA is stored in minute cytoplasmic vesicles in which it is transported along the nigrostriatal tract and then accumulates in these vesicles within varicose presynaptic terminals in the corpus striatum (Fig. 9.7). Neuronal activity in the striatum is regulated by release of DA discharged by the nigrostriatal terminals and finally adsorbed by specific post-synaptic receptors in the striatal neurones (Fig. 9.7). Unused DA is oxidised by mitochondrial monoamine oxidase to an intermediate aldehyde and then to 3,4-dihydroxyphenylacetic acid (DOPAC), and this is finally methylated to

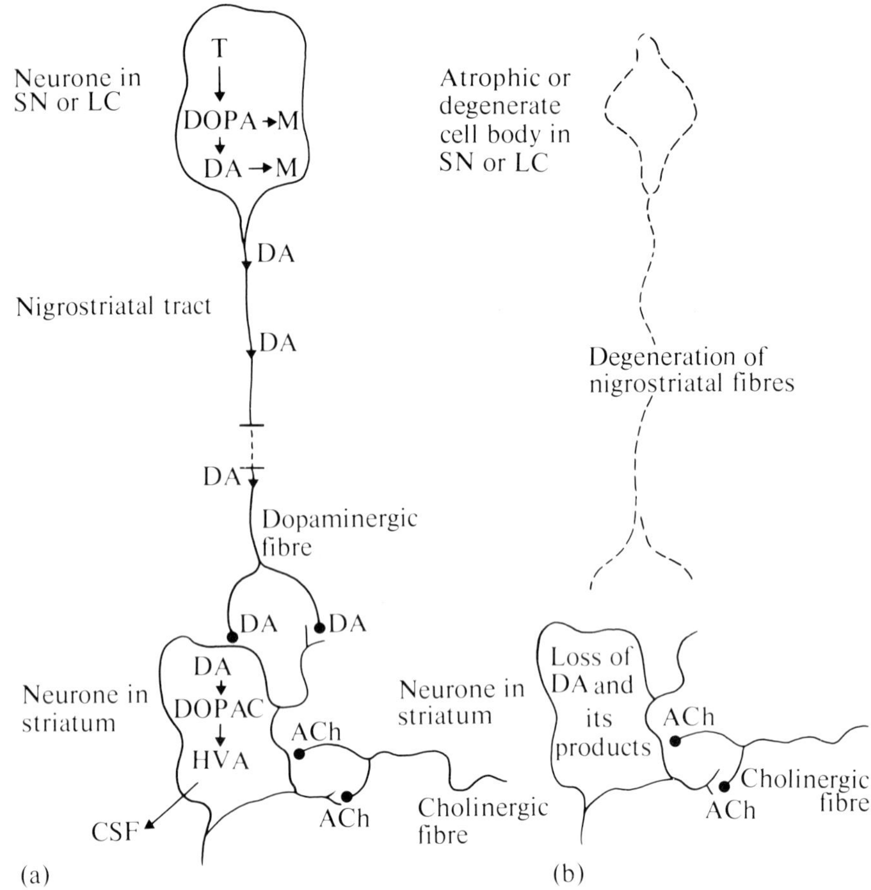

FIG. 9.7 Effects of Parkinson's disease on nigrostriatal system.

a. Normal nigrostriatal mechanisms: DA, formed in neurones of SN or LC, passes along dopaminergic fibres of nigrostriatal tract, is discharged from presynaptic terminals at nigrostriatal synapses, and then acts on dopaminergic receptors in striatal neurones. Other cholinergic receptors are simultaneously activated by ACh.

b. Parkinson's disease caused by atrophy or necrosis of neurones in SN or LC: DA no longer formed and dopaminergic receptors on striatal cells cease to be activated. Cholinergic action then becomes dominant and striatal cells behave abnormally.

SN	substantia nigra		presynaptic varicose terminal
LC	locus caeruleus		axosomatic synapse
T	tyrosine		axodendritic synapse
DOPA	L-3,4-dihydroxyphenylalanine	M	melanin
DA	dopamine		
DOPAC	3,4-dihydroxyphenylacetic acid		
HVA	homovanillinic acid		
ACh	acetylcholine		
CSF	cerebrospinal fluid		

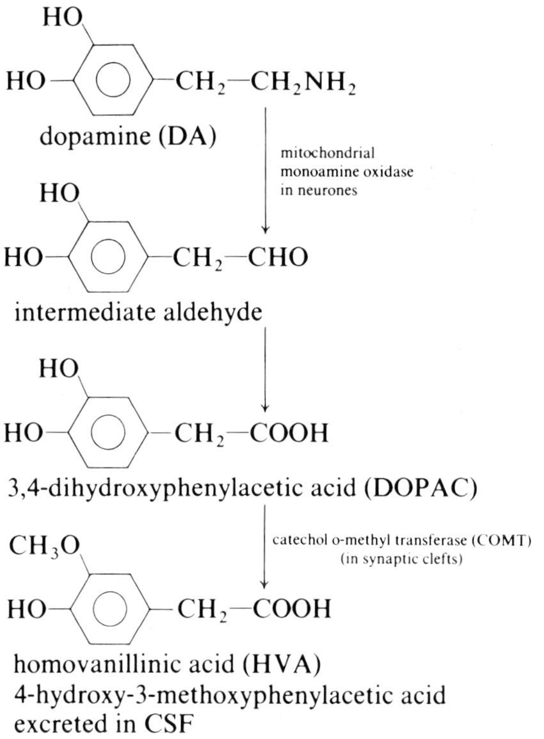

FIG. 9.8 Final inactivation of DA by conversion to HVA which is excreted in CSF.

4-hydroxy-3-methoxyphenyl acetic acid (homovanillic acid, HVA; Fig. 9.8). HVA is finally excreted in the CSF (Figs. 9.7, 9.8).

Coordinated activity of striatal neurones depends on their continuous stimulation by cholinergic terminals along with compensating action of dopaminergic terminals which respectively release acetylcholine (ACh) and DA (Fig. 9.7).

The most important lesion in Parkinson's disease is atrophy and destruction of the pigmented neurones in the brain stem especially in the SN and LC. The darkly coloured cell bodies in these neurones lose their granules of melanin and ultimately shrivel and disappear. At the start of this process concentric hyaline inclusions called Lewy bodies appear in the cytoplasm of some of the pigmented neurones (Fig. 9.9). These eosinophilic bodies visible in the pigmented neurones may herald the subsequent degeneration and atrophy.

Parkinson's disease today mainly occurs in elderly patients and is possibly induced by senile ischaemia; a viral origin is also possible and might account for the Lewy inclusion bodies. Earlier in the present century Parkinsonism with akinesia and rigidity was a dreaded sequel to encephalitis lethargica (sleepy sickness) caused by a then prevalent viral infection of the brain. Mild symptoms

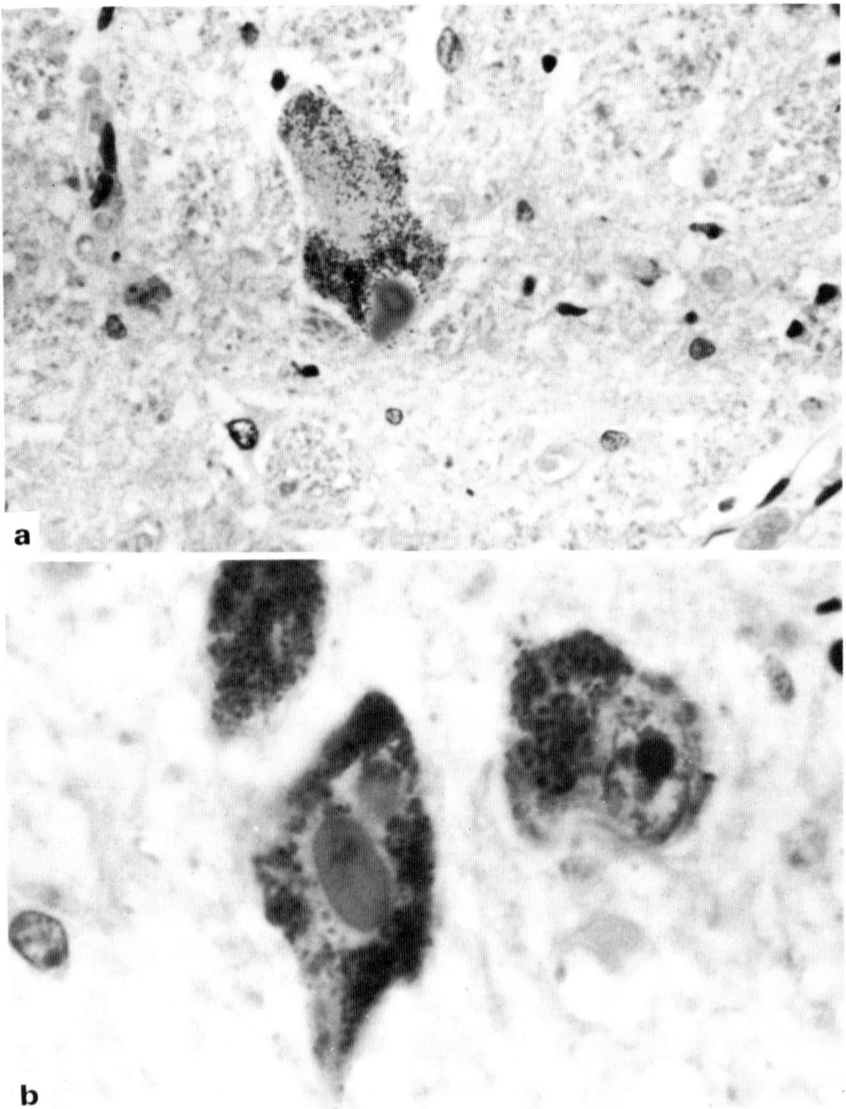

FIG. 9.9 Lewy bodies in pigmented neurones of locus caeruleus in Parkinson's disease. From a woman of 78 with Parkinson's disease diagnosed two years before her death due to heart failure.

a. × 520. Neuronal cell body containing granules of melanin and a hyaline Lewy body at lower pole.

b. × 1440. Cell body in centre contains melanin granules and two hyaline Lewy bodies: cell body on the right shows nucleus and nucleolus and also numerous melanin granules. Section by courtesy of Professor G. A. Gresham.

of striatal defect sometimes also occur in phenylketonuria, presumably owing to fault in conversion of phenylalanine to tyrosine with resultant retardation in formation of DA.

The concentration of DA and HVA in the substantia nigra and in the caudate nucleus and putamen of the corpus striatum is strikingly diminished [34] in all patients dying with signs of Parkinson's disease. The Parkinson syndrome, irrespective of cause, results from deficiency of DA in the corpus striatum. When the neurones of the SN atrophy and disappear their axons in the nigrostriatal tract degenerate and no longer secrete DA. The dopaminergic receptors in the striatum are therefore no longer stimulated and the striatal neurones behave abnormally; this results in tremor, rigidity and akinesia, probably owing to uncompensated stimulation of cholinergic receptors in these cells (Fig. 9.7).

In living patients with Parkinsonism the production of DA is so grossly retarded that the concentration of its principal end product HVA in the CSF is substantially diminished (Fig. 9.7).

Although the disorder of striatal neurones is basically caused by atrophy or necrosis of neurones in SN, its immediate determinant is an *invisible defect* in behaviour and activity of the striatal neurones through *lack of DA*. This concept of the mechanism of Parkinsonism was dramatically confirmed by the observation that a single injection of L-DOPA results in remarkable abolition of akinesia; bedridden patients unable to sit up, or who could not stand, or who when standing could not walk, performed all these acts after treatment with L-DOPA [34].

Defects in secretion of acetylcholine (ACh) in botulism

Comparable deficit in secretion of acetylcholine at cholinergic terminals occurs in botulism (p. 220) owing to the action of the exotoxin of *Clostridium botulinum*. This toxin prevents the release of ACh from cholinergic axonal terminals in striated muscle. Observations by EM on these nerve terminals after exposure to botulinum toxin labelled with ferritin suggest that the toxin blocks the site of release of ACh in the unmyelinated terminals.

Other examples of inhibition of formation and reception of neurotransmitters will be considered in the following section on hepatic encephalopathy.

Hepatic encephalopathy and coma

Disturbance of cerebral function, causing delirium or drowsiness culminating in coma, is a sinister sequel of hepatic disease. Cerebral malfunction of this kind is called hepatic encephalopathy (HE).

HE occurs as a terminal event in acute fulminating viral hepatitis with massive necrosis of the liver, which is usually caused by hepatitis B virus; in this form delirium or mania may precede the onset of coma. HE with more gradual onset or with successive intermittent attacks is usually a consequence of hepatic cirrhosis with portal obstruction caused by prolonged fatty change, alcoholism or chronic viral hepatitis with scarring; this more chronic form is characterised by drowsiness, slurred speech and tremor, also terminating in coma.

After extensive hepatic necrosis harmful substances reaching the liver by the portal blood are no longer detoxicated by the dead hepatic cells, while in cirrhosis with portal obstruction the detoxicating action of the hepatocytes is diminished by hepatic ischaemia, or is annulled when these cells are bypassed by diversion of their principal blood supply. Such portasystemic bypass may occur spontaneously in cirrhosis by development of venous shunts within the liver itself or else by extrahepatic shunts formed by umbilical or oesophageal

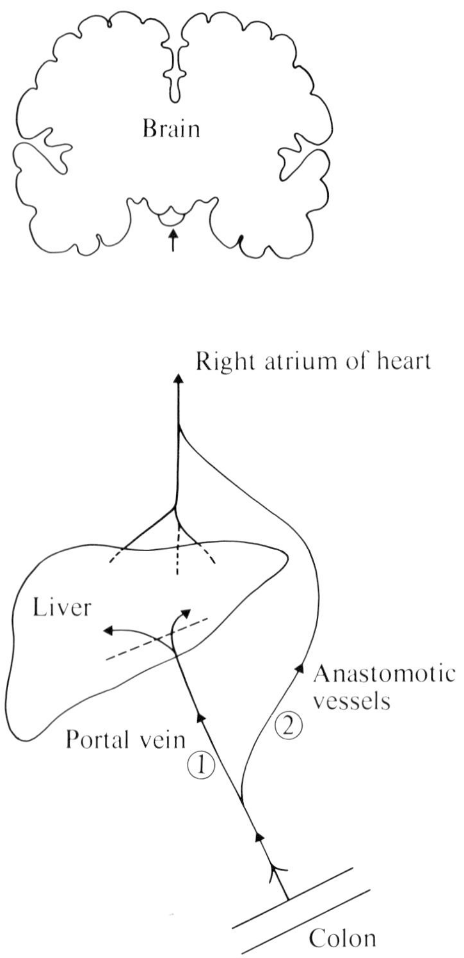

FIG. 9.10 Portacaval shunt and hepatic encephalopathy. Obstruction of hepatic circulation can cause development of anastomotic vessels (2) so that circulation is diverted from portal vein (1) along (2). In this way venous blood from the bowel returns directly to the heart and the brain eventually becomes exposed to blood which has not filtered through the liver.

venous anastomosis; these diversions shunt venous blood returning from the intestines directly to the right side of the heart without any preliminary percolation through the hepatic sinusoids (Fig. 9.10). Thus, when the liver cells are either eliminated or bypassed, the brain becomes exposed to substances absorbed from the intestines which are normally made harmless by the detoxicating metabolism of the hepatic cells.

In HE following cirrhosis with portal obstruction, the level of consciousness is progressively depressed. At first the patient is confused and his speech slurred. His extended wrists and metarcarpal joints may show flapping tremor (asterixis). These signs are followed by progressive drowsiness, stupor and coma. Along with these changes the EEG is altered *pari passu* [35, 36]. The mean frequency of oscillation falls from the normal α-rhythm of 8–13 Hz to <4 Hz, while the amplitude of the waves increases (Fig. 9.11). Later slow triphasic waves of large amplitude develop along with onset of coma. As coma deepens the amplitude decreases and terminally electrical activity disappears (Fig. 9.11).

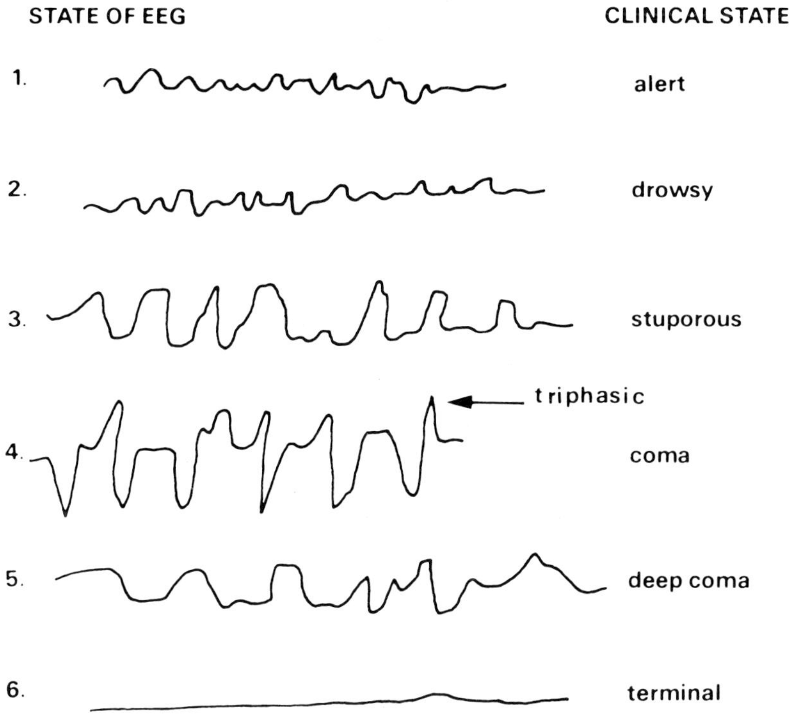

FIG. 9.11 Changes in EEG related to clinical stages in hepatic encephalopathy. Decrease of frequency, increase of amplitude and onset of triphasic waves mark the progression through drowsiness and stupor to hepatic coma. Later, amplitude decreases with deep coma, and terminally electrical activity disappears altogether. Courtesy of Professor Dame Sheila Sherlock. Reproduced from *Brit. J. Hosp. med* (1977), **17**, 144.

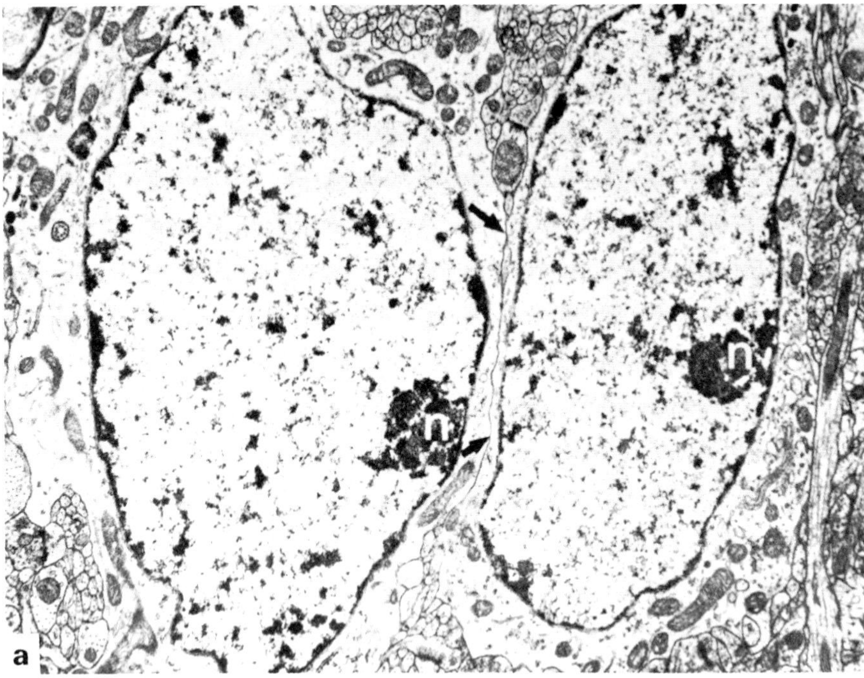

FIG. 9.12 Hypertrophic proliferating astrocytes in cerebral cortex of rats with portacaval anastomosis; these animals developed deep coma on feeding with NH_4^+ in cation exchange resin.

a. Pair of astrocytic nuclei from adjacent daughter cells; each has a prominent nucleolus (n). EM. × 13 000.

This profound cerebral malfunction may not be accompanied by visible changes in neurones or glia in patients who die rapidly with fulminating delirium and coma. But proliferation of glial cells and neuronal disintegration are prominent in the cerebral tissue of patients who die in hepatic coma after more slowly progressive hepatic disease or portasystemic shunting [37]. These changes include multiplication and enlargement of Alzheimer type-2 protoplasmic astrocytes (A-2 glial cells) as well as necrosis of pyramidal cells with microcavitation in cerebral grey matter together with loss of Purkinje cells from cerebellar cortex.

In animals encephalopathy accompanied by similar changes follows artificial portacaval anastomosis [38, 39]. These effects are remarkably accelerated and magnified when NH_4^+ are fed by gastric tube after operation [40, 41]. The A-2 glial cells typically occur in pairs as a result of frequent division (Fig. 9.12a); their cytoplasm appears swollen and vacuolated (as seen by EM) with prominent broad processes extending into the adjacent neuropil (Fig. 9.12b).

The cerebral disability in HE is believed to be caused by exposure of neurones or glia to toxic substances formed in the colon which are normally removed

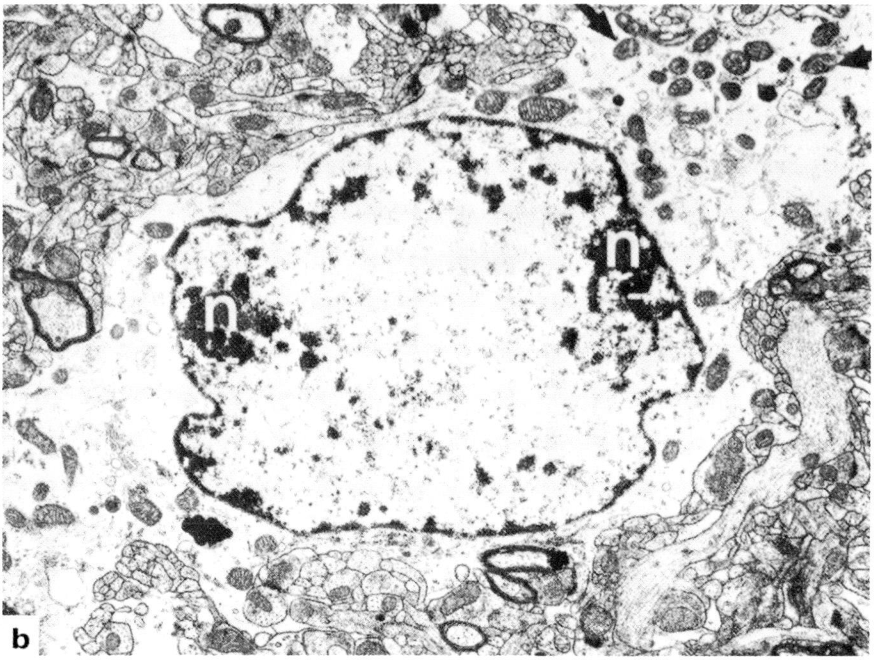

FIG. 9.12 cont.
b. Hypertrophic astrocyte with broad expanded cytoplasmic processes (electron-lucent) extending into the neuropil; two nucleoli (n) in nucleus. EM × 13 000. Courtesy of Dr M. D. Norenberg & Professor L. W. Lapham. Reproduced from *J. Neuropath.* (1974), **33**, 422.

from the portal circulation by the liver. These substances can reach the brain in harmful concentration when the detoxicating action of hepatic cells is eliminated by extensive necrosis or is eluded by portacaval deflection of circulation (Fig. 9.10). Probably many different substances may exert such neurotoxic effects when hepatic activity is either annulled or bypassed (see below). Such substances may include NH_4^+, aromatic amines, and possibly glutamine or its derivatives, which are present in increased concentration in plasma and CSF in both human patients and animals suffering from HE. Exposure of cerebral cells to these toxic substances may be responsible for change in structure as well as the malfunction, which occur in HE; alternatively the cellular damage induced by these substances may determine the disorder of behaviour. Such potential toxigenic action will now briefly be considered.

Ammonia as a cerebral poison

Ammonia is normally formed from urea in the large intestine and is then absorbed into tributaries of the portal vein. In healthy liver cells this ammonia is converted to urea. But when liver cells are destroyed or when their supply of blood is retarded or diverted, as in hepatic cirrhosis, then NH_4^+ accumulate in the blood. Thus the mean level of NH_4^+ in human arterial blood is usually increased about four-fold in patients with hepatic coma and this increase is usually proportional to the depth of coma [42].

The importance of NH_4^+ as a determinant of hepatic coma is further indicated (p. 452) by the extremely toxic action of NH_4^+ fed to rats following portacaval anastomosis. In these animals ingestion of NH_4^+ was followed in a few days by disorders of behaviour, paresis of hind limbs, and terminal coma along with conspicuous proliferation of A-2 glial cells in cerebral cortex [41].

Bessman & Bessman [42] suggested that HE is initiated by entry of NH_4^+ into cerebral tissue where they react with α-ketoglutarate. Glutamate is formed as a result of this reaction:

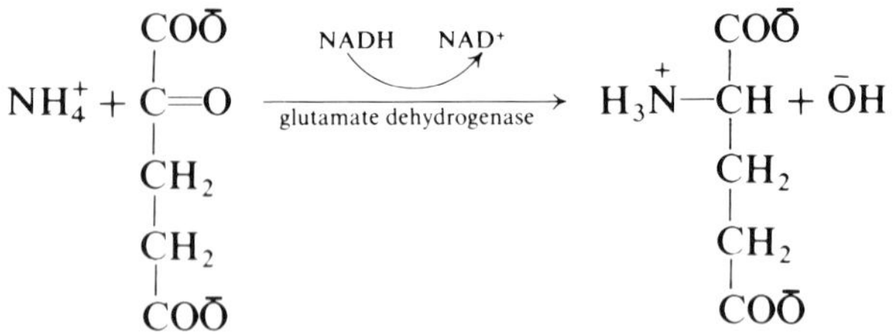

α-ketoglutarate L-glutamate

This glutamate may then react with more NH_4^+ to form glutamine:

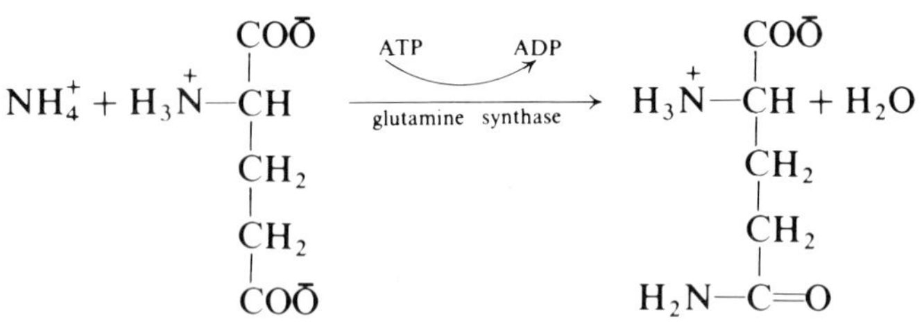

L-glutamate L-glutamine

Thus NH_4^+ can remove α-ketoglutarate and also cause accumulation of glutamine which is constantly found in raised concentration in CSF of patients with hepatic encephalopathy. In this way the neurones may become deprived of α-ketoglutarate which is a principal source of energy for the tricarboxylic acid cycle of aerobic oxidation.

Another possibility is that glutamine formed from NH_4^+ and glutamate (as indicated above) is converted into a toxic agent. In patients with HE the rise in concentration of glutamine in CSF is accompanied by rise in concentration of *α-ketoglaramate* [43]. This metabolite of glutamine, formed by transamination, may possibly exert a neurotoxic action and so contribute to development of hepatic coma.

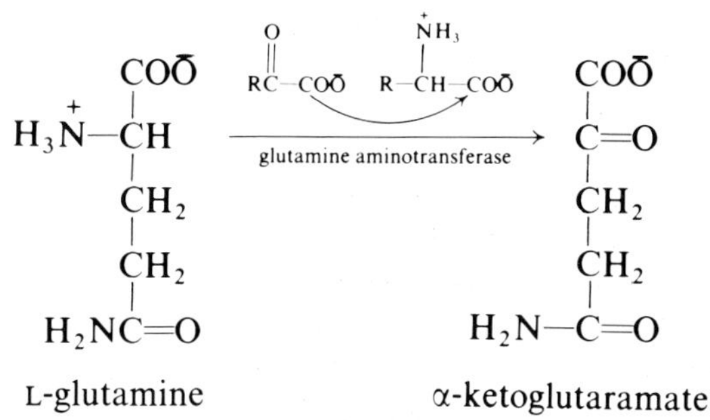

Although the concentration of NH_4^+ in plasma is thus usually raised in patients with hepatic coma, in some cases this effect is not detectable. This may indicate that other noxious substances besides NH_4^+ contribute to development of HE or that excess of NH_4^+ is sometimes evanescent owing to rapidity of its reaction with α-ketoglutarate and glutamate.

Aromatic amines: false transmitters

Other substances formed in the intestine by bacterial action and absorbed into the blood include the aromatic amines tyramine and 2-phenylethylamine, formed from tyrosine and phenylalanine respectively. These substances enter the portal blood and are normally conveyed to the liver where they are converted to harmless aldehydes by monoamine oxidase in the hepatic cells; tyramine is formed and detoxicated as shown in Fig. 9.13.

When the action of hepatic cells is nullified by necrosis or bypass, these amines are not detoxicated and pass directly into the systemic circulation and enter cerebral cells. Within minute granular vesicles of adrenergic neurones the

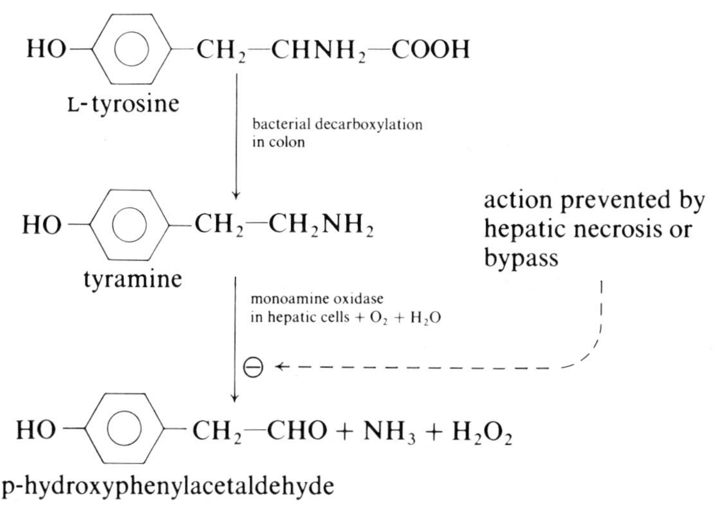

FIG. 9.13 Effect of hepatic injury or bypass in preventing oxidation of toxic amines, such as tyramine, by monoamine oxidase in the liver. These amines can then enter the systemic circulation and act on the brain to cause HE.

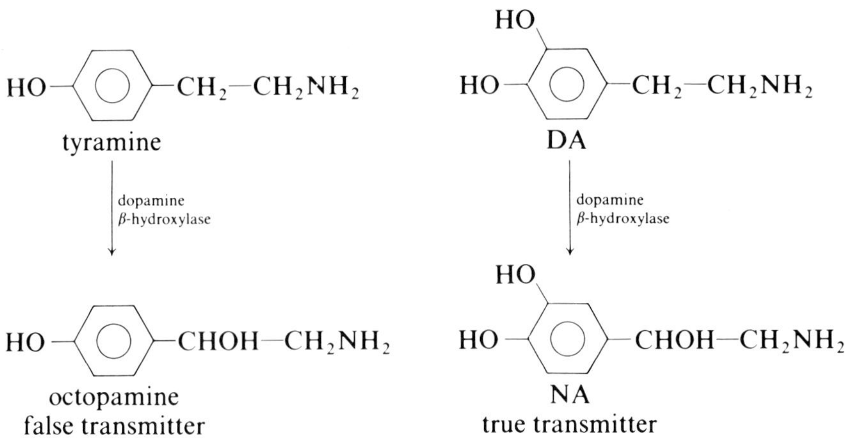

FIG. 9.14 Action of octopamine as a 'false' transmitter. When tyramine is not detoxicated in the liver it may enter presynaptic adrenergic cerebral neurones, where it is converted to octopamine by dopamine β-hydroxylase in the same way as dopamine (DA) is normally converted to noradrenaline (NA). Octopamine may then be discharged from the presynaptic terminals and be absorbed on postsynaptic receptors in the same way as the 'true' transmitter NA. In this way octopamine may act as a 'false' transmitter and block the action of NA and so cause HE and coma. Octopamine may also competitively inhibit oxidation of DA to NA by dopamine β-hydroxylase.

enzyme dopamine β-hydroxylase normally oxidizes dopamine (DA) to noradrenaline (NA); this enzyme can similarly convert other amines to β-hydroxy derivatives which are homologues of NA. Thus tyramine is converted to octopamine in the same way (Fig. 9.14).

In normal brain NA is formed and stored in these vesicles in the presynaptic terminal of adrenergic neurones and is then liberated as a neurotransmitter which traverses the synaptic cleft and activates surface receptors in the postsynaptic neurones. If abnormal β-hydroxy amines such as octopamine are formed by the same process in the presynaptic terminals, they may also be discharged by nervous activity and then be adsorbed on the same receptors, but block them instead of causing stimulation. Such 'false transmitters' may then suppress neurotransmission by NA and so cause HE and coma [44]. Amines such as tyramine may also retard formation of NA by direct competitive inhibition of DA β-hydroxylase.

The operation of these kinds of mechanism in the pathogenesis of hepatic coma correlates with the raised concentration of octopamine both in plasma and urine of human patients with this disorder. Moreover observations on rats during hepatic coma produced by portacaval anastomosis [45] show that:

1. Concentration of octopamine in the brain is increased.
2. This increase *precedes* increase of octopamine in plasma.
3. Concentration of NA in the brain is simultaneously diminished.

These findings indicate that octopamine is formed in the brain during hepatic coma and is associated with fall in concentration of NA. Thus interference with the action of NA in the brain, either by diminution in its rate of formation or by elaboration of false transmitters such as octopamine (Fig. 9.14), may be a potent determinant of cerebral malfunction and coma caused by hepatic disease.

Observations on the effect of feeding L-DOPA (a precursor of NA in the brain) to patients in hepatic coma support the idea that this disorder is determined by interference with the action of NA. Administration of L-DOPA by stomach tube to these comatose patients is followed by arousal along with temporary improvement in mental state and transient restoration in normal frequency of EEG within a few minutes [46]. This effect may be due to an increase in supply of NA (from L-DOPA) and temporary restoration of the NA pathway.

Renal encephalopathy

Drowsiness and coma also occur as sequels to severe renal disease. Cerebral malfunction due to renal failure can conveniently be called renal encephalopathy (RE); the term 'uraemia' is also applied to this condition.

In *chronic renal failure* the number of active nephrons and the rate of glomerular filtration may progressively diminish, so that eventually the concentration of urea in the plasma rises and its pH falls; the patients then become listless and drowsy and may finally lapse into coma; they also suffer from muscular twitching or epileptiform spasms. The EEG shows slowing in frequency with short bursts of activity. Sleepiness and stupor, but with more sudden onset, may also follow *acute renal failure* caused by hypotension from acute haemorrhage and shock; acute renal failure produces oliguria and sometimes terminates in cardiac arrest, but recovery with diuresis follows effective treatment.

The basic cause of RE is undetermined. Chromatolysis, pyknosis and loss of cerebral neurones occur in patients who die with chronic RE; but these changes may be caused by terminal hypoxia due to coincident heart failure. Probably hyperosmolality of plasma, produced by urea and other retained metabolites, contributes to coma. Convulsions in chronic RE and cardiac arrest in acute RE may be related to high $(K^+)/(Ca^{++})$ ratio in plasma. Less is known about the cause of coma in RE than in HE. In both these disorders coma is accompanied by diminution in cerebral uptake of 0_2.

These disorders of behaviour illustrate how profound cerebral malfunction can occur when no directly causative damage is discernible in the affected cells. Possibly these maladies involve cellular changes at macromolecular level which cannot be detected by methods now available. In the next section neoplasia will be considered as an inherent disorder of growth which is similarly not directly determined by overtly visible lesions.

NEOPLASIA

Behaviour of neoplastic cells

Neoplasia consists of unrestrained and uncoordinated cellular growth. This growth involves (1) expansion, (2) infiltration and (3) metastasis. The tumour or mass of cells produced by such growth is termed *benign* if it grows by expansion only, but *malignant* if it also grows by infiltration into surrounding tissues and by metastasis in establishing secondary growths in distant organs. Infiltration and metastasis are hallmarks of malignant neoplasia and on them depend many of the lethal effects of cancer.

Expansion (growth in volume)

A tumour arises from uncoordinated growth of a group of cells which, unlike normal adult differentiated cells, retain the property of repeated mitosis.

In normal adult tissue only stem cells continue to enter mitosis. These stem cells produce by their division:

1. Other stem cells which re-enter mitosis after interphase (G_1 phase).
2. Maturing cells, which do not normally divide, but enter a long or permanent period without mitosis (G_0 phase); these maturing cells only divide if stimulated (e.g. lymphocytes after exposure to phytohaemagglutinin or liver cells after loss of their contiguous neighbours).

The actual rate of doubling in volume by primary tumours in man is not usually as great as that of normal fetal tissue or of adult tissue during regeneration after injury, nor is the mitotic cycle of neoplastic cells any faster than that of stem cells in normal tissue [47]. But the cells of a tumour do not differentiate to form maturing cells and they continue to divide, although sometimes with long intermitotic intervals. Thus mitosis continues in neoplastic cells and their power of maturation is defective. In this sense the cells of tumours are undifferentiated, and they are undifferentiated in other respects also (see below).

This doubling time of tumour volume (DT) varies widely from patient to patient but shows a median value of about two months [48]. DT is substantially diminished owing to loss of tumour cells by necrosis. Kinetic studies on tumour cells exposed to tritiated thymidine, which measure the percentage of labelled mitosis among the cells, indicate that the interval between successive mitoses is very variable and has a mean of about two days; these studies coupled with observations on DT suggest that 70–90 per cent of the new cells produced are lost. The loss by necrosis may help to explain why DT is 30–90 times longer than the duration of the mitotic cycle. This loss is probably one of the main factors in limiting the rate of growth.

Anaplasia, infiltration and metastasis

The cells formed by rapid neoplastic growth are undifferentiated in structure, pattern and behaviour. Such primitive cells are said to show *anaplasia*, i.e. they have lost the specialised structural features of their cells of origin. They have a high nuclear/cytoplasmic volume ratio (Fig. 9.16), and usually show a primitive glycolytic type of metabolism. The latter depends on high activity of glycolytic enzymes such as hexokinase and phosphofructokinase, which results in characteristic aerobic formation of lactic acid from glucose. In contrast the *specialised* metabolic activities of anaplastic cells are decreased. Thus the cells of gastric carcinoma usually produce no pepsin, no HCl, nor intrinsic factor, which are such essential products of normal gastric epithelium. Another primitive characteristic of neoplastic cells, as emphasised above, is their continuing mitosis.

Extreme degrees of anaplasia are typical of malignant tumours. The cells lose their mutual arrangement characteristic of the organ in which they originate. Their growth is uncoordinated and their cells have lost concerted polarity and limitation of growth, on which the normal specialised structure of different tissues depend.

Fig. 9.15 shows this uncoordinated proliferation produced by extreme malignant anaplasia in a rapidly infiltrating carcinoma of the colon. Although the cells show epithelial contiguity and retain the capacity to form tubules, all semblance of colonic mucous glands is lost. The nuclear/cytoplasmic volume ratio is high (Fig. 9.16) and numerous mitoses are visible. The number of mitoses in some malignant tumours may be increased by delay in the process of mitosis produced by gross heteroploidy (p. 38); also the proportion of cells entering mitosis is increased when differentiated cells, which do not divide, are scarce or absent.

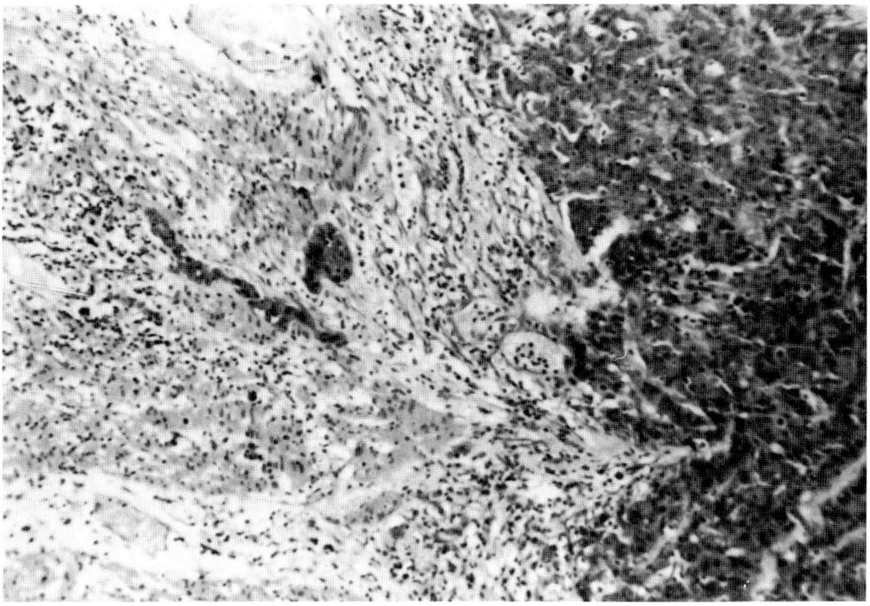

FIG. 9.15. Anaplastic carcinoma of the colon. × 130.

Undifferentiated contiguous epithelial cells, grouped in irregular pseudotubules at right side of figure, have infiltrated into submucosa. Already some tentacles of this neoplasm have extended into the circular muscle coat of the colon and are visible at left side of the figure.

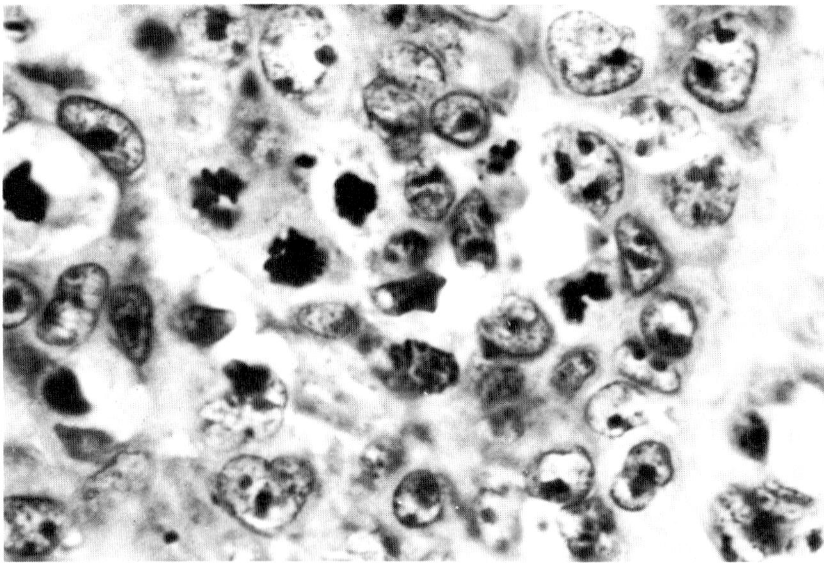

FIG. 9.16. Same anaplastic colonic carcinoma as shown in Fig. 9.15. × 1300. These malignant epithelial cells have high nuclear/cytoplasmic volume ratio and many of them are in mitosis.

Infiltration and metastasis are facilitated by the power of malignant tumours to spread along lymphatic vessels, venules and other natural passages. Permeation of lymphatic vessels by a colonic carcinoma is illustrated in Fig. 9.17. Fig. 9.17a shows normal colonic mucosa with three dilated lymphatics in submucosa immediately subjacent to the muscularis mucosae of the colon. In each of these lymphatics is seen a column of neoplastic cells spreading along the lumen of the vessel. Fig. 9.17b shows, at higher magnification, one of these lymphatics containing a column of malignant cells. More remote extension of this same tumour is shown in Fig. 9.18; here a tubular strand of neoplastic cells is seen growing out into the circular muscle of the colonic wall. Such invasive behaviour is a conspicuous and cardinal characteristic of malignant tumours.

Infiltration is also aided by the capacity of malignant neoplastic cells to utilize the vascular supply of surrounding tissues and to grow and spread through existing or potential tissue spaces without repulsion by adjacent normal cells. Thus both squamous and oat-cell carcinomata of bronchial epithelium grow profusely in cavities provided by pulmonary alveoli, and are lavishly supplied with nutriments by the highly vascular framework formed by interalveolar capillaries. These two highly lethal types of bronchial carcinoma, which so frequently affect the lungs of smokers, can in this way actively proliferate and extend throughout the bronchiolar and alveolar air spaces (Fig. 9.19 and 9.20). More difficult to explain is the power of some malignant cells to invade compact

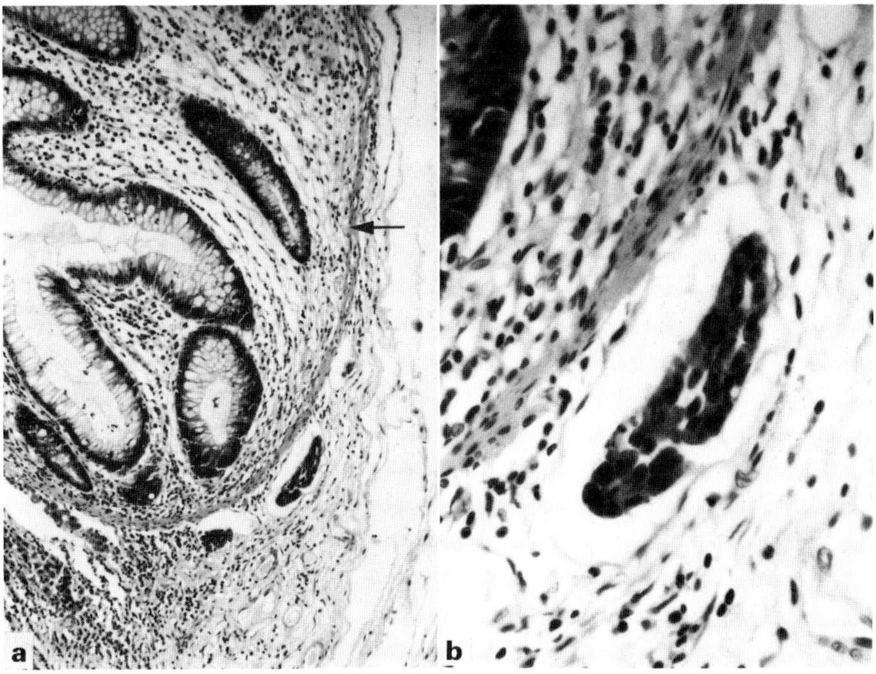

FIG. 9.17 Anaplastic colonic carcinoma; lymphatic permeation.

a. × 130. Normal colonic mucosa (upper left) consists of coordinated tubular glands composed of differentiated goblet cells bounded internally by muscularis mucosae (arrow). Immediately below the muscularis mucosae are visible three dilated lymphatic vessels, each of which contains a pseudotubular column of malignant epithelial cells which have infiltrated along the lymphatics from a colonic carcinoma.

b. × 510. One of the lymphatic vessels enclosing a tubular outgrowth of undifferentiated malignant epithelial cells.

tissue; oat-cell bronchial carcinoma can penetrate bronchial cartilage and spread within its resistant glycoprotein matrix (Fig. 9.21, p. 464).

Much attention has been given to analysing the behaviour of neoplastic cells with the object of discovering the mechanism of infiltration and metastasis. Aberrations of cancer cells *in vitro* which may be concerned with these two principal harmful effects of malignant disease will now be considered.

Decrease in mutual adhesiveness

Coman [49] measured the force required to separate pairs of adherent epithelial cells. He compared in this respect normal cells from human lip and cervix uteri respectively with cells from squamous carcinomata from these two sites and found that malignant cells have less power of mutual adhesiveness than that of

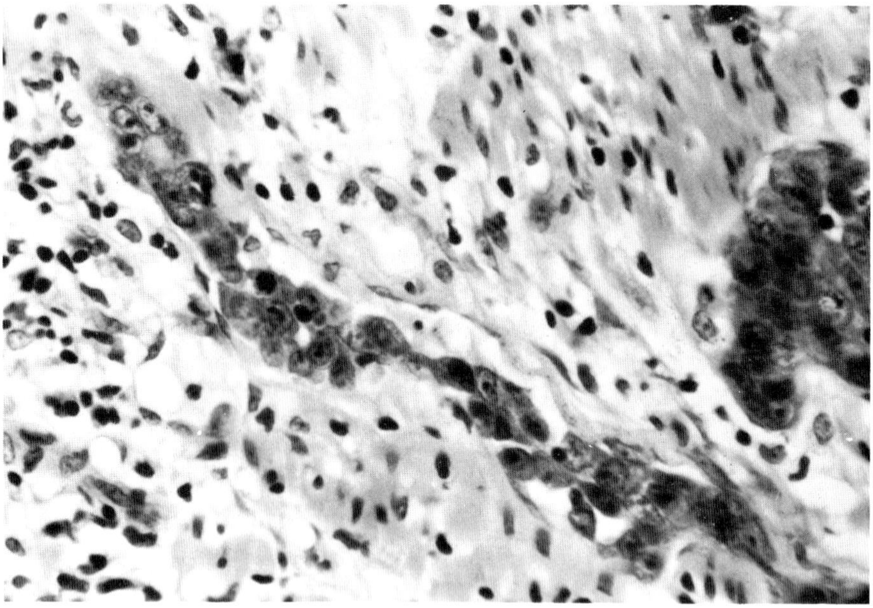

FIG. 9.18 Anaplastic colonic carcinoma penetrating intestinal muscle. × 510. Tubular extensions from main growth (shown in Fig. 9.15) is seen infiltrating between myofibres of circular muscle coat of the intestinal wall; this tentacular outgrowth consists of anaplastic epithelial cells.

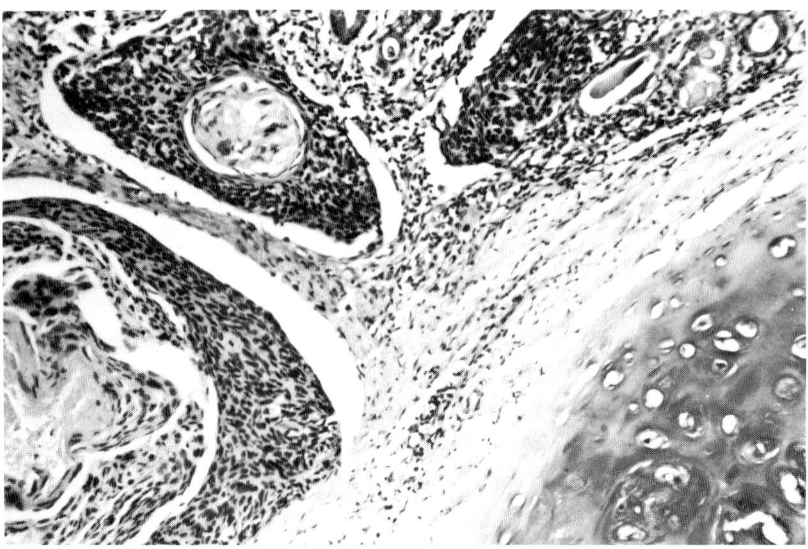

FIG. 9.19 Squamous cell carcinoma of the bronchus; intra-alveolar spread. × 120. This tumour shows squamous metaplasia of bronchial epithelium forming tubular masses of squamous cells with cornified 'cell nests'; the tumour is infiltrating alveolar and bronchiolar spaces and is approaching a plate of bronchial cartilage (bottom right).

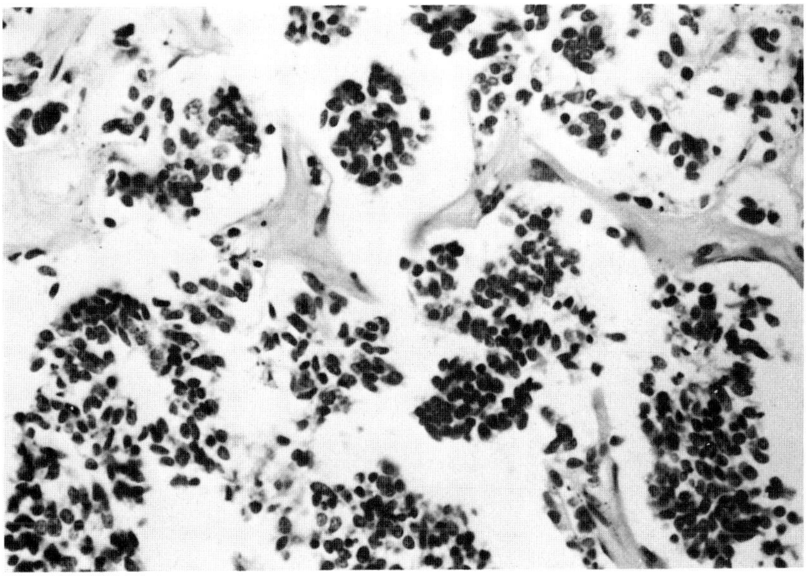

FIG. 9.20 Oat-cell carcinoma of bronchus: intra-alveolar spread. × 330. Acinar masses of undifferentiated epithelial cells growing profusely in the alveolar spaces.

corresponding normal cells. Such decrease in adhesiveness may well account for some of the invasive and metastatic properties of malignant neoplasms.

Increase in stickiness to foreign surfaces

Coman [50] also compared the strength of attachment to glass of benign and malignant cells which had been allowed to become deposited on glass and were then subjected to controlled washing with saline; he found that normal rabbit epidermal cells are much more readily washed away than those of a rabbit carcinoma which stick more permanently to the glass. This power of the rabbit carcinoma cells to stick more firmly to foreign objects contrasts with their *decreased* power of *mutual* adhesiveness which is less than that of comparable rabbit epidermal cells. Stickiness to foreign cells and tissues may also play a part in infiltration by malignant cells.

Loss of contact inhibition of movement

Normal fibroblasts grown in culture show undulating movement which ceases as soon as they touch each other in confluent growth, but sarcoma cells continue movement after contact and grow over each other and also over normal fibroblasts [51]. When a confluent layer of cloned baby hamster kidney (BHK) fibroblasts is wounded by incision to produce a sharp edge, polarised fibroblasts move out from the uninjured cells and migrate at right angles to the edge [52]. In contrast, BHK fibroblasts when transformed by polyoma virus migrate from a similar cut edge in an entirely random fashion with much overlap. These latter

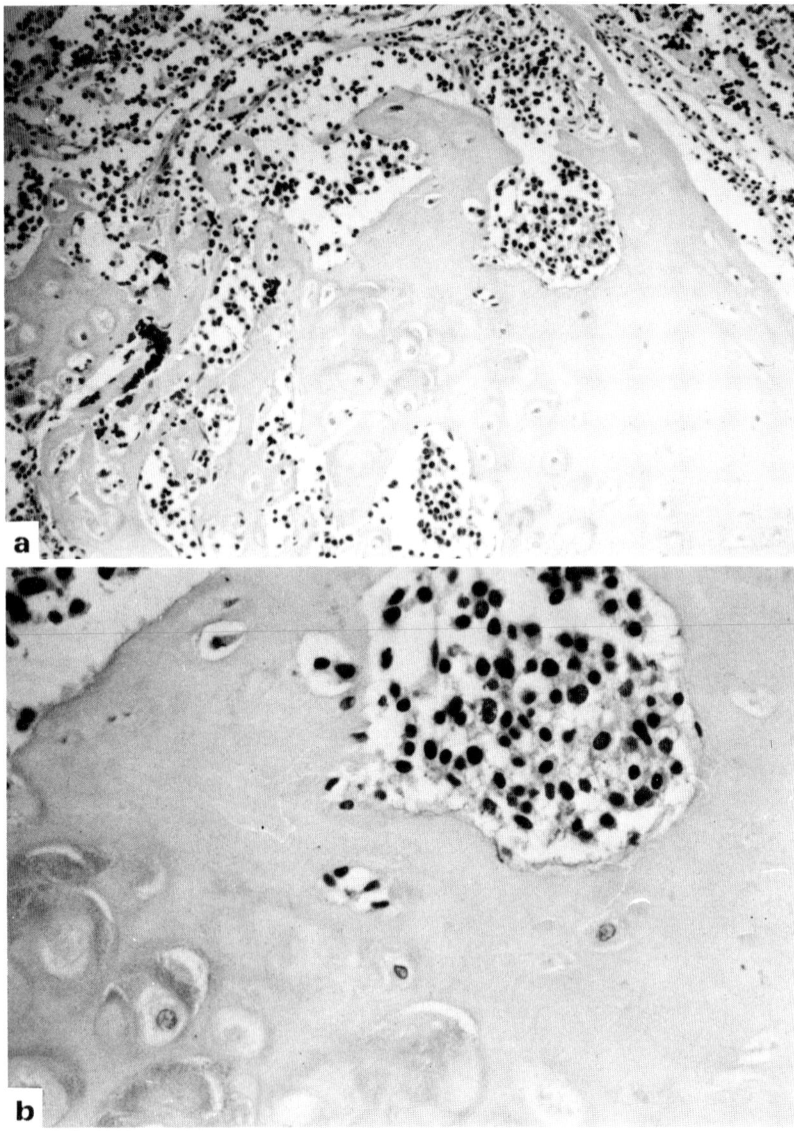

FIG. 9.21 oat-cell carcinoma of bronchus: malignant invasion of cartilage. Irregular masses of anaplastic malignant epithelial cells are infiltrating compact bronchial cartilage.

a. × 120.

b. × 330.

cells are malignant and produce tumours on inoculation into hamsters. The deficiency in contact inhibition of movement and loss of polarity in migration may be extremely important in determining malignant invasion.

Loss of contact inhibition of growth

Normal BHK fibroblasts grow on a glass surface until they become confluent. Cell division then stops in prolonged interphase. When adjacent cells are then wiped away to leave a bare area, other cells migrate on to the bare area and subsequently DNA synthesis is resumed and cell division follows until contact between cells is re-established. BHK cells previously *transformed* by polyoma virus behave very differently; they continue to divide after contact is established by confluence of growth and they then pile up on each other to form a layer many cells thick, in striking contrast to the behaviour of normal fibroblasts [53]. The transformed cells continue to synthesise DNA and to divide after mutual contact. The loss of the effect of mutual cell contact in preventing replication of DNA and cell division may thus be a basic defect which accounts for aberrant growth and infiltration by neoplastic cells.

Epidermal cells from lesions in psoriasis (p. 328) also proliferate excessively and are defective in contact inhibition of growth as well as in mutual adhesion. These aberrations are probably due to local deficiency of glycoprotein in the cell calyx. However, the psoriatic epidermal cells, unlike neoplastic cells, grow in a coordinated and polarised manner to produce mature differentiated cells, which are neither anaplastic nor invasive like the cells of malignant tumours.

Growth of unanchored cells

Normal cells, when suspended unanchored in a viscous medium, cannot divide although they may remain alive [53]. But cells transformed by polyoma virus can divide and form colonies even when isolated from solid surfaces by suspension in viscous media. This power of neoplastic cells to grow and divide, when not attached to any solid surface, may enable such isolated cells to multiply in body fluids and so to set up metastatic growth.

An illuminating contrast between the behaviour of normal and neoplastic cells was made by Stoker by comparing benign BHK 21 fibroblasts with cells from the same clone after transformation to malignant cells by polyoma virus. The benign cells can initiate synthesis of DNA, grow, and divide only when three conditions are satisfied:

1. The cells must have a free edge so as to divide without contact inhibition of growth.
2. They must be anchored.
3. They require soluble factors present in serum.

In contrast the transformed cells which can produce tumours in animals show the following characteristics in culture:

1. They are not affected by contact inhibition of growth, and they grow over each other and divide after mutual contact.

2. They do not require anchorage and form colonies when grown on soft agar.

3. They continue to divide and give a few successive mitoses and also synthesise DNA in the absence of serum factors, but the latter are required for continuous growth.

The properties of neoplastic cells *in vitro* thus account for much of the abnormal behaviour of new growths *in vivo*. But the mechanisms by which basic abnormalities in karyotype can so profoundly alter cellular behaviour and coordination are still unknown.

Alterations of cell surface in neoplastic cells

Aberrations of behaviour displayed by neoplastic cells almost certainly reflect changes in physical and molecular nature of the cell surface. Some of these changes which are probably relevant to neoplastic behaviour are now briefly discussed.

Change in surface charge

Some neoplastic cells show an increase in electrophoretic mobility when compared with normal cells. Thus stilboestrol-induced renal tumour cells of hamsters have a higher mobility towards the anode than normal renal cells. This change may be related to increase in sialic acid density in fucose-containing glycoproteins of the cell calyx which is present in several types of neoplastic cells [52].

Molecular alterations in cell surface

Changes in the glycoproteins and glycolipids of the cell calyx and plasma membrane are also detectable in neoplastic cells. Such changes, although minute in relation to the size of the macromolecules concerned, may profoundly affect biological behaviour. The cell surface is covered by projecting glycosidic chains composing the terminals of glycopeptides and glycolipids of the cell calyx and plasma membrane. These chains may act as specific ligands which bind intensively to foreign proteins from plants or to immunoglobulins for which the glycosides are antigenic. These reactions of surface ligands reveal changes in structure and conformation of cell surface with great sensitivity [54].

Reaction with plant lectins

Proteins extracted from wheat germ and soya bean have remarkable power to agglutinate red cells by combining with specific glycosidic residues on the cell surface; such plant proteins are called phytohaemagglutinins or lectins. Wheat germ lectin agglutinates suspensions of mouse lymphoma cells and other tumour cells but does not agglutinate cells from comparable normal tissues [55, 56]. This reaction is probably caused by ligation of the lectin to specific glycosidic groups on the surface of the tumour cells. This agglutination is inhibited by a glycolipid extractable from carcinomatous tissue which may contain a similar glycosidic ligand.

Concanavalin A, a lectin from soy bean, is bound to the surface glycosides of many kinds of cells. The extent of this ligation can be measured by using concanavalin labelled with ^{63}Ni. Using this technique Inbar and Sachs [57] showed that baby hamster cells, after transformation to neoplastic cells by polyoma virus or by dimethyl nitrosamine, bind more concanavalin than normal cells. But after treatment with trypsin the ligation by normal cells is raised to the high level found in transformed cells. These observations suggest that glycosidic ligands which are hidden in normal cells become exposed on neoplastic transformation or by digestion with trypsin. These transformed cells, after a few days in culture, become agglutinable by concanavalin A; but comparable normal baby hamster cells grown in this way are inagglutinable. The ligand appearing on the surface of the transformed cells is apparently associated with malignant behaviour since the capacity of these cells to produce tumours in hamsters increases as their agglutinability develops in culture [58].

Glycolipids of cell membrane

Transformation to the neoplastic state is associated with decrease in monosialo- and disialo-ceramides in the cell membrane. This change occurs when chick fibroblasts are transformed by Rous sarcoma virus (RSV). The same transformation along with decrease in these same glycolipids in the cell membrane can be effected by a temperature-sensitive strain of RSV grown at 35°. But when such a temperature-sensitive RSV is eliminated by subsequent growth at 41° both the behaviour in culture and the glycolipids of the cell membrane revert to normal [54]. This observation indicates in a particularly cogent manner that neoplastic behaviour may be related to the composition or conformation of the cell surface.

Deep surface changes

Neoplasia may also alter the superficial parts of the cell which are immediately deep to the plasma membrane. In normal cells, which are mobile in culture, EM shows arrayed microfilaments and microtubules orientated in parallel to the surface lying subjacent to the plasma membrane. After malignant transformation these contractile elements are disarrayed; this may correlate to the loss of polarity and assumption of random movement by the transformed cells [52].

Antigens of neoplastic cells

The cells of tumours usually differ from their tissue of origin in their antigenic composition and structure. These differences affect the mozaic of antigens on the cell surface as well as deeper antigens. The changes may involve appearance of new antigenic material (by addition or unmasking), or antigens of the cells of origin may be missing from the tumour cells.

Antigenic proteins of embryonic type are liberated from some neoplastic cells and can be detected by immunological methods in the serum of patients with gastrointestinal tumours (carcinoembryonic antigen) and hepatocellular carcinoma (α_1-fetoproteins). The presence of these antigens in plasma was at one time regarded as a possible screening test for gastrointestinal neoplasm.

Although these substances are undoubtedly formed in relative large amounts by many tumours of bowel and lung, they can also be released from normal tissues and inflammatory lesions so that they are not a specific antigenic constituent of neoplastic cells [59].

Some tumours, however, contain more specific additional antigens which readily evoke production of antibodies. Thus the serum of patients with malignant melanomata frequently contains autoantibodies to these tumours. These autoantibodies can be detected by preliminary incubation of tumour cells *in vitro* with the patient's serum followed by application of fluorescent anti-human globulin which reveals preceding attachment of specific antibody to the cells. By this method two types of autoantibody are found in sera of patients with malignant melanoma:

1. An autologous antibody which reacts with *surface membranes* of the living tumour cells and is specific for each *individual* tumour.
2. A heterologous antibody present in sera of many different patients, which reacts with an *internal cytoplasmic* antigen of killed tumour cells and is apparently present in *all* melanoma cells [60].

Thus the neoplastic cell possesses antigens which are absent or unexposed in normal cells. Tumour-associated antigens, absent from normal cells, are present in several kinds of tumour, including melanoma, osteosarcoma, neuroblastoma and Burkitt's lymphoma. On the other hand, some antigenic constituents of normal cells may be missing from tumours; a gastrointestinal antigen, detectable in the mucoid cells of human gastric and colonic epithelium by indirect fluorescent antiglobulin reaction, is absent from similar cells in human gastric and colonic carcinomata [61].

Initiation and progression of neoplasia

Although the initiating agents for the majority of human neoplasms are unknown, enough is known about factors which influence the occurrence of tumours both in man and animals to enable a partial picture of events to be discerned.

Initiating factors

Genomic instability (p. 329), radiation (p. 129), oncogenic substances (p. 169), endocrine secretions (p. 182) and infection by viruses (p. 262) may each act specifically in determining the incidence of neoplasia. More than one of these factors may act in concert or in succession.

Stages in development of neoplasia

A series of changes, some of which may be *latent*, probably determines the development of highly malignant anaplastic tumours which are both invasive and metastatic. This view is supported by observations on induction of neoplasia in animals as well as on pre-malignant ('precancerous') conditions in man. Some of this evidence will now be considered.

Induction and promotion of neoplasia in animals

Rous and his colleagues [62–65] showed that brief application of tar to the skin of rabbits' ears is followed by latent neoplastic changes which may never reveal themselves. When however tarring is continued for a longer period, papillomata (warts) then appear. If tarring ceases, these warts regress and disappear, but on re-tarring the warts reappear at the original sites and additional warts also develop. After tarring for a short time altered cells may be present in large numbers and persist in a latent state for a considerable period without forming tumours. But the stimulus of wound healing or the application of non-specific irritants, such as turpentine, makes some of these altered cells in the previously tarred skin proliferate and form tumours.

These observations suggested that development of tumours involves several steps initiated by a *latent* change. This latent change is induced by specific initiating agents such as benz(a)pyrene and methylcholanthrene (p. 171), while growth to form tumours is mediated by non-specific promoting agents, once the latent change has been initiated. Such promoting agents include turpentine, croton oil and even wounding followed by healing. Tar exerts both kinds of activity. Promoting agents can also revive papillomata at their original site, after regression, when application of irritant has been interrupted. More recent work showed that even a single application of an initiating agent, such as benz(a)pyrene, to the skin of a mouse is sufficient to cause latent initiation of neoplasia; when this is followed by repeated application of a promoting agent (e.g. croton oil) tumours then develop [66, 67].

Carcinomata occasionally develop from papillomata following continued application of tar to mice. However, once these malignant tumours appear they do not usually regress when the irritant is no longer applied. This final change to a malignant tumour thus apparently involves a more irrevocable step in progression to a primitive anaplastic growth.

The initiating latent injury may be a change in DNA which amounts to a transmissible mutation, and the mutant cells may then be unstable and tend to mutate further if they are stimulated to continue mitosis. These further mutations may ultimately generate frankly malignant neoplastic cells.

Latent stages in development of human neoplasia

Similar sequential changes can occur in the initiation and emergence of human neoplasia. The initial changes may at first be latent or may produce non-invasive cellular proliferation which herald ultimate progression to malignant invasive tumours. Such non-invasive proliferation is called premalignant or precancerous change.

Some premalignant conditions in man are associated with visible abnormality in karyotype. Such disorders include:

1. Multiple polyposis coli or Gardner's disease (p. 39), from which one or more polyps may become a malignant carcinoma.
2. Epithelial dysplasia (carcinoma *in situ*) of uterine cervix (p. 39) which may progress to form an invasive carcinoma.

3. Chronic myeloid leukaemia (p. 41) during which a blastic crisis may occur to produce acute leukaemia.

4. Bloom's syndrome (p. 329). This inherited disorder is characterised by stunted growth and facial telangiectasis, followed by ultimate development of squamous or columnar carcinoma or acute myeloid leukaemia. Mitotic chromosomes have a high incidence of quadriradials formed by the apposition of a pair of homologous chromosomes; this arrangement involves two pairs of chromatids which form a cross by symmetrical apposition of their long arms [68]. Such apposition probably induces exchange of chromatid segments, which may result in more profound heteroploidy at a later mitosis with concomitant development of malignant neoplasia. This hereditary aberration, though latent, is a permanent menace of neoplasia.

Latent precancerous change may also occur in human cells in which either the karyotype has not been studied or else no visible alteration of karyotype has been detected. In these cells abnormal behaviour may depend on invisible molecular changes in genome. Among such abberations are:

1. Senile hyperkeratosis which occurs on skin of face and hands of elderly people; this may progress to locally invasive rodent ulcer or to fully malignant squamous carcinoma.

2. Epidermal papillomata, on the skin of men exposed to oncogenic hydrocarbons (p. 169), which usually regress and disappear if exposure is terminated, but may progress to produce rodent ulcer or squamous carcinoma if exposure continues.

3. Bronchial dysplasia and metaplasia which commonly occur in the bronchial epithelium of smokers and are believed to signify a usual premalignant stage in the emergence of bronchial carcinoma; fortunately these premalignant bronchial lesions regress if smoking is stopped before irreversible transition to malignant neoplasia.

4. Xeroderma pigmentosum (XP). In this inherited recessive defect (p. 137) injury of the skin by UVL is much more severe than in normal persons. Exposure to UVL results in partial epidermal atrophy with irregular proliferation of pigmented cells in the rete mucosum and eventual formation of verrucous nodules, rodent ulcers or squamous carcinoma. This disorder is apparently caused by inherited defect in the process of repair–replication, which first excises pyrimidine dimers formed in DNA chains of nuclei by exposure to UVL (p. 136) and then repairs the broken DNA chains by inserting fresh nucleotide groups. The latter part of the process can be followed by observing rate of incorporation ^{3}H-thymidine into the DNA of interphase nuclei of skin fibroblasts after irradiation with UVL. This incorporation is retarded in the irradiated fibroblasts of patients with XP [69]. It is uncertain, however, at which stage in excision or repair the process is initially interrupted, but ineffective restoration of altered DNA chains may eventually cause emergence of neoplastic mutants.

In all these premalignant states either visible or molecular alteration in karyotype probably causes genomic instability which enables subsequent mutations with ultimate progression to malignant neoplasia to result from relatively minor environmental insult. Also latent changes in karyotype may be present, which enable spontaneous mutation to occur at a later cell division. Thus, lymphocytes previously damaged by radiation (p. 133) may suffer a latent genomic change which only becomes apparent when mitosis is stimulated later in life and visible alterations in the mitotic chromosomes are then revealed. Similar latent changes in thyroid or mammary epithelium may account for an interval of many years between exposure to radiation and appearance of carcinoma, since neoplastic progression can only occur with onset of repeated mitosis.

Somatic mutation

The phases in progression to highly malignant neoplasia may thus involve a sequence of somatic mutations. This view is supported by the fact that somatic mutations occur among malignant tumours themselves. Carcinoma of the prostate, on first appearance, is generally *hormone-dependent* and requires secretion of the male hormones of the testis for continued growth. After suppression of this secretion by orchidectomy or by treatment with stilboestrol, these hormone-dependent tumours regress. But eventually the tumours may reappear in forms which are not affected by treatment with stilboestrol. This change appears to be caused by further mutation to a hormone-insensitive type of cell. Other neoplasms, such as acute myeloblastic leukaemia and Hodgkin's disease, are on initial appearance usually sensitive to radiation or cytotoxic drugs, but sometimes, after temporary regression, insensitive forms of these tumours arise which are unaffected by these therapeutic measures. These insensitive neoplastic cells probably arise by mutation from initially sensitive but unstable cells.

Mutation may also determine 'inappropriate' formation by neoplastic cells of hormones or hormone-receptors not normally found in the cells of origin; thus ACTH may be produced by oat-cell carcinoma of the bronchus and many mammary carcinomas can synthesise receptors for oestradiol [69a]. Such mutations may depend on inactivation of repressors which results in expression of previously masked genes.

Further evidence for mutation as the basis for origin and emergence of neoplastic cells comes from the study of their clonal origin and of their alterations in karyotype.

Monoclonal origin of neoplastic cells

If a neoplasm arises by somatic mutation of one cell, then all the cells derived from it would initially be identical. Evidence from study of a cell marker in tumours suggests that such monoclonal origin is usual. The enzyme glucose-6-phosphate dehydrogenase (G-6-PD) serves as a valuable marker for this purpose (p. 28).

G-6-PD is X-linked and exists in two allelic forms in every female tissue

(p. 379). These two isozymal variants may differ considerably in their electrophoretic mobility. Indeed electrophoretic analysis of tissues from many women show two isozymes with sharply disparate mobilities; for instance 40 per cent of negro women are heterozygous and possess both the common B variant and the fast-moving A form, which are both present in their normal tissues. But when neoplasia occurs in such females only variant A *or* B is found in each individual tumour. Thus although the unaffected tissues (including myometrium) of women with uterine fibroids (leiomyomata) may have both variants A and B, the fibroids contain only A *or* B [70]. This same limitation to variant A or B alone is found in single warts, in tissue from Burkitt's lymphoma, in granulocytes and red cells in chronic myeloid leukaemia, all from women with both A and B variants in their unaffected tissue [71]. Cells from each neoplasm then contain only one isozymic variant, as would be expected if each tumour is a clone of cells derived from one individual mutant.

Change of karyotype

The karyotypes of most human malignant tumours are grossly abnormal (p. 38). Indeed the cells in several human precancerous lesions such as cervical dysplasia, carcinoma *in situ* of cervix and some benign tumours (p. 39) show detectable chromosomal aberrations. This indicates that change of karyotype is a determinant rather than a consequence of neoplastic behaviour; such a view is also supported by the consistent presence of a marker chromosome ($14q^+$) in Burkitt's lymphoma cells from different patients [71a].

Although the cells of some animal tumours on first appearance may show no detectable chromosomal abnormality, these tumours on successive transplantation nearly always become heteroploid. Moreover fibrosarcomas induced in rats by Rous sarcoma virus (p. 42) followed a characteristic karyotypic evolution on transplantation to produce striking non-random patterns of chromosomal aberration associated with development of more primitive anaplastic cell type [72]. An entirely different non-random karyotypic pattern was visible in primary tumours induced by the oncogenic hydrocarbon DMB (p. 186) in the same inbred strain of rats [73]. This suggests that different agents induce different pathways of chromosomal aberration and that extreme diversity of chromosomal patterns in human neoplasms may reflect wide differences in the causal agents.

Similarly BHK cells transformed by polyoma virus may at first be euploid but heteroploidy usually develops in subculture. Moreover human skin fibroblasts when fully transformed by SV_{40} show heteroploidy in nearly every mitosis [74].

It is therefore likely that oncogenic viruses, oncogenic substances and harmful radiation induce change of karyotype which involves alteration in the genome but which may at first be invisible. This change may itself be sufficient to determine neoplastic behaviour. But the initial molecular change also promotes instability of karyotype which results in further mutations. When these are substantial the karyotype becomes visibly altered. Observations on karyotype further indicate a clonal pattern [72], suggesting unicellular origin of each successive stage. If this altered karyotype is viable, anaplasia and invasive behaviour may be obligatory concomitants of such a grossly altered genomic pattern.

Another kind of oncogenic abnormality of karyotype has recently been revealed in *hydatidiform moles* of pregnancy [79]. These rapidly expanding trophoblastic tumours are composed of swollen chorionic villi. Their cells have a karyotype 46,XX and are entirely *paternal* in origin, probably arising from a parent cell formed by duplication of a normal 23,X sperm. This singular genetic composition, with completely homozygous pairs of chromosomes, probably determines the neoplastic behaviour of these trophoblastic cells and also their power of sometimes transforming to a highly malignant chorioncarcinoma.

Vertical transmission of neoplasia

Mammary carcinoma develops in nearly all females of certain inbred strains of mice. Bittner in 1936 discovered that this neoplasm is transmitted by an agent present in the mother's milk to the suckling mice (p. 262). This agent is now known to be a retrovirus which is liberated into the milk from infected cells of the mammary gland. Male mice, infected similarly with this virus, only develop mammary carcinoma if they are treated with oestrogens.

Gross in 1951 discovered that murine lymphatic leukaemia and lymphoma are also caused by a filterable agent. This is directly transmitted from mother to embryo, thus passing from one generation to the next. Gross called this process *vertical transmission.* All mice of some inbred strains (such as Ak) develop this viral leukaemia if they live long enough. In most other strains of mice (such as C3H) leukaemia only rarely becomes apparent. But Gross succeeded in producing leukaemia in C3H mice by inoculating newborn animals with extracts and filtrates from spleen and lymph nodes of leukaemic Ak mice [75].

The transmissible agent of this murine leukaemia is also a retrovirus. Cells infected by this virus form viral particles at their surface by a process of budding. The fully formed particle of Gross' murine leukaemia virus has an electronic dense central core (neucleoid) surrounded by a clear halo covered by a single or double membrane, probably derived in part from the surface membrane of the infected cells. The whole particle has a diameter of 100 nm.

The virus is harboured by many strains of mice which normally do not develop leukaemia. In the cells of these animals the virus normally produces no discernible effect, but is transmitted from mother to embryo in a latent state. When such animals are exposed to radiation or fed with DMB or 3-methylcholanthrene they develop leukaemia. The virus can then be detected in lymphoid cells as budding particles, which are visible by EM, and also by the formation of a group-specific viral antigen. Within a few days after total-body X-ray irradiation of C3H mice, which normally do not develop leukaemia, the typical budding particles become visible by EM at the surface membranes of cells in spleen and lymph nodes [76]; these particles also are consistently present in the organs of mice from this strain when they develop leukaemia following irradiation. Fig. 9.22 shows the particles emerging from splenic and lymphoid cells of these irradiated mice. The fully formed particles have a dense centre,

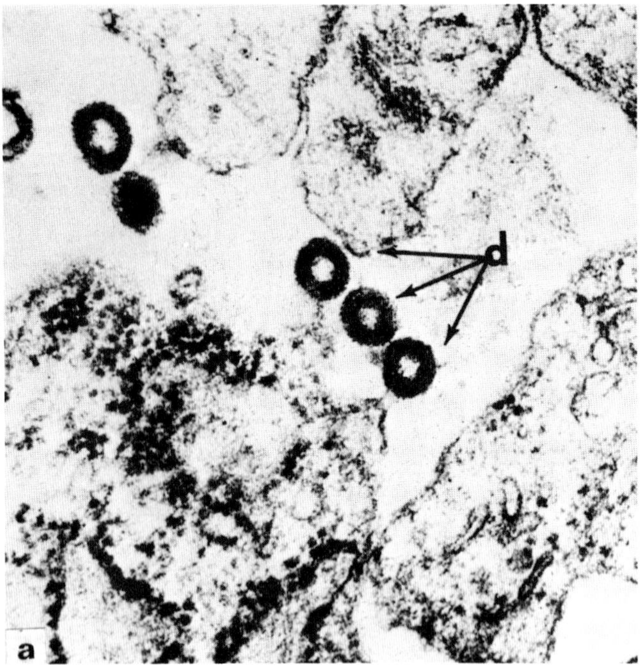

FIG. 9.22 Tissues of mice with lymphatic leukaemia induced by X-irradiation. Particles of Gross' leukaemia virus are seen emerging from surface of cells. × 62 000.

a. Spleen; immature doughnut-like particles (d) budding from a cell membrane, and one free mature particle (with a dense core) beside two other empty immature particles.

but the 'doughnut-like' particles with empty centres are probably immature particles budding from the cell membranes (Fig. 9.22a).

Such latent or masked leukaemia virus is apparently also responsible for the appearance of lymphomata and leukaemia in mice on treatment with dimethylnitrosamine and 3-methylcholanthrene; these lymphomata are then transmissible from cell-free extracts of the initially formed tumours. During the initial chemical induction of lymphomata antibodies to murine leukaemia virus appear in the mice before the onset of overt lymphoma [77]. These observations indicate that unmasking of a latent leukaemia virus may be an indigenous activating cause of overt lymphoma. Since retroviruses replicate by means of complementary DNA (c-DNA) formed from viral RNA by reverse transcriptase, it is likely that the masked viral determinant is held integrated in the cellular genome in the form of c-DNA. In fact infection of animal cells by RNA tumour viruses can result in transcription of c-DNA which becomes covalently bound to host cell chromosomes and can be detected by molecular hybridization technique [77a].

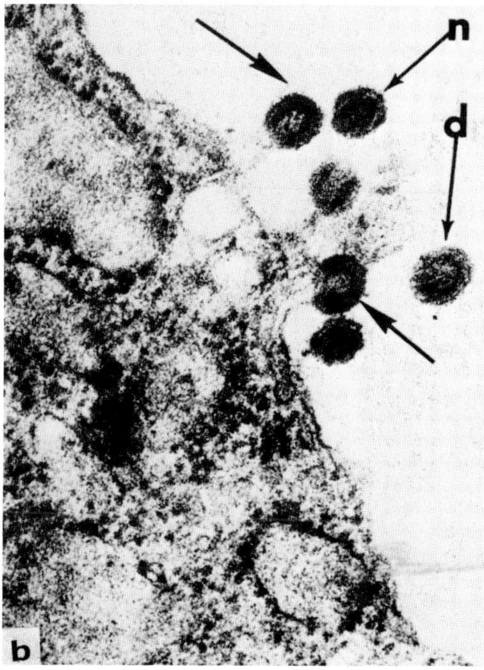

FIG. 9.22 cont.
b. Lymph node; particles budding from cell membrane, mature particle with dense core (n).
Courtesy of Professor L. Gross & Dr Dorothy G. Feldman. Reproduced from *Cancer Res.* (1968), **28**, 1677.

Viral oncogene hypothesis

To unify these observations Todaro & Huebner [78] suggested that vertebrates contain the genetic information for producing these RNA tumour viruses in an unexpressed form both in their somatic and germ cells. This information may have been part of the genetic make up of vertebrates since early evolution. The genes for producing retroviruses (virogenes) and the portion of the virogenes capable of transforming a normal cell to a tumour cell (oncogenes) are supposed to be held in an unexpressed state by repressors in normal cells. Various agents, such as radiation, oncogenic substances and possibly exogenous viruses may initiate neoplasm by triggering this oncogenic genetic code.

Evidence in support of this view comes from study of long term cultures of embryonic cells from strains of mice with a low incidence of leukaemia. Treatment of these cultures with radiation or oncogenic substances can activate formation of virus. Moreover the thymidine analogues 5-bromodeoxyuridine and 5-iododeoxyuridine are highly efficient in this process of induction possibly by causing mutation by inactivating suppressor loci which normally prevent the expression of viral synthesis or cell transformation. If only the oncogenic proviral portion of the virogene becomes expressed then transformation and neoplasia might result even without liberation of infective virus. When the oncogene alone is expressed then a limited messenger RNA sequence would be transcribed which would translate proteins responsible for transformation and neoplastic behaviour.

The view has thus developed that neoplasia is initiated by inactivation of suppressor loci in the genome which normally block the action of proviral genes responsible for transformation. This theory, by suggesting that neoplastic behaviour lies dormant in every cell, surmounts the difficulty of accounting for the embarrassingly wide variety of oncogenic agents which can induce tumours in animals and probably also in man. Once the oncogene becomes expressed, then genomic instability may be established and so lead to further alterations in karyotype DNA along with sequential neoplastic progression.

Although the viral oncogene hypothesis conveniently accounts for activation of similar forms of neoplasia by different agents, it suffers from the possible disadvantage of implying, as Gross [80] has emphasised, that neoplasia is initiated by spontaneous generation of infective agents.

Origin of neoplasia

The onset and progression of tumours clearly indicate that neoplasia, however caused, depends on mutations which impose an altered transmissible genome on the affected cells.

The actual mechanism of mutation is uncertain. Several different mechanisms have been suggested such as:

1. *Direct alteration of transmissible genome by the agent itself.* This implies that the oncogen causes mutation of the cell or cells which themselves form the neoplasm. Inherited transmission of a directly induced mutation almost certainly occurs when cells are transformed by oncogenic viruses to produce neoplasms which carry the viral genome or part of it in their own cells [81]. Possibly oncogenic substances may also initiate mutation by ligating with DNA and causing direct alteration in its strands (p. 173).

2. *Unmasking of a suppressed genomic potentiality.* The power of radiation, DMB or 3-methylcholanthrene to activate latent oncogenic viruses suggests that these agents can enable masked portions of the genomic code to become expressed and thus evoke transmissible neoplastic behaviour which was previously suppressed by a regulator mechanism. The oncogene hypothesis would be included in this kind of explanation.

3. *Selection of spontaneous mutants.* This mechanism may account for tumours induced by inhibition of mitosis. Thus 4-dimethylaminostilbene inhibits mitosis, markedly retards the growth of rats, and also gives rise to malignant tumours [82]. This neoplastic effect may result from emergence of a spontaneous mutant which is released from the influence of the inhibitor. Normally such a mutant might have no chance of survival, but freedom from inhibition of mitosis and growth puts it at an advantage over other cells and enables it to grow in an

environment which is inimical to the parent cell [83]. The mutant then survives, but because its growth is no longer coordinated it may also be released from other controlling influences and so be neoplastic (Haddow's hypothesis). Similar selection of a *spontaneous* mutant, which is hormone-independent and therefore resistant to inhibition of growth by stilboestrol, probably accounts for the emergence of hormone-independent growths in the malignant progression of carcinoma of the prostate.

If neoplasia is initiated in cells by direct alteration of their transmissible genome (1 above), or by unmasking of a suppressed genomic potentiality (2 above), then oncogenesis depends on inheritance of an acquired characteristic in a Lamarckian type of evolution. But if the establishment of a neoplastic clone of cells arises indirectly by selection of spontaneous mutants possessing some inherent advantage over their collaterals (3 above), then neoplasia is the result of survival of the most successful variant in the Darwinian sense. However since the progression to malignant neoplasia almost certainly involves a sequence of steps, the actual mechanism of mutation may differ at these separate steps in the development of even one malignant tumour and thus involve direct action, unmasking or selection at these different points in genomic alteration.

Such a sequence of events in progression to malignant neoplasia may account for the long period which may elapse between exposure to a specific initiating oncogen and the final appearance of an overtly malignant growth. In this way mammary carcinoma may develop many years after exposure to excessive radiation (p. 129). The appearance of clear-celled adenocarcinoma of the vagina in young females, 9–25 years after exposure of their mothers to stilboestrol during pregnancy (p. 183), probably depends on successive mutations possibly evoked by different mechanisms.

Malignant neoplasia thus probably develops by a series of successive mutations, which may either be directly induced by an external oncogenic agent or else selected by the agent from a large number of spontaneous mutants.

REFERENCES

[1] MILNE M. D. (1964) Disorders of amino acid transport. *Brit. med. J.*, **1**, 327.

[2] MATTHEWS D. M. (1971) Experimental approach to chemical pathology. *Brit. med. J.*, **3**, 659.

[3] BUTCHER R. W., SNEYD J. G. T., PARK C. R. & SUTHERLAND E. W. (1966) Effects of insulin on adenosine-3¹, 5¹-monophosphate in the rat epididymal fat pad. *J. biol. Chem.*, **241**, 1651.

[4] BUTCHER R. W., BAIRD C. E. & SUTHERLAND E. W. (1968) Effects of lipolytic and antilipolytic substances on adenosine-3¹, 5¹-monophosphate in isolated fat cells. *J. biol. Chem.*, **243**, 1705.

[5] BORNSTEIN J. AND LAWRENCE R. D. (1951) Two types of diabetes mellitus with and without available plasma insulin. *Brit. med. J.*, **1**, 732.

[6] NEWSHOLME E. A. & START C. (1973) *Regulation in Metabolism.* Wiley, London.

[7] GEPTS W. (1965) Pathological anatomy of the pancreas in juvenile diabetes. *Diabetes*, **14**, 618.

[8] YALOW R. S. & BERSON S. A. (1960) Immunoassay of endogenous plasma insulin in man. *J. clin. Invest.*, **39**, 1157.

[9] CERASI E. & LUFT R. (1970) Pathogenesis of diabetes mellitus: a proposed concept. *Proceedings of the 13th Nobel Symposium, Stockholm*, p. 17. Almquist & Wiskell, Stockholm.

[10] SIPERSTEIN M. D. (1970) The relationship of carbohydrate derangements to the microangiopathy of diabetes. *Proceedings of the 13th Nobel Symposium, Stockholm*, p. 81. Almquist & Wiskell, Stockholm.

[11] SMITH, M. H. J. & TAYLOR K. W. (1956) Blood pyruvate and α-ketoglutarate in normal and diabetic subjects. *Brit. med. J.*, **2**, 1035.

[11a] BUTTERFIELD W. J. H. (1961) Progress in the understanding and treatment of diabetes mellitus. *Brit. med. J.*, **1**, 1705.

[12] RANDLE P. J., GARLAND P. B., HALES C. N. & NEWSHOLME E. A. (1963) The glucose fatty acid cycle: its role in insulin sensitivity and the metabolic disturbances of diabetes mellitus. *Lancet*, **1**, 785.

[13] GARLAND P. B., RANDLE P. J. & NEWSHOLME E. A. (1963) Citrate as an intermediary in the inhibition of phosphofructokinase in rat heart muscle by fatty acids, ketone bodies, pyruvate, diabetes and starvation. *Nature*, **200**, 169.

[14] BIERMAN E. L. DOLE V. P., & ROBERTS T. N. (1957) An abnormality of nonesterified fatty acid metabolism in diabetes mellitus. *Diabetes*, **6**, 475.

[15] FULOP M., TANNENBAUM H. & DREYER N. (1973) Ketotic hyperosmolar coma. *Lancet*, **2**, 635.

[16] FULOP M., ROSENBLAT A., KREITZER S. M. & GERSTENHABER B. (1975) Hyperosmolar nature of diabetic coma. *Diabetes*, **24**, 594.

[17] FISHMAN R. A. (1974) Cell volume, pumps and neurologic function: brain's adaptation to osmotic stress. *Res. Publ. Ass. nerv. ment. Dis.*, **53**, 159.

[18] SULWAY M. J. & MALINS J. M. (1970) Acetone in diabetic ketoacidosis. *Lancet*, **2**, 736.

[19] DILLON E., RIGGS H. E. & DYER W. W. (1936) Cerebral lesions in uncomplicated fatal diabetic acidosis. *Amer. J. med. Sci.*, **192**, 360.

[20] SIPERSTEIN M. D., UNGER R. H. & MADISON L. L. (1968) Studies of muscle capillary basement membranes in normal subjects, diabetic and prediabetic patients. *J. clin. Invest.*, **47**, 1973.

[21] JORDAN S. W. & PERLEY M. J. (1972) Microangiopathy in diabetes mellitus and ageing. *Arch. Path.*, **93**, 261.

[22] SIESJO B. K., JOHANNSSON H., LJUNGGREN B. & NORBERG K. (1974) Brain dysfunction in cerebral hypoxia and ischemia. *Res. Publ. Ass. nerv. ment. Dis.*, **53**, 75.

[23] KETY S. S., POLIS B. D., NADLER C. S. & SCHMIDT C. F. (1948) The blood flow and oxygen consumption of the human brain in diabetic acidosis and coma. *J. clin. Invest.*, **27**, 500.

[24] LASSEN N. A. (1959) Cerebral blood flow and oxygen consumption in man. *Physiol. Rev.*, **39**, 183.

[25] COWAN S. L. (1934) The action of potassium and other ions on the injury potential and action current in Maia nerve. *Proc. roy. Soc. B.*, **115**, 216.

[26] HODGKIN A. L. (1951) The ionic basis of electrical activity in nerve and muscle. *Biol. Rev.*, **26**, 339.

[27] ASHFORD, C. A. & DIXON K. C. (1935) The effect of potassium on the glycolysis of brain tissue with reference to the Pasteur effect. *Biochem. J.*, **29**, 157.

[28] DIXON K. C. (1940) A study of cortical metabolism in relation to cerebral disease. *Brain*, **63**, 191.

[28a] KEYNES R. D. & AIDLEY D. J. (1981) *Nerve and Muscle*, p. 42. Cambridge University Press, Cambridge.

[29] REDFEARN E. R. (1961) Electron transport and oxidative phosphorylation. *A. R. Chem. Soc.*, **57**, 395.

[30] WHITTAM R. (1962) The dependence of the respiration of brain cortex on active cation transport. *Biochem. J.*, **82**, 205.

[31] KETY S. S. (1950) Circulation and metabolism in human brain in health and disease. *Amer. J. Med.*, **8**, 205.

[32] FELDBERG W. (1959) A physiological approach to the problem of general anaesthesia and consciousness. *Brit. med. J.*, **2**, 771.

[33] DIXON K. C. (1967) Neuronal membrane patterns in memory and concussion. *Lancet*, **1**, 27.

[34] HORNKIEWIEZ O. (1973) Dopamine in the basal ganglia: its role and therapeutic applications (including the clinical use of L-Dopa). *Brit. med. Bull.*, **29**, 172.

[35] KENNEDY J., PARBHOO S. P., MACGILLIVRAY B. M. & SHERLOCK S. (1973) Effect of extracorporeal liver perfusion on the electroencephalogram of patients in coma due to acute liver failure. *Quart. J. Med.*, **42**, 549.

[36] SHERLOCK S. (1977) Hepatic encephalopathy. *Brit. J. Hosp. Med.*, **17**, 144.

[37] VICTOR M., ADAMS R. D. & COLE M. (1965) The acquired (non-Wilsonian) type of chronic hepatocerebral degeneration. *Medicine*, **44**, 345.

[38] CAVANAGH J. B. (1972) Cellular abnormalities in the brain in chronic liver disease. In *Scientific Basis of Medicine*, ed. by I. Gilliland & J. Francis. Athlone Press, London. p. 238,

[39] CAVANAGH J. B. (1974) Liver bypass and the glia. *Res. Publ. Ass. nerv. ment. Dis.*, **53**, 13.

[40] NORENBERG M. D. & LAPHAM L. W. (1974) The astrocyte response in experimental portal-systemic encephalopathy: an EM study. *J. Neuropath. exp. Neurol.*, **33**, 422.

[41] NORENBERG M. D., LAPHAM L. W., NICHOLS F. A. & MAY A. G. (1974) An experimental model for the study of hepatic encephalopathy. *Arch. Neurol.*, **31**, 106.

[42] BESSMAN S. P. & BESSMAN A. N. (1955) The cerebral and peripheral uptake of ammonia in liver disease with an hypothesis for the mechanism of hepatic coma. *J. clin. Invest.*, **34**, 622.

[43] DUFFY T. E., VERGARA F. & PLUM F. (1974) α-Ketoglutaramate in hepatic encephalopathy. *Res. Publ. Ass. nerv. ment. Dis.*, **53**, 39.

[44] FISCHER J. E. & BALDESSARINI R. (1971) False neurotransmitters and hepatic failure. *Lancet*, **2**, 75.

[45] FISCHER J. E. (1974) False neurotransmitters and hepatic coma. *Res. Publ. Ass. nerve. ment. Dis.*, **53**, 53.

[46] PARKES J. D., SHARPSTONE P. & WILLIAMS R. (1970) Levadopa in hepatic coma. *Lancet*, **2**, 1341.

[47] LAMBERTON L. F. (1976) In *Scientific Foundations of Oncology*, p. 120, ed. by T. Symington & R. L. Carter. Heinemann, London.

[48] TUBIANA M. & MALAISE E. P. (1976) In *Scientific Foundations of Oncology*, p. 126, ed. by T. Symington & R. L. Carter. Heinemann, London.

[49] COMAN D. R. (1944) Decreased mutual adhesiveness, a property of cells from squamous carcinomas. *Cancer Res.*, **4**, 623.

[50] COMAN D. R. (1961) Adhesiveness and stickiness: two independent properties of the cell surface. *Cancer Res.*, **21**, 1436.

[51] ABERCROMBIE M. & AMBROSE E. J. (1962) The surface properties of cancer cells: a review. *Cancer Res.*, **22**, 525.

[52] AMBROSE E. J. (1975) The surface properties of tumour cells. In *Biology of Cancer*, 2nd Ed., p. 27, ed. by E. J. Ambrose & F. J. C. Roe. Horwood, Chichester.

[53] STOKER M. G. P. (1970) New growth and viruses. *Brit. med. J.*, **3**, 541.

[54] HAKOMORI S. (1973) Glycolipids of tumour cell membrane. *Advanc. Cancer Res.*, **18**, 265.

[55] AUB J. C., TISELAU C. & LANKESTER A. (1963) Reactions of normal and tumor cell surfaces to enzymes. I. Wheat-germ lipase and associated lipopolysaccharides. *Proc. nat. Acad. Sci.* (Wash.), **50**, 613.

[56] AUB J. C., SANFORD B. H. & COTE M. N. (1965) Studies on reactivity of tumor and normal cells to wheat germ agglutinin. *Proc. nat. Acad. Sci.* (Wash.), **54**, 396.

[57] INBAR M. & SACHS L. (1969) Structural differences in sites on the surface membrane of normal and transformed cells. *Nature*, **223**, 710.

[58] INBAR M., BEN BASSAT H. & SACHS L. (1972) Membrane changes associated with malignancy. *Nature new Biol.*, **236**, 3 and 16.

[59] Anonymous (1972) Carcinoembryonic antigen. Brit. med. J., **2**, 600.

[60] LEWES M. G., ILONOPISOV R. L., NAIRN R. C., PHILLIPS T. M., HAMILTON FAIRLEY G., BODENHAM D. C. & ALEXANDER P. (1969) Tumour-specific antibodies in human malignant melanoma and their relation to the extent of the disease. *Brit. med. J.*, **3**, 547.

[61] NAIRN R. C., FOTHERGILL J. E., MCENTAGART M. G. & RICHMOND H. G. (1962) Loss of gastrointestinal-specific antigen in neoplasia. *Brit. med. J.*, **1**, 1791.

[62] ROUS P. & KIDD J. G. (1939) A comparison of virus-induced rabbit tumors with the tumors of unknown cause initiated by tarring. *J. exp. Med.*, **69**, 404.

[63] ROUS P & KIDD J. G. (1941) Conditional neoplasms and subthreshold neoplastic states. *J. exp. Med.*, **73**, 365.

[64] MACKENZIE I. & ROUS P. (1941) The experimental disclosure of latent neoplastic changes in tarred skin. *J. exp. Med.*, **73**, 391.

[65] FRIEDENWALD W. F. & ROUS P. (1944) The initiating and promoting elements in tumor production: an analysis of the effects of tar, benzopyrene and methylcholanthrene on rabbit skin. *J. exp. Med.*, **80**, 101.

[66] MOTTRAM J. C. (1944) A developing factor in experimental blastogenesis. *J. Path. Bact.*, **56**, 181.

[67] BERENBLUM I. & SHUBIK P. (1947) The role of croton oil applications associated with a single painting of a carcinogen in tumour induction in the mouse's skin. *Brit. J. Cancer*, **1**, 379.

[68] GERMAN J. (1974) Bloom's syndrome. In *Chromosomes and Cancer*, p. 601. Wiley, New York.

[69] CLEAVER J. E. (1968) Defective repair replication of DNA in xeroderma pigmentosum. *Nature*, **218**, 652.

[69a] LECLERCQ G., HEUSON J. C., DEBOELM M. C. & MATTHEIEM W. (1975) Oestrogen receptors in breast cancer: a changing concept. *Brit. med. J.*, **1**, 185.

[70] LINDNER D. & GARTLER S. M. (1965) Glucose-6-phosphate dehydrogenase mosaicism: utilization of a cell marker in the study of the leiomyomas. *Science*, **150**, 67.

[71] FIALKOW P. J. (1974) Human genetic markers as tracers of tumour histogenesis. *J. clin. Path.*, **7**, suppl. 27, 11.

[71a] MITELMAN F. (1981) Marker chromosome $14q^+$ in human cancer and leukaemia. *Adv. cancer res.*, **34**, 141.

[72] MITELMAN F. (1972) Predetermined sequential chromosome changes in serial transplantation of Rous rat sarcomas. *Acta path. microbiol. scand.* section A, **80**, 313.

[73] MITELMAN F., MARK J., LEVAN G. & LEVAN A. (1972) Tumor etiology and chromosome pattern. *Science*, **176**, 1340.

[74] HARNDEN D. G. (1974) Viruses, chromosomes and tumours: the interaction between viruses and chromosomes. In *Chromosomes and Cancer*, p. 152, ed. by J. German. Wiley, New York.

[75] GROSS L. (1974) The role of viruses in the etiology of cancer and leukemia. *J. Amer. med. Ass.*, **230**, 1029.

[76] GROSS L. & FELDMAN D. G. (1968) Electron microscopic studies of radiation-induced leukemia in mice: virus release following total-body X-ray irradiation. *Cancer Res.*, **28**, 1677.

[77] IGEL H. J., HUEBNER R. J., TURNER H. C., KOTIN P. & FALK H. J. (1969) Mouse leukaemia virus activation by chemical carcinogens. *Science*, **166**, 1624.

[77a] HILL M. & HILLOVA J. (1976) Genetic transformation of animal cells with viral DNA of RNA tumour viruses. *Adv. Cancer Res.*, **23**, 237.
[78] TODARO G. J. & HUEBNER R. J. (1972) The viral oncogene hypothesis: new evidence. *Proc. nat. Acad. Sci. (Wash.)*, **69**, 1009.
[79] KAJII T. & OHAMA K. (1977) Androgenic origin of hydatidiform mole. *Nature,* **268**, 633.
[80] GROSS L. (1974) Facts and theories on viruses causing cancer and leukemia. *Proc. nat. Acad. Sci. (Wash.)*, **71**, 2013.
[81] STOKER M. G. P. (1963) Neoplastic transformation by polyoma virus and its wider implications. *Brit. med. J.*, **1**, 1305.
[82] HADDOW A. & KON G. A. R. (1947) Chemistry of carcinogenic compounds. *Brit. med. Bull.*, **4,** 314.
[83] HADDOW A. (1947) Mode of action of chemical carcinogens. *Brit. med. Bull.*, **4**, 331.

Postscript

In some diseases therefore the determinant cellular defects are substantially apparent, and in some cases even the order of sequential lesions resulting from these defects can clearly be discerned. But present knowledge can seldom provide that complete and detailed picture of morbid events so vividly imagined by Molière in his remarkable description of consecutive phenomena in the evolution of mortal illness:

Que vous tombiez dans la bradipepsie.
De la bradipepsie dans la dispepsie.
De la dispepsie dans l'apepsie.
De l'apepsie dans la lienterie.
De la lienterie dans la dyssenterie.
De la dyssenterie dans l'hydropsie.
De l'hydropsie dans la privation de la vie.

Le Malade Imaginaire
Acte III, scène 6

Index